CONTEMPORARY VASCULAR SURGERY

Mark K. Eskandari, MD
James S. T. Yao, MD, PhD Professor of Education in Vascular Surgery
Professor of Radiology and Cardiology
Chief, Division of Vascular Surgery
Department of Surgery
Northwestern University
Feinberg School of Medicine
Chicago, IL

Mark D. Morasch, MD
John F. Marquardt, MD, Clinical Research Professor of Vascular Surgery
Division of Vascular Surgery
Department of Surgery
Northwestern University
Feinberg School of Medicine
Chicago, IL

William H. Pearce, MD
Violet R. and Charles A. Baldwin Professor of Vascular Surgery
Division of Vascular Surgery
Department of Surgery
Northwestern University
Feinberg School of Medicine
Chicago, IL

James S. T. Yao, MD, PhD
Professor Emeritus
Division of Vascular Surgery
Department of Surgery
Northwestern University
Feinberg School of Medicine
Chicago, IL

2011
PEOPLE'S MEDICAL PUBLISHING HOUSE—USA
SHELTON, CONNECTICUT

People's Medical Publishing House-USA
2 Enterprise Drive, Suite 509
Shelton, CT 06484
Tel: 203-402-0646
Fax: 203-402-0854
E-mail: info@pmph-usa.com

PMPH-USA

11 12 13/9 8 7 6 5 4 3 2 1

ISBN-13: 978-1-60795-166-7

Printed in China by People's Medical Publishing House
Editor: Jason Malley
Typesetter: Spearhead Global, Inc.
Cover designer: Mary McKeon

Library of Congress Cataloging-in-Publication Data

Contemporary vascular surgery / editors, Mark K. Eskandari ... [et al.].
　　p. ; cm.
Includes bibliographical references and index.
ISBN 978-1-60795-166-7
I. Eskandari, Mark K.
[DNLM: 1. Vascular Surgical Procedures—methods. 2. Cerebrovascular Disorders—surgery. WG 170]
LC classification not assigned
617.4'13—dc23

2011034314

Sales and Distribution

Canada
McGraw-Hill Ryerson Education
Customer Care
300 Water St
Whitby, Ontario L1N 9B6
Canada
Tel: 1-800-565-5758
Fax: 1-800-463-5885
www.mcgrawhill.ca

Foreign Rights
John Scott & Company
International Publisher's Agency
P.O. Box 878
Kimberton, PA 19442
USA
Tel: 610-827-1640
Fax: 610-827-1671
Japan
United Publishers Services Limited
1-32-5 Higashi-Shinagawa
Shinagawa-ku, Tokyo 140-0002

Japan
Tel: 03-5479-7251
Fax: 03-5479-7307
Email: hayashi@ups.co.jp

United Kingdom, Europe, Middle East, Africa
McGraw Hill Education
Shoppenhangers Road
Maidenhead
Berkshire, SL6 2QL
England
Tel: 44-0-1628-502500
Fax: 44-0-1628-635895
www.mcgraw-hill.co.uk

Singapore, Thailand, Philippines, Indonesia
Vietnam, Pacific Rim, Korea
McGraw-Hill Education
60 Tuas Basin Link
Singapore 638775
Tel: 65-6863-1580
Fax: 65-6862-3354
www.mcgraw-hill.com.sg

Australia, New Zealand
Papua New Guinea, Fiji, Tonga,
Solomon Islands, Cook Islands
Woodslane Pty Limited
Unit 7/5 Vuko Place
Warriewood NSW 2102
Australia
Tel: 61-2-9970-5111
Fax: 61-2-9970-5002
www.woodslane.com.au

Brazil
SuperPedido Tecmedd
Beatriz Alves, Foreign Trade
Department
R. Sansao Alves dos Santos, 102 | 7th floor
Brooklin Novo
Sao Paolo 04571-090
Brazil
Tel: 55-16-3512-5539
www.superpedidotecmedd.com.br

India, Bangladesh, Pakistan, Sri Lanka, Malaysia
CBS Publishers
4819/X1 Prahlad Street 24
Ansari Road, Darya Ganj,
New Delhi-110002
India
Tel: 91-11-23266861/67
Fax: 91-11-23266818
Email:cbspubs@vsnl.com

People's Republic of China
People's Medical Publishing House
International Trade Department
No. 19, Pan Jia Yuan Nan Li
Chaoyang District
Beijing 100021
P.R. China
Tel: 8610-67653342
Fax: 8610-67691034
HYPERLINK
"http://www.pmph.com/en/"www.pmph.com/en/

A New Leader

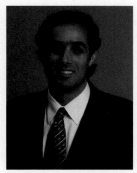

Mark K. Eskandari, MD

This 2011 Northwestern Vascular Symposium is the 36th of our continuing education series sponsored by the Division of Vascular Surgery, Feinberg School of Medicine, Northwestern University. It also marks a change of leadership in the Symposium. Dr. Mark K. Eskandari became the Chief of the Division on September 1, 2010, after Dr. William H. Pearce stepped down as the Chief following more than 12 years of service since January 1, 1998. This year, Dr. Eskandari is also taking over leadership of the Symposium.

Mark Eskandari represents the modern generation of vascular surgeons. He is knowledgeable in vascular disease, fully equipped for open surgical procedures, and skillful in catheter-based endovascular technology. He is a great teacher and also an innovative investigator. Over the past year, Dr. Eskandari has proven himself to be another excellent leader and we look forward to working with him in the coming years.

We thank Dr. William Pearce for his excellent leadership during his tenure as Chief of the Division of Vascular Surgery.

James S .T. Yao

Preface

This year marks the 36th Annual Vascular Symposium sponsored by the Division of Vascular Surgery, Feinberg School of Medicine, Northwestern University. Once again, we have brought together national experts for our 2 ½ day annual meeting to address contemporary topics in vascular surgery. As has been the tradition, presentations cover changes in management of extracranial cerebrovascular disease, new treatment options for lower extremity arterial occlusive disease, novel techniques in hemodialysis access management, as well as recent cutting-edge developments in aortic stent graft repair in the chest and abdomen. Other less common vascular problems including complex venous disease, visceral vessel pathology, and thoracic outlet are also included. In conjunction with the presentations are corresponding chapters found in this hardcover book with more in depth details and "pearls" from the experts. We have again chosen the InterContinental Hotel for our December Symposium as our venue given its prime location in the heart of Chicago along the Magnificent Mile. It is our sincere hope that you will find the contributions in this book valuable to your practice of vascular and endovascular surgery. We thank you for your interest and support of our annual meeting.

Acknowledgment

We thank our esteemed authors who have thoughtfully contributed to this year's book. Their willingness to share their personal expertise and knowledge is what makes our book a success to other practitioners. Special thanks to Sara Minton, administrative secretary, for her hard work in assembling and proofing the chapters and for keeping us on track with the deadlines of the Symposium. Without her, the symposium and book would not have been possible. We would also like to thank W.L. Gore & Associates, Incorporated for their continued generous educational grant which helps support the Symposium and printing of the book.

Contents

Rabih A. Chaer, MD, FACS, RVT

Rafael D. Malgor, MD, RPVI and Nicos Labropoulos, PhD, DIC, RVT

Mark D. Morasch, MD

SECTION II Cerebrovascular Disease II   55

K. Craig Kent, MD

Matthew B. Burruss, MD and Michael C. Stoner, MD, RVT, FACS

9 Contemporary Management of Patients with Concomitant Coronary
   and Carotid Artery Disease   73

Peter H. Lin, MD

10 Primary Extracranial Vertebral Artery Aneurysms   89

Sachin V. Phade, MD and Mark D. Morasch, MD

SECTION III Lower Extremity I   95

11 Endovascular Interventions for TASC II D Lesions   97

Luke Marone, MD and Donald T. Baril, MD

12 The Use of Distal Arterial Access for Femoro-popliteal and Tibial Subintimal Angioplasty   109

Joseph S. Giglia, MD

13 Effect of Immuno-Suppression on Bypass Outcomes   117

Satish C. Muluk, MD and Joseph L. Grisafi, MD

14 Deciding between Major Amputation and Attempts at Limb Salvage   125

Neal R. Barshes, MD, MPH and Michael Belkin, MD

SECTION V EVAR   185

SECTION IX Hemodialysis   383

Contributors

Ali F. AbuRahma, MD, RVT, RPVI
West Virginia University
Charleston, WV

Gorav Ailawadi, MD
University of Virginia Health System
Charlottesville, VA

Jason D. Alder, MD
University of Oklahoma College of Medicine
Tulsa, OK

Praveen R. Anchala, MD
Northwestern University
Feinberg School of Medicine
Chicago, IL

Ali Azizzadeh, MD
University of Texas Medical School
Houston, TX

Donald T. Baril, MD
University of Massachusetts Medical School
Worcester, MA

Neal R. Barshes, MD, MPH
Brigham and Women's Hospital
Boston, MA

Michael Belkin, MD
Brigham and Women's Hospital
Boston, MA

Marshall E. Benjamin, MD
University of Maryland
School of Medicine
Glen Bernie, MD

Matthew B. Burruss, MD
East Caroline University
Brody School of Medicine
Greenville, NC

John Byrne, MCh, FRCSI(Gen)
Albany Medical College
Albany, NY

Timothy G. Canty, Jr., MD
Southern California Permanente Medical
    Group
San Diego, CA

Rabih A. Chaer MD, FACS, RVT
University of Pittsburgh Medical Center
Pittsburgh, PA

Benjamin B. Chang, MD
Albany Medical College
Albany, NY

Kristofer Charlton-Ouw, MD
University of Texas Medical School
Houston, TX

Jason A. Chin, BS
Northwestern University
Feinberg School of Medicine
Chicago, IL

Kenneth J. Cherry, MD
University of Virginia Health System
Charlottesville, VA

Daniel G. Clair, MD
Cleveland Clinic
Cleveland, OH

M.P., Colgan, MD
St. James' Hospital
Dublin, Ireland

R. Clement Darling III, MD
Albany Medical Center Hospital
Albany, NY

M.G. Davies, MD
Methodist DeBakey Heart & Vascular
    Center
The Methodist Hospital
Houston, TX

Kip W. Dorsey, MD
University of Oklahoma College of
    Medicine
Tulsa, OK

Yazan Duwayri, MD
Emory University School of Medicine
Atlanta, GA

Mark K. Eskandari, MD
Northwestern University
Feinberg School of Medicine
Chicago, IL

Anthony L. Estrera, MD
University of Texas Medical School
Houston, TX

Grant T. Fankhauser, MD
Mayo Clinic College of Medicine
Phoenix, AZ

Cindy L. Felty, MSN, CNP, CWS
Mayo Clinic
Rochester, MN

William R. Flinn, MD
University of Maryland
School of Medicine
Glen Bernie, MD

Tanya R. Flohr, MD
University of Virginia Health System
Charlottesville, VA

Antonios P. Gasparis MD, RVT
Stony Brook Medical Center
Stony Brook, NY

Joseph S. Giglia, MD
University of Cincinnati College of
    Medicine
Cincinnati, OH

David L. Gillespie, MD
University of Rochester
School of Medicine & Dentistry
Rochester, NY

Joseph L. Grisafi, MD
Albert Einstein Medical Center
Philadelphia, PA

Thomas S. Huber, MD, PhD
University of Florida College of
    Medicine
Gainesville, Florida

Eric S. Hungness, MD, FACS
Northwestern University
Feinberg School of Medicine
Chicago, IL

William C. Jennings, MD, FACS
University of Oklahoma College of
    Medicine
Tulsa, OK

William D. Jordan, Jr., MD
University of Alabama @ Birmingham
Birmingham, AL

Mark L. Keldahl, MD
Advocate Masonic Medical Center
Chicago, IL

K. Craig Kent, MD
University of Wisconsin School of
    Medicine and Public Health
Madison, WI

John A. Kern, MD
University of Virginia Health System
Charlottesville, VA

E.A. Kheirelseid, MD
St. James' Hospital
Dublin, Ireland

Melina R. Kibbe, MD
Northwestern University
Feinberg School of Medicine
Chicago, IL

Irving L. Kron, MD
University of Virginia Health System
Charlottesville, VA

Nicos Labropoulos, PhD, DIC, RVT
Stony Brook Medical Center
Stony Brook, NY

Samuel S. Leake, BS
University of Texas Medical School
Houston, TX

Cheong Jun Lee, MD
Northwestern University
Feinberg School of Medicine
Chicago, IL

G. Matthew Longo, MD
University of Nebraska Medical Center
Omaha, NE

Alan B. Lumsden, MD
Methodist DeBakey Heart & Vascular
   Center
The Methodist Hospital
Houston, TX

Sean P. Lyden, MD
Cleveland Clinic
Cleveland, OH

Jason N. MacTaggart, MD
University of Nebraska Medical
   Center
Omaha, NE

P. Madhavan, MD
St. James' Hospital
Dublin, Ireland

S. Chris Malaisrie, MD
Northwestern University
Feinberg School of Medicine
Chicago, IL

Rafael D. Malgor MD, RPVI
Stony Brook Medical Center
Stony Brook, NY

Luke Marone, MD, FACS
University of Pittsburgh
Pittsburgh, PA

Marlene Mathews, MD
University of Rochester
School of Medicine & Dentistry
Rochester, NY

William D. McMillan, MD
Minnesota Vascular Physicians
Minnesota Vascular Surgery Center
Plymouth, MN

Manish Mehta, MD, MPH
Albany Medical College
Albany, NY

Douglas Miller, MS
The University of Manchester
Manchester, UK

Samuel R. Money, MD, FACS, MBA
Mayo Clinic College of Medicine
Phoenix, AZ

D.J. Moore, MD
St. James' Hospital
Dublin, Ireland

Mark D. Morasch, MD
Northwestern University
Feinberg School of Medicine
Chicago, IL

A. Moriarty, MD
St. James' Hospital
Dublin, Ireland

Satish C. Muluk, MD
Allegheny General Hospital
Pittsburgh, PA

Shardul B. Nagre, MBBS, MS
University of Alabama @ Birmingham
Birmingham, AL

Peter A. Naughton, MD
St. James' Hospital
Dublin, Ireland

David G. Neschis MD
University of Maryland
School of Medicine
Glen Bernie, MD

S.M. O'Neill, MD
St. James' Hospital
Dublin, Ireland

Michael Park, MD
Northwestern University
Feinberg School of Medicine
Chicago, IL

William H. Pearce, MD
Northwestern University
Feinberg School of Medicine
Chicago, IL

Brian G. Peterson, MD
Saint Louis University
St. Louis, MO

Sachin V. Phade, MD
University of Tennessee at Chattanooga
Chattanooga, TN

B. Ramlawi, MD
Methodist DeBakey Heart & Vascular
  Center
The Methodist Hospital
Houston, TX

M.J. Reardon, MD
Methodist DeBakey Heart & Vascular Center
The Methodist Hospital
Houston, TX

Scott A. Resnick, MD
Northwestern University
Feinberg School of Medicine
Chicago, IL

Heron E. Rodriguez, MD
Northwestern University
Feinberg School of Medicine
Chicago, IL

Thom W. Rooke, MD
Mayo Clinic
Rochester, MN

Hyde M. Russell, MD
Northwestern University
Feinberg School of Medicine
Chicago, IL

Brian G. Rubin, MD
Washington University School of Medicine
St. Louis, MO

Hazim J. Safi, MD
University of Texas Medical School
Houston, TX

Timar P. Sarac, MD
Cleveland Clinic Lerner School of Medicine
Cleveland, OH

Salvatore T. Scali, MD
University of Florida College of Medicine
Gainesville, Florida

Samir K. Shah, MD
Cleveland Clinic
Cleveland, OH

Benjamin W. Starnes, MD
University of Washington
Seattle, WA

William M. Stone, MD
Mayo Clinic College of Medicine
Phoenix, AZ

Michael C. Stoner, MD, RVT, FACS
East Carolina University
Greenville, NC

Shankar M. Sundaram, MD
Harrison Health Partners Thoracic and
Vascular Surgery
Bremerton, WA

Carlos H. Timaran, MD
University of Texas Southwestern
Medical School
Dallas, TX

David E. Timaran, MD
University of Texas Southwestern
Medical School
Dallas, TX

Margaret C. Tracci, MD
University of Virginia Health System
Charlottesville, VA

Nam T. Tran, MD
University of Washington
Seattle, WA

Gilbert Upchurch, Jr., MD
University of Virginia Health System
Charlottesville, VA

Karen Woo, MD
Keck School of Medicine
University of Southern California
Los Angeles, CA

Emily A. Wood, MD
Stony Brook Medical Center
Stony Brook, NY

James S.T. Yao, MD, PhD
Emeritus
Northwestern University
Feinberg School of Medicine
Chicago, IL

Kyle Zanocco, MD
Northwestern University
Feinberg School of Medicine
Chicago, IL

1

Dr. Ben Eiseman and the Accidental Discovery of Gore-Tex® Graft

James S.T. Yao, MD, PhD

Note: This chapter is dedicated to Mr. Jack Hoover and Mr. Don Lass, formerly of W. L. Gore & Associates, Inc. The accidental discovery of Gore-Tex® graft brought to us not only a new prosthetic graft but also a pair of exemplary business representatives of a visionary company. Since 1980, under their leadership, W. L. Gore & Associates, Inc., has provided to the Division of Vascular Surgery an education grant for support of the annual Northwestern Vascular Symposium and the publication of a compendium book at the time of the meeting. This year marks the 36th Northwestern Vascular Symposium. Remarkably, both Hoover and Lass have a perfect attendance record—one more than the author, who missed the 2009 symposium. In these modern days, partnership with industry is essential and we thank W. L. Gore & Associates, Inc., for their support of continuing education at Northwestern.

INTRODUCTION

On February 1, 2011, at the Annual Academic Congress, the Society of University Surgeons bestowed a Lifetime Achievement Award upon Dr. Ben Eiseman, Emeritus Professor of Surgery and Medicine, University of Colorado Medical School, Denver, Colorado. Ben Eiseman served as President of the Society of University Surgeons in 1962 and is universally acknowledged as a great contributor in surgical research. (Figure 1–1) As I remembered vaguely the story of how he discovered Gore-Tex® graft as an arterial substitute, I called him for more detailed information and to congratulate him for the Lifetime Achievement Award. This led to a long interview on the discovery of Gore-Tex® graft. I also called Mr. Jack Hoover and Mr. Don Lass of W. L. Gore & Associates, Inc., for their input. Unfortunately, Mr. Wilbert L. Gore has passed away and, hence, his side of the story will not be available. The telephone interviews with these individuals and also reports in the literature form the basis of this chapter. I found accidental scientific discovery to be

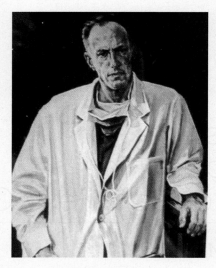

Figure 1–1. Ben Eiseman, M.D.

of great interest. There are many factors governing the success of a discovery and each discovery carries its own interesting story. The story on the discovery the use of PTFE materials as a bypass graft resulted from a friendship between Mr. Wilbert L. Gore and Dr. Ben Eiseman.

WILBERT L. GORE AND BEN EISEMAN

The history of Gore-Tex® started in 1958 when Wilbert Gore identified a market opportunity for polytetrafluoroethylene or PTFE. This is better known as DuPont Teflon®. His idea was to use it as insulation for electronic wires. Mr. Gore and his wife set up shop in the basement of their home to make PTFE insulated ribbon cables. In 1969, Mr. Gore's son, Robert, discovered that PTFE could be stretched to form a strong, porous material. It was patented and has the trademark Gore-Tex®.[1]

Mr. Wilbert Gore was a good friend of Dr. Ben Eiseman and they shared an interest in outdoor athletic activities. Both were avid skiers and mountain climbers. (Figure 1–2) At that time, Eiseman was looking for a graft to replace major veins, in particular the portal vein. Eiseman and his colleague, Dr. Glen Kelly, were also interested in developing an extracorporeal membrane oxygenator. On one of their ski trips to Vail, Colorado, in 1971, Mr. Gore showed up at cocktail hour wearing a tie made of expanded PTFE (polytetrafluoroethylene) material. The white tie with a tinge of gray certainly attracted the attention of Dr. Eiseman. On inquiry about the tie, Mr. Gore explained the nature of PTFE material to Dr. Eiseman. He then did a demonstration of the unique characteristics of PTFE material. He first poured ketchup over the tie and then, using a napkin, wiped the ketchup off. The ketchup came off the tie without a trace. He then repeated the same maneuver and this time he used mustard. Once again, the mustard came off instantly without a trace on the surface of the tie. Mr. Gore then mentioned the tie was made of a new expanded type of Teflon® that they had recently developed. He then removed a sample of the cloth from his pocket

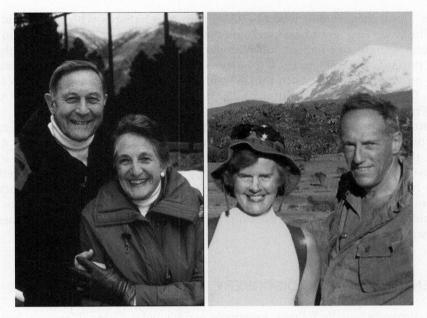

Figure 1–2. Wilbert Gore and his wife (left) and Ben Eiseman and his wife (right).

and demonstrated its water-repellent quality by cupping the material in his hand and pouring water into it. It held water like a dish. He next demonstrated its porosity to air by asking Eiseman to blow out a match held on the opposite side of the cloth. The match went out instantly.[2] This same story on the demonstration by Wilbert Gore was told by James Chandler in a speech entitled "Magical Moments in Vascular Surgery" to the Rocky Mountain Vascular Surgical Society's 31st Annual Meeting, Squaw Valley, California, in July 2010.[3] Dr. Eiseman then examined the tie and thought it was a very sleek material, soft and pliable with a smooth surface and easy handling characteristics. He immediately concluded the expanded PTFE material could be made into a bypass graft to replace major veins or arteries. He asked Mr. Gore to produce some short grafts (3 to 6 cm in length and 6 to 9 mm in diameter) to be used as venous prostheses in animal experiments. Mr. Gore said there would be no problem to make tubular structures with PTFE material because they were using the material for insulating electric cables already.

After the ski trip, Ben Eiseman and his colleagues at University of Colorado (T. Soyer, M. Lempinen, P. Cooper, L. Norton, and G. Kelly) began implanting PTFE grafts from W. L. Gore & Associates, Inc., in the portal vein, inferior vena cava, and external iliac vein in 27 pigs. Figure 1–3 shows the expanded PTFE (Gore-Tex®) tubes used as venous replacement. Of 27 Gore-Tex® vein prostheses, 24 (80%) were patent when examined two hours to six months after insertion. Of those followed two months after insertion, 80% were patent. Several months later, Eiseman became the first surgeon to implant a

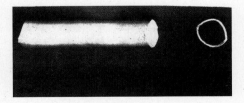

Figure 1–3 Expanded PTFE (Gore-Tex®) tubes used as venous replacement.

Gore-Tex® graft in a human when he used it in two patients with pancreatic carcinoma.[4] The Gore-Tex® graft was used as substitute for portal vein after resection of the tumor. Interestingly, one patient survived the procedure and lived for 32 months with a patent portal Gore-Tex® graft.[5] Dr. Larry Norton of the group then presented their findings on venous prosthesis to the 26th annual meeting of the Society for Vascular Surgery, Carmel, California, June 22-23, 1972. The manuscript, entitled "A New Venous Prosthesis," was published in *Surgery*, December 1972.[4]

Beginning in June 1972, PTFE graft was also performed by Kelly and Eiseman in canine common carotid artery (38 grafts) and common femoral artery (36 grafts). Delayed thrombosis is common in these arterial grafts.[2] Also common is intimal hyperplasia at the arterial anastomotic margin and this finding discouraged Kelly and Eiseman from extensive early clinical trial. Although animal studies are necessary before clinical trial, the small dog model presents harsh experimental challenges to the investigators. One may conclude the only meaningful trial is of prolonged patency in human beings.

ACCIDENTAL SCIENTIFIC DISCOVERY

Scientific discovery usually follows a vigorous experimental design. However, accidental discovery has been reported in many scientific discoveries.[6] Table 1–1 shows the top ten accidental discoveries reported in the literature. Of accidental scientific discoveries, the discovery of penicillin is the most dramatic. In 1928, after a period away from his laboratory at St. Mary's Medical School in London, Alexander Fleming noticed that a mold had infected a dish where he had been growing experimental bacteria. Curiously, the area surrounding the mold growing in the dish was clear, suggesting that the bacteria could not survive near the mold. Fleming concluded that a compound produced by the mold must have an antibacterial action. He called the new chemical "penicillin". Along with other antibiotics, it revolutionized health care and dramatically reduced mortality rates. Fleming was awarded the Nobel Prize in 1945.[7]

Many of the products discovered by accident are important to our everyday lives, including Teflon®, Velcro®, Post-it® notes, nylon, polyethylene, pace-maker, microwave, safety glass, plastics, and many other products. The idea to produce Velcro® came from an accidental observation. In the early 1950s, George deMestral, the

TABLE 1-1. TOP TEN ACCIDENTAL SCIENTIFIC DISCOVERIES

Penicillin
Safety Glass
Pacemaker
Teflon®
X-rays
Microwave
Velcro®
Post-its®
Potato Chips
Coca-Cola®

inventor, went for a walk in the countryside of his native Switzerland. Upon returning home he noticed that his jacket was covered with cockleburs. As he began picking off the burrs, he wondered "What makes them stick so tenaciously?" His curiosity led him to use a microscope to investigate more carefully. He discovered that cockleburs are covered with hooks and the hooks had become embedded in the loops of fabric of his cloth jacket. DeMestral wondered whether a system patterned after the cocklebur could be designed that would be useful. He then set up a company to market his novel product. The rest is history and Velcro® now secures everything from children's shoes to microphones in space shuttles. In the book *Serendipity: Accidental Discoveries in Sciences*, Royston M. Roberts has written extensively about accidental scientific discoveries that changed the world.[6] He used the word "serendipity" to further define the phenomenon. Serendipity is the ability of making accidental but fortuitous discoveries, especially while looking for something entirely unrelated. In other words, serendipity is making a great discovery by complete accident or finding something that they weren't expecting to find. Serendipity also occurs in surgery. One example is the surgical glove developed by William Halsted to prevent his operating room nurse (whom he subsequently married) from developing dermatitis due to the mercury chloride used for asepsis.[7] Halsted asked the Goodyear Rubber Company to fashion thin rubber gloves for her. The decrease in postoperative infections following the use of gloves was a later but much more useful offshoot of this invention. A keen state of mind of the inventor may play a role in the discovery. The French scientist Louis Pasteur famously said, *"In the field of observation, a chance favors only the prepared mind."*[7]

Like the story of penicillin and Velcro®, the discovery of Gore-Tex® graft was purely accidental. Had Eiseman not been exposed to the white tie made of expanded PTFE material, the Gore-Tex® graft may not exist today. When Eiseman first examined the PTFE material, his mind was prepared because he was at that time looking for the ideal graft material for venous replacement. As explained by Roberts[6], besides a prepared mind, there are two other characteristics in accidental discovery: curiosity and perception. For curiosity, the observer must be curious to understand the accident he observes. The best example is the discovery of Velcro® in which the observer was curious about the stickiness of the burrs. With reference to perception, the observer witnesses a phenomenon that is unexpected and he takes note of it rather than dismiss it as trivial. The discovery of PTFE graft is unquestionably due to the keen perception of Dr. Ben Eiseman after the ketchup-mustard demonstration and his high degree of curiosity about the material. Investigators should be taught to keep an open mind when encountering expected or unexpected findings. Above all, it is essential to maintain an insatiable curiosity. Perhaps, Albert Szent Gyogyi said it best: "Discovery consists of seeing what everybody has seen and thinking what nobody has thought."[6]

OTHER FACTORS INFLUENCE SCIENTIFIC DISCOVERY

Besides accidental discovery, the different and sometimes unexpected pathways to medical discoveries have been recently described by Weisse.[7] Some years ago, it was suggested that "The Phoenix Phenomenon" might be a term suitably applied to ideas in science and medicine that, although presented as original concepts, had been proposed in the past and then rejected and forgotten until later arising again like the mythical bird, the Phoenix, from their own ashes.[8] In recent years, Weisse suggested the term might more appropriately be applied to cases in which an investigator suffers a devastating event—perhaps loss of data, the ability to reproduce results, or severe illness—yet moves on to ultimately achieve the treasured final goal. Weisse cited examples of James Collip and insulin and how Collip suddenly lost the ability to reproduce purified insulin and its eventual recovery. Another example is the accidental loss of a manuscript by Thomas Carlyle, the Scottish essayist and historian. For a pioneering cardiac surgeon such as John Kirklin of Mayo Clinic, the loss of four of eight patients created deep grief of the surgeons. Kirklin was known to disappear for a day or two following the loss to grieve, collect himself, and then move on. Weisse also went into great detail to describe the illnesses of Sherwin B. Nuland and Arthur C. Guyton and how it affected their careers.[8] Obviously, the pathway to a successful discovery is not always straight and it may take several turns before it reaches the final goal.

THE GORE-TEX® GRAFT

Following the report on the use of PTFE graft as a new venous prosthesis, W. L. Gore & Associates, Inc., began to introduce reinforced expanded PTFE (Gore-Tex®) graft for arterial circulation. In 1973, Matsumoto and his associates reported excellent patency rates using Gore-Tex® as an arterial substitute in dogs.[9] In 1974, Campbell and colleagues placed Gore-Tex® grafts in the carotid and femoral arteries of dogs to study tissue ingrowths and patency rate.[10] In the USA, the first femoropopliteal graft using reinforced PTFE (Gore-Tex®) graft was performed by Dr. Roger Gregory of Virginia in September 1975, in a patient with critical ischemia.[11] The graft was a femoral to below-knee popliteal artery bypass. The graft was patent for several years and there was no limb loss on follow-up. In 1976, Campbell and his colleagues from University of Pittsburg reported their experience in 15 patients who underwent PTFE graft for limb salvage. They found 13 of 15 patients demonstrated a viable extremity with a result of overall early patency and limb salvage rate of 87%.[12] Since then, PTFE graft has been used extensively for infrainguinal revascularization. At present, over a million PTFE grafts have been used for infrainguinal revascularization.

CONCLUSION

Scientific discovery, whether it is accidental or not, is essential for our future. A high level of curiosity, good perception, a prepared mind, and, certainly, luck may influence the outcome of accidental discovery. The accidental discovery by Mr. W. L. Gore and Dr. Ben Eiseman that Gore-Tex® could be used as a graft to serve as a conduit substitute for veins or arteries is one of the major accidental medical discoveries and has greatly impacted limb salvage in patients suffering from critical limb ischemia.

Acknowledgement

We thank Dr. James Chandler for the provision of the photo of Mr. Wilbert Gore and Dr. Ben Eiseman and their wives. (Figure 1–2)

REFERENCES

1. US Patent 3,962,153. Very highly stretched polytetrafluoroethylene and process therefor. Issued to W. L. Gore and Associates, Inc., June 8, 1976.
2. Kelly GL, Eiseman B. Development of a new vascular prosthetic: Lessons learned. *Arch Surg* 1982;117:1367–1370.
3. Chandler JG. Magical moments in vascular surgery. Rocky Mountain Vascular Surgical Society, 31st Annual Meeting, Squaw Valley, California, July 2010.
4. Soyer T, Lempinen M, Cooper P, Norton L, Eiseman B. A new venous prosthesis. *Surgery* 1972;72:864–872.
5. Norton L, Eiseman B. Replacement of portal vein during pancreatectomy for carcinoma. *Surgery* 1975;77:280–284.
6. Roberts RM. *Serendipity: Accidental discoveries in science.* New York: John Wiley & Sons, 1989.
7. Weisse AB. Medical odysseys: The different and sometimes unexpected pathways to twentieth-century medical discoveries. Piscataway NJ: Rutgers University Press, 1991.
8. Weisse AB. The Phoenix phenomenon in medical research. *Pharos* 2008;71(3)26–33.
9. Matsumoto H, Hasegawa T, Fuse K, Yamamoto M, Saigusa M. A new vascular prosthesis for a small caliber artery. *Surgery* 1973;74:519–523.
10. Campbell CD, Goldfarb D, Roe R. A small arterial substitute: Expanded microporous polytetrafluoroethylene: Patency vs porosity. *Ann Surg* 1975;182:138–143.
11. Gregory R. Personal communication. December 9, 2010.
12. Campbell CD, Brooks DH, Webster MW, Bahnson HT. The use of expanded microporous polytetrafluoroethylene for limb salvage: A preliminary report. *Surgery* 1976;79:485–491.

SECTION **I**

Cerebrovascular
Disease I

2

Recurrent Carotid Stenosis: CAS or CEA

Ali F. AbuRahma, MD

INCIDENCE/ETIOLOGY

The incidence of post-carotid endarterectomy (CEA) restenosis ranges from 1% to 41%, depending on the length of follow-up and reported severity of stenosis.[1] However, only 1–8% of all CEA patients will develop hemodynamically significant restenosis. It has bi-modal occurrence, the first of which is noted between 6 and 24 months after CEA, which is generally caused by intimal hyperplasia. Early recurrence can be caused by local technical factors, e.g. clamp trauma or intimal/medial flaps.[2,3] Other causes include a small internal carotid artery (ICA) (<4 mm), female gender, and primary closure of the arteriotomy site. The second mode is usually noticed after 24 months and is related to systemic factors, such as continued smoking, hypertension, hypercholesterolemia, and diabetes mellitus, which may lead to recurrence of atherosclerosis.[3,4]

Proper identification of the risk factors for recurrent stenosis is important; the ultimate goal being reduction of recurrent stenosis via modification of identified risk factors. It is difficult, however, to draw meaningful conclusions from the data published to date, since the majority of patients who undergo CEA have more than one risk factor present. Conclusions drawn from a simple univariate analysis of risk factors in this population must then be interpreted with great caution. However, multivariate analysis, using multiple linear regression models, allows more definitive conclusions regarding the impact of individual risk factors and excludes confounding effects of other variables.

Technical imperfections at the time of CEA have been implicated in the etiology of early post-CEA restenosis. An analysis of these technical factors revealed that CEAs closed with patch angioplasty had a statistically significantly lower incidence of restenosis when compared to primary closure.[5–7]

Several studies have suggested that female gender may play a significant role in post-CEA restenosis;[3–5] however most of these studies included CEAs with primary

11

closure, which has been demonstrated to have a higher incidence of perioperative stroke and late restenosis.[8]

AbuRahma et al,[4,5] in a prospective randomized trial using multiple linear regression analyses, noted that the occurrence of 50% or more stenosis was more strongly associated with primary closure (p<0.001) and female gender (p=0.0051). Female gender was associated with a 20% incidence of ≥50% stenosis in contrast to 11% for male gender in the whole series (p=0.013). No correlation was found between gender and ≥50% recurrent stenosis in patients with PTFE patching or vein patch closure; however, women with primary closure had a higher recurrent stenosis rate than men (46% versus 23%, p=0.008). The carotid artery diameter at the time of surgery was not significantly associated with recurrent stenosis and neither were hypertension, coronary artery disease, smoking, diabetes mellitus, serum triglyceride or cholesterol concentrations, aspirin therapy, or age. This is presumably due to the fact that these represent risk factors for recurrent atherosclerosis and, therefore, may be implicated in more long-term recurrences than we observed in our follow-up period.

Previous studies have suggested that hypertension may be a significant risk factor for post-CEA recurrent stenosis.[9,10] Because most recurrences occur within two years postoperatively, it is generally believed that they are the result of local intimal hyperplasia. Hypertension is known to cause an exaggerated healing response in experimental models of arterial injury. In our series, hypertension showed significance as a risk factor when the entire population was examined (p=0.0407), however hypertension failed to achieve significance as a risk factor in CEA patients with patch angioplasty. This is logical, since patching may improve the local flow characteristics, thus limiting local arterial injury and subsequent intimal hyperplasia. Also, the increased diameter of the vessel after patching may lessen the effect of intimal hyperplasia, if it should occur. Each of the studies published to date that demonstrated significance of hypertension as a risk factor was composed mainly of patients who underwent primary closure.[10]

A younger age has also been implicated as a risk factor for CEA restenosis.[3,10] Hugl et al[3] studied the effect of age and gender on restenosis after 372 CEAs on 344 patients, and concluded that patients with restenosis were significantly younger (67.8 versus 73.1 years, p=0.005), and that females with restenosis were significantly younger than females without restenosis (66.1 versus 74 years, p=0.001). When they analyzed their data with respect to age 70 years at time of surgery, they detected an incidence of restenosis of 2.8% in males and 6.9% in females over the age of 70; in contrast to 6.6% in males and 25.7% in females younger than 70 years (p=0.003). The authors felt that these findings may be representative of the fact that younger patients with carotid occlusive disease have a particularly more virulent form of atherosclerosis.[3]

MANAGEMENT OF POST-CEA RESTENOSIS

Post-CEA restenosis is being detected more and more frequently with the use of duplex ultrasound surveillance after carotid interventions. Duplex criteria have been developed specifically to measure degrees of restenosis after standard CEA with patching.[11] In spite of the good accuracy of carotid duplex ultrasound in detecting restenosis, other imaging modalities, e.g. CTA and/or carotid angiography are done prior to carotid intervention.

Reoperation for Post-CEA Restenosis

For years, redo CEA has been the standard treatment for post-CEA restenosis. While it is generally agreed upon by most experts that reoperation for significant symptomatic post-CEA restenosis is indicated, there is some controversy regarding the indications for reoperation for asymptomatic restenosis.[12] This is largely due to the inherent risks in any open reintervention in a previously operated field, such as increased scar tissue, which can obscure tissue planes and make identification of anatomic structures and surgical landmarks more challenging. Reoperation can have morbidity and mortality rates as high as 8% to 20%,[12,13] although recent literature suggests that this is improving.[14,15]

O'Donnell et al reported on the results from a meta-analysis of six series that showed a 4.2% stroke rate and a 1% mortality rate for redo carotid surgery, and indicated that the incidence of cranial nerve injury in these patients averaged 8.5%.[12] Hill et al reported a much lower 30-day stroke and death rate of 0% for reoperation versus 1.1% for primary CEA.[15] This study compared only 40 reoperations against 350 primary operations, and the results may simply reinforce the difference in the pathophysiology between atherosclerotic disease found mostly in primary lesions and neointimal fibrous hyperplasia often seen in recurrent disease. A five-year stroke-free survival rate of 92% and a freedom from severe restenosis rate of 89% at five years with redo CEA have been published.[16,17]

We previously reported our experience in redo CEA versus primary CEA.[18] All reoperations for recurrent carotid stenosis performed during a 7-year period by a single vascular surgeon (AFA) were compared with primary CEA. Because all redo CEAs were done with polytetrafluoroethylene (PTFE) or vein patch closure, we only analyzed those primary CEAs that used the same patch closures.

Of 547 primary CEAs, 265 had PTFE or saphenous vein patch closure, and 124 reoperations had PTFE or vein patch closure during the same period. Both groups had similar demographic characteristics. The indications for reoperation and primary CEA were symptomatic stenosis in 78% and 58% of cases and asymptomatic ≥80% stenosis in 22% and 42% of cases, respectively (p<0.001). The 30-day perioperative stroke and transient ischemic attack rates for reoperation and primary CEA were 4.8% versus 0.8% (p=0.015) and 4% versus 1.1% respectively. There was no perioperative death in either group. Cranial nerve injury was noted in 17% of reoperation patients versus 5.3% of primary CEA patients; however, most of these injuries were transient (p<0.001, Table 2–1). The mean hospital stay was 1.8 days for reoperation versus 1.6 days for primary CEA. Cumulative rates of stroke-free survival at 1, 3, and 5 years were 96%, 91%, and 82% for reoperation and 94%, 92%, and 91% for primary CEA. The freedom from ≥50% recurrent stenosis at 1, 3, and 5 years were 98%, 96%, and 95% for reoperation and 98%, 96%, and 96% for primary CEA (no significant differences).

We concluded that reoperation carries higher perioperative stroke and cranial nerve injury rates than primary CEA. However, reoperations are durable and have stroke-free survival rates that are similar to primary CEA.

Carotid Artery Stenting for Post-CEA Restenosis

Carotid artery stenting (CAS) has been advocated by some investigators as an alternative to reoperation for post-CEA restenosis.[19–21] The last decade has seen a rise in the number of CAS procedures performed. One of the approved indications for CAS is post-CEA restenosis. Lanzino et al found no major periprocedural neurologic deficits or deaths with 25 CAS on 21 patients.[19] New et al, in a multicenter study of 358 CAS on 338 patients demonstrated

TABLE 2–1. PERIOPERATIVE COMPLICATIONS AND LATE EVENTS: PRIMARY CEA
VERSUS REOPERATION

	Primary CEA (n=265)	Reoperation (n=124)	P
30-Day Perioperative Events			
Ipsilateral stroke	2 (0.8)*	6 (4.8)**	0.015
Ipsilateral TIAs	3 (1.1)	5 (4)	NS
Perioperative carotid thrombosis	5 (1.9)	3 (2.4)	NS
Myocardial infarction	1 (0.4)	0	NS
Death	0	0	NS
Bleeding	1 (0.4)	1 (0.8)	NS
Cranial nerve injuries (total)	14 (5.3)	21 (17)	<0.001
Transient	13 (4.9)	19 (15.3)	0.001
Permanenet	1 (0.4)***	2 (1.6) ***	NS
Late events			
Ipsilateral stroke	0	0	NS
Ipsilateral TIA	1 (0.4)	1 (0.8)	NS
Deaths	25 (9.4)	15 (12.1)	NS

*Both were in symptomatic patients
**Five were in symptomatic patients and one was in an asymptomatic patient
***All vagal nerve injuries
All values are in n (%)

a 3.7% 30-day stroke and death rate with a minor stroke rate of 1.7%.[20] The major nonfatal stroke was 0.8% and the fatal stroke rate was 0.3%.

REOPERATION VERSUS CAS FOR POST-CEA STENOSIS

In spite of the positive results for CAS in these studies, only a few reports with a small number of patients have directly compared redo CEA to CAS for post-CEA restenosis.[21–24] Hobson et al compared 16 cases treated by carotid reoperation with 15 cases treated with CAS over an eight-year period.[22] No deaths or 30-day strokes were reported and no stent occlusion or restenosis was found in the CAS group over a seven month follow-up period.[22]

Bowser et al compared 52 CAS procedures over a five year period with 27 carotid reoperations over a nine year period.[21] Overall 30-day morbidity was similar between the two groups (12% versus 11%), and the combined stroke and death rate was 5.7% for CAS and 3.7% for reoperation (p>0.1).[21] Stenosis-free ICA patency (defined as <50% diameter reduction by duplex ultrasound) at 36 months was 75% for reoperation and 57% for CAS.[21] Bettendorf et al evaluated outcomes of CAS versus redo CEA in treating recurrent stenosis.[23] Interestingly, they found secondary recurrence to be higher after redo CEA (14% versus 6.1%), however this was not statistically significant.[23]

Recently, Attigah et al, retrospectively evaluated early and midterm results of redo CEA and CAS in 79 consecutive patients (86 arteries), including 41 CEA and 45 CAS procedures.[24] There was one complication in the CAS group and four neurological complications in the CEA group (p=0.13). Wound site and cardiac complication rates were significantly higher in the CEA group (p=0.029), with a median follow-up of 35 months. After 60 months, the overall actuarial survival rate was 83% in the redo CEA group and 100% in the CAS group (p=0.87). Freedom from repeat intervention for re-recurrence was 89% in the redo CEA group and 95% in the CAS group (p=0.52). They concluded that freedom from reintervention and survival was not significantly different between the two groups.

Another issue regarding CAS for post-CEA recurrent stenosis, in comparison to redo surgery, is durability. When recurrent stenosis after CEA is treated with CAS, in-stent restenosis can be as high as 13% at 14 months, as reported by Rockman et al,[25] and up to 24% at 20 months, as described by AbuRahma et al.[16] To be noted, these high in-stent restenosis rates in our earlier experience can be explained by the fact that we used the carotid duplex velocity criteria for native carotids, i.e. these rates are probably falsely high. However, Hobson et al reported no restenosis or stent occlusion at seven months.[22] However, most authorities conclude that CAS for recurrent carotid artery stenosis not only appears technically feasible and reasonably safe, but in-stent recurrent stenosis rates appear high, requiring both early and longer term follow-up surveillance.

OUR CLINICAL EXPERIENCE

We recently compared the outcome of CAS versus carotid reoperation for patients with post-CEA stenosis.[1] This study analyzed 192 patients: 72 had reoperation (Group A) and 120 had CAS for post-CEA stenosis (Group B). Patients were followed prospectively and had duplex ultrasounds at one month, and every 6–12 months thereafter.

Demographic/clinical characteristics were comparable for both groups, except for diabetes mellitus and coronary artery disease, which were significantly higher in Group B. The indications for reoperations were transient ischemic attacks (TIA)/stroke in 72% for Group A versus 57% for Group B (p=0.0328). The mean follow-up was 33 months (range: 1–86) for Group A and 24 months (range: 1–78) for Group B (p=0.0026). The proportion of early (<24 months) carotid restenosis prior to intervention was 51% in Group A versus 27% in Group B (p=0.0013). The perioperative stroke rates were 3% and 1%, respectively (p=0.5573). There were no myocardial infarctions or deaths in either group. The overall incidence of cranial nerve injury was 14% for Group A versus 0% for Group B (p<0.0001). However, there was no statistical difference between the groups relating to permanent cranial nerve injury (1% versus 0%, Table 2–2). The combined early and late stroke rates for Groups A and B were 3% and

TABLE 2–2. 30-DAY PERIOPERATIVE COMPLICATIONS: REOPERATION (GROUP A) VERSUS CAS (GROUP B)

	Group A (N=72)	Group B (N=120)	Total (N=192)	P value
Perioperative ipsilateral strokes	2 (3%)	1 (1%)	3 (2%)	0.5573
Ipsilateral TIA	1 (1%)	3 (3%)	4 (2%)	1
Myocardial infarction	0	0	0	
Death	0	0	0	
Bleeding	1 (1%)			
Total cranial nerve injury	10 (14%)	0	10 (5%)	<0.0001
Transient	9 (13%)	0	9 (5%)	<0.0001
Permanent	1 (1%)	0	1 (1%)	0.375

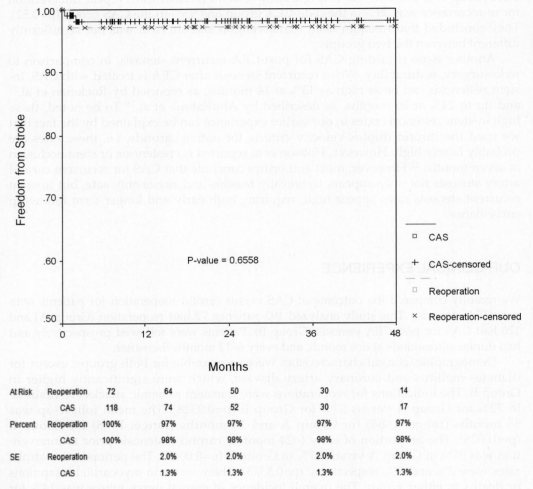

Figure 2–1. Freedom from stroke: Reoperation versus CAS.

2%, respectively (p=0.6347). The stroke-free rates at 1, 2, 3, and 4 years for Groups A and B were 97%, 97%, 97%, and 97%; and 98%, 98%, 98%, and 98%, respectively (p=0.6490, Figure 2–1). The stroke-free survival rates were not significantly different (Figure 2–2). The rates of freedom from ≥50% restenosis at 1, 2, 3, and 4 years were 98%, 95%, 95%, and 95% for Group A versus 95%, 89%, 80%, and 72% for Group B (p=0.0175, Figure 2–3). The freedom from ≥80% restenosis at 1, 2, 3, and 4 years for Groups A and B were 98%, 97%, 97%, and 97%; versus 99%, 96%, 92%, and 87%, respectively (p=0.2281, Figure 2–4). Four patients (one symptomatic) in Group B had reintervention for ≥80% restenosis. The rate of freedom from reintervention for Groups A and B were 100%, 100%, 100%, and 100% versus 94%, 89%, 83%, and 79%, respectively (p=0.0634).

Our study is the largest comparative evaluation of reoperation versus CAS for post-CEA stenosis, analyzed 72 carotid reoperations with 120 CAS. Not only did our

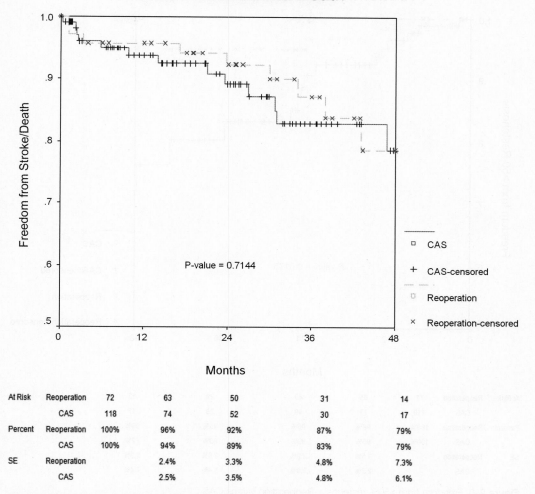

Figure 2–2. Freedom from stroke/death: Reoperation versus CAS.

study reinforce the feasibility of CAS in this situation, but it demonstrated equivalency between CAS and reoperation for post-CEA stenosis. No statistically significant difference was observed between CAS and CEA in regards to the primary end points of perioperative stroke, myocardial infarction, and/or death. However, there was an increased incidence of transient cranial nerve injuries with redo CEA, in contrast to an increased incidence of ≥50% in-stent restenosis in patients who underwent CAS. Meanwhile, the freedom from ≥80% restenosis at four years was equivalent in both groups.[1]

In conclusion, 1–8% of all CEA patients will develop hemodynamically significant restenosis, which can be treated with CAS and seems to be at least as safe as carotid reoperation. Redo CEA has a higher incidence of transient cranial nerve injury; however, CAS has a higher incidence of ≥50% in-stent restenosis.

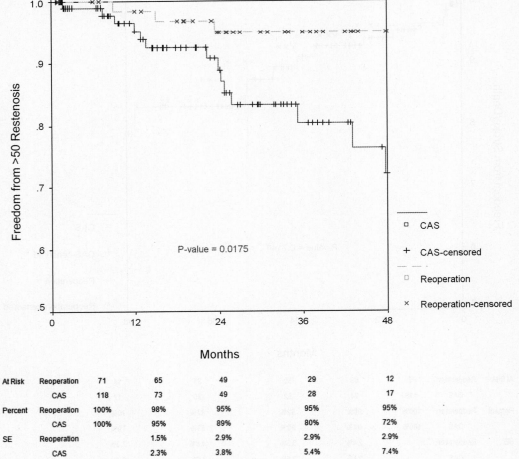

At Risk	Reoperation	71	65	49	29	12
	CAS	118	73	49	28	17
Percent	Reoperation	100%	98%	95%	95%	95%
	CAS	100%	95%	89%	80%	72%
SE	Reoperation		1.5%	2.9%	2.9%	2.9%
	CAS		2.3%	3.8%	5.4%	7.4%

Figure 2–3. Freedom from ≥50% restenosis: Reoperation versus CAS.

REFERENCES

1. AbuRahma AF, Abu-Halimah S, Hass SM, Nanjundappa A, Stone PA, Mousa A, Lough E, Dean LS. Carotid artery stenting outcomes are equivalent to carotid endarterectomy outcomes for patients with post-carotid endarterectomy stenosis. *J Vasc Surg* 2010;52:1180–7.
2. Ouriel K, Green RM. Clinical and technical factors influencing recurrent carotid stenosis and occlusion after endarterectomy. *J Vasc Surg* 1987;5:702–6.
3. Hugl B, Oldenburg WA, Neuhauser B, Hakaim AG. Effect of age and gender on restenosis after carotid endarterectomy. *Ann Vasc Surg* 2006;20:602.8.
4. AbuRahma AF, Robinson PA, Richmond BK. Reanalysis of factors predicting recurrent stenosis in a prospective randomized trial of carotid endarterectomy comparing primary closure and patch closure. *Vasc Surg* 2000;34:319–29.
5. AbuRahma AF, Robinson PA, Saiedy S, Khan JH, Boland JP. Prospective randomized trial of carotid endarterectomy with primary closure and patch angioplasty with saphenous vein, jugular vein, and polytetrafluoroethylene: Long-term follow-up. *J Vasc Surg* 1998; 27:222–32; discussion 233–4.

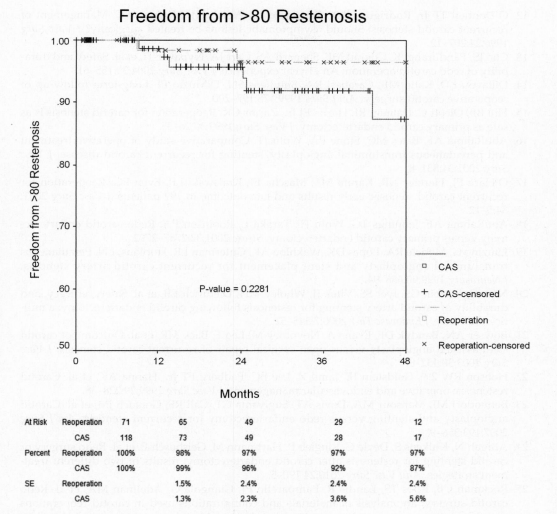

Figure 2–4. Freedom from ≥80% restenosis: Reoperation versus CAS.

6. AbuRahma AF, Robinson PA, Saiedy S, Richmond BK, Khan J. Prospective randomized trial of bilateral carotid endarterectomies: Primary closure versus patching. *Stroke* 1999;30: 1185–89.

7. Bond R, Rerkasem K, Naylor AR, AbuRahma AF, Rothwell PM. Systematic review of randomized controlled trials of patch angioplasty versus primary closure and different patch materials during carotid endarterectomy. *J Vasc Surg* 2004; 40:1126–35.

8. Akbari CM, Pulling MC, Pomposelli FB, et al. Gender and carotid endarterectomy: does it matter? *J Vasc Surg* 2000;31:1103–1109.

9. Arramovic JR, Fletcher JP. The incidence of recurrent carotid stenosis after carotid endarterectomy and its relationship to neurological events. *J Cardiovasc Surg* 1992;33:54–58.

10. Clagett PG, Rich NM, McDonald PT, et al. Etiologic factors for recurrent carotid artery stenosis. *Surgery* 1983;93:313–318.

11. AbuRahma AF, Stone PA, Deem S, Dean LS, Keiffer T, Deem E. Proposed duplex velocity criteria for carotid restenosis following carotid endarterectomy with patch closure. *J Vasc Surg* 2009;50:286–91.

12. O'Donnell TF Jr, Rodriguez AA, Fortunato JE, Welch HJ, Mackey WC. Management of recurrent carotid stenosis: Should asymptomatic lesions be treated surgically? *J Vasc Surg* 1996;24:207–12.
13. Cho JS, Pandurangi K, Conrad MF, Shepard AS, Carr JA, Nypaver TJ, et al. Safety and durability of redo carotid operation: An 11 year experience. *J Vasc Surg* 2004;39:155–61.
14. Dillavou ED, Kahn MB, Carabasi RA, Smullens SN, DiMuzio PJ. Long-term follow-up of reoperative carotid surgery. *Am J Surg* 1999;178:197–200.
15. Hill BB, Olcott C, Dalman RI, Harris EJ Jr., Zarins CK. Reoperation for carotid stenosis is as safe as primary carotid endarterectomy. *J Vasc Surg* 1999;30:26–35.
16. AbuRahma AF, Bates MC, Stone PA, Wulu JT. Comparative study of operative treatment and percutaneous transluminal angioplasty/stenting for recurrent carotid disease. *J Vasc Surg* 2001;34:831–8.
17. O'Hara PJ, Hertzer NR, Karafa MT, Mascha EJ, Krajewski LP, Even EG. Reoperation for recurrent carotid stenosis: early results and late outcome in 199 patients. *J Vasc Surg* 2001; 34:5–12.
18. AbuRahma AF, Jennings TG, Wulu JT, Tarakji L, Robinson PA. Redo carotid endarterectomy versus primary carotid endarterectomy. *Stroke* 2001;32:2787–2792.
19. Lanzino G, Mericle RA, Lopes DK, Wakhloo AK, Guterman LR, Hopkins, LN. Percutaneous transluminal angioplasty and stent placement for recurrent carotid artery stenosis. *J Neurosurg* 1999;90:688–94.
20. New G, Roubin GS, Iyer SS, Vitek JJ, Wholey MH, Diethrich EB, et al. Safety, efficacy, and durability of carotid artery stenting for restenosis following carotid endarterectomy: a multicenter study. *J Endovasc Ther* 2000;7:345–52.
21. Bowser AN, Bandyk DF, Evans A, Novotney M, Leo F, Back MR, et al. Outcome of carotid stent-assisted angioplasty versus open surgical repair of recurrent carotid stenosis. *J Vasc Surg* 2003;38:432–8.
22. Hobson RW 2nd, Goldstein JE, Jamil Z, Lee BC, Padberg FT Jr., Hanna AK, et al. Carotid restenosis: operative and endovascular management. *J Vasc Surg* 1999;29:228–38.
23. Bettendorf MJ, Mansour MA, Davis AT, Sugiyama GT, Cali RF, Gorsuch JM, et al. Carotid angioplasty and stenting versus redo endarterectomy for recurrent stenosis. *Am J Surg* 2007;193:356–9.
24. Attigah N, Kulkens S, Deyle C, Ringleb P, Hartmann M, Geisbusch P, et al. Redo surgery or carotid stenting for restenosis after carotid endarterectomy: results of two different treatment strategies. *Ann Vasc Surg* 2010;24:190–5.
25. Rockman CB, Riles TS, Landis R, Lamparello PJ, Giangola G, Adelman MA, et al. Redo carotid surgery: an analysis of materials and configurations used in carotid reoperations and their influence on perioperative stroke and subsequent recurrent stenosis. *J Vasc Surg* 1999;29:72–81.

3

Role and Utility of Virtual Histology Intravascular Ultrasound for Carotid Stenting

Carlos H. Timaran, MD and David E. Timaran, MD

Carotid artery stenting (CAS) is an established treatment option for carotid stenosis.[1] Although initially restricted to high-surgical-risk patients, particularly those with significant comorbidities or a hostile neck from previous surgical procedures or radiation, recent randomized clinical trials have revealed that CAS may also be used for standard risk patients.[2, 3] Among symptomatic patients, however, CAS has been equivalent to CEA only for patients younger than 70 years.[3] The higher risk of stroke among older patients favors endarterectomy as the treatment of choice in patients 70 years or older.

Because stroke represents the main complication of CAS despite the development and widespread use of embolic protection devices (EPDs), carotid plaque composition has been investigated as a means to identify vulnerable plaques and prevent embolization of plaque debris to the brain and subsequent stroke.[4] Plaques with a large lipid and necrotic core size have, in fact, been associated with an increased risk of distal embolization during carotid interventions.[4–6] Whether determining plaque morphology and composition may predict the emboligenic potential of carotid lesions remains to be elucidated. Virtual histology intravascular ultrasound (VH-IVUS) has been used to determine plaque composition in the coronary and carotid arteries.[6–8] The role of VH-IVUS during carotid interventions has not been established, particularly with the routine use of EPDs during CAS.

In a recent study, we investigated the relationship between atherosclerotic plaque composition determined with VH-IVUS and the occurrence of cerebral embolization after carotid stenting.[9] The amount of lipid and necrotic core was specifically assessed as a predictor for distal embolization.

VIRTUAL HISTOLOGY INTRAVASCULAR ULTRASOUND (VH-IVUS) AND DETERMINATION OF CAROTID PLAQUE COMPOSITION & CEREBRAL EMBOLIZATION

VH-IVUS images are usually obtained using a 2.9-F, 20-MHz Eagle Eye Gold catheter s(Volcano Corp., Rancho Cordova, CA) with an incorporated 20-MHz phased-array transducer beginning from the distal vessel, at least 10 mm distal to the culprit lesion, and progressing in a retrograde direction to the most distal common carotid artery free of disease.[5,6,10] Deployment of an embolic protection device (EPD) is usually required prior to the IVUS exam. Given the potential risk of embolization during the advancement and withdrawal of the IVUS catheter, this needs to be advanced through the carotid lesion before this can be examined. Although manual catheter pullback may be used, motorized pullback at a rate of 1.0 mm/s is preferable, particularly to determine plaque volumes. The image frames need to be analyzed by experienced observers. Vessel and lumen area are calculated for each frame, using previously published methods.[11] Plaque burden is calculated as [(external elastic membrane$_{area}$–lumen$_{area}$/external elastic membrane$_{area}$) × 100]. Virtual histology analysis is performed for each frame, and the area of each plaque constituent (fibrous, fibrofatty, calcific, and necrotic core) is determined in an automated fashion using Volcano S5 software (Volcano Corp., Rancho Cordova, CA). Planar VH-IVUS analysis is performed at the site of the minimal luminal area and the site of the largest necrotic core. Volumetric VH-IVUS analysis is performed in those cases in which a motorized pullback has been used along the length of the lesion using Simpson's rule.[11] VH-IVUS analyses are reported in absolute amounts and as percentages (relative amounts) of plaque area and volume.

Although several predictors of adverse outcomes after CAS have been identified, the effects of plaque composition, including type of plaque and amount of necrotic core, on neurologic adverse events have not been established. Diffusion-weighted magnetic resonance imaging (DW-MRI) and transcranial Doppler (TCD) are imaging techniques frequently used to detect subclinical cerebral embolization during carotid interventions.[12–14] Because adverse neurologic events after CAS are rare in high volume practices, quantification of cerebral embolization using DW-MRI and TCD monitoring may be used as surrogate endpoint of postprocedural ischemic brain injury.[15] In a recent study, we assessed the relationship between atherosclerotic plaque composition determined with VH-IVUS and the occurrence of cerebral embolization after carotid stenting.[9] Specifically, the amount of lipid and necrotic core was assessed as a risk factor for distal embolization.

TRANSCRANIAL DOPPLER PROTOCOL

Transcranial Doppler signals, using a portable digital 2-MHz PMD/spectral TCD unit (PMD150, Spencer Technologies, Seattle, WA) may be recorded from bilateral middle cerebral arteries via transtemporal windows.[16] Monitoring is started before CAS and continued for 30 minutes after the procedure. A head frame is usually used for ultrasound probe fixation and continuous flow assessment in M1 segment of the middle cerebral artery (MCA). Several TCD parameters may be recorded: MES counts and microemboli shower detection during the different steps of the procedure, initial MCA mean velocity, mean MCA velocity during CAS, and final mean MCA velocity. MES are identified according to the recommended guidelines.[17]

DIFFUSION-WEIGHTED MRI EXAMS

DW-MRI scans of the brain obtained immediately prior to CAS and 18 to 24 hours after CAS may be used to assess acute ischemic brain injury related to the procedure. Post-procedural DW-MRI studies are compared to preprocedural studies to identify new proce-dure-related ischemic cerebral lesions. DW-MRI with echo-planar imaging sequence (B0 = 1000) and fluid-attenuated inversion recovery (FLAIR) images are usually obtained in axial and coronal sections. On the postprocedural MRI, acute embolic lesions are defined as focal hyperintense areas with restricted diffusion signal, which are confirmed by appar-ent diffusion coefficient mapping to rule out artifacts.[14] New postprocedural cerebral lesions consistent with microemboli are recorded in terms of location and number for all DW-MRI exams performed. In our study, DW-MRI was obtained using standard head coils on 1.5 Tesla Siemens scanners (Siemens Avanto or Magnetom Sonata, Siemens, Erlangen, Germany).[9]

CAROTID PLAQUE COMPOSTION DETERMINED WITH VH-IVUS AND RISK OF CEREBRAL EMBOLIZATION DURING CAROTID STENTING

In a recent series of 24 CAS procedures, we assessed target lesions with VH-IVUS at the time of CAS and obtained transcranial Doppler (TCD) monitoring during CAS and pre- and 24-hour postprocedural diffusion-weighted magnetic resonance imaging (DW-MRI) scans of the brain.[9] For the entire group, VH-IVUS revealed a plaque area of 25.8 mm^2 (IQR, 21.8–31) at the minimum luminal area site and 21.6 mm^2 (IQR, 17.4–25) at the largest necrotic core site. Plaque volume was 342.5 mm^3 (IQR, 187–488) for the entire lesion length. Seventeen patients (71%) demonstrated new acute cerebral emboli in DW-MRI. Of these, all revealed ipsilateral lesions and 12 (50%) had also contralateral lesions. The median ipsi-lateral TCD MES counts were 227 (IQR, 143–315). For the entire study group, the median number of ipsilateral cerebral microemboli was 1 (IQR, 0–3) and the median total number of DW-MRI acute lesions was 2 (IQR, 0.25 to 4).

In our study, the association between plaque components and the frequency of TCD-detected MES counts during CAS and the incidence and location of acute post-procedural embolic lesions detected with DW-MRI were assessed with bivariate statis-tical tests, scatter plots and Pearson or Spearman rank correlation coefficients, as appropriate.[9]

None of the plaque components as assessed in planar VH-IVUS analysis at the site of minimal luminal area and largest necrotic core site was significantly associated with the presence of ipsilateral cerebral embolization as determined by DW-MRI. Volumetric VH-IVUS analysis revealed that there was a trend for larger median dense calcium volume in patients with new ipsilateral cerebral microemboli compared to patients without acute lesions as detected with DW-MRI (33.2 ± 24.5 mm^3 vs. 11.4 ± 6.1 mm^3, P = .08). The mean proportion of dense calcium volume was, in fact, larger in patients with cerebral microemboli (9.9 ± 5.2% vs. 5.5 ± 0.8%, P =.09). Plaque volume (410.9 ± 239.3 mm^3 vs. 238.9 ± 91.4 mm^3, P = .28) and necrotic core volume (71.9 ± 38.1 mm^3 vs. 40.3 ± 14.4 mm^3, P = .22) were also larger in patients with ipsilateral acute mi-croemboli, but these differences did not reach statistical significance. Ipsilateral acute microemboli in DW-MRI did not correlate with either the volume or proportion of fibrotic and fibrofatty plaque components.

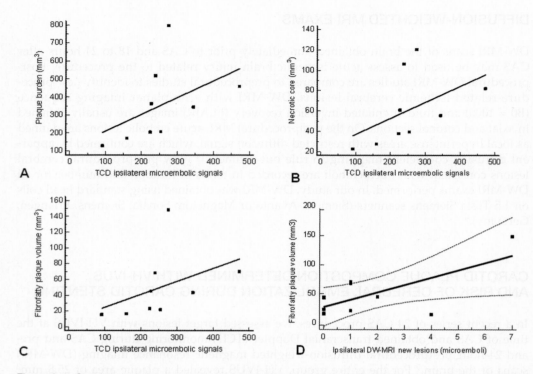

Figure 3–1. Correlation of plaque components and subclinical cerebral embolization detected with transcranial doppler (TCD) and diffusion-weighted MRI (DW-MR).

Scatter plots of plaque components and cerebral microemboli as detected with TCD revealed statistically significant correlation between the volumes of plaque burden (Spearman $r = 0.71$, $P = .03$), necrotic core (Spearman $r = 0.71$, $P = .03$), fibrofatty (Spearman $r = 0.73$, $P = .025$) and fibrous (Spearman $r = 0.68$, $P = .04$) plaque components and MES counts (Figure 3–1A, 1B & 1C). No correlation was found between the areas of plaque components at the minimum lumen and largest core sites and MES counts. There was statistically significant correlation between fibrofatty plaque volume (Spearman $r = 0.49$, $P = .016$) and number of new ipsilateral lesions detected in DW-MRI (Figure 3–1D). There was also statistically significant correlation between the areas of fibrofatty plaque at the minimum lumen site (Pearson $r = 0.6$, $P = .002$) and the largest necrotic core site (Person $r = 0.7$, $P = .04$) and the number of microemboli. No significant correlation was demonstrated between necrotic core and dense calcium areas and volumes and the number of microemboli.

SIGNIFICANCE OF VIRTUAL HISTOLOGY INTRAVASCULAR ULTRASOUND FINDINGS DURING CAROTID STENTING

A clinical need exists to develop methods to determine carotid plaque composition as a means of treatment stratification for patients with carotid artery stenosis and to define if carotid endarterectomy, carotid stenting, or medical treatments are indicated. Moreover, identification of carotid plaques prone to cerebral embolization during carotid interventions could result in better methods of embolic protection and choice of therapy. VH-IVUS uses spectral analysis of radiofrequency ultrasound backscatter signals from the IVUS images to define the 4 specific plaque components, i.e. fibrous, fibro-fatty, dense calcific, and necrotic core areas and volumes within the plaque.[7] The correlation between VH-IVUS and histological examination of carotid plaques removed during CEA with respect to plaque compositions has only been assessed in one study.[6] A strong correlation between VH-IVUS plaque composition and histology examination of the same plaques was observed in 15 patients. Extensive evaluation of plaque composition of the coronary arteries using VH-IVUS has, however, reported inconsistent results.[8, 18] Although some studies have histologically validated VH-IVUS findings for coronary lesions, plaque characterization using VH-IVUS do not consistently correlate with histology as to the accurate identification of plaque components, thereby raising concerns about the accuracy and utility of this imaging technique.[7, 19, 20] Moreover, the role of VH-IVUS to discern when embolic protection is indicated during percutaneous coronary interventions (PCIs) has particularly been questioned because VH-IVUS is not reliable for the detection of intravascular thrombus, the single most important predictor for distal embolization during PCIs.[20]

The relationship between plaque composition determined with VH-IVUS and the frequency of distal embolization after PCIs in patients with ST-segment elevation myocardial infarction (STEMI) or angina, as assessed in 2 small studies, has shown that necrotic core size in the culprit lesion is the major direct correlate and independent predictor of distal embolization.[21, 22] No embolic protection was used for PCI in any of these 2 studies. Contrary to these reports, the results of our study did not reveal a significant association between necrotic core size and distal embolization during CAS.[9] The different anatomic location and possible type II statistical error due to sample size, the routine use of embolic protection in our study and the presence of disrupted plaques in the coronary studies may account for the dissimilar results. All CAS procedures in our study were performed with a filter device for embolic protection. Whether the use of embolic protection effectively prevents distal embolization in plaques with large necrotic cores, as may be suggested by our findings, remains to be established. Unfortunately, no quantification of the amount of debris recovered in the filters was performed. Although 42% of the patients in our study were symptomatic, none presented with acute symptoms, which represents a significant difference with the types of lesions treated in the series reported by Kawaguchi et al,[21] which required mechanical thrombectomy before VH-IVUS examination could be performed.

Conventional IVUS has been used as an adjunct imaging modality during CAS.[23] IVUS provides accurate vessel measurements and may assist in assessing stent sizing and expansion. To date, however, the use of VH-IVUS to determine plaque composition and the potential risk of cerebral embolization during CAS has not been systematically evaluated. Our study is one of the first that attempts to assess plaque composition using VH-IVUS and its association with subclinical cerebral embolization during CAS.[9] We failed to demonstrate that carotid plaques with a large necrotic core size are definitely associated with a higher incidence of subclinical cerebral embolization. Moreover, necrotic core areas and volumes failed to correlate with the number of cerebral microemboli detected on postprocedural DW-MRI. Our data, therefore, does not support the use of covered stents or endografts or the avoidance of CAS with embolic protection with filters for carotid lesions with large necrotic core size detected in VH-IVUS.

Extensive calcification of the carotid plaques may be considered an ominous risk factor for CAS, not only because circumferential calcification may result in inadequate stent expansion and distal embolization, but also because our data supports the association between the presence of large dense calcium volume and distal embolization during CAS. Similarly, large fibrofatty areas and volume are associated with the number of ipsilateral microemboli detected in DW-MRI after CAS performed under embolic protection. Very likely, firm plaque fragments, such as the ones that may originate in plaques with large fibrofatty and dense calcium components, may result in microemboli that may pass through the pores of a filter. Conversely, filters may effectively catch fragments that consist of necrotic core. Whether different filters and other types of embolic protection may be more or less effective in preventing distal embolization remains to be established.

Volumetric analyses revealed that carotid plaque burden and the extent of necrotic core, fibrofatty and fibrous components correlate with TCD MES counts during CAS. Although higher MES counts may be associated with increased risk of ischemic stroke in several medical conditions, such association in patients undergoing CAS has not been established and the significance of MES counts seen during CAS remains to be elucidated. Because fibrofatty plaque volume correlates with the number of ipsilateral microemboli detected in DW-MRI and the MES counts, this component better predicts the frequency of subclinical cerebral embolization during and after CAS.

In summary, carotid plaque composition, as determined by VH-IVUS, only weakly correlates with the degree of subclinical cerebral embolization after carotid stenting. Specifically, there is a trend for an increased incidence of cerebral embolization after CAS in patients with a higher volume and proportion of dense calcium and a significant correlation between fibrofatty volume and the number of new lesions detected in DW-MRI. Conversely, and despite being considered the main component of unstable or vulnerable plaques, necrotic core size is not definitely associated with subclinical cerebral embolization after CAS under embolic protection. According to our results, the role of VH-IVUS in evaluating plaque composition during CAS remains to be established and warrant further investigation. Moreover, the clinical significance of subclinical cerebral embolization after CAS, the effectiveness of distal protection devices in preventing embolization and the ultimate impact of reducing distal embolization on the frequency of stroke remain uncertain and also should be further investigated.

REFERENCES

1. Furie KL, Kasner SE, Adams RJ, Albers GW, Bush RL, Fagan SC, et al. Guidelines for the Prevention of Stroke in Patients With Stroke or Transient Ischemic Attack: A Guideline for Healthcare Professionals From the American Heart Association/American Stroke Association. *Stroke* 2011;42:227–76.
2. Brott TG, Hobson RW, 2nd, Howard G, Roubin GS, Clark WM, Brooks W, et al. Stenting versus endarterectomy for treatment of carotid-artery stenosis. *N Engl J Med* 2010;363: 11–23.
3. Short-term outcome after stenting versus endarterectomy for symptomatic carotid stenosis: a preplanned meta-analysis of individual patient data. *The Lancet* 2010;376:1062–73.
4. Spagnoli LG, Mauriello A, Sangiorgi G, Fratoni S, Bonanno E, Schwartz RS, et al. Extracranial thrombotically active carotid plaque as a risk factor for ischemic stroke. *JAMA* 2004; 292:1845–52.

5. Diethrich EB, Irshad K, Reid DB. Virtual histology and color flow intravascular ultrasound in peripheral interventions. *Semin Vasc Surg* 2006;19:155–62.
6. Diethrich EB, Pauliina MM, Reid DB, Burke A, Ramaiah V, Rodriguez-Lopez JA, et al. Virtual histology intravascular ultrasound assessment of carotid artery disease: the Carotid Artery Plaque Virtual Histology Evaluation (CAPITAL) study. *J Endovasc Ther* 2007;14: 676–86.
7. Nair A, Kuban BD, Tuzcu EM, Schoenhagen P, Nissen SE, Vince DG. Coronary plaque classification with intravascular ultrasound radiofrequency data analysis. *Circulation* 2002;106: 2200–6.
8. Hong MK, Mintz GS, Lee CW, Suh J, Kim JH, Park DW, et al. Comparison of virtual histology to intravascular ultrasound of culprit coronary lesions in acute coronary syndrome and target coronary lesions in stable angina pectoris. *Am J Cardiol* 2007;100:953–9.
9. Timaran CH, Rosero EB, Martinez AE, Ilarraza A, Modrall JG, Clagett GP. Atherosclerotic plaque composition assessed by virtual histology intravascular ultrasound and cerebral embolization after carotid stenting. *J Vasc Surg* 2010;52:1188–94.
10. Timaran CH, Rosero EB, Higuera A, Ilarraza A, Modrall JG, Clagett GP. Randomized clinical trial of open-cell vs closed-cell stents for carotid stenting and effects of stent design on cerebral embolization. *J Vasc Surg* 2011; In Press, Corrected Proof.
11. Mintz GS, Nissen SE, Anderson WD, Bailey SR, Erbel R, Fitzgerald PJ, et al. American College of Cardiology Clinical Expert Consensus Document on Standards for Acquisition, Measurement and Reporting of Intravascular Ultrasound Studies (IVUS). A report of the American College of Cardiology Task Force on Clinical Expert Consensus Documents. *J Am Coll Cardiol* 2001;37:1478–92.
12. Tedesco MM, Lee JT, Dalman RL, Lane B, Loh C, Haukoos JS, et al. Postprocedural microembolic events following carotid surgery and carotid angioplasty and stenting. *J Vasc Surg* 2007;46:244–50.
13. Rubartelli P, Brusa G, Arrigo A, Abbadessa F, Giachero C, Vischi M, et al. Transcranial Doppler monitoring during stenting of the carotid bifurcation: Evaluation of two different distal protection devices in preventing embolization. *J Endovasc Ther* 2006;13:436–42.
14. Bonati LH, Jongen LM, Haller S, Flach HZ, Dobson J, Nederkoorn PJ, et al. New ischaemic brain lesions on MRI after stenting or endarterectomy for symptomatic carotid stenosis: a substudy of the International Carotid Stenting Study (ICSS). *Lancet Neurol* 2010;9: 353–62.
15. Bonati LH, Fraedrich G. Age Modifies the Relative Risk of Stenting versus Endarterectomy for Symptomatic Carotid Stenosis - A Pooled Analysis of EVA-3S, SPACE and ICSS. *Eur J Vasc Endovasc Surg* 2011;41:153–8.
16. Garami ZF, Bismuth J, Charlton-Ouw KM, Davies MG, Peden EK, Lumsden AB. Feasibility of simultaneous pre- and postfilter transcranial Doppler monitoring during carotid artery stenting. *J Vasc Surg* 2009;49:340–4, 5.
17. Ringelstein EB, Droste DW, Babikian VL, Evans DH, Grosset DG, Kaps M, et al. Consensus on microembolus detection by TCD. International Consensus Group on Microembolus Detection. *Stroke* 1998;29:725–9.
18. Surmely JF, Nasu K, Fujita H, Terashima M, Matsubara T, Tsuchikane E, et al. Coronary plaque composition of culprit/target lesions according to the clinical presentation: a virtual histology intravascular ultrasound analysis. *Eur Heart J* 2006;27:2939–44.
19. Granada JF, Wallace-Bradley D, Win HK, Alviar CL, Builes A, Lev EI, et al. In vivo plaque characterization using intravascular ultrasound-virtual histology in a porcine model of complex coronary lesions. *Arterioscler Thromb Vasc Biol* 2007;27:387–93.
20. Porto I, Selvanayagam JB, Van Gaal WJ, Prati F, Cheng A, Channon K, et al. Plaque volume and occurrence and location of periprocedural myocardial necrosis after percutaneous coronary intervention: insights from delayed-enhancement magnetic resonance imaging, thrombolysis in myocardial infarction myocardial perfusion grade analysis, and intravascular ultrasound. *Circulation* 2006;114:662–9.

21. Kawaguchi R, Oshima S, Jingu M, Tsurugaya H, Toyama T, Hoshizaki H, et al. Usefulness of virtual histology intravascular ultrasound to predict distal embolization for ST-segment elevation myocardial infarction. *J Am Coll Cardiol* 2007;50:1641–6.

22. Kawamoto T, Okura H, Koyama Y, Toda I, Taguchi H, Tamita K, et al. The relationship between coronary plaque characteristics and small embolic particles during coronary stent implantation. *J Am Coll Cardiol* 2007;50:1635–40.

23. Irshad K, Millar S, Velu R, Reid AW, Diethrich EB, Reid DB. Virtual histology intravascular ultrasound in carotid interventions. *J Endovasc Ther* 2007;14:198–207.

4

Determinants of Adverse Neurologic Outcomes in Elderly Patients Undergoing Carotid Angioplasty and Stenting

Rabih A. Chaer, MD, FACS, RVT

INTRODUCTION

Stroke ranks third among all causes of death, only behind heart disease and cancer, and is a leading cause of serious long-term disability in the US. Each year nearly 795,000 patients experience a stroke, 87% being ischemic in nature. Of those, between 10 and 30% are due to emboli from the carotid arteries and are secondary to extracranial carotid stenosis.[1–3]

The management of carotid occlusive disease is in evolution. Carotid endarterectomy (CEA), first introduced in the 1950s, has been the established gold standard for the treatment of carotid stenosis for many years. More recently, carotid angioplasty and stenting (CAS) emerged as a minimally invasive alternative, and several trials ensued to determine its safety, efficacy, and the indications for its use. While CAS has proven to be feasible and relatively safe, the appropriate clinical setting for its preferential use over CEA continues to be the subject of ongoing clinical trials and also of frequent debates in day-to-day clinical practice.

Only recently has attention focused on identification of patients who are at greater risk for adverse outcomes during and after CAS, in an effort to refine indications for its use.[4,5] One clear limitation has become evident so far, namely, the higher rate of adverse outcomes in octogenarians. Older patients, most notably octogenarians, represent a subset at especially high risk for complications with CAS. Several studies have demonstrated increased rates of stroke and death among elderly patients with carotid stenosis treated with CAS.[6–8] Although many studies focused on patients in their 80s, evidence suggests an increased risk even with advanced age over 70.[9,10] The purpose of this chapter is to review the outcomes of CAS in elderly patients treated for carotid stenosis, and the determinants of adverse outcomes in this patient group.

CLINICAL EVIDENCE

Although agreement is far from universal, the evidence is nearly overwhelming that advanced age is associated with increased adverse events with CAS. Several studies have demonstrated increased rates of stroke and death among octogenarians. The Carotid Revascularization Endarterectomy versus Stenting Trial (CREST) lead-in phase reported a 30-day stroke and death rate of 12.1% for octogenarians compared with 3.2% among nonoctogenarians (P<.0001), leading to caution in enrollment of patients 80 years of age and older in the study.[6] Similarly, results from Stanziale and associates indicated that CAS in octogenarians was associated with a statistically significantly higher rate of adverse events at 30 days and at 1-year follow up.[7] More recently, a subgroup analysis of the Stent-Supported Percutaneous Angioplasty of the Carotid Artery versus Endarterectomy (SPACE) trial also found that the rate of complications was significantly associated with age in the CAS group; on the other hand, patients in the CEA group had homogenous event rates across all age groups.[9]

The etiology of increased adverse event risk for CAS in the elderly remains incompletely understood. It has been suggested that adverse vascular anatomy and lesion characteristics that have the potential to increase the technical complexity of CAS may account for this finding, since recent studies have suggested that some of these complex anatomic features are more prevalent among older patients.[11,12] Lin and coworkers found that aortic arch calcification, common carotid and innominate artery stenosis, and tortuosity of the common and internal carotid arteries were significantly more severe in patients greater than 80 years old.[11] Likewise, in addition to the features mentioned earlier, others have also found unfavorable arch elongation, severe lesion stenosis greater than 85%, and plaque ulceration to be significantly more common among patients age 80 years and older.[13] (Table 4–1).

Other variables that have been associated with increased risk of adverse events include abnormal arch anatomy,[14] vessel tortuosity,[15] long stenotic lesions (>15 mm),[16] involvement of the internal carotid ostium, and plaque echolucency.[17] However, it is important to also note that, although these anatomic and lesion characteristics are thought to be more common in the elderly population, younger patients may also have similar unfavorable risk factors since long stenoses and ostial involvement can be associated with increased risk of stroke independent of octogenarian status.[16]

TABLE 4–1. PREVALENT HIGH RISK PREDICTORS OF ADVERSE NEUROLOGIC OUTCOMES OF CAS IN ELDERLY PATIENTS

Anatomic high risk	Physiologic high risk
Aortic arch elongation	Decreased cerebral reserve
Aortic arch calcification	
Common carotid and innominate stenosis	
Carotid tortuosity	
Severe lesion stenosis	
Plaque ulceration/vulnerability	

Recent studies have also focused on the relationship between aortic arch anatomy and age. Using high resolution magnetic resonance angiography (MRA), age related morphologic changes of the aortic arch were analyzed.[18] Arch imaging of 105 patients was reviewed and showed increased incidence of Type II/III arch morphology to be associated with age>60. In addition, arch branch vessel angle was increasingly acute with advanced age. These findings suggest increased arch elongation in older patients, and may adversely affect the outcomes of CAS in this patient group.

EFFECT OF HIGH RISK ANATOMIC CRITERIA

Aortic Arch

Arch elongation is a significant deterrent to safe and simple access sheath or guide placement during CAS. The arch is considered a Type I arch if the branches originate at the top of the arch, Type II if they originate within a couple cm inferior to a line drawn across the top of the arch, and Type III if the branches originate along the upslope of the arch, substantially inferior to the top of the arch. As the arch just proximal to the descending aorta becomes elongated a peak or a focal point is created at the upper inner aspect of the arch. With increased arch tortuosity, this point becomes a fulcrum over which the catheter must work and over which the carotid access sheath must pass to enter the common carotid artery. This raises the difficulty of great vessel cannulation, as more catheter and wire manipulation in the aortic arch may be required, potentially increasing the risk of embolization and adverse neurologic events.

Internal Carotid Artery

Carotid tortuosity can increase the difficulty of crossing the target lesion and can complicate the delivery of sheaths and catheters. It may also make the landing zone for the filter too short or may present a situation where stenting is not possible because the stent is unable to conform to the tortuous bifurcation and distal internal carotid artery. Tortuosity of the artery is not alleviated by stent placement and may in fact be worsened by stenting, by propagating the tortuosity to another segment of non-stented artery. This can result in hemodynamically significant kinks or instent stenosis.

Lesion Characteristics

In addition to ostial lesions, and long (>15mm) lesions, high risk lesions for CAS include those with circumferential calcification, heavy plaque burden, highly echogenic plaque, and those that are symptomatic, especially if there has been a recent stroke or a series of TIAs.

Patients with symptomatic carotid stenosis treated with CAS have a higher incidence of stroke compared with asymptomatic patients or patients treated with CEA. While the etiology of adverse neurologic events may be multifactorial, including a higher propensity for embolization of a soft necrotic core, symptomatic patients also appear to have a higher incidence of platelet activation in filter debris as evaluated by electron microscopy. This could represent a consequence of the increased plaque thrombogenicity and vulnerability noted in elderly symptomatic patients, and may explain the increased rate of neurologic complications.

Cerebral Reserve

The effect of cerebral reserve (CR) on outcomes of carotid interventions for occlusive disease remains poorly defined, especially in older patients who might have intracranial occlusive disease as well as various degrees of brain atrophy that may limit their tolerance for minor emboli. CAS is well known to result in frequent subclinical microemboli detected as filling defects on early diffusion MRI.[19, 20] It is plausible that compromised cerebral reserve in the elderly may unmask the subclinical nature of these events, accounting for the increased rate of clinically significant symptomatic neurologic events.

Several techniques have been used experimentally to study the ability of the cerebral vessels to vasodilate. The measurement of cerebral blood flow (CBF) can be performed by various techniques including carotid duplex evaluation,[21] transcranial Doppler (TCD),[22] perfusion-weighted magnetic resonance imaging (PWI),[23] and xenon brain scanning.[24] Using a combination of these techniques, various investigators have demonstrated that certain patients lose the ability to autoregulate their intracerebral vessels and may be intolerant to microembolization.

Although compromised cerebral blood flow is a known predictor of stroke in patients with carotid artery occlusive disease,[25–27] the effect of age on cerebral reserve in this setting remains poorly defined, and may explain the poor outcomes associated with CAS in this patient population. Stable xenon computed tomography (Xe/CT) CBF mapping had been readily available in the US and continues to be used widely overseas, offering a valuable technique for measuring CBF. It allows CR to be easily be assessed by the response to a cerebral vasodilator challenge, acetazolamide (ACZ). Findings using this imaging modality were recently analyzed to evaluate whether older patients may have compromised intracranial collaterals and CR as measured by stable Xe/CT and thus are possibly less tolerant to otherwise clinically silent emboli that are generated during CAS.[28]

The records of all patients evaluated with a Xe/CT CBF mapping before and after ACZ administration between 1991 and 2001 were retrospectively reviewed. Stable xenon ceased to be readily available for clinical use in 2001 as mandated by the FDA, therefore limiting the study period. Out of 1024 patients identified, only 916 had studies that were deemed suitable for analysis. The entire cohort was analyzed initially and then stratified by the presence or absence of carotid stenosis. Information on the status of the carotid vasculature was available for the review in 780 patients (85%) and was based on duplex imaging, computed tomography, or magnetic resonance angiography. Patients were stratified by the presence or absence of carotid stenosis, defined as the presence of a >50% internal carotid stenosis. Two categories of carotid stenosis were therefore used in the analysis model, and patients with carotid occlusion were separately analyzed.

Because compromised cerebral hemodynamics are associated with maximum vasodilatation, CBF response to a vasodilatory challenge should provide a better assessment of vascular reserves or reactivity. ACZ induces maximal cerebral vasodilatation caused by tissue acidosis and can unmask any areas of diminished reserve. Whereas the normal response to ACZ is a 20% to 40% augmentation of flow in all vascular territories, areas with poor perfusion and limited reserve show a decrease in CBF akin to cardiac stress testing with nuclear imaging. Although CBF may change little in areas of basal vasodilatation with moderate collateral compromise, it may actually drop in territories with severe compromise of collaterals representing a "steal" phenomenon.

CBF changes were categorized as normal or abnormal and were analyzed by age, gender, cerebral symptoms, and by the presence of intracranial, carotid or vertebral artery disease. Logistic regression was used to determine the effect of age on CR in the entire group, as well as patients with carotid occlusion, and a subgroup of 179 patients with significant carotid stenosis of >50%. Carotid occlusion was predictive of decreased reserve (OR, 3.9; P=.03) regardless of age. There was also a trend toward lower reserve with severe carotid stenosis >70% (OR, 3) and in women (OR, 1.8; P=.08). Age >70 had no effect on reserve in the overall heterogeneous population that included patients with and without carotid disease; neither did a history of stroke, carotid, or intracranial stenosis.[28]

In a subgroup of 179 patients with significant >50% carotid stenosis, old age>70 was strongly predictive of poor CR (OR, 2.7 [1.1–6.5]; P=.03). This association remained significant, regardless of the severity of stenosis. The presence of peripheral vascular disease (PVD) was also associated with poor CR (OR, 3.7 [1.1–12.7]; P=.03). A trend toward poor CR was also observed in women (OR, 2.3 [0.9–5.7]; P=.08) but did not quite reach statistical significance.[28]

Diminished cerebral reserve may be particularly important during CAS. Embolization during CAS is not uncommon but not always clinically significant.[19,20] It can occur at different stages of the procedure, including aortic arch navigation, during positioning, and even after deployment of cerebral protection devices.[29–31] The current generation of commercially available filters have pore sizes of 100 to 150 µm. Meanwhile, a high-volume of microemboli <60 µm have been demonstrated in experimental models at all stages of the procedure, including the initial wire passage. In addition, routine use of cerebral protection devices has been associated with a significant number of diffusion-weighted magnetic resonance imaging defects, especially octogenarians.[19] This may therefore affect an already diminished cerebral reserve in this group of patients with compromised collateral circulation, and can partially account for the adverse neurologic outcomes seen with CAS in elderly patient.

Although other modalities have been proposed as a tool to evaluate cerebral reserve, the sensitivity of Xe/CT appears to be superior in detecting areas of negative reactivity, and may therefore be the optimum method for assessing cerebral hemodynamic compromise in patients with carotid occlusive disease, particularly when compared to less invasive modalities such as transcranial Doppler imaging.[27] However, the lack of availability of Xe/CT testing currently limits the practical clinical value of this technique.

Cerebrovascular reserve assessed by examining the quantitative response of flow by Xe/CT in patients with carotid occlusive disease can identify high-risk subgroups.[25,26] Patients with symptomatic carotid disease who have significantly compromised CBF vasoreactivity even despite normal baseline CBF appear to have a substantial risk for stroke. In addition, old age >70 in patients with >50% carotid stenosis appears to have a significant association with abnormal cerebral reserve when compared with younger patients and was not affected by the presence of stroke or TIA.[28] Diminished CR is a marker of compromised cerebral collateral circulation, and these patients may therefore be intolerant to minor otherwise silent emboli generated during the different stages of CAS. These findings suggest that elderly patients with carotid stenosis, regardless of symptom status, may be at a higher risk of stroke with CAS because of diminished baseline reserve. It is therefore possible that the combination of adverse lesion pathology and arch anatomy, as well as poor reserve, places the elderly at a particularly high risk of neurologic adverse events during CAS.

Despite the fact that Xe/CT is not currently available for routine clinical use, measuring cerebral reserve in patients being considered for treatment of carotid stenosis is attractive, and may give an insight on the expected functional and cognitive outcomes anticipated with revascularization. Evaluation of reserve could also prove to be beneficial in treatment algorithms for carotid occlusive disease and may guide the choice of the optimal revascularization technique for each individual patient.

CONCLUSIONS

Elderly patients with carotid occlusive disease seem to have prevalent anatomic and physiologic predictors of adverse neurologic outcomes with CAS. Age >70 is also associated with poor cerebral reserve in patients with significant carotid stenosis. Elderly patients could therefore be at a higher risk of stroke during CAS non-withstanding hostile anatomy, and should be considered for alternative treatment modalities. Though anatomic considerations such as carotid tortuosity, proximal stenosis, or hostile arch characteristics, may be the culprits rather than age itself, the role of depleted cerebral reserve and increased plaque vulnerability is increasingly recognized, cautioning the use of CAS in elderly patients.

REFERENCES

1. Chaturvedi S, Bruno A, Feasby T, et al; Therapeutics and Technology Assessment Subcommittee of the American Academy of Neurology. Carotid endarterectomy—an evidence-based review: report of the Therapeutics and Technology Assessment Subcommittee of the American Academy of Neurology. *Neurology* 2005; 65:794–801.
2. Howell GM, Makaroun MS, Chaer RA. Current management of extracranial carotid occlusive disease. *J Am Coll Surg* 2009; 208:442–453.
3. Barnett HJ, Gunton RW, Eliasziw M, et al. Causes and severity of ischemic stroke in patients with internal carotid artery stenosis. *JAMA* 2000; 283:1429–1436.7.
4. Chaer RA, Makaroun MS. Carotid artery stenosis: what is left to surgery? *J Cardiovasc Surg (Torino)*. 2009;50(1):39–47.
5. Chaer RA, Makaroun MS. Current indications for carotid angioplasty and stenting. *Perspect Vasc Surg Endovasc Ther* 2008;20(3):239–44.
6. Hobson RW 2nd, Howard VJ, Roubin GS, Brott TG, Ferguson RD, Popma JJ, et al; CREST Investigators. Carotid artery stenting is associated with increased complications in octogenarians: 30-day stroke and death rates in the CREST lead-in phase. *J Vasc Surg* 2004;40: 1106–11.
7. Stanziale SF, Marone LK, Boules TN, Brimmeier JA, Hill K, Makaroun MS, Wholey MH. Carotid artery stenting in octogenarians is associated with increased adverse outcomes. *J Vasc Surg* 2006;43:297–304.
8. Roubin GS, New G, Iyer SS, Vitek JJ, Al-Mubarak N, Liu MW, et al. Immediate and late clinical outcomes of carotid artery stenting in patients with symptomatic and asymptomatic carotid artery stenosis: a 5-year prospective analysis. *Circulation* 2001;103:532–7.
9. Stingele R, Berger J, Alfke K, Eckstein HH, Fraedrich G, Allenberg J, et al. Clinical and angiographic risk factors for stroke and death within 30 days after carotid endarterectomy and stent-protected angioplasty: a subanalysis of the SPACE study. *Lancet Neurol* 2008; 7:216–22.

10. Yadav JS, Wholey MH, Kuntz RE, Fayad P, Katzen BT, Mishkel GJ, et al; Stenting and Angioplasty with Protection in Patients at High Risk for Endarterectomy Investigators. Protected carotid-artery stenting versus endarterectomy in high-risk patients. *N Engl J Med* 2004;351:1493–501.

11. Lin SC, Trocciola SM, Rhee J, Dayal R, Chaer R, Morrissey NJ, et al. Analysis of anatomic factors and age in patients undergoing carotid angioplasty and stenting. *Ann Vasc Surg* 2005;19:798–804.

12. Lam RC, Lin SC, DeRubertis B, Hynecek R, Kent KC, Faries PL. The impact of increasing age on anatomic factors affecting carotid angioplasty and stenting. *J Vasc Surg* 2007;45:875–80.

13. Kastrup A, Gröschel K, Schnaudigel S, Nägele T, Schmidt F, Ernemann U. Target lesion ulceration and arch calcification are associated with increased incidence of carotid stenting-associated ischemic lesions in octogenarians. *J Vasc Surg* 2008;47:88–95.

14. Faggioli GL, Ferri M, Freyrie A, Gargiulo M, Fratesi F, Rossi C, et al. Aortic arch anomalies are associated with increased risk of neurological events in carotid stent procedures. *Eur J Vasc Endovasc Surg* 2007;33: 436–41.

15. Faggioli G, Ferri M, Gargiulo M, Freyrie A, Fratesi F, Manzoli L, Stella A. Measurement and impact of proximal and distal tortuosity in carotid stenting procedures. *J Vasc Surg* 2007; 46:1119–24.

16. Sayeed S, Stanziale SF, Wholey MH, Makaroun MS. Angiographic lesion characteristics can predict adverse outcomes after carotid artery stenting. *J Vasc Surg* 2008;47:81–7.

17. Biasi GM, Froio A, Diethrich EB, Deleo G, Galimberti S, Mingazzini P, et al. Carotid plaque echolucency increases the risk of stroke in carotid stenting: the Imaging in Carotid Angioplasty and Risk of Stroke (ICAROS) Study. *Circulation* 2004;110:756–62.

18. DeRubertis BG, Alktaifi A, Finn JP, Farley S, Saleh RS, Moore WS, Lawrence PF Anatomic Assessment of the Aortic Arch: Relationship between Arch Anatomy and Age. Presented at the Society for Vascular Surgery Annual Meeting, Chicago, IL, June 2011.

19. Barbato JE, Dillavou E, Horowitz MB, Jovin TG, Kanal E, David S, Makaroun MS. A randomized trial of carotid artery stenting with and without cerebral protection. *J Vasc Surg* 2008;47:760–5.

20. Coggia M, Goëau-Brissonnière O, Duval JL, Leschi JP, Letort M, Nagel MD. Embolic risk of the different stages of carotid bifurcation balloon angioplasty: an experimental study. *J Vasc Surg* 2000;31: 550–7.

21. Ascher E, Markevich N, Schutzer RW, Kallakuri S, Jacob T, Hingorani AP. Cerebral hyperperfusion syndrome after carotid endarterectomy: predictive factors and hemodynamic changes. *J Vasc Surg* 2003;37:769–777.

22. Muller M, Voges M, Piepgras U, Schimrigk K. Assessment of cerebral ultrasound and breath holding. A comparison with acetazolamide as vasodilatory stimulus. *Stroke* 1995;26: 96–100.

23. Fukuda T, Ogasawara K, Kobayashi N, et al. Prediction of cerebral blood volume measured by perfusion weighted MR imaging compared with single-photon emission CT. *AJNR* 2007;28:737–742.

24. Riegel MM, Hollier LH, Sundt TM, Piepgras DG, Sharbrough FW, Cherry KJ. Cerebral hyperperfusion syndrome: a cause of neurologic dysfunction after carotid endarterectomy. *J Vasc Surg* 1987;5:628–634.

25. Webster MW, Steed DL, Yonas H, Latchaw RE, Wolfson SK Jr., Gur D. Cerebral blood flow measured by xenon-enhanced computed tomography as a guide to management of patients with cerebrovascular disease. *J Vasc Surg* 1986;3:298–304.

26. Webster MW, Makaroun MS, Steed DL, Smith HA, Johnson DW, Yonas H. Compromised cerebral blood flow reactivity is a predictor of stroke in patients with symptomatic carotid artery occlusive disease. *J Vasc Surg* 1995;21:338–44.

27. Pindzola RR, Balzer JR, Nemoto EM, Goldstein S, Yonas H. Cerebrovascular reserve in patients with carotid occlusive disease assessed by stable xenon-enhanced ct cerebral blood flow and transcranial Doppler. *Stroke* 2001;32:1811–7.

28. Chaer RA, Shen J, Rao A, Cho JS, Abu Hamad G, Makaroun MS. Cerebral reserve is decreased in elderly patients with carotid stenosis. *J Vasc Surg*. 2010;52(3):569–74; discussion 574–5.

29. Gossetti B, Gattuso R, Irace L, Faccenna F, Venosi S, Bozzao L, et al. Embolism to the brain during carotid stenting and surgery. *Acta Chir Belg* 2007;107:151–4.

30. Hellings WE, Ackerstaff RG, Pasterkamp G, De Vries JP, Moll FL. The carotid atherosclerotic plaque and microembolisation during carotid stenting. *J Cardiovasc Surg (Torino)* 2006;47:115–26.

31. Macdonald S. Is there any evidence that cerebral protection is beneficial? Experimental data. *J Cardiovasc Surg (Torino)* 2006;47:127–36.

5

Asymptomatic Carotid Artery Stenosis Risk Stratification

Rafael D. Malgor, MD, RPVI and
Nicos Labropoulos, PhD, DIC, RVT

BACKGROUND

Stroke is an important economic and social burden in the US.[1-2] The most common cause of stroke is embolism. A carotid artery atherosclerotic plaque (carotid atheroma) is a significant source of embolization as it is responsible for about a third of all embolic strokes. Patients bearing carotid atheromas are either symptomatic presenting with transient ischemic attack (TIA), amaurose fugax (AF), stroke or have no symptoms. Asymptomatic carotid artery disease (ACAD) is responsible for about 8% of all strokes.

The annual risk of developing any cerebrovascular event in patients with a carotid atheroma is 1-2% based on the Asymptomatic Carotid Atherosclerosis Study (ACAS) and the Asymptomatic Carotid Surgery Trial (ACST).[3-4] Regardless of the plaque characteristics, patients in these two large trials were treated based on degree of stenosis. At that time the medical treatment was significantly different from the current. In the nonsurgical arm of ACAS, patients received 325mg of aspirin and were educated about risk factors such as diabetes, hypertension and tobacco use prior to enrollment.[3] The use of anti-platelets, lipid-lowering and anti-hypertensive drugs were utilized by the ACST investigators but relied on each center's discretion. Furthermore, the amount of ACST patients who were on the lipid-lowering medications greatly increased over time and therefore it became difficult to analyze the impact of medical treatment.[5]

A systematic review of ACAD trials over a 22-year period including 3,724 patients demonstrated decreasing rates of cerebrovascular events related to the improvement of medical therapy.[6] In a prospective analysis of 101 patients with ACAD who were routinely treated with anti-platelets, statins and anti-hypertensive medications if blood pressure (BP) > 130/80mmHg in the Oxford area the annual risk of ipsilateral events was 0.34% (95% CI, 0.01 to 1.87).[7] This was the first prospective study focusing on the current medical therapy over the last 10 years.

In the US, unless the patients can be stratified properly the best medical treatment will remain an alternative option. Therefore, at the present time the most challenging question for those who deal with ACAD patients is when to operate. A great deal of data available on the treatment of ACAD derives from large trials evaluating the treatment performed by either carotid endarterectomy (CEA) or stenting (CAS).[3–4, 8] The only criterion used in those trials was the degree of stenosis. The proven deficiency of using one aspect of the plaque to define who would benefit of any sort of treatment is the simplistic concept that only flow reduction to the brain counts for tissue ischemia. In a subset analysis of 3,007 ACST patients a reduced vessel diameter distal to the area of stenosis was protective showing a low risk of ipsilateral stroke. This rose the concern that the degree of stenosis alone should not always justify an intervention in asymptomatic patients.[9]

Several authors have investigated the importance of plaque components and its instability causing either embolization of plaque fragments or in-situ thrombosis due to exposure of its components.[10] The likelihood of plaques that are uniformly echogenic and have a fibrotic cap have less embolization than those with hypoechoic material.[10] Furthermore, clinical features including cardiovascular risk factors and lifestyle habitus such as smoking, hypertension and hyperlipidemia coupled with plaque morphology and degree of stenosis are also important factors accounting to increased risk of disease progression and adverse outcomes such as TIA and stroke.[11]

Pertinent presentation of the results of studies on ACAD available in the literature, natural history and specific risk factors involved in the risk stratification are discussed.

NATURAL HISTORY OF ACAD

Two different extremes of the same disease exist in symptomatic and asymptomatic patients with atherosclerotic carotid disease. Whilst the outcomes in the symptomatic group are poor if not treated in a timely fashion, the course of ACAD has a low event rate and therefore a much better prognosis. The natural history of ACAD has been extensively studied over the past three decades.[10, 12–20]

Patients with ACAD are indentified from the presence of cervical bruits, during investigation of nonspecific signs and symptoms and prior to pre-operative evaluation for cardiac or other major surgery. The first imaging study utilized to rule out any cerebral ischemic event is a CT scan of the head and a duplex ultrasound (DU) of the carotid artery. Evaluation with DU relies on determining the degree of carotid stenosis. The plaque characteristics are not taken into account routinely and are not reported on a standardized fashion.

Patients with abnormally elevated DU velocities or ratios are stratified as having a mild, moderate or severe stenosis. Accordingly, those patients are stratified and therefore offered a procedure or place on medical therapy if a non-high grade stenosis is found. After the publication of the ACAS in 1995, there was an increase in the accrual number of CEA in the US. The number of asymptomatic patients treated based on DU velocities found in a national and statewide databases demonstrated that the majority of CEAs are performed to treat patients with ACAD.[21] The rationale of treating ACAD was the slightly lower rate of cerebrovascular events in patients who underwent CEA in the ACST and ACAS when compared to the control group receiving medical treatment. However, the stroke-free incidence found in the ACAS and ACST indicate that more than 94% of the procedures were perhaps unnecessary.[22] Moreover, the patients enrolled in the ACST that were managed with best medical treatment had risk of any or ipsilateral stroke of about 12% and 5% at 5-year that was reduced to 7% and 4% at 10-year period.

Certain plaque morphology characteristics such as ulceration and echolucent material are known to have a more active cellular turnover making the plaque prone to rupture and embolize. Recent research on the plaque morphology and its components graded using grayscale median (GSM), white areas and the area of the plaque have assisted in gauging the "benign" versus unstable plaques from cerebral and retinal ischemic embolic events.[10] The largest prospective study on patients with ACAD enrolled 1,121 consecutive patients as part of the Asymptomatic Carotid Stenosis and Risk of Stroke (ACSRS) Study Group.[10] All patients had DU assessment of internal carotid artery stenosis and plaque morphology that were correlated to clinical characteristics and followed for a mean period of 4 years. The degree of stenosis of the ICA was found to be correlated with the outcomes. An increasing risk of ipsilateral cerebrovascular events was demonstrated in patients with severe stenosis (> 90% to 99% ECST criteria[23]) compared to those who had mild or moderate stenosis (≤ 89% ECST). However, estimated risk of developing any ipsilateral ischemic cerebral event in a 5-year period was estimated to be high in only 9% of the patients who had a stable carotid plaque despite ≥70% stenosis using the ECST criteria.

The implications of risk stratification found by the ACSRS collaborators and other prospective studies[11, 19] provide evidence that the vast majority of patients are better off with conservative treatment. Also patients at higher risk could be identified and offered operative treatment. However, validation of predicted risk in that study was limited since it was done for the same group of patients on whom the score was developed. These findings need to be validated in prospective studies using current best medical therapy.

RISK STRATIFICATION

Several factors have been associated with ipsilateral events to carotid plaque (Figure 5–1). The evidence for each of these factors is discussed below.

Degree of Stenosis

The degree of stenosis remains the mainstay criterion upon which vascular interventionalists use to decide who should have a carotid artery intervention. The importance of the degree of carotid stenosis and its correlation to cerebrovascular events has been demonstrated by several studies.[3,10,17,23] Treatment is often indicated for ACAD when a >60% stenosis is detected.[3–4, 23]

The shortcoming of relying only upon the degree of stenosis alone is that not all plaques that generate a vessel stenosis are unstable enough to prompt distal embolization or trigger an episode of in-situ thrombosis with subsequent occlusion of the vessel. Spence et al investigating 319 ACAD patients with >60% stenosis demonstrated

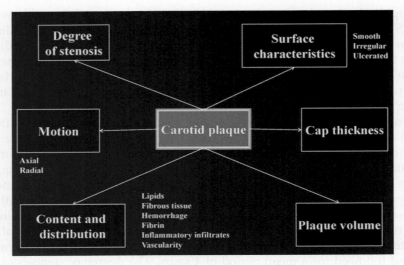

Figure 5–1. Plaque characteristics associated with cerebrovascular events.

that <1% of them developed stroke if there were no high intensity transient signals (microemboli) on transcranial Doppler (TCD).[11] In the ACSRS patients with moderate to severe stenosis had more cerebral ischemic events than those with <50% stenosis. However, only 9% of patients with ≥70% stenosis were deemed to be high-risk for cerebral or retinal events based on other risk factors such as absence of contralateral TIA or stroke, no discrete white areas (DWAs), plaque area and GSM. In addition, Kakkos at al analyzing data of 462 ACAD patients with 60–99% stenosis showed that silent CT embolic infarcts have doubled the risk for developing a stroke compared to those without infarction.[24] Therefore, the degree of stenosis alone may no longer reflect or predict the group of patients who will have a stroke and may benefit from carotid artery intervention.

Plaque Morphology

The study of plaque morphology includes the following: surface characteristics, echogenicity, distribution of plaque content, volume and plaque kinetics. These have been studied by several methods such as DU, MRI, CT and histology. Prospective studies supporting the role of plaque morphology are displayed on Table 5–1.

Surface

The surface of the plaque is defined as the linen that covers the plaque contents. The surface is defined as smooth, irregular and ulcerated. Arteriographic and histological analysis provided by endarterectomy specimens has been utilized to detect surface abnormalities of the plaque.[25] Ulceration has often been characterized as a depression of >1mm in width and depth[25] however its real definition is loss of endothelial lining. In patients with asymptomatic carotid stenosis who are not always candidates for a procedure a noninvasive imaging evaluation using DU, CT or MR is more adequate reserving catheter-based angiogram for endovascular interventions and rarely for diagnostic purposes.[26]

TABLE 5–1. PROSPECTIVE STUDIES SUPPORTING THE ROLE OF PLAQUE MORPHOLOGY ON DEVELOPING IPSILATERAL CEREBROVASCULAR EVENTS

	Year of Publication	N	Follow-up, months (range)	Institution
Johnson et al[13]	1985	297	36	Single-center
Sterpetti et al[32]	1988	214	34 (26–39)	Single-center
Langsfeld et al[33]	1989	289	22 (3–48)	Single-center
Bock et al[14]	1993	242	28 (n/a)	Single-center
CHS[34]	1998	104	40 (0.3–49)	Multi-center
Tromsø study**[35]	2001	223	36	Multi-center
Nadareishvili et al[20]	2002	106	120 (60–216)	Multi-center
Grønholdt et al[36]	2002	246	53 (36–70)	Multi-center
ACRCS[10]	2010	1121	48 (6–96)	Multi-center

*297 carotid arteries in 297 patients were follow-up for 3 years; 6 died but it is not reported if other patients were lost; CHS, Cardiovascular Health Study; ACSRS, Asymptomatic Carotid Stenosis and Risk of Stroke (Study Group); **All patients were followed up for 36 months.

The sensitivity and specificity of the DU on detecting ulceration has improved over the years. Both B-mode imaging and flow disturbance originated by ulceration can be used to identify surface abnormalities on DU. The improvement of ultrasound imaging and possibility of 3D format certainly will assist in increasing the likelihood of ulcer detection. A high-resolution MR imaging and multidetector CT angiography have also shown very good results of ulceration detection.[27]

The plaque ulceration might be included in the risk stratification due to its importance of generating embolic and thrombotic events. Frequently, surface abnormalities such as ulceration are found in symptomatic patients but can be found in up to 60% of the asymptomatic patients.[25] The risk of stroke in patients with carotid stenosis and ulcerated plaque was found to be doubled among patients with >70% stenosis compared to those without plaque ulceration. In addition, asymptomatic carotid artery plaques that are ulcerated or have surface thrombi were found to be associated with higher cerebral embolization rate up to 53% when stenotic plaques are present.

Another important surface feature is the neovascularization and adventitial vasa vasorum of the plaque. Neovascularization of an atheroma was initially described in patients with coronary artery disease triggering myocardial ischemic events.[28] Investigation of the adventitial hyperplastic network in patients with carotid disease has also been performed utilizing MR, CT or DU with contrast. The latter is of great interest in vascular practice due to wide availability, short learning curve and anatomic access due to relative superficial location of carotid artery. Vicenzini and colleagues studying 23 patients with ACAD demonstrated that neovascularization is constantly present underneath ulcerated areas rendering the plaque potentially more vulnerable.[29] In addition, the angiogenesis network was identified coming from the adventitia toward the inner layers of the plaque but this pattern was not detected in hyperechoic plaques with acoustic shadow (calcified) nor in those with advance inflammatory changes such as hypoechoic necrotic plaques.[29] Regression of the adventitial vasa vasorum in a patient upon initiation of treatment with statins was reported suggesting a potential role for treatment monitoring.[30]

Plaque cap thickness has been correlated with plaque vulnerability. In a study of 22 patients who underwent carotid endarterectomy greater number of plaques with cap thickness defined as <200μm was found to be associated with cerebrovascular events (P=.01).[31] In another study, histological analysis of 105 plaques in asymptomatic and symptomatic patients demonstrated that the presence of an echogenic cap was four times more frequent in symptomatic patients compared to those with asymptomatic plaques (P<0.05).[32] In addition, the echolucent region juxtaluminal was more often present in symptomatic plaques (67% versus 33%; P<0.01).[32]

Plaque Content and Its Distribution

The amount of lipid and its characteristic is variable and related to oxidative reactions led by inflammation and misbalanced production and scavenging of free radicals. The vulnerability of the plaque is directly linked to amount of core necrosis and intra-plaque hemorrhagic events.[25, 33] Distinct nomenclature is already utilized to characterize the plaque morphology (i.e. echolucent versus echogenic, soft versus dense, complicated versus uncomplicated). Plaques have been classified in 4 or 5 types based on their echogenicity. The morphologic classification and the corresponding ultrasound images are shown on Figure 5–2. In addition to the macroscopic ultrasonic evaluation of echogenicity, the GSM defined as a score is obtained using computer software as a surrogate marker of plaque vulnerability. In fact, lipid-rich plaque core is seen in the DU as echolucent and fibrotic components as echogenic. The association of GSM and discrete white areas (DWAs) with the homogeneity of the plaque was also described by Nicolaides at al in a study of 1,121 asymptomatic patients showing that plaques with DWAs and lower GSM (<15) are more prone to generate cerebral and retinal events.[10]

The association of macrophages and plaque lipid content and hemorrhage has been established.[34] In a study of 106 patients who had DU and subsequently underwent endarterectomy with plaque histology analysis, a higher concentration of macrophages in the plaque was related to more echolucent plaques.[34] The use of aspirin was associated with decreased number of macrophages and therefore inflammatory changes.[34] Interestingly, echolucent plaques are more commonly found in women than men with carotid stenosis >50% and triglyceride-rich lipoproteins. Other blood lipid fraction misbalances such as low levels of high-density lipoprotein (HDL) were also associated with echolucent plaques.

In the Tromso study a total of 223 patients with carotid artery stenosis were compared to 215 age-gender matched control patients demonstrating that 28% who had a stenotic plaques and predominantly or completely echolucent plaques had an ipsilateral cerebrovascular event.[35] By contrast, in the same study only 4% of patients with predominantly echogenic or completely echogenic plaques had ipsilateral cerebrovascular events.[35]

Volume

Volume analysis can be achieved using ultrasound, CT or MR imaging. Frequently, the method utilized in CT and MR is the demarcation of the regions of interest in multiple planes generating the area of the plaque that are added together creating a 3D image. The ultrasonic assessment of the plaque volume is achieved using a real-time cine-loop recording application that utilizes the sequential 2D gray scale imaging.

The sex differences related to the plaque volume was evaluated in a study 131 asymptomatic carotid plaques using a 3.0-Tesla MR showing that an increased volume of LRNC is more prevalent in men. Underhill at al analyzing predictors of surface disruption and subsequent cerebral ischemic event also using MR in a cohort of 180

Plaque type

Type 1. Uniformly echolucent (black): Only 15% of the pixels in the plaque area were occupied by pixels with grayscale values >25

Type 2. Mainly echolucent: pixels with grayscale values >25 occupy 15% to 50% of the plaque area

Type 3. Mainly echogenic: pixels with grayscale values >25 occupy 50% to 85% of the plaque area

Type 4. Uniformly echogenic: pixels with grayscale values >25 occupy > 85% of the plaque area.

Type 5. Dense plaque calcification that does not allow characterization of the content.

Carotid plaque with significant surface disruption indicating the presence of an ulcer.

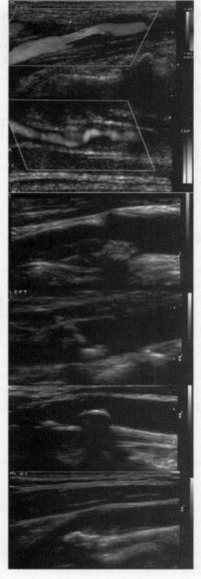

Figure 5–2. Classification of plaque morphology by ultrasound.

asymptomatic patients with carotid stenosis between 50-79% demonstrated that a larger percentage of lipid-rich necrotic core volume (LRNC) (16.1 ± 14.9 versus 3.1 ± 7.1%, respectively; P < .001) was associated with surface disruption.[33]

The actual limitations of the plaque volume studies are the relative small number of studies with small number of patients, a variety of measuring methods and poor long-term prospective follow-up to define the cutoffs to assist in selecting patients at risk of an ischemic cerebral event. Nonetheless, as availability of high-quality imaging data expands the use of plaque volume analysis in patients with ACAD will certainly provide vascular specialists with another parameter to define vulnerable plaques.

Plaque Motion

A proposition of changing in plaque motion following medical treatment was made by Lenzi and Vicenzini. In the evaluation of two asymptomatic patients the carotid plaque and vessel wall move in the opposite direction of the blood flow.[36] The motion pattern described was hypothesized to be a potential cause of external plaque layer disruption creating a thrombogenic surface with exposure of the plaque material and embolization of plaque fragments.

Clinical association of plaque motion was assessed in a study of 242 stroke and 336 transient ischemic attack (TIA) patients showing that presence of longitudinal plaque motion tripled the risk of developing a TIA (P=0.02).[37] Regardless some evidence and delineation of the plaque kinetics underpinnings, it remains an evolving concept that need more clinical grounding assessments but certainly will be added to the risk stratification of ACAD patients in the future.

CONTRALATERAL ISCHEMIC BRAIN ATTACK

The association of contralateral symptomatic carotid stenosis with an ipsilateral asymptomatic carotid stenosis was demonstrated in the ACST.[4] In this trial, patients with contralateral ischemic brain events secondary to carotid plaque were found to have more ipsilateral strokes than those patients with ipsilateral carotid stenosis and no significant or asymptomatic contralateral disease (35 *vs.* 11, p=0·0004).[4]

The results of the ACST are in agreement with those found in the ACSRS trial conducted by Nicolaides et al.[10] In the latter, 1,121 patients with asymptomatic carotid plaque who had a history of contralateral TIAs or stroke had an increased risk of ipsilateral cerebrovascular or retinal ischemic event (Hazard ratio (HR) 2.35; CI 95% 1.60–3.43) and ipsilateral stroke (HR 3.03; CI 95% 1.77–5.20).[10]

BASELINE INFARCTS ON CT SCAN/MRI

Embolic activity of carotid plaque can be indirectly stated in the absence of cardioembolism by finding a silent brain infarct in a CT or MRI. A reasonable number of patients with a high-grade asymptomatic carotid stenosis will develop a silent embolic infarct that may perhaps be predictive of a future TIA or stroke.[24]

In a large prospective multicenter study of 821 patients, 17% had a CT scan showing cortical, subcortical and basal ganglia brain infarcts in patients with ≥60% asymptomatic carotid artery stenosis. In that study the cumulative stroke-free rate was 0.92 (1.0% annual stroke rate) in the absence of embolic infarcts and 0.71 (3.6% annual stroke rate) in their presence (P < .002; HR, 3.0; 95% CI, 1.46–6.29).[24] The findings of silent brain infarcts in patients combined to other factors herein discussed may assist in selecting high-risk asymptomatic patients for treatment. Evaluation with CT or MR during follow-up of asymptomatic patients is warranted.

Transcranial Doppler

Transcranial Doppler (TCD) has been described as an important tool in the assessment of patients with ACAD. The evaluation of cerebral vasoreactivity response and identification of plaque fragments traveling through the brain circulation can be done by the TCD. The embolic debris originated from a carotid artery plaque can be detected as embolic signals insonating the middle cerebral or ophthalmic artery.[11] The cerebral vasoreactivity is tested by asking the patients to inspire 6% carbon dioxide or by injecting acetazolamide to estimate the vasodilatory effects in the cerebral blood flow.

The Asymptomatic Carotid Emboli Study (ACES), a prospective observational study that recruited 482 patients to assess the embolic activity of carotid plaques demonstrated that about 16% of the patients had a positive TCD signal compatible with plaque fragments embolization.[38] In those who had emboli signals the risk of ipsilateral stroke and TIA was higher compared with those without emboli signals (HR=2.54, 95% CI 1·20–5·36; p=0·015) as well as the risk of ipsilateral stroke alone (HR=5.57, 95% CI 1·61–19·32; p=0·007).[38]

Spence at al following a cohort of 319 for a 2-year period reported incidence of 10% of patients with ACAD with positive embolic signals. Those patients with negative TCD for embolic signals had lower risk of stroke during the first year of follow-up (15.6%, 95% CI, 4.1 to 79; versus 1%, 95% CI, 1.01 to 1.36; $P < 0.0001$). As stated above the risk of stroke was nearly 1% in asymptomatic patients. This raised concern as endarterectomy or stenting have a higher risk. In a subsequent prospective study (n= 468 patients) the same authors demonstrated that the trends of embolic signals rate throughout a 7-year period decreased. This probably was due to plaque stabilization secondary to an expanding number of patients on best medical therapy.[39]

A subset analysis of the 106 patients participating in the ACES found that there was no association between impaired cerebral vasoreactivity and recurrent ischemic events but the study was unpowered; however, a meta-analysis performed by the authors did show association between impaired vasoreactivity and future ischemic cerebral events.[40] In reality, the ACES collaborators advocated that vasoreactivity measurement will require further data to be supported as a diagnostic tool in the risk stratification algorithm in patients with ACAD.

CONCLUSION

Asymptomatic carotid artery stenosis risk stratification remains a complex and evolving subject in Vascular Surgery. The past concept of degree of carotid plaque stenosis alone in asymptomatic patients justifying a massive number of procedures has been slowly put in dispute. Carotid plaque characteristics such as type of the plaque, plaque surface and volume, history of contralateral TIAs and stroke, evaluation of silent embolic strokes by CT or MR and assessment of embolic particles by transcranial Doppler must be combined at the final patient assessment whenever available in order to offer the best treatment tailored to each patient specifics.

REFERENCES

1. Qureshi AI, Suri MF, Nasar A, Kirmani JF, Ezzeddine MA, Divani AA, et al. Changes in cost and outcome among US patients with stroke hospitalized in 1990 to 1991 and those hospitalized in 2000 to 2001. *Stroke* 2007 Jul;38(7):2180–4.
2. Reed SD, Blough DK, Meyer K, Jarvik JG. Inpatient costs, length of stay, and mortality for cerebrovascular events in community hospitals. *Neurology* 2001 Jul 24;57(2):305–14.

3. Endarterectomy for asymptomatic carotid artery stenosis. Executive Committee for the Asymptomatic Carotid Atherosclerosis Study. *JAMA* 1995 May 10;273(18):1421–8.

4. Halliday A, Mansfield A, Marro J, Peto C, Peto R, Potter J, et al. Prevention of disabling and fatal strokes by successful carotid endarterectomy in patients without recent neurological symptoms: randomised controlled trial. *Lancet* 2004 May 8;363(9420):1491–502.

5. Halliday A, Harrison M, Hayter E, Kong X, Mansfield A, Marro J, et al. 10-year stroke prevention after successful carotid endarterectomy for asymptomatic stenosis (ACST-1): a multicentre randomised trial. *Lancet* 2010 Sep 25;376(9746):1074–84.

6. Abbott AL. Medical (nonsurgical) intervention alone is now best for prevention of stroke associated with asymptomatic severe carotid stenosis: results of a systematic review and analysis. *Stroke* 2009 Oct;40(10):e573–83.

7. Marquardt L, Geraghty OC, Mehta Z, Rothwell PM. Low risk of ipsilateral stroke in patients with asymptomatic carotid stenosis on best medical treatment: a prospective, population-based study. *Stroke* 2010 Jan;41(1):e11–7.

8. Silver FL, Mackey A, Clark WM, Brooks W, Timaran CH, Chiu D, et al. Safety of stenting and endarterectomy by symptomatic status in the Carotid Revascularization Endarterectomy Versus Stenting Trial (CREST). *Stroke* 2011 Mar;42(3):675–80.

9. Rothwell PM, Warlow CP. Low risk of ischemic stroke in patients with reduced internal carotid artery lumen diameter distal to severe symptomatic carotid stenosis: cerebral protection due to low poststenotic flow? On behalf of the European Carotid Surgery Trialists' Collaborative Group. *Stroke* 2000 Mar;31(3):622–30.

10. Nicolaides AN, Kakkos SK, Kyriacou E, Griffin M, Sabetai M, Thomas DJ, et al. Asymptomatic internal carotid artery stenosis and cerebrovascular risk stratification. *J Vasc Surg* 2010 Dec;52(6):1486–96 e1–5.

11. Spence JD, Tamayo A, Lownie SP, Ng WP, Ferguson GG. Absence of microemboli on transcranial Doppler identifies low-risk patients with asymptomatic carotid stenosis. *Stroke* 2005 Nov;36(11):2373–8.

12. Bock RW, Gray-Weale AC, Mock PA, App Stats M, Robinson DA, Irwig L, et al. The natural history of asymptomatic carotid artery disease. *J Vasc Surg* 1993 Jan;17(1):160–9; discussion 70–1.

13. Chambers BR, Norris JW. Outcome in patients with asymptomatic neck bruits. *N Engl J Med* 1986 Oct 2;315(14):860–5.

14. Hennerici M, Hulsbomer HB, Hefter H, Lammerts D, Rautenberg W. Natural history of asymptomatic extracranial arterial disease. Results of a long-term prospective study. *Brain* 1987 Jun;110 (Pt 3):777–91.

15. Norris JW, Zhu CZ, Bornstein NM, Chambers BR. Vascular risks of asymptomatic carotid stenosis. *Stroke* 1991 Dec;22(12):1485–90.

16. Zhu CZ, Norris JW. A therapeutic window for carotid endarterectomy in patients with asymptomatic carotid stenosis. *Can J Surg* 1991 Oct;34(5):437–40.

17. Mackey AE, Abrahamowicz M, Langlois Y, Battista R, Simard D, Bourque F, et al. Outcome of asymptomatic patients with carotid disease. Asymptomatic Cervical Bruit Study Group. *Neurology* 1997 Apr;48(4):896–903.

18. Nadareishvili ZG, Rothwell PM, Beletsky V, Pagniello A, Norris JW. Long-term risk of stroke and other vascular events in patients with asymptomatic carotid artery stenosis. *Arch Neurol* 2002 Jul;59(7):1162–6.

19. Goessens BM, Visseren FL, Kappelle LJ, Algra A, van der Graaf Y. Asymptomatic carotid artery stenosis and the risk of new vascular events in patients with manifest arterial disease: the SMART study. *Stroke* 2007 May;38(5):1470–5.

20. Johnson JM, Kennelly MM, Decesare D, Morgan S, Sparrow A. Natural history of asymptomatic carotid plaque. *Arch Surg* 1985 Sep;120(9):1010–2.

21. Woo K, Garg J, Hye RJ, Dilley RB. Contemporary results of carotid endarterectomy for asymptomatic carotid stenosis. *Stroke* 2010 May;41(5):975–9.

22. Naylor AR, Gaines PA, Rothwell PM. Who benefits most from intervention for asymptomatic carotid stenosis: patients or professionals? *Eur J Vasc Endovasc Surg* 2009 Jun;37(6):625–32.

23. MRC European Carotid Surgery Trial: interim results for symptomatic patients with severe (70–99%) or with mild (0–29%) carotid stenosis. European Carotid Surgery Trialists' Collaborative Group. *Lancet* 1991 May 25;337(8752):1235–43.

24. Kakkos SK, Sabetai M, Tegos T, Stevens J, Thomas D, Griffin M, et al. Silent embolic infarcts on computed tomography brain scans and risk of ipsilateral hemispheric events in patients with asymptomatic internal carotid artery stenosis. *J Vasc Surg* 2009 Apr;49(4):902–9.

25. Park AE, McCarthy WJ, Pearce WH, Matsumura JS, Yao JS. Carotid plaque morphology correlates with presenting symptomatology. *J Vasc Surg* 1998 May;27(5):872–8; discussion 8–9.

26. Homburg PJ, Plas GJ, Rozie S, van der Lugt A, Dippel DW. Prevalence and calcification of intracranial arterial stenotic lesions as assessed with multidetector computed tomography angiography. *Stroke* 2011 May;42(5):1244–50.

27. Tartari S, Rizzati R, Righi R, Deledda A, Capello K, Soverini R, et al. High-Resolution MRI of Carotid Plaque With a Neurovascular Coil and Contrast-Enhanced MR Angiography: One-Stop Shopping for the Comprehensive Assessment of Carotid Atherosclerosis. *AJR Am J Roentgenol* 2011 May;196(5):1164–71.

28. Kumamoto M, Nakashima Y, Sueishi K. Intimal neovascularization in human coronary atherosclerosis: its origin and pathophysiological significance. *Hum Pathol* 1995 Apr;26(4): 450–6.

29. Vicenzini E, Giannoni MF, Puccinelli F, Ricciardi MC, Altieri M, Di Piero V, et al. Detection of carotid adventitial vasa vasorum and plaque vascularization with ultrasound cadence contrast pulse sequencing technique and echo-contrast agent. *Stroke* 2007 Oct;38(10):2841–3.

30. Feinstein SB. Contrast ultrasound imaging of the carotid artery vasa vasorum and atherosclerotic plaque neovascularization. *J Am Coll Cardiol* 2006 Jul 18;48(2):236–43.

31. Faggioli GL, Pini R, Mauro R, Pasquinelli G, Fittipaldi S, Freyrie A, et al. Identification of carotid 'vulnerable plaque' by contrast-enhanced ultrasonography: correlation with plaque histology, symptoms and cerebral computed tomography. *Eur J Vasc Endovasc Surg* 2011 Feb;41(2):238–48.

32. Pedro LM, Pedro MM, Goncalves I, Carneiro TF, Balsinha C, Fernandes e Fernandes R, et al. Computer-assisted carotid plaque analysis: characteristics of plaques associated with cerebrovascular symptoms and cerebral infarction. *Eur J Vasc Endovasc Surg* 2000 Feb;19(2): 118–23.

33. Underhill HR, Yuan C, Yarnykh VL, Chu B, Oikawa M, Dong L, et al. Predictors of surface disruption with MR imaging in asymptomatic carotid artery stenosis. *AJNR Am J Neuroradiol* 2010 Mar;31(3):487–93.

34. Gronholdt ML, Nordestgaard BG, Bentzon J, Wiebe BM, Zhou J, Falk E, et al. Macrophages are associated with lipid-rich carotid artery plaques, echolucency on B-mode imaging, and elevated plasma lipid levels. *J Vasc Surg* 2002 Jan;35(1):137–45.

35. Mathiesen EB, Bonaa KH, Joakimsen O. Echolucent plaques are associated with high risk of ischemic cerebrovascular events in carotid stenosis: the tromso study. *Circulation* 2001 May 1;103(17):2171–5.

36. Lenzi GL, Vicenzini E. The ruler is dead: an analysis of carotid plaque motion. *Cerebrovasc Dis* 2007;23(2-3):121–5.

37. Iannuzzi A, Wilcosky T, Mercuri M, Rubba P, Bryan FA, Bond MG. Ultrasonographic correlates of carotid atherosclerosis in transient ischemic attack and stroke. *Stroke* 1995 Apr;26(4): 614–9.

38. Markus HS, King A, Shipley M, Topakian R, Cullinane M, Reihill S, et al. Asymptomatic embolisation for prediction of stroke in the Asymptomatic Carotid Emboli Study (ACES): a prospective observational study. *Lancet Neurol* 2010 Jul;9(7):663–71.

39. Spence JD, Coates V, Li H, Tamayo A, Munoz C, Hackam DG, et al. Effects of intensive medical therapy on microemboli and cardiovascular risk in asymptomatic carotid stenosis. *Arch Neurol* 2010 Feb;67(2):180–6.

40. King A, Serena J, Bornstein NM, Markus HS. Does impaired cerebrovascular reactivity predict stroke risk in asymptomatic carotid stenosis?: a prospective substudy of the asymptomatic carotid emboli study. *Stroke* 2011 Jun;42(6):1550–5.

6

Technique for Subclavian to Carotid Transposition, Tips and Tricks

Mark D. Morasch, MD

Cervical reconstruction via transposition is the surgical technique of choice for single proximal occlusive lesions involving the subclavian arteries. In addition, with the advent of thoracic endovascular therapy, surgical manipulation of the supra-aortic trunks to prepare patients with thoracic and thoracoabdominal aortic aneurysms, dissections, or traumatic tears for an endovascular stent-graft repair has become accepted and commonplace. Subclavian artery reconstruction is now commonly performed in order to preserve vertebral and left upper extremity flow while extending the proximal neck "landing zone" prior to endograft deployment (Figure 6–1). We have taken an aggressive approach to pre-endograft revascularization of the left subclavian in order to optimize posterior brain, spinal cord and upper extremity circulation. Not only is preservation of the vertebral artery critical, but it is equally important to mobilize and preserve the valuable internal mammary artery.[1] When there is a usable ipsilateral "source vessel" an arterial transposition should be the first choice. When performed properly, transposition not only preserves arm, vertebral and mammary flow, it obviates the need for proximal subclavian ligation or

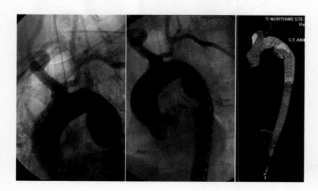

Figure 6–1. Images before and after endograft deployment in a patient who has had subclavian transposition.

transcatheter embolization to prevent large retrograde Type II endoleaks. Transposition procedures carry very low risk for complication. The long-term patency rate for arterial transposition, when performed by surgeons with experience, is virtually 100%.[4–6]

Arterial transpositions are completed through a short, transverse cervical incision above the clavicle. The surgical dissection is carried out between the two heads of the sternocleidomastoid muscle. This is an important contradistinction to bypass which is carried out lateral to the entire sternocleidomastoid muscle. After dividing the omohyoid muscle between ligatures or with electrocautery, the jugular vein is reflected laterally and the common carotid is reflected medially with the vagus nerve. The carotid is mobilized circumferentially with the dissection carried out deeply toward the mediastinum. On the left side, the thoracic duct and small identifiable lymphatics are identified, ligated, and divided (Figure 6–2). On the right, multiple cervical lymphatic channels must also be tied. After dividing the vertebral vein (Figure 6–3), the subclavian artery and its proximal branches can be identified behind the clavicle. If the vessel is patent, digital palpation can help with localization. Care must be taken when isolating and controlling the vertebral artery as it takes origin from an awkward position on the posterior aspect of the subclavian artery. The medial aspect of the anterior scalene muscle may be encountered with more lateral dissection of the subclavian artery. Again, in contradistinction from bypass, the anterior scalene never required division for a transposition. Only slight lateral reflection of this muscle may be necessary in order to obtain control of the subclavian vessel distal to the thyrocervical trunk. The subclavian artery is dissected as far proximal as possible, also well into the mediastinum. It is possible to enter the pleural space anteriorly. This can be avoided by keeping the dissection close to the arterial wall. Care is also taken to avoid disrupting sympathetic branches which cross anterior to the subclavian and ascend in the neck along side the vertebral artery. Once heparin has been administered, the subclavian and its proximal branches are controlled. The vertebral, mammary and thyrocervical trunk are temporarily occluded with microbulldog-type clamps. The distal subclavian

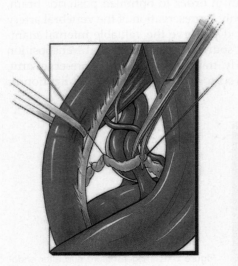

Figure 6–2. Ligation and division of the thoracic duct.

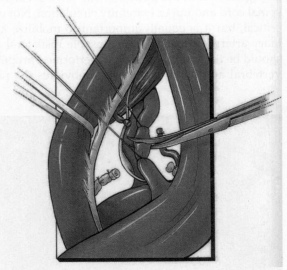

Figure 6–3. Ligation and division of the vertebral vein.

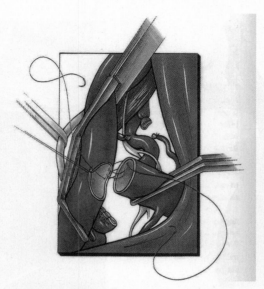

Figure 6–4. Subclavian stump and transposition
suture line.

can be controlled with loops or, preferably with a profunda clamp. The proximal subclavian is then transected beyond a right angled clamp or stapled with a vascular load
stapler. It is important to secure the proximal stump immediately after the diseased
artery has been divided; if control of the transected stump is lost in the chest or mediastinum, the consequences clearly can be devastating. At this point, the carotid is
slightly rotated to expose the posterior aspect and then clamped proximally and distally. A punch arteriotomy is created in the side of the donor carotid and the end-to-
side anastomosis completed without tension (Figure 6–4). Occasionally some
redundant subclavian must be resected to avoid a kink. The anastomosis is facilitated
by using parachute technique and by starting the suture-line on the posterior wall.
Rarely is the subclavian too short to reach to the side of the carotid. If this problem is
encountered, more carotid can be mobilized to swing it further lateral to the subclavian. Clamps are removed and flow is re-established into the vertebral artery last
(Figure 6–5). A drain is useful to collect lymphatic fluid and the wound is closed.

Occasionally, it is not feasible to do a straightforward arterial transposition so
the use of a bypass conduit becomes necessary. Long-term patency rates are commonly reported to be 10–15% poorer than for transposition. Arterial transposition is
not possible when the vertebral artery takes off early from the subclavian artery or
when the atherosclerotic process extends far distally beyond the vertebral origin.
Another indication for carotid-subclavian bypass is subclavian disease or anticipation
of subclavian coverage with an endograft in a patient with a patent internal mammary
artery graft. With the use of a cervical bypass, the arterial clamps can be placed beyond the atherosclerosis or, in the case of a LIMA, beyond the internal mammary
artery to avoid myocardial ischemia. Bypasses are performed, most expediently,
through dissection just lateral to the clavicular head of the sternocleidomastoid muscle. The jugular vein is reflected medially to expose the common carotid. The subclavian artery is identified more distally than during transposition by dividing the

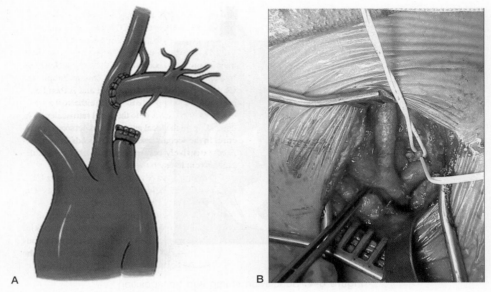

Figure 6–5. A & B-Completed transposition.

anterior scalene muscle. Care must be taken to avoid injury to the phrenic nerve during this more lateral approach. The bypass is completed to or from the retroscalene portion of the subclavian artery, usually using prosthetic conduit rather than vein, by performing sequential clamping and serial anastomoses (Figure 6–6). In this position, prosthetic conduits clearly out-perform autogenous vein with regard to long term patency.[2,3]

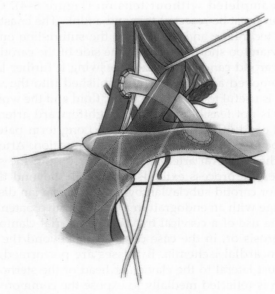

Figure 6–6. Carotid to subclavian bypass.

REFERENCES

1. Peterson BG, Eskandari MK, Gleason TG, Morasch MD. Utility of left subclavian artery revascularization in association with endoluminal repair of acute and chronic thoracic aortic pathology. *J Vasc Surg* Mar 2006;43(3):433–439.
2. Morasch M, Berguer R. Supra-aortic Trunk revascularization. In: Yao JST PW, ed. <u>Modern Vascular Surgery</u> New York: McGraw-Hill; 2000:137.
3. Ziomek S, Quinones-Baldrich WJ, Busuttil RW, Baker JD, Machleder HI, Moore WS. The superiority of synthetic arterial grafts over autologous veins in carotid-subclavian bypass. *J Vasc Surg* Jan 1986;3(1):140–145.
4. Berguer R, Morasch MD, Kline RA, Kazmers A, Friedland MS. Cervical reconstruction of the supra-aortic trunks: a 16-year experience. *J Vasc Surg* Feb 1999;29(2):239–246; discussion 246–238.
5. Cina CS, Safar HA, Lagana A, Arena G, Clase CM. Subclavian carotid transposition and bypass grafting: consecutive cohort study and systematic review. *J Vasc Surg* Mar 2002;35(3):422–429.
6. Schardey HM, Meyer G, Rau HG, Gradl G, Jauch KW, Lauterjung L. Subclavian carotid transposition: an analysis of a clinical series and a review of the literature. *Eur J Vasc Endovasc Surg* Nov 1996;12(4):431–436.

SECTION **II**

Cerebrovascular Disease II

7

Results of Carotid Artery Stenting in Symptomatic/ Asymptomatic Patients

K. Craig Kent, MD

There are few medical interventions as controversial as carotid artery stenting (CAS). Although CAS utilizes innovative technology, the introduction of this technology has been complex for a variety of reasons. First, CAS replaces a durable and very straight-forward surgical procedure, Carotid Endarterectomy (CEA) that has been the status quo for treating carotid artery stenosis for multiple years. CEA is a superficial operation that can be performed under local anesthesia with minimal morality and morbidity. Moreover, CEA requires only an over-night hospital stay and patients recover rapidly and are back to their usual state of health within two weeks of surgery. Endovascular technology has transformed the treatment of many types of vascular disease by replacing complex and morbid open operations with minimally invasive interventions. Open repair of abdominal aortic aneurysm or femoral tibial bypass for lower extremity vascular ischemia are examples of where minimally invasive treatments have provided great benefit. In comparison, the differential between CAS and CEA in terms of complexity and patient risk is much less significant. Adding to the controversy have been a number of external factors that are unrelated to patient care. There is an obvious advantage to industry if carotid stenting is the preferred treatment of carotid artery disease, and thus industry has been a motivational force in moving this technology forward. There is controversy amongst interventionalists that perform these techniques. Surgeons more often perform CEA, and cardiologists and radiologists perform CAS. The consequence has been inherent prejudices in the support for CAS by various specialists (both positive and negative) based upon having access to only one of the tools to treat carotid disease. There is little doubt that "turf" has played a significant role in the development, testing, and acceptance of carotid stenting.

These issues aside, there have been multiple attempts over the years to evaluate CAS and to compare CAS to CEA. In comparing two interventions there are a variety of techniques that can be used. These range from single institutional studies to large multi-center prospective randomized trials. Although the latter is considered the gold standard for evaluating comparative effectiveness, randomized clinical trials do have draw-backs. The institutions that are chosen for these clinical trials are typically centers of excellence for the technique that is being evaluated. Often the expertise found in these centers is not available to the population at large. Moreover, in prospective clinical trials, there are exclusion criteria that often eliminate from study many patients who eventually receive treatment in the community setting. Thus, complimenting the findings of prospective studies with those derived from large data-sets can often be helpful in confirming the utility of medical treatments.

It is disappointing that our understanding of the utility of CAS is less robust than one might anticipate considering that this technology has been available for almost 15 years. There are thousands of studies that have been published regarding outcomes for CEA, as well as CAS, with some of these evaluations being comparative. The purpose of this chapter is not to review these studies or to provide a summary of the current available randomized data on CAS versus CEA. Rather, the intent is to present yet another approach to evaluating outcomes of these two techniques with a population-based approach using comprehensive data from two large states.[1]

TECHNIQUES FOR EVALUATING LARGE DATA SETS

There are a number of large data-sets that are currently available that can be used to evaluate comparative outcomes for vascular interventions. These include national data-sets such as Medicare and the National In-Patient sample. Also inclusive are state databases. Almost every state has some type of method of recording health care outcomes, although some are more robust than others. Inclusive in these data-sets are outcomes for every patient treated for a particular intervention. For example, available in the Medicare data-set are the outcomes of all Medicare beneficiaries (usually above the age of 65) that have had treatment with CEA or CAS. Thus, national or state data-sets allow access to the outcomes of large numbers of patients. Moreover, the outcomes that are derived from large data-sets reflect prevailing practice in the community and across the country rather than from just specialized centers. Consequently, large data-sets provide data that is reflective of "real world" outcomes. There are limitations to analyses derived from large data-sets. Inevitably, there are coding inaccuracies. Moreover, evaluation of these data-sets requires a detailed knowledge of hospital and patient codes. Although data regarding comorbidities is available, the data is not always granular making risk adjustment difficult. For example, a patient that is given a code for congestive heart failure may have an ejection fraction of 45%, or alternatively 25%. A patient who is coded as having renal insufficiency may have a creatinine of 5.0 or 1.6. Thus, risk adjustment of large data-sets using comorbidities is not always precise.

In this analysis we have used both the New York as well as the California State datasets. The reason that these states were chosen is that the differentiation between a pre- and post-operative stroke can be definitively made using these data-sets. Differentiating between a stroke that leads to a carotid intervention versus one that is a consequence of a procedure is a critical issue in these types of analyses. For both New York as well as California there is a flag included in the data set for "present on admission". Thus, if a stroke is "present on admission" we know that the stroke led to carotid intervention. However, if the "present on admission" flag is not coded, we can assume that the stroke was a post-operative event.

Another issue with large data-sets in terms of performing comparative evaluations is that the patient cohorts that have had differing interventions are not always identical. Since its introduction, CAS has been used preferentially for high-risk patients and it would not be surprising to find that the cohort of patients receiving stents is significantly different in terms of comorbidities and demographics than those receiving carotid endarterectomy. Thus, a direct comparison of these two cohorts is not valid and would lead to little beneficial information. In the evaluation that follows we used the technique of propensity matching, where "like" patients receiving CAS and CEA are compared. Although there have been previous studies of CAS versus CEA using large data-sets, most of these have not adequately dealt with the issue of perioperative stroke nor have the patient cohorts been matched.

CAS VS. CEA IN ASYMPTOMATIC PATIENTS

All patients treated in New York or California with CEA or CAS from 2005-2007 were included in this analysis. A total of 43,236 patients with asymptomatic carotid disease were evaluated. Using the raw cohorts before a propensity matching, the outcomes of CAS were inferior to those of CEA. However, when the comorbidities of these two patient cohorts were compared it was clear that those that received stents were much higher risk and more often symptomatic than those that received CEA. Thus, propensity matching was a useful tool in creating two equivalent groups of patients for comparison.

After propensity matching, we found that the rate of stroke, the mortality, as well as the composite endpoint of stroke and mortality were equivalent for the two interventions. This data is displayed in Table 7–1. The risk of death in both groups was around 0.5% and the risk of stroke was equivalent at approximately 2%. Moreover, the overall rate of complication was reasonably equivalent between the two groups. CEA patients more frequently had respiratory or urinary complications or cranial neuropathy whereas those undergoing CAS more often developed iatrogenic hypotension. For those patients who did not have a post-procedural stroke, the length of stay was slightly greater for CEA than for CAS.

TABLE 7–1. OUTCOMES IN CAROTID ARTERY STENTING (CAS) OR CAROTID ENDARTERECTOMY (CEA) DURING 2005 TO 2007 IN NEW YORK AND CALIFORNIA[1]

Outcome	Number[a]	CAS (%)	CEA (%)
Asymptomatic	4353		
Death		0.55	0.39
Stroke		2.04	1.75
Stroke/death		2.37	1.93
Symptomatic	543		
Death		3.68	1.29
Stroke		5.71	4.05
Stroke/death		8.29	4.60

[a] Matched pairs by propensity analysis.

These findings are of potentially great significance to those who embrace CEA as the preferred method of treating carotid disease. It is worth noting the majority of patients treated in this country with intervention for carotid disease are asymptomatic. In this evaluation almost 90% of treated patients treated were asymptomatic. In other series the percentage ranges from 75%–90%. If CAS becomes the preferred treatment for asymptomatic carotid artery disease, the impact nationally on the number of patients treated with CEA could be substantial.

Using our understanding of the pathophysiology of stroke related to carotid artery disease one might be able to rationalize these findings. In an asymptomatic patient with carotid stenosis the plaque is often stable. The absence of symptoms significantly lessens the likelihood that the intraluminal plaque is friable and/or prone to embolization. Thus, intraluminal manipulation of this type of plaque is likely to carry a significantly diminished risk of embolization compared to an unstable and/or friable plaque that might be found in a symptomatic patient. Thus, it is not surprising that the outcomes of carotid stenting in asymptomatic patients are quite favorable and equivalent to those of CEA.

The question is how to best interpret these findings. If an invasive intervention is compared to one that is minimally invasive and the outcomes are equivalent, the minimally invasive intervention usually becomes the preferred approach. The analysis of course, is not always that simple. Cost, at least in years to come, has the potential to be a significant factor. The availability of well-trained interventionalists is also an important issue. It is clear that there is a learning curve for CAS with less favorable outcomes early in an interventionalist's experience. These issues aside, currently in the community CAS outcomes appear to be equivalent to those of CEA, suggesting that stenting may become the preferred method of treatment.

CAS VS. CEA IN SYMPTOMATIC PATIENTS

In the raw cohort of symptomatic patients before propensity matching, we found significant advantage of CEA over CAS in terms of stroke, mortality, as well as the combined endpoint. However, converse to our findings with asymptomatic disease, after matching the advantage of CEA for all 3 outcomes persisted. In the CAS cohort the overall mortality in symptomatic patients was 3.7%, whereas the mortality in the carotid endarterectomy cohort was 1.3%. The rate of stroke following CAS in symptomatic patients was near 6%, whereas the rate of stroke in the carotid endarterectomy cohort was 4%. For combined stroke and mortality, the rate in CAS patients was 8.3%, which was considerably inferior to an incidence of 4.6% found in patients treated with CEA. In terms of complications, the rates between the two interventions were equivalent. However, numerically as was found with asymptomatic patients, there was a higher rate of cranial neuropathy with CEA and transient hypotension in the patients treated with CAS. Length of stay was equivalent for both groups.

These findings are similar to those that reported by the EVA 3S investigators.[2] In this comparative trial, which was terminated prematurely, 527 patients with symptomatic carotid disease were randomized to CEA or CAS. At 30 days, the incidence of stroke or death was 3.9% after endarterectomy and 9.6% after stenting. The rate of disabling stroke or death was 1.5% after CEA and 3.4% after CAS. The advantage of CEA persisted for 6 months at which time the incidence of stroke or death was 6.1% for patients treated with CEA and 11.7% for those treated with CAS. Although this study has been criticized for a number of reasons including the "lack of experience" of those performing CAS, it is important to note that the findings of this randomized trial are near identical to ours reported using large U.S. datasets.

The recently reported results of CREST offer a somewhat different perspective.[3] In CREST 2,502 patients were randomized to either stenting or endarterectomy and 4 year outcomes were reported. Using the primary endpoint of death, stroke, and myocardial infarction the outcomes of CAS and CEA were equivalent at 7.2% vs. 6.8%. Using a composite outcome that included only stroke and death, the incidence associated with CAS was 6.4% as opposed to an incidence of 4.7% with CEA, a difference that was statistically significant. The symptomatic and asymptomatic cohorts were then analyzed separately. In *symptomatic* patients, at four years, the incidence of stroke and death was 8% in patients that received CAS versus 6.4% in those that received CEA, a difference that was not statistically significant. The rate of stroke and death at 4 years for *asymptomatic* patients was at 4.5% for stent versus 2.7% for CAS, a difference that was also not statistically significant. Thus, CREST did demonstrate a relative advantage of CEA over CAS with regard to stroke and death, however, dissimilar to the findings in our analysis there was not a significant differential in outcome between symptomatic and asymptomatic patients.

Although it is difficult to understand why the findings of our study and those of EVA 3S differ so greatly from those of CREST, it may well have been that the expertise of the interventionalists performing carotid stenting was a key factor. Those interventionalists that participated in CREST were highly experienced. Perhaps they performed CAS at a level that was superior to those interventionalists performing CAS in the community setting reflected in our population base evaluation, or those interventionalists involved in EVA 3S. In our analysis, we evaluated volume of CAS versus outcome and found a continuous improvement in the incidence of stoke and mortality with increasing volume of CAS. Moreover, we found in California and New York at least at the point of this evaluation, the majority of CAS procedures was performed in low-volume hospitals. In fact, fewer than 25 carotid artery stents were performed annually in 82% of hospitals in California and 54% of hospitals in New York where carotid stenting was offered. We also found in our dataset that patients greater than the age of 80 faired poorly with carotid stenting. This is not a unique finding. In fact this observation has been made by multiple investigators. A reasonable number of elderly patients were treated in our community-based study, and this factor might also explain the differences we observed.

Unfortunately, despite a plethora of available data, the preferred treatment of carotid stenosis is still not fully clear. There is much more that needs to be learned. However, the data that is available suggests that when it comes to the treatment of carotid disease, one size does not fit all. There will be patients that are better served by CAS and alternatively others that are better served by CEA. One can conclude from all of the available data that CAS is here to stay and is likely to play an important role in the treatment of patients with asymptomatic carotid stenosis. Our data, however, do suggest that caution should be exercised when using CAS in symptomatic patients. It may be that in this patient cohort, the experience of the interventionalist performing CAS is a critical factor in determining outcome.

REFERENCES

1. Giacovelli JK, Egorova N, et al. Outcomes of carotid stenting compared with endarterectomy are equivalent in asymptomatic patients and inferior in symptomatic patients. *J Vasc Surg* 2010;52:906–13, 913.e1–4.
2. Mas JL, Chatellier G, et al. Endarterectomy versus Stenting in Patients with Symptomatic Severe Carotid Stenosis. *N Engl J Med* 2006; 355:1660–1671.
3. Brott TG, Hobson RW, et al. Stenting versus Endarterectomy for Treatment of Carotid-Artery Stenosis. *N Engl J Med* 2010; *363:11–23*, July 1, 2010

8

Pharmacotherapies that can Improve Patient Outcomes from Carotid Endarterectomy

Matthew B. Burruss, MD and Michael C. Stoner, MD, RVT, FACS

INTRODUCTION

Carotid endarterectomy (CEA) has been well established as the preferred treatment for flow-limiting stenoses of the carotid artery in both symptomatic and asymptomatic patients. The stroke/death rate metrics that are used today were established in the early 1990's by large-scale randomized trials. Achievement of these outcomes has been replicated outside of clinical trials, and two recent large-scale database studies in fact compare favorably to these. Vascular surgeons strive to always perform the perfect operation by minimizing any complications. Some of these complications can be minimized or negated by perioperative medical management. Medical therapies in the perioperative period have proven to significantly influence at least the short term outcomes of CEA.

All attempts need to be made to optimize the outcomes of CEA surgery since it is a risk-reduction operation. Because CEA represents a risk-reduction procedure, all attempts should be made to improve the safety profile of the procedure. The purpose of this manuscript is to elicit the optimal perioperative medical therapies to ensure the best patient outcomes and reduce neurological and non-neurological adverse events (Table 8–1).

CARDIAC RELATED EVENTS AFTER CEA

About a decade after the landmark 1954 operation by Eastcott and collegues, DeBakey and other authors described myocardial infarction as the principle non-neurological immediate and long-term adverse event associated with CEA.[1] In addition longitudinal studies after CEA indicated that associated coronary artery disease was the principle cause of late

TABLE 8–1. SUMMARY OF PHARMACOTHERAPIES FOR PATIENTS UNDERGOING CAROTID ENDARTERECTOMY

Therapy	Benefits
Beta-blockade	• May Reduce myocardial injury rates following surgery up to 10-fold
	• Low-risk patients likely do not derive a benefit if not already on a beta blocker
	• May be associated with adverse events at higher doses or if used indiscriminately
ACE Inhibitor/ARB	• Reduces cardiovascular mortality in patients with atherosclerosis by up to 25%
	• Stabilizes carotid plaque and improve vessel wall biology
	• Appropriate long-term agent for patients without contraindication
Statin	• Reduces acute and long-term stroke risk, reduces cardiovascular event rate, associated with long-term survival
	• Multiple mechanisms of action including lipid profile and plaque stabilization
	• Reasonable agent for all patient undergoing vascular surgery
Antiplatelet	• Associated with an up to 7% absolute reduction in early stroke following CEA
	• Low-dose aspirin efficacious
	• No clear benefit to dual therapy or high-dose therapy in patients undergoing CEA

mortality in patients with or without overt cardiac disease at the time of endarterectomy.[2] Subsequently, the association between carotid and coronary disease has been repeatedly demonstrated. Anatomical coronary artery disease has been demonstrated in 73% of patients undergoing carotid revascularization with up to 26% having severe correctable coronary artery disease.[3]

In contemporary practice, the incidence of Q-wave MI following CEA is typically less than 2%, but represents almost half of the major adverse events associated with carotid revascularization in asymptomatic patients.[4,5] It is hard to know but one can conclude that the incidence of minimal myocardial injury is probably higher. It is not a surprise that the data indicates that individuals undergoing carotid revascularization have a significant atherosclerotic disease burden.

CARDIAC RISK STRATIFICATION

Much of the prodigious literature on cardiac risk stratification was developed in vascular surgery patients. The groundbreaking work looking into noninvasive physiologic testing (nuclear stress test) to predict cardiac events was reported in a series of vascular surgery patients.[6]

Despite a prevalence of anatomical coronary disease as high as 73%, the past literature did not support coronary revascularization in patients with either stable angina or occult disease.[7] Prophylactic myocardial revascularization has only an anecdotal benefit in the most recent reviews, and has not been demonstrated to be of benefit in any randomized trial. An example of this is the randomized CARP trial that failed to demonstrate any benefit to prophylactic coronary revascularization undergoing elective vascular surgery.[8] With no realized benefit to coronary revascularization for elective vascular surgery, specific coronary workup is not routinely recommended in patients undergoing CEA. There is evidence that patients who have symptomatic carotid disease undergoing CABG benefit from CEA.

TABLE 8–2. CLASSIFICATION OF RECOMMENDATIONS

Classification of Recommendations	
Class I	Conditions for which there is evidence for and/or general agreement that the procedure or treatments is beneficial, useful, and effective.
Class II	Conditions for which there is conflicting evidence and/or divergence of opinion about the usefulness/efficacy of a procedure or treatment.
Class IIa	Weight of evidence/opinion is in favor of usefulness/efficacy.
Class IIb	Usefulness/efficacy is less well established by evidence/opinion.
Class III	Condition for which there is evidence and/or general agreement that the procedure/treatment is not useful/effective, and in some cases may be harmful.

The current American College of Cardiology/American Heart Association guidelines consider carotid endarterectomy as an intermediate risk surgical procedure. The ACC/AHA guidelines provide Class I (Table 8–2) data to support non-invasive stress testing in patients with active cardiac conditions: unstable coronary syndrome, decompensated heart failure, significant arrhythmias or severe valvular disease.[8]

Other indications for non-invasive testing may be appropriate in select patients, but are not supported with Class I data. The DECREASE (Dutch Echocardiographic Cardiac Risk Evaluation Applying Stress Echo)-II study showed that if patients were appropriately beta-blocked, the perioperative cardiac event rate was reduced regardless of preoperative non-invasive testing. The cardiac death and MI rate at 30 days in patients with no testing was 1.8% vs. 2.3%. Cardiac testing delayed surgery for more than three weeks.[9] Based on the lack of data to support coronary revascularization to reduce myocardial injury risk, there are likely few cases which will benefit from expanded indications. Medical optimization of myocardial risk remains the cornerstone of treatment for patients undergoing carotid endarterectomy.

BETA BLOCKADE

Beta adrenergic receptor antagonists (beta blockers, β-blockers) were originally brought to clinical fruition in the 1960s, and have been used for a variety of approved indications including angina pectoris, hypertensive control, cardiac arrhythmia management, post-coronary revascularization mortality reduction and post-myocardial infarction risk reduction. The classically described mechanism of action is a sympatholytic one, with a resultant negative inotropic and chronotropic effect. Beta blockade also leads to a decreased production of renin, which provides an antihypertensive effect.

Perioperative β-blockade has become standard therapy in the prevention of myocardial infarction in patients undergoing vascular surgery. This enthusiasm arose after two landmark publications showed a significant improvement in cardiovascular complications and mortality in patients undergoing non-cardiac vascular surgery. Mangano et al randomized 200 patients to receive atenolol or placebo in the perioperative period. It was surmised that the prevention of cardiac deaths in the first six to eight months led to a survival advantage at two years.[10] Poldermans' study randomized patients to bisoporol or standard of care in patients undergoing vascular surgery. This study showed a 10-fold reduction in the perioperative cardiovascular event rate amongst the patients who received bisoprolol.[9]

A number of follow-up studies have been performed comparing beta-blockers with placebo in non-cardiac vascular surgery with mixed results. Unfortunately, the dramatic benefits seen in the studies cited above have not been universally reproduced. The POISE trial looked at 8,351 patients who received a single preoperative does of 100 mg of extended release metoprolol followed by 200mg daily for 30 days.[11] There were 4174 patients in the treatment arm and 4177 patients in the placebo group. The rate of myocardial infarction was lower in the treatment group vs. the placebo group. However; there were more deaths in the metoprolol group than in the placebo group. It is important to note that clinically significant hypotension and bradycardia was higher in the metoprolol group. It seems that an overly aggressive dose of metoprolol may negate the beneficial effects of cardiac protection that is goal.

A recent meta-analysis of 33 randomized controlled trials has raised a cautionary flag with respect to the ubiquitous application of perioperative β-blockers.[12] In this study β-blockers were not associated with any significant reduction in the risk of all-cause mortality, cardiovascular mortality or heart failure but did reduce the incidence of non fatal myocardial infarction and myocardial at the expense of an increase in non fatal strokes. The POISE trial was a major component in this meta-analysis and therefore caution must be used when interpreting this data, again because of the relatively high dose beta-blockade.

Heart rate control remains a contentious issue in perioperative beta blocker management. The optimal heart rate has not been confirmed as of yet. Rate control of less than 75 beats per minute was not significant for efficacy outcomes other than non-fatal myocardial infarction.[12] These data, which do not refute the potential protective benefits of beta-blockers, do however urge caution in their unfettered use because of potential consequences and an ill-defined therapeutic window.

The American College of Cardiology and American Heart Association (ACC/AHA) currently recommends β-blockers for non-cardiac surgery (inclusive of CEA) in a number of clinical situations:[13]

1. Continue in patients already on therapy for defined indication i.e. hypertension, arrhythmia or angina. Initiate therapy in patients that have ischemia on preoperative testing. (Class I)
2. Patients that are undergoing vascular surgery who are high-risk; congestive heart failure or more than one clinical risk factor for cardiac disease recognized on preoperative evaluation. (Class IIa)
3. Patients undergoing vascular surgery with one or more clinical risk factors for cardiac disease. (Class IIb)

The issue is looming on the horizon as a performance measure despite the unanswered questions about β-blockade including optimal target heart rate, duration, timing of administration and efficacy.

ANGIOTENSIN BLOCKADE

ACE inhibitors impart cardiovascular protection through a variety of mechanisms, including: hypertensive control, inhibition of platelet aggregation, reduced oxidative stress, nitric oxide stimulation, and enhancing endogenous fibrinolysis. They also are hypothesized to stabilize vascular plaques, which has a direct implication on the management of carotid surgery patients. The role of ACE in the pathogenesis of inflammation and rupture of atherosclerotic plaque has led to a myriad of studies that demonstrated ACE-inhibitor related carotid plaque stabilization, and improved vessel wall histopathology. Evolving data indicates that a similar protective benefit can be attributed to angiotensin receptor antagonist, although the volume of evidence is not as compelling. Furthermore, there is biological evidence that angiotensin blockade coupled with antiplatelet (aspirin) therapy, may have a synergistic effect on plaque inflammatory markers, adding a scientific background to the role of multi-agent medical therapy for patients with atherosclerosis.[14,15]

The risk reduction attributed to ACE inhibition is significant. The 2004 HOPE trial was a large-scale trial designed to examine the effects of ramipril on cardiovascular events in patients with peripheral arterial occlusive disease.[16] The study demonstrated a 25% mortality rate reduction, irrespective of hypertensive status.

The ACC/AHA guidelines recommend treating all patients with atherosclerotic disease with an ACE inhibitor, unless there is a contraindication.[17] This recommendation is based on the myocardial risk reduction attributed to these agents, and patients with both coronary and non-coronary vascular disease. The study reported a 0.12% rate of renal dysfunction following the initiation of ACE inhibitor therapy. These data contradict the classical concern that renal artery stenosis is a contraindication to angiotensin blockade.

HMG COA REDUCTASE INHIBITORS (STATINS)

Statins are competitive inhibitors of 3-hydroxy 3-methylglutaryl coenzyme A (HMG CoA) reductase, the rate limiting step in cholesterol biosynthesis. This enzyme converts HMG-CoA into mevalonic acid, which is a cholesterol precursor. The end result is a 25–50% reduction in the level of circulating LDL cholesterol as well as a reduction in the total cholesterol and triglyceride levels and an elevation in high density lipoprotein level.

The ability of statins to affect perioperative outcomes appears to be related to effects other than simply lowering cholesterol, and is referred to as pleiotropic effects. One of the most important effects in the prevention of perioperative events is its ability to stabilize atheromatous plaque that is at risk of rupture resulting in thrombosis or embolism and acute ischemic events. This is achieved by decreased matrix metalloproteases, lipid oxidation, and inflammation that destabilize atherosclerotic plaques. Statins also can increase the levels of collagen and inhibitors of matrix metalloproteases that lead to plaque stabilization. Patients on statins were also less likely to have spontaneous cerebral embolization detected by Doppler during carotid endarterectomy.[18] The expanding list of lipid profile-independent effects strongly supports the use of statins in patients with peripheral vascular disease, and certainly expands their indication to include all patients undergoing CEA.

There is a growing body of literature that demonstrates that statins reduce baseline and perioperative mortality, myocardial infarction and stroke rates in vascular patients. One of the largest studies to evaluate the benefit of statins in patients with CAD or peripheral vascular disease was the Heart Protection study. All-cause mortality was significantly reduced over a five year period, irrespective of the initial cholesterol level, with 12.9% deaths among 10,269 allocated simvastatin vs. 14.7% among 10,267 allocated placebo; P = 0.0003). This protective effect was attributed to a highly significant 18% relative reduction in the coronary death rate, a marginally significant reduction in other vascular deaths, and a non-significant reduction in non-vascular deaths.[19]

The StaRRS study looked at patients undergoing major vascular surgery including carotid endarterectomy, aortic surgery and lower extremity revascularization with the primary outcome measure being death, myocardial infarction, ischemia, congestive heart failure, and ventricular tachyarrhythmias occurring during the index hospitalization. These data showed significantly fewer patients reached the primary endpoint who were taking statins vs. patients who were not on a statin. The benefit arose primarily from a reduction in the rate of myocardial infarction and congestive heart failure. With a risk-adjusted model, statins still provided a protective effect.[20] The recent SPARCL study has also demonstrated a benefit to statin therapy in terms of both primary and secondary stroke prevention, in addition to protection from major cardiac events.[21]

Current recommendations by the AHA/ACC for perioperative statin use for non-cardiac vascular surgery are as follows:[13]

1. Patients who are on statins preoperatively should have them continued. (Class I)
2. Patients undergoing vascular surgery with or without clinical risk factors; statin use is reasonable. (Class II)

There are a number of retrospective studies looking at statin use and endarterectomy. One of the largest studies comes from a Canadian administrative database reviewing carotid endarterectomy in 3,360 patients. In patients treated for symptomatic disease there was a protective effect of statin use in perioperative death, perioperative stroke and death, but not to cardiovascular outcomes. These protective effects were largely driven by the symptomatic CEA cases, with no statistically significant benefit seen in asymptomatic cases.[22]

A 10-year review from the Johns Hopkins University Hospital demonstrated a stroke-risk reduction benefit and improved peri-procedural outcomes.[23] There was an insignificant trend towards a lower rate of perioperative myocardial infarction.

A second 10-year retrospective study from LaMuraglia demonstrated an association between statin therapy and restenosis after CEA.[24] The authors examined 2,127 carotid endarterectomy cases, and conducted a multivariate analysis for correlates of both early and late anatomical failure. Female gender, renal insufficiency and elevated cholesterol were all found to be correlates of restenosis. Lipid-lowering pharmacotherapy was protective for both early and late recurrent carotid disease. The fact that drug therapy modulates restenosis at both time points, suggests that statin therapy has a beneficial effect to both intimal hyperplasia remodeling and recurrent atherosclerosis after CEA.

Despite all the benefits of statin therapy, longer term compliance after carotid endarterectomy still remains low. Widespread use of statin drugs in this patient population has the potential to improve both neurological and non-neurological adverse events associated with CEA, and the long term vascular health of this patient population. The long-term adoption of statin therapy has obvious advantages, especially when evaluated within the context of a stroke-risk reduction operation.

ANTIPLATELET THERAPY

The causes of stroke after carotid endartectomy are multifactorial. Intra-operative stroke tends to follow inadvertent technical error such as intra-operative embolization, carotid dissection or creation of an intimal flap. Post-operative stroke can be the result of hyperperfusion or hemorrhage. Transcranial doppler (TCD) is a validated method to evaluate patients undergoing carotid endarterectomy. It has been noted that approximately 50% of patients with a sustained high-rate of embolization will progress toward thrombotic stroke. Patients who thrombose after carotid reconstruction may have a 1 to 2 hour period of increasing cerebral embolization that precedes the onset of symptoms, which has been detected with TCD.[25]

Antithrombotic therapy is an intuitive adjuvant for patients undergoing carotid endarterectomy. Immediately following CEA, the endarterectomy bed represents a thrombogenic nidus. In fact, tagged platelet studies have demonstrated a decreased platelet adherence to the carotid endarterectomy site in patients treated with antiplatelet therapy.

Several trials have demonstrated a cardiovascular benefit to antiplatelet therapy in patients with coronary and non-coronary vascular disease. The literature has shown that antiplatelet therapy reduced combined vascular events by one quarter, non-fatal myocardial infarction by one-third, non-fatal stroke was reduced by one-quarter, and vascular mortality by one-sixth. The absolute benefits outweighed the risks of bleeding.[26]

The CAPRIE study compared aspirin (325 mg once daily) vs. clopidogrel (75 mg once daily) in reducing the risks of a composite outcome of stroke, myocardial infarction, or vascular death.[27] The patients studied had an atherosclerotic disease manifested by: recent stroke, recent myocardial infarction or symptomatic peripheral arterial disease. Over a mean follow-up of almost 2 years, patients taking clopidogrel had an annual 5.32% risk of stroke, myocardial infarction, or vascular death vs. 5.83%.[68] While a relative risk reduction of 8.7% was realized, the longitudinal use of a relatively expensive drug may not justify the cost efficacy vis a vis a modest absolute risk reduction of less than 1%.

A 1999 study randomized over 2,700 patients to varying doses of aspirin (81 – 1300 mg daily) and examined stroke, myocardial infarction and death at 30 and 90 days after carotid revascularization. Using a composite endpoint, aspirin doses of 325 mg or less were associated with improved outcomes at both the 30 day (5.4% vs. 7.0%) and 90 day (6.2% vs. 8.4%) time points, compared to the higher dose regimen. Cervical hematoma rate and systemic bleed complications did not differ between treatment groups. While caution must be exercised when concluding that higher-dose regimens are deleterious, these data demonstrate the non-inferiority of lower dose regimens.

A publication from the Cochrane Collaboration reviewed randomized trials looking at the use of antiplatelet medication after carotid endarterectomy.[28] Six trials fit the criteria for entry into this meta-analysis. Antiplatelet therapy was found to be significantly protective for the occurrence of stroke. This study estimated that three out of 100 patients treated with antiplatelet therapy could be saved from stoke within the follow up period.

A retrospective study reviewing 260 consecutive patients undergoing CEA showed that patients taking clopidogrel are at a much higher risk of developing post operative neck hematomas compared to patients that are on low dose ASA for antiplatelet therapy. Of the patients taking clopidogrel a Dacron patch repair had a higher rate of neck hematoma then an eversion endarterectomy (35% vs. 4.2%).[29]

Based on the rationale that antiplatelet therapy reduces procedural stroke rate, myocardial infarction rate, and provides a long-term cardiovascular event risk reduction, the American College of Chest Physicians recommends perioperative low-dose aspirin and lifelong therapy for patients undergoing CEA. The role of other agents and multi-agent therapy is unclear, and thus far only a theoretical advantage has been proposed. Despite the recommendations, up to one third of patients undergoing CEA are not placed on antiplatelet therapy preoperatively.[30]

CONCLUSION

Carotid endarterectomy remains the gold standard for stroke-risk reduction in patients with hemodynamically significant carotid artery disease. With the adoption of evidence-based medical therapy, there exists an avenue to optimize the care of patients with carotid disease, to both improve the stroke-risk reduction benefit and the short and long-term cardiovascular event rate of patients undergoing carotid endarterectomy. Although the exact dosages have not been elicited on all the therapies there has been evidence that the medical therapies discussed above do reduce the post-operative neurological and non-neurological complications.

REFERENCES

1. Debakey ME, Crawford ES, Cooley DA, et al. Cerebral Arterial Insufficiency: One to 11-year results following arterial reconstructive operation. *Ann Surg* 1965;161:921–945.
2. Mackey WC, O'Donnell TF Jr, Callow AD. Cardiac risk in patients undergoing carotid endarterectomy: impact on perioperative and long-term mortality. *J Vasc Surg* 1990;11(2): 226–233; discussion 233–234.
3. Hertzer NR, Young JR, Beven EG, et al. Coronary angiography in 506 patients with extracranial cerebrovascular disease. *Arch Intern Med* 1985;145(5):849–852.
4. Sidawy AN, Zwolak RM, White RA, et al. Risk-adjusted 30-day outcomes of carotid stenting and endarterectomy: results from the SVS Vascular Registry. *J Vasc Surg* 2009;49(1): 71–79.
5. LaMuraglia GM, Brewster DC, Moncure AC, et al. Carotid endarterectomy at the millennium: what interventional therapy must match. *Ann Surg* 2004;240(3):535–544; discussion 544–546.
6. Brewster DC, Okada RD, Strauss HW, et al. Selection of patients for preoperative coronary angiography: use of dipyridamole-stress–thallium myocardial imaging. *J Vasc Surg* 1985; 2(3):504–510.
7. Yeager RA, Moneta GL, McConnell DB, et al. Analysis of risk factors for myocardial infarction following carotid endarterectomy. *Arch Surg* 1989;124(10):1142–1145.
8. McFalls EO, Ward HB, Moritz TE, et al. Clinical factors associated with long-term mortality following vascular surgery: outcomes from the Coronary Artery Revascularization Prophylaxis (CARP) Trial. *J Vasc Surg* 2007;46(4):694–700.
9. Poldermans D, Boersma E, Bax JJ, et al. The effect of bisoprolol on perioperative mortality and myocardial infarction in high-risk patients undergoing vascular surgery. Dutch Echocardiographic Cardiac Risk Evaluation Applying Stress Echocardiography Study Group. *N Engl J Med* 1999;341(24):1789–1794.
10. Mangano DT, Layug EL, Wallace A, Tateo I. Effect of atenolol on mortality and cardiovascular morbidity after noncardiac surgery. Multicenter Study of Perioperative Ischemia Research Group. *N Engl J Med* 1996;335(23):1713–1720.
11. Devereaux PJ, Yang H, Yusuf S, et al. Effects of extended-release metoprolol succinate in patients undergoing non-cardiac surgery (POISE trial): a randomised controlled trial. *Lancet* 2008;371(9627):1839–1847.
12. Bangalore S, Wetterslev J, Pranesh S, et al. Perioperative beta blockers in patients having non-cardiac surgery: a meta-analysis. *Lancet* 2008;372(9654):1962–1976.

13. Fleisher LA, Beckman JA, Brown KA, et al. ACC/AHA 2007 guidelines on perioperative cardiovascular evaluation and care for noncardiac surgery: executive summary: a report of the American College of Cardiology/American Heart Association Task Force on Practice Guidelines (Writing Committee to Revise the 2002 Guidelines on Perioperative Cardiovascular Evaluation for Noncardiac Surgery). *Anesth Analg* 2008;106(3):685–712.

14. Mukherjee D, Yadav JS. Carotid artery intimal-medial thickness: indicator of atherosclerotic burden and response to risk factor modification. *Am Heart J* 2002;144(5):753–759.

15. Sattler KJE, Woodrum JE, Galili O, et al. Concurrent treatment with renin-angiotensin system blockers and acetylsalicylic acid reduces nuclear factor kappaB activation and C-reactive protein expression in human carotid artery plaques. *Stroke* 2005;36(1):14–20.

16. Yusuf S, Sleight P, Pogue J, et al. Effects of an angiotensin-converting-enzyme inhibitor, ramipril, on cardiovascular events in high-risk patients. The Heart Outcomes Prevention Evaluation Study Investigators. *N Engl J Med* 2000;342(3):145–153.

17. Smith SC Jr, Blair SN, Bonow RO, et al. AHA/ACC Scientific Statement: AHA/ACC guidelines for preventing heart attack and death in patients with atherosclerotic cardiovascular disease: 2001 update: A statement for healthcare professionals from the American Heart Association and the American College of Cardiology. *Circulation* 2001;104(13):1577–1579.

18. Molloy KJ, Thompson MM, Schwalbe EC, et al. Comparison of levels of matrix metalloproteinases, tissue inhibitor of metalloproteinases, interleukins, and tissue necrosis factor in carotid endarterectomy specimens from patients on versus not on statins preoperatively. *Am J Cardiol* 2004;94(1):144–146.

19. Anon. MRC/BHF Heart Protection Study of cholesterol lowering with simvastatin in 20,536 high-risk individuals: a randomised placebo-controlled trial. *Lancet* 2002;360(9326):7–22.

20. Lonn EM, Gerstein HC, Sheridan P, et al. Effect of ramipril and of rosiglitazone on carotid intima-media thickness in people with impaired glucose tolerance or impaired fasting glucose: STARR (STudy of Atherosclerosis with Ramipril and Rosiglitazone). *J Am Coll Cardiol* 2009;53(22):2028–2035.

21. Amarenco P, Goldstein LB, Sillesen H, et al. Coronary heart disease risk in patients with stroke or transient ischemic attack and no known coronary heart disease: findings from the Stroke Prevention by Aggressive Reduction in Cholesterol Levels (SPARCL) trial. *Stroke* 2010;41(3):426–430.

22. Kennedy J, Quan H, Buchan AM, Ghali WA, Feasby TE. Statins are associated with better outcomes after carotid endarterectomy in symptomatic patients. *Stroke* 2005;36(10):2072–2076.

23. McGirt MJ, Perler BA, Brooke BS, et al. 3-hydroxy-3-methylglutaryl coenzyme A reductase inhibitors reduce the risk of perioperative stroke and mortality after carotid endarterectomy. *J Vasc Surg* 2005;42(5):829–836; discussion 836–837.

24. LaMuraglia GM, Stoner MC, Brewster DC, et al. Determinants of carotid endarterectomy anatomic durability: effects of serum lipids and lipid-lowering drugs. *J Vasc Surg* 2005;41(5):762–768.

25. Gaunt ME, Smith JL, Ratliff DA, Bell PR, Naylor AR. A comparison of quality control methods applied to carotid endarterectomy. *Eur J Vasc Endovasc Surg* 1996;11(1):4–11.

26. Lennard N, Smith JL, Hayes P, et al. Transcranial Doppler directed dextran therapy in the prevention of carotid thrombosis: three hour monitoring is as effective as six hours. *Eur J Vasc Endovasc Surg* 1999;17(4):301–305.

27. Anon. A randomised, blinded, trial of clopidogrel versus aspirin in patients at risk of ischaemic events (CAPRIE). CAPRIE Steering Committee. *Lancet* 1996;348(9038):1329–1339.

28. Engelter S, Lyrer P. Antiplatelet therapy for preventing stroke and other vascular events after carotid endarterectomy. *Cochrane Database Syst Rev* 2003;(3):CD001458.

29. Rosenbaum A, Rizvi AZ, Alden PB, et al. Outcomes related to antiplatelet or anticoagulation use in patients undergoing carotid endarterectomy. *Ann Vasc Surg* 2011;25(1):25–31.

30. Assadian A, Eidher U, Senekowitsch C, et al. Antiplatelet therapy prior to carotid endarterectomy–still room for improvement. *VASA*. 2006;35(2):96–100.

9

Contemporary Management of Patients with Concomitant Coronary and Carotid Artery Disease

Peter H. Lin, MD

INTRODUCTION

Cardiovascular disease is one of the most common causes of death in developed countries, including the United States (U.S.). It is estimated that nearly 40% of all cardiovascular-related fatalities in the U.S. is due to myocardial ischemia caused by atherosclerotic coronary artery disease.[1] As the result of systemic atherosclerotic progression, many patients with coronary artery occlusive disease are similarly inflicted with carotid artery occlusive disease. It is reported that stroke due to carotid artery atherosclerosis accounts for 18% of all cardiovascular-related fatalities in the U.S.[1]

The presence of systemic atherosclerosis involving coronary artery or carotid artery occlusive disease is a common phenomenon in patients undergoing either coronary artery bypass grafting (CABG) or carotid endarterectomy (CEA). Among the patients undergoing CEA, it has been shown that 28% had severe coronary artery disease which was indicated for CABG.2 Similarly, hemodynamically significant carotid artery occlusive disease with greater than 80% luminal stenosis can be found in 12% of patients undergoing coronary revascularization.[1,2] Post-operative neurological complication following CABG is one of the most feared surgical complications, and frequency of postoperative stroke among patients undergoing CABG has been shown to range between 0.5% – 7%.[3] It is well reported that carotid artery occlusive disease is an independent predictor of perioperative stroke in patients undergoing CABG.[1,3]

Although numerous studies have convincingly demonstrated the efficacy and safety of preventive CEA for reducing the risk of stroke before CABG, controversy exists regarding the benefit of prophylactic CEA in patients with asymptomatic carotid stenosis. Several researchers have suggested that CEA for asymptomatic carotid disease does not necessarily reduce the risk of stroke in patients undergoing CABG.

These conflicting perspectives may have been the result of heterogeneity of the patient population and their disease patterns, particularly related to factors including the severity of carotid stenosis and operative variables associated with coronary revascularizations.

Due in part to the complex factors contributing to the neurological complication, the management of carotid arterial stenosis in patients who undergo CABG remains has been a subject of debate. Commonly utilized treatment strategies have included simultaneous CEA-CABG, staged CEA followed by CABG, and staged CABG followed by CEA. Recent studies have highlighted the role of carotid artery stenting (CAS) before CABG, and the use of off-pump CABG as a means to reduce perioperative ischemic stroke.[4] Despite theoretical benefits of each therapeutic approach, there remain no uniformly accepted treatment guidelines among physicians or surgeons who provide care to these patient cohorts.

The purpose of this article is to review various treatment strategies in patients who undergo CEA and CABG. Advances in endovascular treatment for carotid artery disease as well as surgical techniques with off-pump CABG have similarly increased the therapeutic armamentarium for these patients who require CEA and CABG. Rationales for these various treatment strategies as well as current literature to support their clinical applications are discussed. A proposed treatment algorithm encompassing these various treatment strategies is also provided.

PUBLISHED TREATMENT GUIDELINES ON CEA AND CABG

Although current literatures are inundated with studies with conflicting outcomes using various treatment strategies for patients requiring CEA and CABG, the American Heart Association (AHA) issued guidelines regarding the appropriateness of combined or synchronous CABG and CEA in 1998.[5] Specifically, this treatment guideline addressed CABG patients with asymptomatic occlusive carotid disease. It is noteworthy that this guideline reflected a consensus view of experts who advocated that synchronous CEA and CABG is "acceptable but not proven" in patients with unilateral asymptomatic carotid lesions greater than 60% luminal stenosis where there is a proven operative stroke and death risk of less than 3%. For institutions where the operative stroke and death risk rates are greater than 3%, on the other hand, the clinical benefits and treatment efficacy of synchronous CEA and CABG were described as "uncertain" according to the AHA guidelines.[5]

The published guidelines by the AHA, however, did not fully resolve the controversy regarding the ideal treatment strategy for patients with high-grade carotid artery disease who require coronary revascularization. Debates continued regarding how to screen and identify patients with carotid occlusive disease before undergoing coronary revascularization. The American College of Cardiology (ACC) and American Heart Association (AHA) issued guidelines for CABG in 2004, which recommended a screening carotid ultrasound for those older than 65 years, individuals with left main coronary stenosis, peripheral vascular disease, or those with history of smoking, transient ischemic attack, stroke, or for the presence of carotid bruit on examination.[1] This carotid screening guideline would detect severe carotid stenosis (greater than 80%) in approximately 95% of patients undergoing CABG.[1] In spite of the publication of this screening guideline, controversy abounds as authors conceded that these recommendations are based on a few observational studies and expert consensus, rather than any randomized studies. Many questioned the cost-effectiveness of screening carotid ultrasound in CABG patients for stroke prevention. Furthermore, the benefit of carotid screening in perioperative stroke or mortality reduction in the CABG population has not been proven in a large scale clinical study.[1]

PREVALENCE AND ETIOLOGY OF NEUROLOGICAL COMPLICATIONS FOLLOWING CARDIAC SURGERY

Ischemic stroke is by far one of the most feared complications following any surgical procedure, particularly cardiac operations. Neurological complications following CABG is associated with a mortality of 24.8% and mean hospital stay of 28 days for stroke survivors.[1,2] Studies have identified multiple risk factors for stroke in patients undergoing CABG, which include age, preoperative neurologic symptoms, aortic arch disease, carotid bruit, diabetes, and degree of carotid stenosis. These widely ranged risk factors underscore the complex multifactorial etiologies which contribute to post-CABG neurological complications.

It is noteworthy the incidence of neurological complications varies depending on the type of cardiac interventions. It is estimated that stroke occurs in 0.3% to 5.2% of patients undergoing cardiac surgery, 1.3% after cardiac catheterization, 0.3% following percutaneous transluminal coronary angioplasty, 1.4%–11.0% following percutaneous transluminal aortic valvuloplasty, 3.2%–4.2% after percutaneous mitral valvuloplasty, and 9.0% after cardiac transplantation.[6,7] Specifically among patients who are older than 75 years of age, the risk of stroke can reach as high as 9% following CABG, and 16% following valve replacement. In a prospective multicenter trial, Wolman and colleagues reported that ischemic stroke occurred in one out of every six patients who underwent coronary revascularization combined with intracardiac operation.[8]

Utilizing a prospective database on 16,184 consecutive patients undergoing cardiac surgery, Bucerius and associates reported an overall incidence of stroke was 4.6% but varied depending on the surgical procedures.[9] Specifically, the incidence of stroke was 3.8% following CABG, 1.9% following beating heart CABG, 4.8% following aortic valve surgery, 8.8% following mitral valve surgery, 9.7% following double or triple valve surgery, and 7.4% following CABG and valve surgery. Other researchers conducted prospective studies of consecutive patients undergoing CABG, and reported that the risk of major ischemic stroke ranged between 1%–6%.[10] Using multivariate analysis, these authors have identified multiple factors which were associated with an increased risk of stroke in patients undergoing cardiac surgery. These factors include: age older than 60 years, greater than 50% carotid stenosis, prior stroke or transient ischemic attack, history of congestive heart failure, valvular disease, repeat heart surgery, postoperative atrial fibrillation, bypass time of more than 2 hours, and prior myocardial infarction.

Regarding possible pathogenic mechanisms of stroke during cardiac surgery, researchers have postulated various causes. These mechanisms include cerebral flow compromise due to intraoperative hypotension with concomitant carotid artery occlusive disease, atheromatous emboli during aortic manipulation either during aortic cannulation or during application of the aortic side biting clamps for performing the aorto-coronary saphenous vein graft anastomosis, air emboli, hemodynamic instability during cardiopulmonary bypass or inadequate intracerebral cross-perfusion. Despite the heterogeneity of these pathogenic mechanisms, many researchers believed that the stroke risk during CABG is related to the degree of carotid stenosis. In a meta-analysis, Naylor and associates reported that patients with no significant carotid disease had a 1.9% risk of stroke following CABG.[11] The risk of stroke increased to 3% in neurologically asymptomatic patients with unilateral 50–99% carotid stenosis, 5% in those with bilateral 50–99% carotid stenoses, and 7–11% in patients with carotid occlusion.[11] Although these authors suggested an association between significant carotid disease and post-CABG stroke, their study did not provide information regarding the laterality of cerebral ischemic events in relation to carotid stenosis. In patients who underwent CABG including left main stem coronary artery revascularization, the incidence of carotid artery disease and postoperative cerebrovascular complications were higher.

Contrary to these findings, other authors have proposed different mechanisms for post-CABG neurological complications which were not related to the severity of carotid disease.[12] Analyzing their institutional data of 1,179 patients regarding post-CABG neurological events, Ricotta and associates reported a discrepancy between stroke distribution and site of carotid stenosis.[12] Additionally, most strokes occurred later than 24 hours following CABG operation, suggesting other potential causes such as atrial fibrillation or postoperative hypotension may have played a crucial role in post-CABG stroke. Other researchers have found that proximal aortic calcification to be a predictor for post-CABG ischemic stroke irrespective of carotid disease, due in part to plaque embolization during aortic manipulation. Additionally, radiological findings including aortic atheroma protrusion based on computed tomography (CT) scan or mobile aortic atheroma as detected by transesophageal echocardiography have also been shown to be associated with a 14% incidence of perioperative stroke. Lastly, Schoof and colleagues reported that, in patients with severe carotid stenosis or occlusion, the presence of an impaired cerebral autoregulatory reserve may contribute to increased stroke risk during cardiac surgery.[13] While these available data do not uniformly underscore a single pathogenic mechanism for post-CABG neurological complications, multiple randomized trials analyzing the efficacy of CEA have demonstrated that removing carotid plaque burden by CEA in patients with hemodynamically significant carotid disease will reduce the risk of ischemic stroke, including those who require coronary revascularization.[14]

POTENTIAL TREATMENT STRATEGIES FOR CEA AND CABG

Various treatment strategies have been proposed to decrease the risk of post-CABG neurological complications in patients who require both carotid and coronary revascularization. Considering that carotid artery stenting has become an accepted treatment option for endovascular revascularization, this represents a potential treatment strategy for these patient cohorts. Consequently, available treatment strategies include the following options:

1. Combined or synchronous CABG and CEA during the same anesthetic setting,
2. Staged CEA first, followed by CABG,
3. Staged CABG first, followed by CEA,
4. Staged CAS first, followed by CABG,
5. CEA with off-pump CABG.

Despite multiple studies demonstrating the feasibility and safety of each of these treatment modalities, controversy exists as to which strategy can optimally reduce the risk of neurological adverse events following coronary revascularization. There are no randomized prospective studies with level 1 evidence to support the ideal treatment strategy. Although the consensus statement released by the American Heart Association acknowledged increased perioperative complications with synchronous carotid and coronary revascularization, it did not provide any recommendation for alternative management strategy for this subgroup of patients.[1,15] Ongoing debates continue regarding the optimal timing and sequence of staged operations, particularly for those who require urgent reconstructions for either symptomatic carotid or coronary lesions during the same hospitalization.

RATIONALE FOR SYNCHRONOUS CEA AND CABG

The combined or synchronous approach, first reported by Bernhard and colleagues in 1972, involves performing CEA which was immediately followed by CABG under the same anesthesia.[16] Clinical studies have shown that advantages of the synchronous approach include: a) decreased incidence of stroke and operative mortality for patients with symptomatic coronary and carotid artery diseases, b) decreased hospital cost and surgical procedural cost, c) shorter hospital length of stay, d) acceptable operative morbidity and mortality, and e) lower stroke risk on long term follow up.

The synchronous approach is generally reserved for patients with severe symptoms involving both carotid and coronary vascular territories, such as those with severe stenosis (greater than 90% luminal stenosis) or bilateral carotid occlusion. Van Der Grond and colleagues postulated that these patient cohorts are most likely to have impaired cerebral autoregulation due to chronic cerebral ischemia.[17] The authors suggested that when the cerebral autoregulation is impaired, the synchronous treatment with CEA and CABG should be considered as this subset of patients with cerebral hypoperfusion and ischemic metabolic changes distal to severe carotid stenosis are probably at high risk for stroke during CABG. This hypothesis, however, has not been validated by any clinical study.

RATIONALE FOR STAGED CEA AND CABG

Numerous studies have found that combined or synchronous treatment of CEA and CABG resulted in higher stroke and death rates, due in part to several reasons.[18] One factor is that synchronous CEA and CABG procedures are more technically challenging, from both a surgical and an anesthesia stand point, thereby resulting in greater perioperative complications. Another factor may be that combined operations result in excessive physiological and cardiovascular stress, resulting in greater hemodynamic fluctuations or instability during relatively long operative procedures. This notion was supported by a systemic review of 94 clinical studies which noted that synchronous treatment carried a relative high morbidity and mortality rates with death or major stroke rate of 11.5%.[19,20]

Many researchers favored the staged approach with CEA prior to CABG, due to perceived advantage of reduced operative time and minimize surgical complexity of two surgical procedures. This approach is generally reserved for patients with stable coronary symptoms who can undergo the initial CEA procedure followed by a variable time interval of recovery before undergoing coronary revascularization.

ROLE OF CAROTID ARTERY
STENTING IN PATIENTS UNDERGOING CABG

Percutaneous stenting of carotid artery stenosis has emerged as an attractive treatment option compared to CEA. The clinical efficacy of CAS has been proven in several randomized trials to be equivalent to CEA.[21] Many have proposed that staged CAS followed by CABG may represent an acceptable treatment option to either staged or synchronous CEA and CABG. The theoretical advantages of CAS are related to the minimally invasiveness and avoidance of general anesthesia, which may reduce cardiac complications.

With regards to incorporating CAS treatment in patients who require CABG, there are three potential treatment strategies which include: 1) CAS followed by CABG several days or weeks later (staged procedures with separate anesthesia approach; 2) CAS under local anesthesia followed by CABG on the same day (same day procedures with two anesthesia approach); and 3) CAS followed by CABG in the same operating room under general anesthesia (same day procedures under general anesthesia approach). Most published results utilized the staged approach in which CABG was performed several weeks following the initial CAS, as this staged approach allows for safe withholding of the anti-platelet agent prior to CABG. Patients undergoing the same day CAS and CAS requiring immediate anti-platelet regimens as soon as CABG is completed. Because an endovascular operating room is needed to allow CAS and CABG to be performed synchronously under the same anesthesia, only limited clinical series are available for such a treatment strategy.

Since there are no randomized trials comparing CAS to CEA for patients who require coronary revascularization, there are several observational studies which compared staged CAS plus CABG with a CEA plus CABG strategy.[22,23] Van der Heyden and associates analyzed 356 patients who underwent CAS followed by CABG, with a mean interval of 22 days. All patients were neurologically asymptomatic and an embolization protection device was used in only 40% of patients. At 30 days post-CABG, the stroke and death rate was 4.8%, myocardial infarction (MI) was 2% and the combined stroke, MI and death rate was 6.7%.[23] Long-term durability and a high rate of freedom from death and stroke were noted during the 5-year follow-up.[23] Another study similarly reported low peri-procedural complication rates in staged CAS followed by CABG.[22] Due to the favorable outcomes with percutaneous carotid stenting prior to CABG, these authors advocated CAS as a preferred treatment strategy compared to CEA prior to coronary revascularization.[22,23]

In a clinical study encompassing a five-year institutional experience which compared CAS followed by open heart surgery (OHS) to combined CEA–OHS, Ziada and associates reported fewer strokes or MI at 30 days with the CAS–OHS approach (5% vs 19%, p=0.02) despite the use of embolization protection device in only 14% of the patients.[24] The favorable outcome with CAS was further underscored by the fact that patients who underwent CAS had a higher risk profile with more unstable or severe angina (52% vs 27%, p=0.002) and had a higher prevalence of symptomatic carotid disease (46% vs 23% p=0.002).[24] A recent meta-analysis of 11 published studies on CAS followed by CABG procedures reported similar 30-day risks for any stroke (4.2%), MI (1.8%) and combined stroke, MI and death (9.4%) when compared to the results from CEA–CABG strategies.[25] While these data showed comparable CAS-CABG outcomes compared to CEA-CABG cohorts, the author cautioned that the majority of patients who received CAS were largely asymptomatic neurologically (87%) and had unilateral carotid artery stenosis (82%).[25]

Utilizing the National Inpatient Sample database, Timaran and colleagues examined nationwide trends and outcomes of 27,084 procedures which comprised of combined CEA–CABG (96.7%) and CAS–CABG (3.3%) procedures.[26] The risk of postoperative stroke was significantly higher in the CEA–CABG group (3.9%) compared to the CAS–CABG group (2.4%), although no difference in the risk of combined stroke and death or in-hospital death was noted (5.2% vs. 5.4%).[26] The authors concluded that CAS might provide a safer carotid revascularization option for patients who require CABG.[26] Although CAS unquestionably has gained popularity due to its minimally invasiveness and perceived less anesthetic risks compared to traditional CEA, a consensus guideline published by the European Society for Vascular Surgery in 2009 underscored an important principle of this treatment modality, in which it recommended that CAS for carotid stenosis should only be performed for high risk patients in high-volume institutions with proven low procedural complication rates.[27]

ROLE OF OFF-PUMP CABG IN PATIENTS WITH CAROTID ARTERY DISEASE

Clinical evidence has suggested that the most important single cause of post-CABG stroke is thrombotic embolization from the aortic arch debris. As the result, many physicians have refined surgical strategies and operative techniques to reduce the risk of embolization during aortic dissection, cannulation, and aortic cross-clamping. In a review article which analyzed 12 studies encompassing 324 synchronous CEA plus off-pump CABG procedures, these patient cohorts had better outcomes of stroke, MI or death (3.6%) compared to those who were treated with either combined or staged CEA and on pump CABG. The operative mortality for synchronous CEA plus off-pump CABG was only 1.5% and the risk of death or any stroke significantly reduced at 2.2%.[28] In a study which reported 38 patients who underwent synchronous CEA and off-pump CABG, the authors reported remarkable outcome with no postoperative neurological complications and an in-hospital death rate of 3%.[29] The clinical efficacy of synchronous CEA and off-pump CABG was similarly underscored by Chen and associates who reported their experience in 51 patients, who did not suffer any postoperative neurological or cardiac complications.[30] With a mean follow up of 39 months, the operative mortality was 1.96%.[30] Several factors may have accounted for the clinical outcome of these studies. Off-pump CABG has been shown to result in reduced incidence of stroke compared to on-pump CABG due to decreased risk of embolization from aortic manipulation. Additionally, the devoid of extracorporeal circulation in off-pump CABG potentially minimizes the likelihood of systemic hypotension and possibly averts cerebral hypoperfusion.

In the study by Mishra and associates, synchronous CEA plus either on-pump or off-pump CABG were performed in 358 patients, which included 166 patients who had off-pump CABG and 192 patients with on-pump coronary revascularization.[4] The authors reported no differences in mortality or stroke between the two CABG approaches, with mortalities of 1.2% in the off-pump group and 1.6% in the on-pump group. Postoperative stroke rates of the off-pump and on-pump patients were 0% and 0.5%, respectively. Although these results suggest no significant difference in outcomes with either on-pump or off-pump CABG, the observed mortality and neurological morbidity rates in this study were lower than the published literature.[31] Several recent studies which analyzed the effect of off-pump CABG versus on-pump CABG in patients undergoing synchronous CEA and coronary revascularization have similarly noted the reduced incidence of postoperative stroke rate in off-pump CABG patients compared to on-pump CABG cohorts.

CONTEMPORARY STUDIES BASED ON MULTI-INSTITUTIONAL DATABASE

In an effort to answer the question of whether patients should undergo staged versus synchronous carotid and coronary revascularization, various authors reported several studies analyzing contemporary large database.[32-34] Analyzing the Nationwide Inpatient Sample database during a recent 10 year period ending in 2007, Gospaldas from our institution compared the outcome of 6,153 patients who underwent staged CEA and CABG versus 16,639 patients who underwent synchronous or combined procedures.[32] Within the synchronous approach, off-pump was performed in 5,280 patients (31.7%) while 2,004 patients (32.5%) underwent off-pump CABG in the staged group. While both staged and synchronous groups shared similar age, perioperative mortality and neurological complication rates, higher perioperative morbidities were noted in staged patients when compared to synchronous cohort, which included greater cardiac, wound, respiratory, and renal complications. When analyzing hospital length of stay, staged approach was independently associated with a longer hospital stay by 3.1 days (p < 0.001). This study was unique as it also analyzed treatment cost. Cost analysis using inflation-adjusted hospital charges showed that staged and synchronous strategy incurred a mean cost of $118,801 ± 78,644 and $98,106 ± 80,053, respectively (< 0.001). Further assessment using risk-adjusted models indicated that staged procedures were independently associated with a $23,328 higher hospital charge.[32] While this analysis showed no difference in mortality or neurological complications between the two groups, the study revealed greater benefits in the synchronous approach due to lower risk for overall complications and reduced hospital charges compared to the staged approach. Additionally, on-pump CABG was associated with greater stroke rates compared to off-pump CABG in the synchronous patients, a finding which was consistent with several other studies.

In a similar clinical report which analyzed a large sample database, Prasad and colleagues examined the Society of Thoracic Surgeons (STS) database which included 745,769 patients who underwent CABG during a recent five-year period.[34] Among them, 5,732 patients had synchronous CEA and CABG while 24,167 patients had staged CEA followed by CABG. The authors also identified a cohort of 15,757 patients who underwent CABG and had ultrasound-proven > 75% carotid stenosis, but without any carotid intervention. The study revealed that synchronous approach yielded a significantly higher hospital length of stay, operative mortality, and in-hospital complications including stroke compared to those who either received staged CEA plus CABG or no carotid intervention. The negative operative treatment outcome for synchronous approach from this study was in contrast to other published series.[30,31,35,36] Recognizing the potential weaknesses of this database analysis which included retrospective observational assessment of a large sample size without long term data variables, the authors underscored the importance of better patient selection when considering synchronous approach for carotid and coronary revascularizations.[34]

STUDIES BASED ON SYSTEMIC
LITERATURE REVIEWS OR META-ANALYSIS

The ideal treatment strategy for patients with carotid and coronary occlusive disease has been a subject of detailed analysis by many researchers in past decades.[11,25,33,34] In one of the early meta-analysis of 56 studies which reviewed three operative strategies in patients with concomitant coronary and carotid artery diseases including: a) simultaneous CEA and CABG, b) CEA followed by CABG, and c) CABG followed by CEA.[14] The authors reported a 10% perioperative stroke rate in patients who underwent CABG first followed by CEA. The stroke rate for patients undergoing combined CEA and CABG was reduced to 6%. For patients treated with CEA followed by CABG, their stroke rate was reduced even further to 5%. However, CEA followed by CABG showed the highest rates for perioperative myocardial infarction (11%) and death (9%), whereas those who underwent simultaneous CEA and CABG and CABG followed by CEA showed lower rates for perioperative myocardial infarction (5% and 3%, respectively) and death (6% and 4%, respectively).[14] The report of this meta-analysis which demonstrated a potential beneficial role for combined treatment strategy was in contrast to a meta-analysis reported by Borger and associates who analyzed 16 studies including a total of 844 patients treated with combined CABG and CEA and 920 patients treated with staged approach.[37] The authors found a significantly higher risk in the composite endpoint, stroke, or death for patients undergoing combined CABG and CEA operations. Specifically, the crude event rates for stroke were 6.0% versus 3.2% for combined versus staged procedure, 4.7% versus 2.9% for death, and 9.5% versus 5.7% for stroke and death.[37] This report underscored the potential higher risk of stroke or death rate in the combined treatment strategy for CABG and CEA procedures. This finding was consistent with several other reviews which revealed that staged CEA followed by coronary revascularization has lower stroke rates compared to those undergoing synchronous CEA and CABG.[38]

Naylor and associates have performed several literature reviews as well as meta-analysis regarding patients undergoing carotid and coronary revascularization.[11,19,20,25] In one of their reports encompassing 59 studies before the year 2000, the authors observed that 91% of screened CABG patients did not have significant carotid occlusive disease, and the stroke risk in these patient cohorts was less than 2%.[11] In patients undergoing CABG who had asymptomatic unilateral 50-99% carotid stenosis, the risk of stroke was increased to 3%. The risk of stroke for patients with bilateral 50-99% carotid disease or unilateral carotid artery occlusion was increased to 5% and 7-11%, respectively.[11] The authors also analyzed 10 studies for a total of 111 patients who suffered stroke after CABG. Among them, 48% of these patients did not have particularly significant disease in either carotid (<50% stenosis), 20% had 50-99% unilateral stenosis, 20% had 50-99% bilateral stenosis, 7% carotid occlusion with <50% contralateral stenosis, and 4% an occlusion with >50% contralateral stenosis and 1% bilateral occlusion.[11] These data, together with those from CT scans and autopsy findings, suggest that only 50% of strokes in CABG patients may be attributed to carotid artery disease. The authors highlighted the importance of understanding the condition of aortic calcification, the choice of site and aortic clamping technique, and to use the off-pump surgical method, with the purpose of reducing non-carotid related neurological complications.[11]

In their subsequent literature review of 97 articles encompassing 8,972 patients undergoing either staged or synchronous carotid and coronary revascularizations, treatment outcomes following these two treatment modalities were analyzed.[19] Approximately 60% of patients undergoing either staged or synchronous procedures were neurologically asymptomatic, while 30–37% had bilateral 50–99% stenosis or contralateral carotid occlusion. The majority of patients in the synchronous treatment group (72%) were New York Heart Association grade 3 or 4, and 39% of these cohorts were classed as "urgent" while left main coronary artery disease was present in 25% of cases. The authors reported that synchronous approach had the highest operative mortality rate of 4.6% while those treated with reversed staged approach (CABG followed by CEA) had the highest risk of ipsilateral stroke (5.8%) and stroke in general (6.3%).[19] The risk of any operative stroke was lowest following staged approach (CEA followed by CABG, 2.7%). Myocardial infarction (MI) had the lowest perioperative risk in patients who underwent the reverse staged procedure (CABG followed by CEA, 0.9%), and the highest in those who underwent synchronous CEA and CABG treatment (6.5%). Death and any stroke were highest in patients undergoing synchronous CEA and CABG treatment (8.7%) and lowest following staged approach (CEA followed by CABG, 6.1%). The authors noted that, however, the benefit conferred by staging the operation was reduced when the risk of myocardial infarction was subsequently included in the analysis (synchronous=11.5%, staged CEA-CABG=10.2%). In a separate literature review by the same author group, it was demonstrated that recent CABG patients without significant carotid artery disease (<50% stenosis) had an operative stroke risk of approximately 1.8%. Unilateral (50–99%) and bilateral (50–99%) stenosis resulted in a 3.2% and 5.2% stroke risk, respectively.[19] Taken these results together, the authors concluded there were no statistically significant differences between staged or synchronous strategies.[19] Additionally, these reviews suggest that carotid stenosis, by itself, may be a marker for other conditions, such as atherosclerotic disease of the aorta, which also may contribute to stroke risk during CABG surgery.

A multistate population based study was reported by Brown and colleagues who assessed both the community wide outcomes of combined CEA and CABG and the risk for adverse events.[2] In their study, 10,561 CEAs were randomly selected using the Medicare database, of which 226 procedures were performed in combination with CABG in the same operative event. Only 12% of patients undergoing combined CEA and CABG had recent ipsilateral stroke or TIA, while 56% had had an asymptomatic carotid stenosis. The combined stroke and death rate was 17.7%.[2] Proximal aortic arch atherosclerosis and symptomatic carotid stenosis were associated with perioperative neurological events. The authors identified several risk factors for higher mortality which included female sex, emergent CABG procedure, redo CABG operation, prolonged total pump time during CABG, presence of left main disease, and number of diseased coronary arteries. The study showed that strokes appeared to be associated with operative events. However, the patency of the carotid artery following stroke was not routinely assessed, and most strokes did not occur in the ipsilateral hemisphere of the CEA.[2] In an article by Das and colleagues who analyzed various strategies for the treatment of concomitant coronary artery disease and asymptomatic carotid artery stenosis as defined by greater than 50% luminal stenosis, the authors assessed four possible treatment strategies: 1) CABG in the presence of carotid stenosis, 2) synchronous CEA and CABG, 3) reverse (CABG followed by CEA in less than 3 months) and 4) prior staged (CEA followed by CABG in less than 3 months).[39] The authors reported a significant reduction in stroke for prior versus combined procedures (1.5% v 3.9%).

The stroke rate in the prior stage also remained significantly lower compared with the other two groups but when total risks for stroke and death were analyzed, similar results were found among the groups: prior 7.4%, reverse stage 7.2%, combined 8.4% and 11.5% in CABG in the presence of carotid stenosis.[39]

Based on these literature reviews and meta-analysis, the vast majority of CABG patients with asymptomatic unilateral carotid stenosis can safely undergo coronary revascularization without any prophylactic carotid intervention. Undoubtedly more data is needed to better identify patients with asymptomatic unilateral carotid stenosis who will benefit from prophylactic carotid intervention.

PROPOSED TREATMENT PARADIGM IN PATIENTS WITH CAROTID AND CORONARY ARTERY DISEASE

Considering available data from published reports, the treatment indication for carotid artery stenosis in patients who require coronary revascularization must weigh in the status of neurological symptoms. While further clinical evidence is needed to support the ideal treatment approach for patients with coronary and carotid disease, we provide the following recommendations based on published literature:

- In patients with unilateral asymptomatic internal carotid artery disease (>60%) who require CABG, combined CABG and CEA is an acceptable but unproven treatment strategy. Patient life expectancy of at least 5 years or greater and perioperative stroke and death risk of less than 3% are needed to justify the combined treatment approach.
- In patients with bilateral internal carotid artery stenosis (>60%) who require coronary revascularization, combined CEA (on the side of the more severe stenosis) and CABG is an acceptable but unproven treatment modality. Greater than 5 years of life expectancy and less than 3% of perioperative stroke and death risk are needed to justify the combined procedures.
- In patients with internal carotid artery stenosis (>60%) and contralateral carotid occlusion who require CABG, there is no available data to support prophylactic CEA or CAS prior to coronary revascularization.
- In patients with symptomatic internal carotid artery stenosis (>60%) who require coronary revascularization for stable coronary disease, CAS is an acceptable but unproven treatment option. Procedural related stroke rate of less than 3% is needed to justify this treatment strategy.

Figure 9–1 outline the various treatment strategies for patients with coronary and carotid disease for consideration of either staged or combined interventions. For those patients with symptomatic carotid artery stenosis who require CABG, a staged treatment approach of CEA followed by CABG may be considered in the setting of stable angina while a combined strategy of CEA and CABG should be reserved for those with acute coronary syndrome. For patients with asymptomatic unilateral carotid stenosis who requires coronary revascularization for stable coronary disease, various carotid treatment strategies including medical therapy alone or CAS can also be considered. For patients with acute coronary syndrome or unstable coronary disease, immediate coronary revascularization with either subsequent staged carotid intervention or combined carotid intervention should be offered. Given the increased availability of

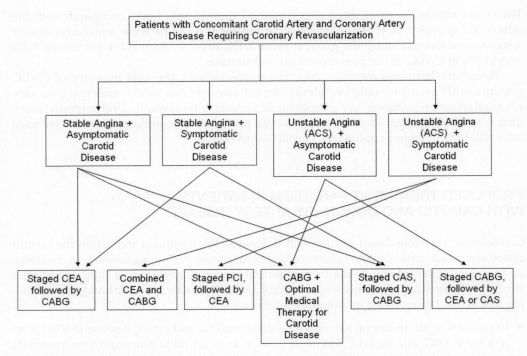

Figure 9–1. Treatment strategies for patients with concomitant carotid artery and coronary artery disease (ACS: acute coronary syndrome, PCI: percutaneous coronary intervention; CAS: carotid artery stenting; CABG: coronary artery bypass surgery).

endovascular hybrid operating suite in many institutions, synchronous treatment strategies for coronary and carotid revascularization can be expanded to CAS or CEA treatment in conjunction with CABG or percutaneous coronary intervention (PCI).

CONCLUSIONS

The ideal treatment strategy for severe carotid and coronary artery disease remains elusive based to current published data. The majority of patients who require coronary and carotid interventions have unilateral carotid disease that are asymptomatic neurologically. It remains a subject of debate whether prophylactic carotid interventions can definitively benefit the survival rate. Ongoing controversy also exists regarding the optimal timing of carotid revascularization in patients with concomitant coronary and carotid disease. Recent advances in endovascular technologies have supported the utility of carotid stenting as an acceptable treatment strategy for carotid revascularization. This percutaneous carotid intervention has become a latest armamentarium for physicians in treating patients who require coronary and carotid revascularization. The role of optimal medical therapy with risk factor modification must also be considered when treating patients with coronary and carotid occlusive disease. Given these multitudes of therapeutic considerations, a randomized clinical trial is undoubtedly needed to address the optimal treatment modality for patients with these concomitant diseases.

REFERENCES

1. Eagle KA, Guyton RA, Davidoff R, Edwards FH, Ewy GA, Gardner TJ, et al. ACC/AHA 2004 guideline update for coronary artery bypass graft surgery: a report of the American College of Cardiology/American Heart Association Task Force on Practice Guidelines (Committee to Update the 1999 Guidelines for Coronary Artery Bypass Graft Surgery). *Circulation* 2004; 110:e340–437.
2. Brown KR, Kresowik TF, Chin MH, Kresowik RA, Grund SL, Hendel ME. Multistate population-based outcomes of combined carotid endarterectomy and coronary artery bypass. *J Vasc Surg* 2003;37:32–9.
3. Lloyd-Jones D, Adams R, Carnethon M, De Simone G, Ferguson TB, Flegal K, et al. Heart disease and stroke statistics—2009 update: a report from the American Heart Association Statistics Committee and Stroke Statistics Subcommittee. *Circulation* 2009;119:e21–181.
4. Mishra Y, Wasir H, Kohli V, Meharwal ZS, Malhotra R, Mehta Y, et al. Concomitant carotid endarterectomy and coronary bypass surgery: outcome of on-pump and off-pump techniques. *Ann Thorac Surg* 2004;78:2037-42; discussion 2042–3.
5. Biller J, Feinberg WM, Castaldo JE, Whittemore AD, Harbaugh RE, Dempsey RJ, et al. Guidelines for carotid endarterectomy: a statement for healthcare professionals from a Special Writing Group of the Stroke Council, American Heart Association. *Circulation* 1998; 97:501–9.
6. Davidson CJ, Mark DB, Pieper KS, Kisslo KB, Hlatky MA, Gabriel DA, et al. Thrombotic and cardiovascular complications related to nonionic contrast media during cardiac catheterization: analysis of 8,517 patients. *Am J Cardiol* 1990;65:1481–4.
7. Holmes DR, Jr., Nishimura RA, Reeder GS, Wagner PJ, Ilstrup DM. Clinical follow-up after percutaneous aortic balloon valvuloplasty. *Arch Intern Med* 1989;149:1405–9.
8. Wolman RL, Nussmeier NA, Aggarwal A, Kanchuger MS, Roach GW, Newman MF, et al. Cerebral injury after cardiac surgery: identification of a group at extraordinary risk. Multicenter Study of Perioperative Ischemia Research Group (McSPI) and the Ischemia Research Education Foundation (IREF) Investigators. *Stroke* 1999;30:514–22.
9. Bucerius J, Gummert JF, Borger MA, Walther T, Doll N, Onnasch JF, et al. Stroke after cardiac surgery: a risk factor analysis of 16,184 consecutive adult patients. *Ann Thorac Surg* 2003;75:472–8.
10. Coffey CE, Massey EW, Roberts KB, Curtis S, Jones RH, Pryor DB. Natural history of cerebral complications of coronary artery bypass graft surgery. *Neurology* 1983; 33:1416–21.
11. Naylor AR, Mehta Z, Rothwell PM, Bell PR. Carotid artery disease and stroke during coronary artery bypass: a critical review of the literature. *Eur J Vasc Endovasc Surg* 2002;23: 283–94.
12. Ricotta JJ, Faggioli GL, Castilone A, Hassett JM. Risk factors for stroke after cardiac surgery: Buffalo Cardiac-Cerebral Study Group. *J Vasc Surg* 1995; 21:359–63; discussion 364.
13. Schoof J, Lubahn W, Baeumer M, Kross R, Wallesch CW, Kozian A, et al. Impaired cerebral autoregulation distal to carotid stenosis/occlusion is associated with increased risk of stroke at cardiac surgery with cardiopulmonary bypass. *J Thorac Cardiovasc Surg* 2007;134: 690–6.
14. Moore WS, Barnett HJ, Beebe HG, Bernstein EF, Brener BJ, Brott T, et al. Guidelines for carotid endarterectomy. A multidisciplinary consensus statement from the Ad Hoc Committee, American Heart Association. *Circulation* 1995;91:566–79.
15. Eagle KA, Guyton RA, Davidoff R, Ewy GA, Fonger J, Gardner TJ, et al. ACC/AHA guidelines for coronary artery bypass graft surgery: executive summary and recommendations: A report of the American College of Cardiology/American Heart Association Task Force on Practice Guidelines (Committee to revise the 1991 guidelines for coronary artery bypass graft surgery). *Circulation* 1999;100:1464–80.
16. Bernhard VM, Johnson WD, Peterson JJ. Carotid artery stenosis. Association with surgery for coronary artery disease. *Arch Surg* 1972;105:837–40.

17. van der Grond J, Balm R, Kappelle LJ, Eikelboom BC, Mali WP. Cerebral metabolism of patients with stenosis or occlusion of the internal carotid artery. A 1H-MR spectroscopic imaging study. *Stroke* 1995;26:822–8.

18. Khaitan L, Sutter FP, Goldman SM, Chamogeorgakis T, Wertan MA, Priest BP, et al. Simultaneous carotid endarterectomy and coronary revascularization. *Ann Thorac Surg* 2000;69:421–4.

19. Naylor AR, Cuffe RL, Rothwell PM, Bell PR. A systematic review of outcomes following staged and synchronous carotid endarterectomy and coronary artery bypass. *Eur J Vasc Endovasc Surg* 2003;25:380–9.

20. Naylor R, Cuffe RL, Rothwell PM, Loftus IM, Bell PR. A systematic review of outcome following synchronous carotid endarterectomy and coronary artery bypass: influence of surgical and patient variables. *Eur J Vasc Endovasc Surg* 2003;26:230–41.

21. Lal BK, Brott TG. The Carotid Revascularization Endarterectomy vs. Stenting Trial completes randomization: lessons learned and anticipated results. *J Vasc Surg* 2009;50:1224–31.

22. Mendiz O, Fava C, Valdivieso L, Dulbecco E, Raffaelli H, Lev G, et al. Synchronous carotid stenting and cardiac surgery: an initial single-center experience. *Catheter Cardiovasc Interv* 2006;68:424–8.

23. Van der Heyden J, Suttorp MJ, Bal ET, Ernst JM, Ackerstaff RG, Schaap J, et al. Staged carotid angioplasty and stenting followed by cardiac surgery in patients with severe asymptomatic carotid artery stenosis: early and long-term results. *Circulation* 2007; 116:2036–42.

24. Ziada KM, Yadav JS, Mukherjee D, Lauer MS, Bhatt DL, Kapadia S, et al. Comparison of results of carotid stenting followed by open heart surgery versus combined carotid endarterectomy and open heart surgery (coronary bypass with or without another procedure). *Am J Cardiol* 2005;96:519–23.

25. Naylor AR. Does the risk of post-CABG stroke merit staged or synchronous reconstruction in patients with symptomatic or asymptomatic carotid disease? *J Cardiovasc Surg (Torino)* 2009;50:71–81.

26. Timaran CH, Rosero EB, Smith ST, Valentine RJ, Modrall JG, Clagett GP. Trends and outcomes of concurrent carotid revascularization and coronary bypass. *J Vasc Surg* 2008;48: 355–360; discussion 360–1.

27. Liapis CD, Bell PR, Mikhailidis D, Sivenius J, Nicolaides A, Fernandes e Fernandes J, et al. ESVS guidelines. Invasive treatment for carotid stenosis: indications, techniques. *Eur J Vasc Endovasc Surg* 2009;37:1–19.

28. Fareed KR, Rothwell PM, Mehta Z, Naylor AR. Synchronous carotid endarterectomy and off-pump coronary bypass: an updated, systematic review of early outcomes. *Eur J Vasc Endovasc Surg* 2009;37:375–8.

29. Beauford RB, Saunders CR, Goldstein DJ. Off pump concomitant coronary revascularization and carotid endarterectomy. *J Cardiovasc Surg (Torino)* 2003;44:407–15.

30. Chen XJ, Chen X, Xie DH, Shi KH, Xu M. Preliminary results of combined carotid endarterectomy and off-pump coronary artery bypass grafting in patients with coexistent carotid and coronary artery diseases. *Chin Med J (Engl)* 2009;122:2951–5.

31. Kougias P, Kappa JR, Sewell DH, Feit RA, Michalik RE, Imam M, et al. Simultaneous carotid endarterectomy and coronary artery bypass grafting: results in specific patient groups. *Ann Vasc Surg* 2007;21:408–14.

32. Gopaldas RR, Chu D, Dao TK, Huh J, LeMaire SA, Lin P, et al. Staged versus synchronous carotid endarterectomy and coronary artery bypass grafting: analysis of 10–year nationwide outcomes. *Ann Thorac Surg* 2011;91:1323–9; discussion 1329.

33. Li Y, Walicki D, Mathiesen C, Jenny D, Li Q, Isayev Y, et al. Strokes after cardiac surgery and relationship to carotid stenosis. *Arch Neurol* 2009; 66:1091–6.

34. Prasad SM, Li S, Rankin JS, O'Brien SM, Gammie JS, Puskas JD, et al. Current outcomes of simultaneous carotid endarterectomy and coronary artery bypass graft surgery in North America. *World J Surg* 2010;34:2292–8.

35. Chiti E, Troisi N, Marek J, Dorigo W, Innocenti AA, Pulli R, et al. Combined carotid and cardiac surgery: improving the results. *Ann Vasc Surg* 2010;24:794–800.

36. Venkatachalam S, Gray BH, Mukherjee D, Shishehbor MH. Contemporary management of concomitant carotid and coronary artery disease. *Heart* 2011;97:175–80.
37. Borger MA, Fremes SE, Weisel RD, Cohen G, Rao V, Lindsay TF, et al. Coronary bypass and carotid endarterectomy: does a combined approach increase risk? A metaanalysis. *Ann Thorac Surg* 1999;68:14–20; discussion 21.
38. Zacharias A, Schwann TA, Riordan CJ, Clark PM, Martinez B, Durham SJ, et al. Operative and 5-year outcomes of combined carotid and coronary revascularization: review of a large contemporary experience. *Ann Thorac Surg* 2002;73:491-7; discussion 497–8.
39. Das SK, Brow TD, Pepper J. Continuing controversy in the management of concomitant coronary and carotid disease: an overview. *Int J Cardiol* 2000;74:47–65.

10

Primary Extracranial Vertebral Artery Aneurysms

Sachin V. Phade, MD and Mark D. Morasch, MD

INTRODUCTION

With approximately 25% of strokes originating from the vertebrobasilar system, the etiology of most vertebral artery pathology is either related to atherosclerotic disease, fibromuscular disease, arteritis, trauma, and dissections.[1] Vertebral artery aneurysms are uncommon, accounting for only 1% of vertebral artery lesions.[2] The majority of vertebral artery aneurysms noted in the literature involve the intracranial segment, and most cervical vertebral aneurysms are truly traumatic or dissection-related pseudoaneurysms. Herein, we report a multi-institutional series of primary extracranial vertebral artery aneurysms, with their presentations, management, and outcomes.

METHODS

Prospectively collected databases from the Divisions of Vascular Surgery at Northwestern University, University of Michigan, Wayne State University, and University College Hospital Galway were used to identify patients who underwent extracranial vertebral artery interventions between January 1, 2000, and January 1, 2011. Those who underwent open, endovascular, or hybrid intervention for primary cervical vertebral artery aneurysms were selected.

Patient demographics and presentations, aneurysm locations and morphology, details of medical and surgical management, and outcomes were recorded. Specifically, personal or family history of connective tissue disorders or other hereditary disorders, aneurysms, and trauma were obtained. The side on which the aneurysm developed, the segments involved in the aneurysm, and concurrent cerebrovascular occlusive or aneurysmal disease were noted. The operative approaches and conduits were examined. Perioperative morbidities and mortalities were recorded along with mid-term follow-up.

RESULTS

Over the 11 year period, 7 patients with 9 extracranial vertebral artery aneurysms were identified. Patients with true vertebral aneurysms that were treated medically, without any intervention, could not be identified due to the constructs of the databases. Three (43%) were male, and mean age was 39 (range 12-56). All patients had a personal history of connective tissue or other hereditary disorder including 2 (28.5%) with Ehler-Danlos, 2 (28.5%) with Marfan's disease, 2 (28.5%) with neurofibromatosis, and 1 (14.5%) with an unspecified connective tissue abnormality. Two (28.5%) had a family history of a connective tissue disorder or premature death of unknown etiology. Notably, 5 (71.4%) had other cerebrovascular disease, including 1 prior stroke, 1 transient ischemic attack, 2 dissections, and 1 with multiple cerebrovascular aneurysms that had previously been ligated. Four (51.7%) patients had other aneurysms, including internal carotid, external carotid, common carotid, anterior cerebral, subclavian, thoracoabdominal, and splenic aneurysms. All four had concurrent cerebrovascular aneurysms, including 2 (28.5%) patients with bilateral vertebral artery aneurysms. Four (51.7%) patients were symptomatic upon presentation, with symptoms including transient ischemic attacks, dizziness and headaches, and tender neck masses.

Of the nine aneurysms, 6 (66.7%%) were on the left side. The segmental distribution was as such: 4 (51.7%) V1 and 7 (77.8%) V2, including two aneurysms involving both the V1 and V2 segments. No aneurysms involved the V3 segment. Of the eight aneurysms in which the aneurysm size was documented, the mean and median sizes were 25.9mm and 13.5mm, respectively (range 7-90mm). Two patients had vertebral arteries that originated from the aortic arch rather than the subclavian artery, one of which was aneurysmal.

Of the 9 aneurysms, 8 were managed operatively. One patient with Ehlers-Danlos and bilateral vertebral artery aneurysms required intraoperative vertebral ligation after failed bypass; the contralateral aneurysm has been managed medically. Similarly, one patient with Marfan's disease underwent attempted external carotid artery autograft, but ultimately required vertebral artery ligation because of anastamotic disruption. The remaining reconstructions were performed as bypasses with autologous venous conduit (3), distal vertebral to internal carotid artery transpositions (2), and aneurysmorrhaphy (1). Two patients underwent successful hybrid repair of their aneurysms. One required coil embolization of the V2 segment after proximal control was lost. The other had a covered stent placed within the subclavian artery to endovascularly exclude the proximal vertebral artery. Additionally, the patient with bilateral vertebral aneurysms who required vertebral ligation for a failed anastamosis underwent transcatheter embolization to halt antegrade flow proximal to the aneurysm. No patients underwent isolated endovascular treatment with embolization or exclusion with covered stents. The patient who underwent vertebral aneurysmorrhaphy required concurrent repair of an arteriovenous fistula involving the vertebral artery and innominate vein. Along with a carotid to vertebral artery bypass, one patient had an ipsilateral common carotid aneurysm repaired with a venous interposition graft.

Perioperative complications were noted in 4 patients. There were no deaths or strokes. The patient who underwent staged bilateral vertebral to carotid transpositions developed left vocal cord paralysis. Meanwhile, the patient who underwent aneurysmorrhaphy and arteriovenous fistula repair developed a large hematoma that necessitated evacuation. As previously noted, two other patients required vertebral artery ligation after failed bypass. At follow-up, one patient was noted to have a vein bypass occlusion at 2 years; the remaining reconstructions were patent at 1, 1.2, 1.5, 4, and 5 year follow-up.

DISCUSSION

Vertebral artery aneurysm surgery was first described in the 1800s, with Stubbs performing the first aneurysm surgery and Matas performing the first vertebral artery bypass.[3,4] Crawford performed the first vertebral artery reconstruction in 1957, and Berguer reported the first vertebral artery bypass with venous conduit in 1976.[5,6] Vertebrobasilar disease subsequently was recognized to primarily be an atherosclerotic disease. Not only was vertebrobasilar insufficiency found to account for approximately one quarter of all strokes, but a series of 100 consecutive vertebral revascularizations demonstrated that 90% of reconstructions are performed for ischemia.[7]

Most cerebrovascular aneurysms are intracranial and involve the anterior circulation. In fact, intracranial vertebrobasilar aneurysms account for less than 3% of intracranial aneurysms, and prophylactic procedures are performed to prevent embolization and rupture, usually into the subarachnoid space.[2] There are reports of extracranial vertebral artery aneurysms, but most are really pseudoaneurysms; despite their protected location within the transverse foramina, these false aneurysms result from trauma or dissection. As such, true extracranial vertebral aneurysms are extremely rare.

Review of the literature reveals few case reports and series of cervical vertebral artery aneurysms. When patients with aneurysmal dilatation after obvious dissection or trauma are excluded, little more than a dozen cases remain. In a previous publication with Sultan et al, we reported a 46 year old Ehlers-Danlos patient who was found to have a 20mm right vertebral artery aneurysm within the V2 segment during evaluation for headaches and dizziness.[2] In a series of 100 distal vertebral artery revascularizations with Berguer et al, we included one cervical vertebral artery aneurysm.[7] In 1986, Rifkinson-Mann et al described a 31 year old female with an extracranial vertebral aneurysm that required ligation.[8] One year later, the same group ligated a 7mm vertebral artery aneurysm in a 31 year old male. Kendi et al found multiple cerebrovascular aneurysms, including a 4mm left vertebral artery aneurysm in the V2 segment, in a patient with migraine headaches.[9] Habozit et al reported a spontaneous vertebral aneurysm in a patient with spinal malformation, but it is unclear whether it resulted from chronic trauma.[10] Likewise, Bartnik et al evaluated a patient with a neck mass and found a vertebral aneurysm.[11] as the patient had rheumatoid cervical spine disease, it is unclear whether the aneurysm resulted from chronic trauma or inflammation. Buerger et al discovered a walnut-sized nontraumatic vertebral artery aneurysm near the atlas arch and ligated it proximally without consequence.[12] A 48 year old neurofibromatosis patient of Ohkata et al had resolution of left upper extremity weakness and numbness when her left cervical vertebral artery aneurysm was ligated.[13] Kim et al recently described an 18 year old male with Ehlers-Danlos who presented with cervical radiculopathy resulting from a vertebral artery aneurysm that extended from C2 to C5.[14] After diagnostic angiography resulted in arterial dissection, the patient was deemed to be of prohibitive risk for further intervention. Finally, Peyre et al presented a case report and literature review of type I neurofibromatosis patients with extracranial vertebral artery aneurysms. While few patients in this review underwent observation or surgical intervention, most were treated with detachable balloons and coils. Results were mixed, with improvement in patient symptoms and aneurysm size in some, continued enlargement or symptoms in others, and death in two.[15]

Several lessons can be learned by collectively examining the presentation, management, and outcomes of the nine vertebral artery aneurysms in this series and comparing them with existing case reports. Upon reviewing the demographics of these patients, it is apparent that primary extracranial aneurysms occur in patients with underlying connective tissue or other hereditary disorders. The most common disorders include Ehlers-Danlos, Marfan's, and neurofibromatosis, although some patients have unspecified disorders. Other cerebrovascular disease is often present. The connective tissue disorders, but not vertebral artery aneurysms, may be hereditary. Most patients in our experience have other concurrent aneurysms; as expected, some are cerebrovascular aneurysms. Both genders are affected. Although there is a wide age range, the diagnosis is typically made in young to middle-aged adults; patients within the extremes of age were not noted in our series, but Pentecost et al reported a 1 year old girl with neurofibromatosis who developed a vertebral aneurysm in the cervical segment.[16]

Presentation is variable. Some are asymptomatic, with the aneurysms noted incidentally. Symptomatic patients can present with neck masses, dizziness, headaches, and neurologic deficits from cerebral ischemia or nerve compression. One patient from our series and others from prior reports had arteriovenous fistulae. Few cases of rupture have also been reported. Although the review by Peyre suggests that most patients are symptomatic, many of our patients' aneurysms were noted incidentally.[15] Vertebral aneurysms can occur on either side, and two patients in our series had bilateral aneurysms. All aneurysms in our series and almost all in the literature involved the V2 segment. Two of our patients also involved the V1 segment. One patient from a prior series involved the V3 segment. Imaging revealed enlargement of transverse foramina to accomodate the V2 aneurysms. Size varies tremendously, and the 90mm aneurysm from our series is the largest reported to date.

As the natural history is unknown, vertebral artery management has been variable. In prior reports, some patients have remained stable with observation.[17] In others, it has led to aneurysm growth, worsening of symptoms, and even death.[16,18] As such, others have elected to observe the aneurysms that they perceive to be of low risk of rupture and embolization; others have selected nonoperative management after diagnostic workup or other procedural complications have made the patients appear high risk for intervention. In our series, a patient with bilateral aneurysms underwent observation for one aneurysm after a disrupted vertebral bypass on the contralateral side resulted in vertebral ligation. Most other aneurysms from the isolated case reports have been ligated or occluded without consequence in short-term follow-up. On the contrary, most aneurysms from our series have been managed with aneurysm exclusion with distal revascularization with open or hybrid techniques.

Although small series have demonstrated that unilateral vertebral artery ligation may be safe,[19, 20] coexisting cerebrovascular disease in patients with vertebral aneurysms can increase this risk. Hence, we have successfully revascularized the distal vertebral artery in all but two of our patients. Certainly, tissue fragility in part guided others away from vertebral revascularization; however, unfamiliarity with the exposure and bypass techniques probably also played a role in the decision to ligate the aneurysms. As such, the approaches to vertebral artery aneurysm repair are worthy of review.

There are several methods of vertebral artery aneurysm repair. The simplest is primary ligation of the inflow and outflow to eliminate antegrade and retrograde flow into the sac. The most complex methods involve vertebral revascularization by distal vertebral to internal carotid transposition, carotid to vertebral bypass with a venous or synthetic conduit, and autologous external carotid to vertebral bypass. Aneurysmorraphy can be performed for aneurysms in the extraosseus segment of the artery. Finally, endovenous balloon and coil embolization have been described, but simple exclusion with covered stents has not been reported.

Regardless of the repair method, gentle manipulation of the tissue is essential in open vertebral artery aneurysm repair. The vessels, in particular, are frail because of the underlying connective tissue disorders. To mitigate against this, the surgeon should consider performing the anastamoses with interrupted mini-pledgeted sutures, especially in Ehlers-Danlos patients. Also, when selecting a conduit for bypass, one must remember that other arteries and veins may be compromised by the connective tissue disorder. Finally, shunts should be avoided, as they can destroy the delicate vessels.

Endoluminal treatment of primary vertebral artery aneurysms has been described with mixed results, and thus, they may be of high risk. Regardless of whether detachable balloons or coils are employed, embolization without revascularization could result in a stroke. Covered stent exclusion of the artery may not be possible because of vessel caliber and tortuosity. Furthermore, wire, catheter, and stent manipulation can result in embolization or dissection and can lead to access site complications.

Nonetheless, endoluminal adjuncts were used to control the proximal vertebral artery in two of our patients. In one, transcatheter embolization was performed emergently when proximal control of the artery was lost; in the other, a covered subclavian stent was used to exclude the vertebral origin, since the 90mm aneurysm made proximal vertebral artery exposure difficult and hazardous.

CONCLUSIONS

Primary extracranial vertebral artery aneurysms are rare and are associated with connective tissue disorders. The natural history is unknown, but open repair should be considered in patients with large or symptomatic aneurysms. Repair can be performed with open and hybrid techniques with low morbidity and mortality.

REFERENCES

1. Morasch MD. Vertebral artery disease. In: Cronenwett JL, Johnston KW, editors. *Rutherford's Vascular Surgery*, Vol. 2. 7th ed. Elsevier. 2010: pp.1557–1574.
2. Sultan S, Morasch M, Colgan MP, Madhavan P, Moore D, Shanik G. Operative and endovacular management of extracranial vertebral artery aneurysm in Ehlers-Danlos syndrome: a clinical dilemma – case report and literature review. *Vasc Endovas Surg* 2002 Sept-Oct (36)5: 389–392.
3. Stubbs H. Aneurysm of the vertebral artery. Ligature of the carotid. *Liverpool Medico-Chir J* 1857 1:110–113.
4. Matas R. Traumatisms and traumatic aneurysms of the vertebral artery and their surgical treatment, with the report of a cured case. *Ann Surg* 1893 Nov 18(5):477–516.
5. Crawford ES, Debakey ME, Fields WS. Roentgenographic diagnosis and surgical treatment of basilar artery insufficiency. *JAMA* 1958 Oct 4;168(5):509–514.
6. Berguer R, Andaya LV, Bauer RB. Vertebral artery bypass. *Arch Surg* 1976 Sep; 111(9): 976–979.

7. Berguer R, Morasch M, Kline R. A review of 100 consecutive reconstructions of the distal vertebral artery for embolic and hemodynamic disease. *J Vasc Surg* 1998 May;27(5):852–859.

8. Rifkinson-Mann S, Laub J, Haimov M. Atraumatic extracranial vertebral artery aneurysm: case report and review of the literature. *J Vasc Surg* 1986 Sep;4(3):288–293.

9. Kendi AT, Brace JR. Vertebral artery duplication and aneurysms: 64-slice multidetector CT findings. *Br J Radiol* 2009 Nov;82(983):e216–218.

10. Habozit B, Battistelli JM. Spontaneous aneurysm of the extracranial vertebral artery associated with spinal osseous anomaly. *Ann Vasc Surg* 1990 Nov;4(6):600–603.

11. Bartnik W, Zapalski S, Bartnik-Krystalska A. *Otolaryngol Pol* 1998;52(4):491–494.

12. Buerger T, Lippert H, Meyer F, Halloul Z. Aneurysm of the vertebral artery near the atlas arch. *J Cardiovasc Surg (Torino)* 1999 Jun;40(3):387–389.

13. Ohkata N, Ikota T, Tashiri T, Okamoto K. A case of multiple extracranial vertebral artery aneurysms associated with neurofibromatosis. *No Shinkei Geka* 1994 Jul;22(7):637–641.

14. Kim HS, Choi CH, Lee TH, Kim SP. Fusiform aneurysm presenting with cervical radiculopathy in Ehlers-Danlos syndrome. *J Korean Neurosurg Soc* 2010 Dec;48(6):528–31.

15. Peyre M, Ozanne A, Bhangoo R, et al. Pseudotunoral presentation of a cervical extracranial vertebral artery aneurysm in neurofibromatosis type 1: case report. *Neurosurgery* 2007 Sep;61(3):E658.

16. Pentecost M, Stanley P, Takahashi M, Isaacs H Jr. Aneurysms of the aorta and subclavian and vertebral arteriesin neurofibromatosis. *Am J Dis Child* 1981 May;135(5):475–477.

17. Schievink WI, Piepgras DG. Carvical vertebral artery aneurysms and arteriovenous fistulae in neurofibromatosis type 1: case reports. *Neurosurgery* 1991 Nov;29(5):760–765.

18. Uranishi R, Ochiai C, Okuno S, Nagai M. Cerebral aneurysms associated with von Recklinghausen neurofibromatosis: report of two cases. *No Shinkei Geka* 1995 Mar;23(3): 237–242.

19. Hoshino Y, Kurokawa T, Nakamura K, et al. A report on the safety of unilateral vertebral artery ligation during cervical spine surgery. *Spine* 1996 Jun 15;21(12):1454–1457.

20. Drake CG. Ligation of the vertebral (unilateral or bilateral) or basilar artery in the treatment of intracranial aneurysms. *J Neurosurg* 1975 Sep;43(3):255–274.

Lower Extremity I

11

Endovascular Interventions for TASC II D Lesions

Luke Marone, MD and Donald T. Baril, MD

INTRODUCTION

The prevalence of peripheral arterial disease (PAD) is nearly 30% for all Americans over the age of 70, resulting in symptoms which may range from claudication to gangrene.[1–2] Treatment of PAD has traditionally consisted of conservative management for symptoms of claudication and surgical management of patients with critical limb ischemia (CLI). In recent years, the development of endovascular techniques to treat PAD and their success has led to a more aggressive posture in the treatment of PAD. Reported initial technical success of greater than 90% and secondary patency rates of greater than 80% at 2 years have been published regarding the treatment of shorter segment femoropopliteal occlusive disease.[3–6] Current Trans-Atlantic Inter-Society Consensus Document on Management of Peripheral Arterial Disease (TASC) recommendations advocate traditional surgical therapy for the treatment of more complex TASC II D lesions.[7] These lesions involve long femoropopliteal segments, an independent predictor for endovascular treatment failure, and anatomically challenged regions (popliteal) which traditionally do not lend themselves to stenting. Secondary to these concerns, endovascular techniques have not acquired significant support in the treatment of these lesions. However, advances in endovascular techniques including the utilization of the subintimal technique, and advances in technology, specifically, the development of re-entry devices and more flexible nitinol stents have significantly contributed to overcoming these technical limitations, making it possible to treat even the most complex occlusive lesion with interventional techniques.

Patients with more complex TASC D lesions often present with CLI and suffer from significant co-morbid medical conditions placing them at high risk for traditional open surgical bypass.[8–9] Our group has previously reported acceptable results in the interventional treatment of TASC B and C lesions with a mean lesion length of 12 cm, assisted primary patency of 87% and secondary patency of 94% at 2 years.[6]

With this background in mind and the fact that no large series had been published evaluating the results of endovascular therapy for the treatment of TASC II D femoropopliteal lesions we sought to conduct a retrospective analysis of our results in this setting.

All patients undergoing endovascular interventions for femoropopliteal occlusive disease between July 2004 and July 2009 were retrospectively identified from a prospectively maintained physician databases. A total of 585 limbs underwent endovascular interventions. Out of this cohort, 74 patients with 79 TASC D lesions were identified. TASC II D lesions were defined as chronic total occlusions of the SFA >20 cm and involving the popliteal artery or chronic total occlusions of the popliteal artery and proximal trifurcation vessels.[7] (Figure 11–1) These patients represented the basis of our report. Indications for intervention were either life style limiting claudication (Rutherford 2/3) or limb salvage (Rutherford 4/5). Therapy for the individual patient was dictated at the preference of the attending surgeon based upon clinical presentation, non-invasive laboratory findings and findings at the time of angiography.

Patient data which were collected included: patient demographics, co-morbidities, pre- and post- procedure ankle-brachial indices (ABI), duplex velocity data and the utilization of adjuvant medical therapy. Additionally, all angiograms and corresponding angiographic reports were reviewed to determine TASC II classification of the treated lesions and to determine the status of the runoff vessels.

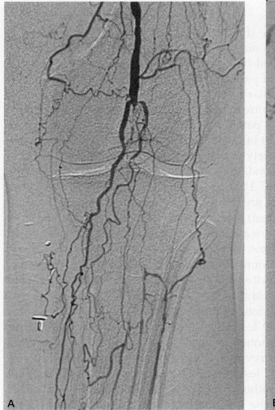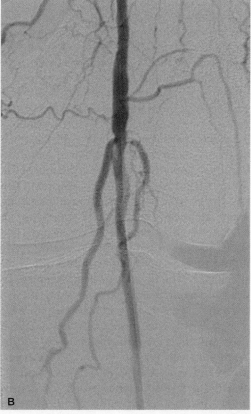

Figure 11–1. a. Pre-intervention angiogram demonstrating popliteal artery occlusion **b.** Angiogram following successful popliteal artery recanalization.

TECHNIQUE

Procedures were performed in either a fixed-imaging hybrid operating room or in the interventional angiography suite by vascular surgeons. All procedures were performed with patients receiving local anesthesia in addition to conscious sedation. Standard digital subtraction techniques were employed to maximize image quality while minimizing use of contrast agent. Patients with preoperative renal insufficiency (baseline SCr>1.5mg/dl) were routinely treated peri-procedurally with oral N-acytelcysteine and intravenous hydration. Arterial access was performed via the common femoral artery through a contralateral retrograde approach or an ipsilateral antegrade approach using 5F or 6F sheaths. A standard aortogram and unilateral or bilateral runoff was performed utilizing a power injector.

Interventions were performed following the administration of systemic heparin (40-100U/kg). Lesions were crossed with a 0.035-inch wire. For complete occlusions a soft or stiff 0.035 inch glide wire (Terumo Medical Corp, Somerset, NJ) and a 4 or 5 Fr glide catheter (Terumo Medical Corp, Somerset, NJ) or other support catheter were utilized to cross in a planned subintimal fashion. When necessary a re-entry device, Outback LTD (Cordis Endovascular, Warren, NJ) was employed to gain access to the flow lumen. Re-entry was confirmed with contrast injection prior to intervention. Balloon angioplasty was subsequently performed with a non-compliant balloon (various manufacturers) for calcified superficial femoral artery lesions or a semi compliant balloon (various manufacturers) for popliteal artery lesions. Balloon diameter was selected based on the angiographic measurements of the non-diseased artery proximal and distal to the lesion. Nominal inflations were maintained for a minimum of one minute. Stents were implanted following balloon angioplasty for the treatment of flow-limiting dissections or residual stenosis of >30% after angioplasty or at the discretion of the operating surgeon. All stents utilized were nitinol self-expanding stents (various manufacturers). Whenever multiple stents were utilized, a minimum overlap zone of 0.5-1.0 cm was achieved. Access site closure was performed using manual compression or with a closure device (various manufacturers) following access site arteriography. All patients were administered a 300-mg loading dose of clopidogrel immediately following the procedure and subsequently maintained on 75 mg daily for a minimum of six months. Patients who had previously been intolerant of clopidogrel secondary to allergic reactions or bleeding complications were administered 325 mg of aspirin and maintained on 325 mg/d.

RESULTS

During the time period reviewed, a total of 79 limbs in 74 patients were treated with TASC D lesions. Twenty-three (29.1%) of these limbs were Rutherford classification 2/3, while the remaining 56 (70.9%) were Rutherford classification 4/5. Of the 56 limbs that were treated for critical limb ischemia, 14 were for rest pain and 42 were for tissue loss. The mean age was 76.5 ± 11.9 years. A slight male predominance (53%) was noted and the typical co-morbid features associated with peripheral arterial disease were identified. (Table 11–1)

Mean pre-procedural ABI was 0.54 ± 0.28. Twenty-three patients had unobtainable ABIs preoperatively secondary to inaudible Doppler signals at the ankle or due to vessel incompressibility. Forty limbs (50.6%) had single-vessel runoff, 27 (34.2%) had

TABLE 11–1. PATIENT AND LESION CHARACTERISTICS

Characteristic	%
Male sex	53%
Cerebrovascular disease	14%
Chronic renal insufficiency	18%
On hemodialysis	4%
Coronary artery disease	63%
Congestive heart failure	15%
Diabetes mellitus	38%
Hypercholesterolemia	65%
Hypertension	82%
Previous bypass	11%
Tobacco use	
Active	19%
Prior	52%
< 2 infrapopliteal runoff vessels	51%

two-vessel runoff, and 12 limbs (15.2%) had three-vessel runoff. Mean lesion length was 188.6 ± 115.6 mm.

Immediate Outcomes

Technical success (<20% residual stenosis) was achieved in 89% of patients who underwent endovascular treatment of TASC D lesions. Four limbs (5.1%) required an antegrade approach to facilitate successful recanalization. Nine limbs (11.4%) necessitated the use of a re-entry device. Popliteal artery stents (including all levels) were placed in 38 limbs (48.1%). There was one peri-procedural death. This occurred in a 91-year-old female patient with multiple comorbidities who presented with advanced gangrenous changes in the involved limb. One day following a successful endovascular intervention, the next of kin decided to withdraw care and the patient subsequently expired. Immediate complications occurred following five interventions (6.3%). Three patients had intra-procedural complications. This included distal embolization in a patient who was successfully treated with thrombolysis at the time of the procedure, a peroneal artery perforation treated with coil embolization, and an extraluminal recanalization treated at a second intervention with covered stents. Two patients had post-procedural complications including a congestive heart failure exacerbation necessitating a one-day intensive care unit stay and one patient who developed access site hemorrhage requiring operative repair.

Mean follow-up length was 10.7 months (range 1-35 months), excluding 5 patients who were lost to follow-up and the one patient who expired in the hospital. A total of 18 patients (24.3%) died during follow-up. Mean immediate increase in ABI (measured within 1 month following intervention) was 0.49 ± 0.35. This included patients who pre-procedure did not have an audible Doppler signal at the ankle and post-procedure had a value which could then be obtained.

Thirty-seven patients whose initial indication for intervention was tissue loss were followed. Thirty-three (89.2%) of these patients demonstrated significant or complete wound healing. Twelve patients (15.2%) underwent amputations either pre-

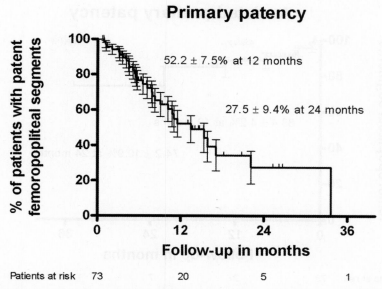

Figure 11-2. Survival curve analysis demonstrating primary patency following endovascular intervention.

or post-procedure. Included in this cohort were 5 patients who underwent planned transmetatarsal amputations and 7 patients who underwent planned toe amputations. There were no major amputations during the follow-up period.

During the follow-up period, 30 limbs (38%) experienced restenosis (21) or occlusions (9). Thirty limbs (38%) underwent reintervention. By survival curve analysis, primary patency was 52.2 ± 7.5% at 12 months and 27.5 ± 9.4% at 24 months. (Figure 11-2) Twenty-nine limbs (36.7%) underwent reintervention during the follow-up time. All patients had duplex findings consistent with restenosis or occlusion prior to reintervention. The one exception to this was the patient who inadvertently underwent extraluminal recanalization and was treated with covered stents. The mean time to reintervention was 7.5 months. Nine limbs (11.4%) required multiple reinterventions including 5 limbs which underwent 2 reinterventions, 3 limbs which underwent 3 reinterventions, and 1 limbs which underwent 4 reinterventions. Assisted-primary patency rates by survival curve analysis were 88.4 ± 4.2% at 12 months and 74.2 ± 10.9% at 24 months. (Figure 11-3)

Of the 9 limbs which suffered occlusion, 4 underwent successful endovascular salvage, 2 were observed following complete wound healing in the affected limb, and 3 went on to surgical bypass. Among the patients who underwent surgical bypass, there were 2 femoral to below-knee popliteal artery bypasses performed for early occlusions (at 1 month and 3 months), and 1 femoral-anterior tibial bypass with prosthetic conduit performed after 3 endovascular reinterventions. Secondary patency rates by survival curve analysis were 92.6± 3.8% at 12 months and 88.9 ± 5.1% at 24 months. (Figure 11-4) There was no significant difference in primary, assisted-primary or secondary patency between patients who underwent their initial intervention for claudication vs. patients who underwent intervention for critical limb ischemia.

Significant predictors or restenosis/occlusion on multivariate analysis included; the presence of cerebrovascular disease (OR 6.25, 95% CI 1.31-29.90, P = 0.02),

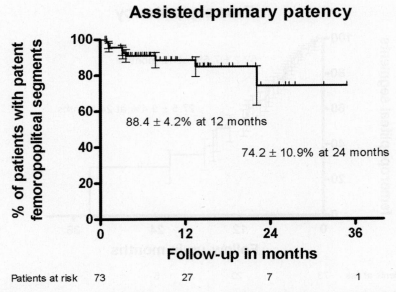

Figure 11–3. Survival curve analysis demonstrating assisted-primary patency following endovascular intervention.

hypercholesterolemia (OR 4.85, 95% CI 1.35-17.38, P= 0.015), the presence of a popliteal stent (OR 4.28, 95% CI 1.24-14.73, P = 0.02), and patients who were current or former smokers (OR 4.50, 95% CI 1.41-14.40, P = 0.01). (Table 11–2) Less than 2 infrapopliteal runoff vessels trended towards being a predictor of restenosis/occlusion (OR 2.52, 95% CI 0.84-7.58, P= 0.098).

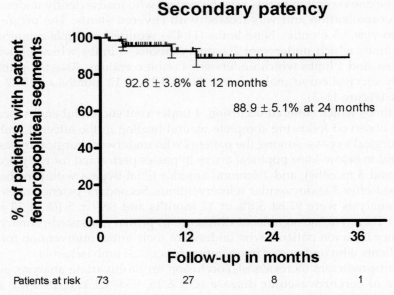

Figure 11–4. Survival curve analysis demonstrating secondary patency following endovascular intervention.

TABLE 11–2. UNIVARIATE AND MULTIVARIATE ANALYSIS OF FACTORS ASSOCIATED WITH RESTENOSIS/OCCLUSION

Risk factor	Hazard ratio	95% confidence interval	P-value
Univariate analysis			
Claudication	1.85	0.70 – 4.86	0.21
Critical limb ischemia	0.80	0.30 – 2.13	0.66
Cerebrovascular disease	2.20	0.61 – 7.97	0.23
Chronic renal insufficiency	0.60	0.17 – 2.12	0.43
Congestive heart failure	0.79	0.22 – 2.88	0.72
Current smoker	1.56	0.50 – 4.86	0.44
Diabetes mellitus	1.81	0.71 – 4.59	0.22
Former smoker	1.70	0.68 – 4.26	0.26
Hypercholesterolemia	2.27	0.82 – 6.28	0.12
Hypertension	1.13	0.34 – 3.74	0.85
Male sex	1.56	0.62 – 3.92	0.34
Popliteal stent	1.74	0.70 – 4.36	0.24
< 2 infrapopliteal runoff vessels	1.56	0.62 – 3.92	0.34
Multivariate analysis			
Cerebrovascular disease	6.25	1.31 – 29.80	0.02
Current or former smoker	4.50	1.41 – 14.40	0.01
Hypercholesterolemia	4.85	1.35 – 17.38	0.02
Popliteal stent	4.28	1.24 – 14.73	0.02
< 2 infrapopliteal runoff vessels	2.53	0.84 – 7.58	0.10

DISCUSSION

Conventional treatment of advanced PAD in patients presenting with lifestyle-limiting claudication and CLI has been risk factor medication and surgical intervention, respectively. However, with advances in endovascular techniques and equipment, the treatment paradigm for patients with PAD has shifted. In particular, patients with anatomically favorable lesions have demonstrated excellent outcomes with endovascular therapy.[3–7] However, enthusiasm for endovascular therapy has been tempered by significant rates of restenosis and occlusion particularly for more advanced lesions. Concomitantly, patients with such complex lesions typically have multiple comorbidities including advanced coronary artery disease and cerebrovascular disease, making them high-risk for surgical intervention. As such, the optimal treatment for patients with TASC D femoropopliteal lesions remains ill-defined.

The treatment of TASC D lesions relies upon particular techniques as well as equipment to optimize technical success. In particular, these lesions, by definition are often quite long, which may require the use of stiff wires to optimize the ability to push across these lesions. Furthermore, as demonstrated in this series, an antegrade approach can also assist in generating greater force to cross longer lesions. In addition to crossing ability, TASC D lesions are more complex with regards to endovascular therapy in that re-entry may be difficult in the setting of heavily calcified lesions or due to a less than optimal anatomic location. Nine limbs in this series required the use of re-entry devices. Our overall technical success, selectively utilizing the aforementioned techniques was 89%. This is less than our previous reported 98% technical success for

TASC B and C lesions. However, this is not dissimilar from other studies which have looked at combined outcomes of endovascular treatment of TASC C and D lesions. Setacci et al. reviewed 145 patients with TASC II C and D lesions who were treated with subintimal angioplasty and selective use of a re-entry device and reported a technical success rate of 83.5% with a 16.5% usage rate of a re-entry device. Rabellino et al. reviewed 234 limbs, 52% of which were TASC II D lesions and reported initial technical success of 97%.

Limb salvage in our series was excellent, with no major amputations during the follow-up time. There was a 15% rate of minor amputations, not unexpected given the extent of arterial disease treated. Furthermore, 89% of patients who presented with tissue loss went on to significant or complete wound healing during follow-up. It should be noted that this study was not reviewed in an intention-to-treat manner, and select patients who failed endovascular intervention initially did go on to have primary major amputations. Regardless, following successful endovascular recanalization, adequate limb salvage rates can be achieved. As with traditional surgical bypass, this is in large part due to the immediate hemodynamic improvement following successful recanalization, as demonstrated by the mean ABI increase of 0.49.

During a follow-up period with a mean of approximately 11 months, nearly one-fourth of the population expired. This highlights the fact that patients with advanced PAD are at very high-risk for death from cardiovascular events, not only perioperatively but in the months to years following their diagnosis of PAD as well. Data from the REACH dataset established that patients with known PAD had a 21.1% incidence of cardiovascular death, myocardial infarction, stroke, or hospitalization for an atherothrombotic event compared to 15.2% for patients with a diagnosis of coronary artery disease alone or 14.5% for patients with a diagnosis of cerebrovascular disease alone in the first year following their initial diagnosis.[12] Furthermore, these event rates increased with the number of symptomatic arterial disease locations, starting at 12.6% for patients with 1 involved arterial bed to 26.3% for patients with 3 symptomatic arterial disease locations. In addition to the immediate post-operative risk in patients with advanced PAD, consideration must be given to the long-term risk and outcomes in such patients. Particularly, the impact of a major operation such as an infrainguinal bypass and the time required for recovery should be incorporated into the decision tree when treating a patient with advanced PAD. Unlike bypass, endovascular intervention may be performed with minimal physiologic impact on this often critically ill patient population. In our current series, there was only one systemic complication directly related to the procedure with an overall peri-procedural complication rate of 6.3%. Conversely, in a recent review of data obtained through the National Surgical Quality Improvement Program (NSQIP) on patients undergoing infrainguinal bypass, major complications occurred in 18.7% patients, including a 9.4% rate of wound infections.[13] Furthermore, major systemic complications occurred in 5.9% of patients. Clearly, an endovascular approach obviates the need for incisions, which often create new wound issues in these compromised extremities.

Restenosis and occlusion continue to complicate endovascular interventions in nearly all arterial beds. Previous studies have demonstrated worse outcomes with more advanced TASC classification and TASC D classification alone has been shown to be a predictor of restenosis.[5-6, 14-15] Although not directly comparable given the retrospective nature of the two studies, our previously reported data on TASC B and C femoropopliteal lesions demonstrated assisted-primary patency rates of 89.3% at 12 months and 87.1% at 24 months and secondary patency rates of 94.0% at 12 months and 94.0% at 24 months. Comparatively, for the TASC D limbs in this series, the assisted-primary and secondary patency rates were 88.4% at 12 months and 74.2% at 24 months and 92.6% at 12 months and 88.9% at 24 months, respectively. Given the long length of these lesions and/or their anatomically unfavorable (popliteal) location such patency rates are not unexpected. However, it should be noted that the majority of these restenoses can be treated using endovascular techniques to achieve assisted primary patency. Additionally, a significant number of the limbs that go on to occlusion can be salvaged through an endovascular approach to achieve secondary patency

Although physical exam and symptomatology can help diagnose patients with failed lower extremity endovascular interventions, they have limited value in the prediction of patients who are developing significant restenotic lesions and in our experience the majority of these patients have mild or no symptoms prior to progressing to high grade lesions and/or occlusions. While ABI measurements assist in the evaluation of the clinical picture, the correlation of ABI with angiographic stenosis is not strong and our previously reported data suggests that a significant decrease in ABI (>0.15) may not be present until a >60% stenosis exists. Additionally, ABIs are affected by proximal and distal disease and thus are less useful in the localization of disease. Duplex surveillance after endovascular intervention provides much more valuable anatomic and hemodynamic data which enables recognition of restenosis at previously treated arterial segments. This is of particular value in TASC D lesions which have a relatively reduced primary patency compared to TASC A, B and C lesions. Furthermore, detection of significant restenosis prior to progression to occlusion allows for the restoration of assisted primary patency which can be completed with a high rate of technical success and reduced patient risk as compared to the achievement of secondary patency (after occlusion of a previously stented vessel). Our previously published report has delineated PSV and velocity ratio (VR) criteria which are predictive of both 50% and 80% in stent stenosis. The set point which discriminates between these degrees of stenosis is very distinct which is additionally helpful in the management of these patients; PSV> 190cm/s and VR >1.5 predictive of 50% in stent stenosis whereas PSV>275cm/s and VR>3.5 predictive of >80% in stent stenosis[17].

Predictors of restenosis/occlusion in this study were cerebrovascular disease, hypercholesterolemia, the presence of a popliteal stent, and patients who were current or former smokers. The exact cause-effect relationship of cerebrovascular disease on restenosis is unclear and can only be postulated to be a predictor of more advanced systemic atherosclerotic disease. Similarly, hypercholesterolemia may be another marker of more aggressive disease. We have previously demonstrated hypercholesterolemia to be a predictor of restenosis in TASC B and C lesions, but the exact mechanism remains ill-defined.[6] Given the significant contribution of tobacco use to atherosclerotic disease, it is not surprising that smokers were at higher risk for restenosis and occlusion as has been previously demonstrated.[16] The presence of a stent in the popliteal segment places a rigid stent at an area of repetitive motion and stress, leading to an increased rate of restenosis, with or without the presence of a stent fracture. Although prospective, randomized data regarding this is lacking, from our experience and others, avoidance of extending stents into the distal SFA and proximal popliteal appears to be beneficial in reducing restenosis. However, it should be noted that "next generation" more flexible and crush resistant nitinol stents such as Supera (IDEV) were not utilized in this study and may offer some benefit in the popliteal location.

This study has a number of limitations, the most important of which is its retrospective nature. Patient selection and treatment modality were not standardized.

Furthermore, although data has been derived based on survival curve analysis, the follow-up time is limited, and longer-term follow-up will be necessary to determine the durability of these interventions.

CONCLUSION

Endovascular interventions for TASC II D lesions can be safely performed with excellent hemodynamic improvement and limb salvage rates in this often medically unfit population. Restenosis is not uncommon in these complex, typically lengthy lesions which mandate strict follow-up utilizing non-invasive arterial studies to help guide timing of reintervention and thus maintain assisted primary patency. Further follow-up is necessary to determine the long-term cost and efficacy of these interventions.

REFERENCES

1. Bhatt DL, Steg PG, Ohman EM, Hirsch AT, Ikeda Y, Mas JL, et al. International prevalence, recognition, and treatment of cardiovascular risk factors in outpatients with atherothrombosis. *JAMA* 2006 Jan 11;295(2):180–9.
2. Hirsch AT, Criqui MH, Treat-Jacobson D, Regensteiner JG, Creager MA, Olin JW, et al. Peripheral arterial disease detection, awareness, and treatment in primary care. *JAMA* 2001 Sep 19;286(11):1317–24.
3. Krankenberg H, Schlüter M, Steinkamp HJ, Bürgelin K, Scheinert D, Schulte KL, et al. Nitinol stent implantation versus percutaneous transluminal angioplasty in superficial femoral artery lesions up to 10 cm in length: the femoral artery stenting trial (FAST). *Circulation* 2007 Jul 17;116(3):285–92.
4. Schillinger M, Sabeti S, Loewe C, Dick P, Amighi J, Mlekusch W, et al. Balloon angioplasty versus implantation of nitinol stents in the superficial femoral artery. *N Engl J Med* 2006 May 4;354(18):1879–88
5. Conrad MF, Cambria RP, Stone DH, Brewster DC, Kwolek CJ, Watkins MT, et al. Intermediate results of percutaneous endovascular therapy of femoropopliteal occlusive disease: a contemporary series. *J Vasc Surg* 2006 Oct;44(4):762–9.
6. Baril DT, Marone LK, Kim J, Go MR, Chaer RA, Rhee RY. Outcomes of endovascular interventions for TASC II B and C femoropopliteal lesions. *J Vasc Surg* 2008 Sep;48(3):627–33.
7. Norgren L, Hiatt WR, Dormandy JA, Nehler MR, Harris KA, Fowkes FG; TASC II Working Group. Inter-Society Consensus for the Management of Peripheral Arterial Disease (TASC II). *J Vasc Surg* 2007 Jan;45 Suppl S:S5–67.
8. Criqui MH, Langer RD, Fronek A, Feigelson HS, Klauber MR, McCann TJ, et al. Mortality over a period of 10 years in patients with peripheral arterial disease. *N Engl J Med* 1992 Feb 6;326(6):381–6.
9. Murabito JM, Evans JC, Nieto K, Larson MG, Levy D, Wilson PW. Prevalence and clinical correlates of peripheral arterial disease in the Framingham Offspring Study. *Am Heart J* 2002 Jun;143(6):961–5.
10. Setacci C, Chisci E, de Donato G, Setacci F, Iacoponi F, Galzerano G. Subintimal angioplasty with the aid of a re-entry device for TASC C and D lesions of the SFA. *Eur J Vasc Endovasc Surg* 2009 Jul;38(1):76–87.
11. Rabellino M, Zander T, Baldi S, Garcia Nielsen L, Aragon-Sanchez FJ, Zerolo I et al. Clinical follow-up in endovascular treatment for TASC C-D lesions in femoro-popliteal segment. *Catheter Cardiovasc Interv* 2009 Apr 1;73(5):701–5.

12. Steg PG, Bhatt DL, Wilson PW, D'Agostino R Sr., Ohman EM, Röther J, et al. One-year car-diovascular event rates in outpatients with atherothrombosis. *JAMA* 2007 Mar 21;297(11): 1197–206.

13. LaMuraglia GM, Conrad MF, Chung T, Hutter M, Watkins MT, Cambria RP. Significant pe-rioperative morbidity accompanies contemporary infrainguinal bypass surgery: an NSQIP report. *J Vasc Surg* 2009 Aug;50(2):299–304, 304.e1–4.

14. Ihnat DM, Duong ST, Taylor ZC, Leon LR, Mills JL Sr., Goshima KR, et al. Contemporary outcomes after superficial femoral artery angioplasty and stenting: the influence of TASC classification and runoff score. *J Vasc Surg* 2008 May;47(5):967–74. Epub 2008 Apr 18.

15. Dearing DD, Patel KR, Compoginis JM, Kamel MA, Weaver FA, Katz SG. Primary stenting of the superficial femoral and popliteal artery. *J Vasc Surg* 2009 Sep;50(3):542–7.

16. Schillinger M, Exner M, Mlekusch W, Haumer M, Sabeti S, Ahmadi R, et al. Effect of smok-ing on restenosis during the 1st year after lower-limb endovascular interventions. *Radiology* 2004 Jun;231(3):831–8.

17. Baril DT, Rhee RY, Kim J, Makaroun MS, Chaer R, Leers SA, Marone LK. Duplex Criteria for Determination of Significant In-stent Stenosis after Angioplasty and Stenting of the Superficial Femoral Artery. *J Vasc Surg* 2009;49:133–139.

12

The Use of Distal Arterial Access for Femoro-popliteal and Tibial Subintimal Angioplasty

Joseph S. Giglia, MD

INTRODUCTION

Peripheral catheter-based intervention has largely replaced open surgical bypass as the first line therapy for treatment of infrainguinal arterial occlusive disease. Subintimal angioplasty is a common type of peripheral intervention that requires reentry into the true lumen distal to an occlusion. A variety of commercial devices have been developed to increase the success of reentering the true lumen, but each has its own inherent drawbacks. Distal arterial access has been developed to increase the success rate of reentering the true lumen following traversal of chronic atherosclerotic occlusions. It is inexpensive, the tools are readily available and there is minimal morbidity.

This chapter will describe the technique of retrograde distal arterial access for subintimal balloon angioplasty of the femoro-popliteal and tibial segments. Its role in the overall management of patients with lower extremity atherosclerotic disease will be discussed.

HISTORICAL BACKGROUND

Arterial access for angiography dates back to the early 1940's. Its scope was limited by the requirement for surgical access to a vessel and ligation or repair following the procedure. In 1953 Seldinger revolutionized the field when he reported a procedure that greatly simplified arterial access for angiography[1]. His technique allowed safe, repetitive arterial access and opened the door for a vast array of arterial and venous interventions.

Initially the field was limited to diagnostic studies due to the size and ridigity of the devices. Eventually Dotter pioneered therapeutic angiography with his serial dilation of a superficial femoral artery lesion, which was soon followed by balloon angioplasty. The era of percutaneous treatment of arterial disease had begun, and the field continues to progress rapidly to this day.

STANDARD BALLOON ANGIOPLASTY

Retrograde contralateral femoral arterial access is the standard approach to lower extremity antegrade angiography with intervention. In certain circumstances, antegrade ispilateral femoral access is required. It is commonly used if the aortic bifurcation is altered from its natural configuration by the presence of aortic endografts or aortoiliac stents.[2] Upper extremity (usually left brachial) access is occasionally used for cases of severe aortoiliac disease but its utility for infrainguinal disease is limited by device length. Regardless of the access site, successful traversal of the atherosclerotic segment with a guidewire is required prior to undertaking a catheter-based intervention.

SUBINTIMAL BALLOON ANGIOPLASTY

Traversal of the atherosclerotic lesion in the lumen is not always possible. Occluded arteries were initially typically treated with catheter-directed thrombolysis. Following lysis, additional attempts were undertaken to cross the lesion while maintaining an intraluminal position. This technique, however, was associated with increased duration, cost, significant morbidity and even mortality. In 1989 Bolia described the technique of intentional subintimal passage of a guidewire across an occluded femoro-popliteal segment in order to perform a catheter-based intervention.[3] This dramatic breakthrough allowed treatment of arterial occlusion without catheter-directed thrombolysis and its inherent drawbacks and significantly increased the number of patients amenable to infrainguinal percutaneous intervention. In addition, it allowed treatment of many patients with limb-threatening ischemia who were not candidates for surgical bypass due to prohibitive risk or lack of suitable venous conduit.

The technique involves standard arterial access as describe above. Specific devices and device manufactures are mentioned as examples and are those that the author utilizes most frequently. Comparable devices are available and effective. Contralateral retrograde femoral access is obtained, and a 5 F sheath is placed. The contralateral iliac system is cannulated with a 5 F OminFlush® catheter and braided wire is advanced to the level of the common femoral artery. The 5F sheath is then exchanged for a long sheath (Terumo Destination® Sheath). The sheath is positioned just proximal to the occlusion to maximize the fidelity of catheter manipulation at the working end. A 45 cm sheath is typically used for proximal superficial artery occlusions and 60 cm or even 90 cm sheaths for more distal disease. A hydrophilic exchange length (260cm) non-stiff guidewire (Glidewire®, Terumo) is advanced initially through a hydrophilic catheter (Glidecatheter®). Often stiffer catheters are required (Cordis® JR4 or MPA) to advance the tip of the wire into the subintimal plane. The tip of the wire assumes a J configuration when properly located in the subintimal plane. It is important to advance the wire and catheter in a controlled fashion. The loop at the leading end of the wire should be no longer than 2–3 cm. This maneuver increases the chance of reentry into the true lumen at a level just distal to the occlusion. Reentry into the true lumen just distal the occlusion is beneficial because it minimizes the length of the subintimal passage that needs to be treated (balloon angioplasty or balloon and stent placement), and it preserves an untouched surgical target if needed.

Dilute contrast (1:2 with heparinized saline 2 units/ml) is injected into the catheter at various points during the process. Opacification of the subintimal plane with prompt filling of the adjacent venous plexus, is an expected finding, although it can be initially unsettling. This angiographic finding confirms the appropriate location of the catheter tip in the subintimal plane and has no significant adverse implication.

The catheter and wire are advanced to the level just distal to the occlusion as demonstrated on the diagnostic angiogram. Care is taken to not proceed significantly past this level until reentry is confirmed. Often the J configuration of the wire is released, and the wire straightens and advances into the distal true lumen. A straight non-stiff hydrophilic wire is helpful at this stage of the procedure.

While usually effective, subintimal intervention is associated with an inability to reenter the true lumen approximately 17 % of the time.[4] Densely calcified bulky lesions, that are often encountered in patients with end stage renal disease on hemodialysis, increase the possibility of failure. A variety of reentry devices[5] are available to increase the number of patients that can be treated in this manner. These devices significantly increase the cost of the procedure and are associated with some risk of perforation. These are beyond the scope of this discussion and will not be discussed further.

Subintimal balloon angioplasty from an antegrade approach has become more widely disseminated, and with increased experience, reentry success rates continue to improve.[6] However, the addition of distal arterial access further increases the opportunity to successfully perform subintimal angioplasty.

GENERAL CONCEPT OF THROUGH-AND-THROUGH WIRE ACCESS

The idea of through-and-through wires is not unique to distal limb occlusive disease cases. It is commonly used in other areas of vascular surgery and by other specialties. Modern vascular surgeons are very familiar with the concept of through-and-through wire access for placement of abdominal and thoracic endografts in patients with difficult iliac anatomy and for treatment of aortoiliac occlusions.[7] Urologists utilize proximal and distal wires to address difficult lesions in the upper urinary tract and esophageal lesions are sometimes approached with a through-and-through technique.

DISTAL ARTERIAL ACCESS FOR LOWER
EXTREMITY SUBINTIMAL ANGIOPLASTY

Simultaneous antegrade and retrograde access for subintimal angioplasty via the popliteal artery was first reported by McCullough in 1993.[8] It was not until 2003 that several reports of distal tibial access for antegrade and retrograde subintimal angioplasty were reported.[9–10] The technique has been referred to as Subintimal Arterial Flossing with Antegrade and Retrograde Intervention or the SAFARI Technique.[11] As experience grew, follow-up reports have been published. Regardless of the site of access or name, the technique is utilized to increase the success rate of subintimal balloon angioplasty for chronic limb ischemia.

GENERAL CONCEPTS

An initial attempt using a standard antegrade approach via the contralateral femoral approach as describe above is attempted. If unsuccessful, distal access for subintimal balloon angioplasty is considered. It is often reserved for those with limb-threatening ischemia, rest pain or ulceration. Patients who are not surgical candidates secondary to prohibitive risk or lack of distal targets are especially well suited for this approach.

Anti-platelet agents are continued without interruption. Patients on chronic oral anticoagulation may have their dose held for 1–2 days prior to the procedure, but it is not required. Patients with mechanical heart valves remain on oral anticoagulation or are bridged with low molecular weight heparin. Routine pre-angiography intravenous fluids are started, and conscious sedation with Versed® and Fentanyl® is administered with appropriate monitoring. If attempts to perform antegrade subintimal angioplasty are unsuccessful, then distal access is considered. Distal access may be performed at the time of the first angiogram if there is a clinical need or if there is an increased likelihood of failure such as in a patient with dense calcification or end-stage renal disease on hemodialysis.

Ultrasound guidance is utilized to aid with access to the vessels. The depth setting is set at 1.9 cm for vessels at the ankle and deeper for more proximal targets. A micro puncture kit or a standard-thin walled 18 g needle may be used. Once access is obtained, a wire is advanced retrograde, and 4F catheter is placed without the use of a sheath for the distal tibial vessels. Figures 12–1 and 12–2. A sheath is used for popliteal access.

Often the distal wire will readily advance into the true lumen proximal to the obstruction. Figure 12–3. When it does not, simultaneous or sequential balloon angioplasty can be utilized to alter the plaque morphology and facilitate reentry.

Branches can be used to facilitate reentry. A wire followed by a catheter is advanced into a branch. If an injection with dilute contrast confirms intraluminal location, the wire is replaced and manipulated. The natural thinning of the plaque at the orifice often allows reentry.

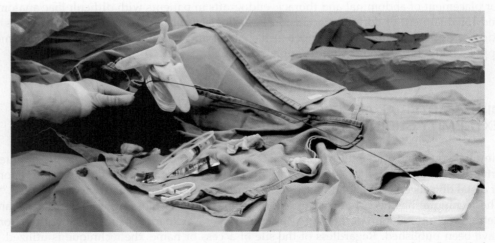

Figure 12–1. Right dorsalis pedis access with a 4 F catheter. Note the blood return from the end of the catheter.

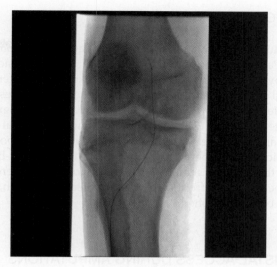

Figure 12–2. Following right dorsalis pedis access an 0.018 inch wire and 4 F catheter have been advanced retrograde to the above knee popliteal artery. Notice the calcification of the vessel.

The popliteal artery can be an effective access site for retrograde subintimal angioplasty.[12] While most favor a prone approach to the popliteal artery for retrograde subintimal angioplasty[13], a technique with the patient supine has been described.[14] Popliteal access for antegrade intervention is an option in select cases.[15] Hemostatic control of the access site is a concern with this approach. Usually manual compression is sufficient, but use of a closure device has been reported.[16] For the distal tibial vessels, simple gentle manual compression at the completion of the procedure is all that is required.

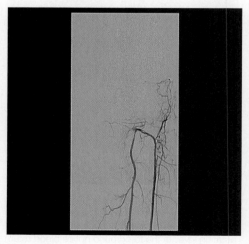
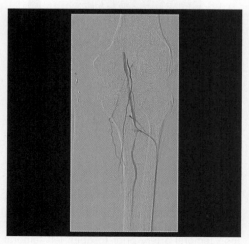

Figure 12–3. Retrograde angiogram from left dorsalis pedis access. B-Repeat angiogram following successful traversal of the distal below knee popliteal artery occlusion.

SPECIAL SITUATIONS

Open surgical procedures can be combined with distal access for subintimal angioplasty in selected situations. Patients with femoropopliteal and tibial occlusion without adequate venous conduit for bypass who have concomitant bulky common femoral disease can be treated with a hybrid open and endovascular technique. Distal access is obtained via the dorsalis pedis or posterior tibial artery, and a wire is advanced retrograde to the ipsilateral common femoral artery. Figure 12–4. A standard common femoral thromboendarterectomy is performed, and the wire is retrieved. Antegrade femoropopliteal and/or tibial subintimal intervention is then performed. Following the catheter-based intervention, a patch angioplasty of the common femoral artery is performed. If there is concomitant iliac disease, a wire can be advanced from a contralateral femoral sheath, and retrograde iliac intervention can also be accomplished.

RETROGRADE DISTAL ACCESS DURING AMPUTATIONS

Certain patients present with irreversible advanced ischemia and require a major amputation. Open distal access and subintimal balloon angioplasty during an amputation is a useful technique to increase the probability of healing or of even preserving an amputation level in patients with marginal perfusion. Figure 12–5. The procedure can be performed in one stage, but typically an open below knee amputation has already been performed to control sepsis. Any of the tibial vessels can be used, with the selection guided by the findings on antegrade angiography. The exposed vessel is retracted distally and punctured with

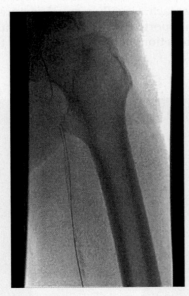

Figure 12–4. Contralateral right femoral wire and a retrograde ipsilateral left DP wire in the left common femoral artery prior to open left femoral thromboendarterectomy and antegrade subintimal angioplasty.

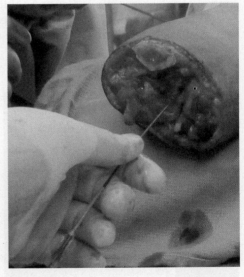

Figure 12–5. In selected circumstances open distal access can be used for subintimal balloon angioplasty to aid healing or even preserve an amputation level. In the foreground notice blood return from the catheter in the transected left anterior tibial artery.

an entry needle, or the open end of the vessel is directly cannulated. The proximal access site can be either common femoral, and a percutaneous or open approach may be utilized.

COMPLICATIONS

Complications related to the combined antegrade and retrograde subintimal angioplasty are not fundamentally different from a simple antegrade approach . Arteriovenous fistulae may occur,[17] but they can often be treated endovascularly at the time of their occurrence. Hemorrhage is not an issue from the distal tibial sites but may occur with a popliteal approach.

RESULTS

Standard antegrade subintimal intervention has been shown to be successful and safe and effective for limb salvage in a large meta analysis.[18] Several smaller series have likewise observed that the addition of distal access to an antegrade subintimal approach is safe and effective for limb salvage.[19-24]

SUMMARY

Distal arterial access using the dorsalis pedis, posterior tibial, anterior tibial and popliteal arteries for combined antegrade and retrograde subintimal angioplasty is a safe effective technique to increase the proportion of patients with chronic limb ischemia who can be treated percutaneously. The materials and skill set required are already available in centers performing state of the art antegrade subintimal interventions. Patients with chronic limb ischemia without other options should be considered for this technique to attempt limb salvage.

REFERENCES

1. Seldinger, S.I., Catheter replacement of the needle in percutaneous arteriography; a new technique. *Acta radiol* 1953;39(5):368–76.
2. Timmons, G., et al., Retrograde vs. Antegrade Puncture for Infra-Inguinal Angioplasty. CardioVascular and Interventional Radiology, 2003;26(4):370–374.
3. Bolia, A., J. Brennan, and P.R. Bell, Recanalisation of femoro-popliteal occlusions: improving success rate by subintimal recanalisation. *Clin Radiol* 1989;40(3):325.
4. Schmidt, A., et al., Retrograde Approach for Complex Popliteal and Tibioperoneal Occlusions. *J Endovasc Ther* 2008;15(5):594–604.
5. Bozlar, U., et al., Outback catheter-assisted simultaneous antegrade and retrograde access for subintimal recanalization of peripheral arterial occlusion. *Clin Imaging* 2008;32(3): 236–40.
6. Meier, G.H., Tips, tricks and bail out strategies for subintimal angioplasty. *Ital J Vasc Endovasc Surg* 2010;17(1):15–21.

7. Saibil, E.A. and R. Maggisano, Combined antegrade-retrograde catheterization of the occluded common iliac artery prior to angioplasty. *Can Assoc Radiol J* 1988;39(3):228–9.

8. McCullough, K.M., Retrograde transpopliteal salvage of the failed antegrade transfemoral angioplasty. *Australas Radiol* 1993;37(4): 329–31.

9. South, S., et al., Percutaneous retrograde tibial access in limb salvage. *J Endovasc Ther* 2003; 10(3):614–618.

10. Spinosa, D.J., et al., Simultaneous antegrade and retrograde access for subintimal recanalization of peripheral arterial occlusion. *J Vasc Interv Radiol* 2003;14(11):1449–54.

11. Pampana, E., et al., The "Safari" Technique to Perform Difficult Subintimal Infragenicular Vessels. *Cardiovasc Intervent Radiol* 2007;30(3):469–473.

12. Evans, C., et al., Five-year retrograde transpopliteal angioplasty results compared with antegrade angioplasty. *Ann R Coll Surg Engl* 2010;92(4):347–52.

13. Noory, E., et al., Retrograde transpopliteal recanalization of chronic superficial femoral artery occlusion after failed re-entry during antegrade subintimal angioplasty. *J Endovasc Ther* 2009;16(5):619–23.

14. Kawarada, O. and Y. Yokoi, Retrograde 3-French Popliteal Approach in the Supine Position After Failed Antegrade Angioplasty for Chronic Superficial Femoral Artery Occlusion. *J Endovasc Ther* 2010;17(2):255–258.

15. Glasby, M.J. and A. Bolia, Subintimal Angioplasty of a Crural Vessel via an Antegrade Popliteal Artery Puncture. *Eur J Vasc Endovasc Surg* 2007;34(3):347–349.

16. Branzan, D., et al., Arterial puncture closure using a clip device after transpopliteal retrograde approach for recanalization of the superficial femoral artery. *J Endovasc Ther* 2008; 15(3):310–314.

17. Ananthakrishnan, G., et al., The occurrence of arterio-venous fistula during lower limb subintimal angioplasty: treatment and outcome. *Eur J Vasc Endovasc Surg* 2006;32(6):675–9.

18. Bown, M.J., A. Bolia, and A.J. Sutton, Subintimal angioplasty: meta-analytical evidence of clinical utility. *Eur J Vasc Endovasc Surg* 2009;38(3):323–37.

19. Cage, D., et al., Subintimal Arterial Flossing with Antegrade-Retrograde Intervention (SAFARI) for Subintimal Recanalization to Treat Chronic Critical Limb Ischemia. *JVIR* 2005;16(1):37–44.

20. Biamino, G., et al., Retrograde approach for complex popliteal and tibioperoneal occlusions. *J Endovasc Ther* 2008;5(5):94.

21. Mirowska, K.K., et al., Insights Into Endovascular Revascularization in Limb Salvage Procedures: "Antegrade-Retrograde" Technique in Chronic Total Occlusion. *Rev Cardiovasc Med* 2011;12(1):42–47.

22. Ko, Y.L., et al., Dual vascular access for critical limb ischemia: Immediate and follow-up results. *Catheter Cardiovasc Interv* 2011;77(2):296–302.

23. Garcia, J.A., et al., Retrograde approach to recanalization of complex tibial disease. *Catheter Cardiovasc Interv* 2011;7(6):915–925.

24. Marinescu, V., et al., Insights into endovascular revascularization in limb salvage procedures: "antegrade-retrograde" technique in chronic total occlusion. *Rev Cardiovasc Med* 2011;2(1):42–7.

13

Effect of Immuno-Suppression on Bypass Outcomes

Satish C. Muluk, MD and Joseph L. Grisafi, MD

Our inchoate understanding of the human immune system is a consequence of its marvelous complexity. The influence of the immune system is exerted over seemingly divergent phenomena like cancer, infection, and wound healing. It is no surprise then that atherosclerosis and other blood vessel disorders are impacted by immune mechanisms. Moreover, balloon angioplasty and arterial bypass procedures aimed at preserving threatened extremities have outcomes that are vulnerable to immune mediated responses. With a limb loss rate of over 90% experienced by patients with untreated critical limb ischemia, the gravity of treatment failure is obvious.

The failure of bypass grafts and endovascular interventions such as balloon angioplasty can generally be attributed to technical problems, increased thrombogenicity, intimal hyperplasia, or some combination of these three factors. In this chapter, we will focus on intimal hyperplasia, the factor that is most likely to be affected by immunosuppressive therapy. Intimal hyperplasia is the pathologic process within an artery whereby medial smooth muscle cells (SMCs) abnormally migrate to the tunica intima, proliferate, and deposit excessive amounts of extracellular ground substance. It is the most common cause of peripheral arterial bypass failure occurring between the 2nd and 3rd postoperative years. Our understanding of this process has grown exponentially since Carrel's first description over a century ago. Grondin elucidated the role of intimal hyperplasia in the process of coronary vein graft occlusion in 1971. Great effort is now taken to detect the subclinical manifestations of intimal hyperplasia in peripheral bypass surgery through surveillance duplex ultrasonography. The cellular and molecular mechanisms involved coincide with innate immune pathways. Our understanding of these mechanisms, while still limited, has led to targeted pharmacotherapy in the treatment of intimal hyperplasia.

Understanding the physiologic response of an artery to injury is a logical starting point of discussion since any vascular manipulation, whether via open surgery or endovascular intervention, involves a controlled injury. With these modalities, the endothelial lining of the intima is disrupted and underlying collagen is exposed to blood. Circulating von Willebrand factor, produced by vascular endothelium, facilitates platelet adhesion to the denuded surface and aggregation by way of platelet membrane glycoprotein receptors (GPR). GPR expression on the surface of SMCs has been demonstrated to be regulated in part by platelet derived growth factor (PDGF), a substance released from activated platelets and found in the arterial wall after injury.

Activated platelets are instrumental in hemostasis, but they also recruit SMCs to the site of injury through the release of chemotactic substances. Neutrophils and monocytes are also recruited to the injury site after the arrival of platelets.

Numerous pharmacologic agents have been used to treat intimal hyperplasia. It is useful to separate them into five major classes of drugs: (1) anti-platelet agents; (2) glucocorticoids; (3) calcineurin inhibitors; (4) mammalian target of rapamycin (mTOR) inhibitors; and (5) phosphodiesterase-3 (PDE-3) inhibitors. The drugs in classes 2–4 have well-known immunosuppressive effects, whereas the drugs in classes 1 and 5 do not directly cause immunosuppression. It is nevertheless useful to discuss the effects of all five drug types on the outcomes of vascular interventions.

ANTIPLATELET AGENTS

Because of the role of GPR expression on both platelets and SMCs (described earlier), GPR inhibition is a rational strategy to reduce thrombogenicity and prevent SMC migration. GPR inhibitors (e.g. abciximab) have been shown to ameliorate the process of intimal hyperplasia.[1] These agents are routinely used in percutaneous coronary interventions and have proven survival benefits and reduced thrombotic complications.[2]

In the EPIC trial, an early clinical study with the abciximab, a reduced rate of clinical restenosis at 6 months after coronary intervention was found.[3] This was consistent with the results of animal studies that implicated GPRs in the process of intimal hyperplasia.[4] Subsequent clinical trials failed, however, to show efficacy in reducing the need for repeat revascularization or degree of intimal hyperplastic stenosis.[5,6] Kokubo and colleagues suggest specific drug affinity for alpha subunit species of various GPR heterodimers may be responsible for conflicting reports. Another factor is that GPRs are up-regulated at sites of intimal hyperplasia lesions for nearly 3 weeks. The relatively short infusion times of abciximab and eptifibatide involved in these clinical studies means that sufficient quantity of drug may not have been delivered at the appropriate time to be effective in preventing intimal hyperplasia.

No prospective trials have been conducted pertaining to the effects of GPR antagonists on restenosis in the periphery. Caution should be exercised when extrapolating coronary data to outcomes for peripheral arterial interventions. Future investigation is needed and should focus on rational study design, inclusion of periprocedural thrombosis and late restenosis as endpoints, and adherence to the reporting standards of the Society for Vascular Surgery.

The benefits of the anti-platelet drug acetylsalicylic acid, commonly known as aspirin, are numerous, and have earned it the moniker 'wonder drug'. The compound's controversial history has been critically reviewed by Sneader.[7] Aspirin exploits a well described inflammatory pathway that begins with arachadonic acid (AA). AA is the precursor of the prostaglandins and thromboxanes, two substances integral to the function of vascular endothelium and platelets. AA is synthesized from the essential fatty acid linoleate, and resides in cell membranes attached to glycerol. The cellular milieu varies by tissue type and enzyme expression. Enzymes specific to activated platelets lead to the synthesis of thromboxane A2, a potent vasoconstrictor and promotor of platelet aggregation. Specific signal transduction pathways liberate AA to the cytosol via the activity of phospholipases. There it is acted upon by the enzyme cyclooxygenase (COX) in the first step of becoming a prostaglandin or thromboxane. It is at this step where aspirin exerts its effect by irreversibly inhibiting COX.

There are at least two isoforms of COX. The constitutively expressed isoform, COX-1, is present in many cell types and the only isoform expressed in platelets, while COX-2 is considered inducible at sites of active inflammation. The avidity of aspirin is 50 to 100 times greater for COX-1 than COX-2. Inhibition of the COX-1 pathway with aspirin has been shown to reduce thrombotic complications associated with coronary and vascular interventions. Aspirin also indirectly prevents local inflammation that otherwise would have been initiated by the kinin, coagulation, and complement systems. Investigations of the effect of aspirin on intimal hyperplasia in animal models of vascular disease have provided mixed results. Clinical reports have clearly demonstrated that aspirin leads to enhanced peripheral arterial bypass patency with prosthetic conduit. The same benefit has not been shown for autogenous vein grafts[8] However, it is widely accepted that aspirin should be administered to all patients with peripheral arterial disease because of the drug's well-documented coronary benefits.

The effect of aspirin on restenosis is less clear. Minar and associates examined the impact of high and low dose aspirin on platelet deposition at femoropopliteal balloon angioplasty sites and followed the patients for restenosis.[9] They found no association between platelet deposition and subsequent restenosis. More recently, Horrocks and company reported similar findings from their placebo controlled trial.[10] The available body of evidence supports that the clinical efficacy of aspirin is primarily due to antithrombotic properties over anti-inflammatory effects.

The inducible role of COX-2 in inflammation would suggest another rational therapeutic target; however, this view has been recently challenged. Attention is being focused on the *constitutive* expression of COX-2 in vascular endothelium, where its role is chiefly the production of the platelet inhibitor, prostacyclin (PGI_2). This insight suggests a mechanism for the observation of increased cardiovascular events with the use of rofecoxib, a COX-2 inhibitor used in the prevention of colorectal adenoma. Rofecoxib was recently withdrawn from the market because of concern about coronary events.

Thienopyridines are a class of antiplatelet agents that include clopidogrel and ticlopidine. These medications inactivate the adenosine diphosphate (ADP) receptor found on platelet surfaces by covalently bonding to it. ADP normally serves as the ligand to the ADP receptor, which signals platelet activation and degranulation via G-protein coupled signal transduction. Two platelet granule types are recognized. First, alpha (α) granules contain PDGF, platelet factor 4, factors V and VIII, transforming growth factor β, fibronectin, and fibrinogen. Second, dense bodies, named for their appearance on electron microscopy, also called delta (δ) granules, contain serotonin, histamine, ADP, calcium, and epinephrine. Granule contents are released during degranulation. Additionally, membrane bound receptors that were internalized within the granules, become expressed on the platelet surface.

Conceptually, blockade of the platelet ADP receptor should depress the process of intimal hyperplasia. Promising animal studies have generated enthusiasm. Herbert and colleagues reported ticlopidine and clopidogrel significantly inhibited intimal hyperplasia in a rabbit model, where aspirin was ineffective.[11] Waksman and company demonstrated, also in rabbits, clopidogrel reduced inflammation and intimal hyperplasia compared to sham treatment.[12] Goncu and associates made similar observations of limited intimal hyperplasia with ticlopidine and clopidogrel compared to placebo.[13] Further, they found reduced expression of PDGF and basic fibroblast growth factor (b-FGF) in the intima of the thienopyridine treated groups.

The pathophysiology of atherosclerotic human arteries is not completely reproduced in animal models, and study medication dosages are substantially greater than routinely prescribed to humans. Even so, this research provides important insight for human studies. In fact, in a randomized controlled clinical trial, Becquemin and investigators compared ticlopidine to placebo in 243 patients with infrainguinal saphenous vein bypass grafts and found that it significantly improved long term patency.[14] Unfortunately, a serious side effect of ticlopidine is neutropenia, and as a result, its use has been supplanted by clopidogrel. More recently, Belch and others found that clopidogrel and aspirin did not improve below knee bypass outcomes compared to aspirin alone; however, subgroup analysis indicated a benefit from clopidogrel and aspirin among prosthetic graft recipients.[15] No study on the effect of thienopyridines on restenosis in peripheral vascular interventions has been reported to date.

GLUCOCORTICOIDS

As noted earlier, neutrophils and monocytes follow platelets in the cellular response to tissue injury. These leukocytes play an important role in clearing debris from the damaged area and promote cell growth and differentiation through the release of cytokines. Glucocorticoids are cholesterol derivatives that are potent anti-inflammatory agents acting on multiple cell types. These lipophilic molecules cross cell membranes and are ligands to cytosol receptors, whereby they are transported to the nucleus to act on regulatory regions of DNA and effect transcription of cytokines among numerous other genes. They also markedly depress the number of circulating lymphocytes. Glucocorticoids, therefore, are anti-inflammatory molecules that may potentially reduce intimal hyperplasia associated with vascular procedures. These drugs are also widely used among transplant recipients because of their immunosuppressive effect.

Despite the theoretical potential of glucocorticoids, Pepine's report from a placebo controlled trial involving 915 patients failed to show a difference in rate of restenosis when pulsed dose methylprednisolone was given prior to coronary angioplasty[16] However, Colburn demonstrated that dexamethasone, when given preinjury and for 8 weeks subsequently, decreased intimal hyperplasia in a dose dependent fashion while improving patency in a balloon catheter injury model of rabbit carotid artery.[17] This is consistent with the current understanding that wound healing is a dynamic response that is active over time, and would seem to suggest that glucocorticoid therapy given through that time span may be more effective than a single dose at or around the time of insult. Schepers and associates evaluated the effect of dexamethasone given over 7 days on intimal thickening of carotid artery venous interposition grafts in hypercholesterolemic mice, and found a significant reduction when compared to placebo.[18] Further, the authors limited treatment to 7 days because of the negative consequences of long term steroid use. Glucocorticoids are known to delay wound healing and increase susceptibility to infection as well as promote hyperglycemia. While these data encourage further investigation, enthusiasm should be tempered. The side effects could promote limb loss or sepsis in patients with ischemic ulcers. The rodent response to exogenous corticosteroids induces apoptosis of lymphocytes. It should be recognized that this does not occur in human physiology. This serves as a reminder once again that results obtained from animal models may not extrapolate to human disease states. Well designed clinical trials are needed to further explore the potential benefits of these medications in peripheral vascular interventions.

CALCINEURIN INHIBITORS

Calcineurin inhibitors are another class of medications that have potent immunosuppressant properties. Cyclosporin A (CsA) belongs to this class and works by binding to cyclophilin in the cytosol of immunocompetent T-cells. This complex then prevents calcineurin, a phosphatase enzyme, from activating the transcription factor NF-AT that leads to the production of interleukin 2 (IL 2). CsA has been used with great success in human transplantation since the 1970's. Jonasson and colleagues discovered that atherosclerotic plaque in humans contains large numbers of T-cells and recognized that CsA may be of therapeutic value. They went on to show that in a rat model, CsA dramatically reduced the development of intimal hyperplasia.[19]

A small number of retrospective clinical studies evaluating the outcomes of coronary and vascular interventions in renal transplant recipients on immunosuppressant medical regimens have been reported. Arruda reported a lower than predicted rate of restenosis after coronary stenting compared to historical reports.[20] McArthur and others found that infrainguinal bypass after renal transplantation resulted in 7% mortality and 78% primary graft patency at 1 year.[21] In contrast, Grisafi and associates compared transplant recipients to hemodialysis patients requiring bypass and found a mortality of 44% vs. 20% and primary patency of 40% vs. 100% at 1 year, respectively.[22] This study, despite being limited by small sample size and other factors, suggests that immunosuppression may lead to worse outcomes for bypass surgery patients.

MTOR INHIBITORS

Nephrotoxicity is a significant side effect of calcineurin inhibitors. The discovery of sirolimus, the first of a new drug class known as mammalian target of rapamycin (mTOR) inhibitors, and its favorable renal profile has resulted in great interest. Sirolimus, like the calcineurin inhibitors, binds to a receptor in the cytosol. This complex then inhibits the mTOR protein, rendering the cell unresponsive to IL 2 stimulation. An in vitro study using rat and human cell cultures demonstrated that sirolimus prevented SMC proliferation where tacrolimus, a calcineurin inhibitor, did not.[23] The same group later reported that sirolimus, but not tacrolimus, stopped SMC migration in both in vitro and in vivo systems by inhibiting the effects of PDGF. Concern for potential side effects of systemic immunosuppression led to the idea of local therapy by way of drug eluting stents (DES). Randomized controlled trials have proven the efficacy of these stents over bare metal stents in reducing rates of restenosis in coronary arteries with a statistically lower rate of overall major cardiac events.[24] The same effect has not been shown outside the heart. Duda and company compared sirolimus eluting to bare metal stents in superficial femoral artery occlusive disease and found no difference between the groups at 24 months for in-stent stenosis.[25]

No randomized controlled trial of oral sirolimus in peripheral vascular disease has been conducted. The side effects of potent immunosuppressive agents may include accelerated atherosclerosis and aneurysm expansion through both direct and indirect mechanisms.[26,27] Additionally, more serious complications may include nephrotoxicity, malignancy, and infection. Therefore, future study design should consider a minimal effective dose and duration of treatment since the stimulus for the hyperplastic response is understood to be transient.

PDE-3 INHIBITORS

While the phosphodiesterase-3 (PDE-3) inhibitor, cilostazol, is not used to prevent allograft rejection after transplantation, it is utilized in the treatment of claudicants to improve upon limited walking distance. Somewhat surprising is the drug's ability to attenuate the proliferation of SMCs. It was also shown to decrease intimal hyperplasia after stenting in the iliac arteries of dogs.[28] Douglas and colleagues conducted a randomized controlled trial evaluating cilostazol with placebo in patients receiving bare metal coronary stents. They found cilostazol reduced the incidence of restenosis.[29] Morishita suggests the mechanism of action involves cyclic adenosine monophosphate accumulation resulting from PDE 3 inactivity that results in upregulation of p53 and apoptosis of SMCs[30]. Additional investigation of this familiar and well-tolerated drug is certainly warranted.

SUMMARY

Antiplatelet agents have a clear, beneficial role in the treatment of patients after bypass grafts or endovascular interventions. These agents have both anti-thrombotic and anti-intimal-hyperplasia effects. Early data also suggest that PDE-3 inhibition may reduce intimal hyperplasia. The role of immunosuppressive drugs (glucocorticoids, calcineurin inhibitors, mTOR inhibitors) is less clear, despite good theoretical basis for the belief that these drugs can reduce intimal hyperplasia. Systemic immunosuppression does not have any proven benefit in humans, possibly because the negative side effects of immunosuppression outweigh any potential amelioration of intimal hyperplasia. Local delivery of mTOR inhibitors (e.g. sirolimus) has positively impacted coronary stent outcomes, but this benefit has not carried over to peripheral applications.

The details of molecular pathways governing the inflammatory response are still being elucidated. Adding to the complexity is variability of gene expression among cells so that a stimulatory signal in one location is an inhibitory message elsewhere. Further research is needed; however, human persistence and information sharing will undoubtedly accelerate discovery and lead to novel findings.

REFERENCES

1. Choi ET, Engel L, Callow AD, et al: Inhibition of neointimal hyperplasia by blocking alpha V beta 3 integrin with a small peptide antagonist GpenGRGDSPCA. *J Vasc Surg* 1994;19: 125–134.

2. Lincoff AM, Califf RM, Moliterno DJ, et al: Complementary clinical benefits of coronary-artery stenting and blockade of platelet glycoprotein IIb/IIIa receptors. Evaluation of Platelet IIb/IIIa Inhibition in Stenting Investigators. *N Engl J Med* 1999;341:319–327.

3. Topol EJ, Califf RM, Weisman HF, et al: Randomised trial of coronary intervention with antibody against platelet IIb/IIIa integrin for reduction of clinical restenosis: results at six months. The EPIC Investigators. *Lancet* 1994;343:881–886.

4. Srivatsa SS, Fitzpatrick LA, Tsao PW, et al: Selective alpha v beta 3 integrin blockade potently limits neointimal hyperplasia and lumen stenosis following deep coronary arterial stent injury: evidence for the functional importance of integrin alpha v beta 3 and osteopontin expression during neointima formation. *Cardiovasc Res* 1997;36:408–428.

5. ERASER Investigators: Acute platelet inhibition with abciximab does not reduce in-stent restenosis (ERASER study). The ERASER Investigators. *Circulation* 1999;100:799–806.

6. IMPACT Investigators: Randomised placebo-controlled trial of effect of eptifibatide on complications of percutaneous coronary intervention: IMPACT-II. Integrilin to Minimise Platelet Aggregation and Coronary Thrombosis-II. *Lancet* 1997;349:1422–1428.

7. Sneader W: The discovery of aspirin: a reappraisal. *BMJ* 2000;321:1591–1594.

8. McCollum C, Alexander C, Kenchington G, Franks PJ, Greenhalgh R: Antiplatelet drugs in femoropopliteal vein bypasses: a multicenter trial. *J Vasc Surg* 1991;13:150–161.

9. Minar E, Ahmadi A, Koppensteiner R, et al: Comparison of effects of high-dose and low-dose aspirin on restenosis after femoropopliteal percutaneous transluminal angioplasty. *Circulation* 1995;91:2167–2173.

10. Horrocks M, Horrocks EH, Murphy P, et al: The effects of platelet inhibitors on platelet uptake and restenosis after femoral angioplasty. *Int Angiol* 1997;16:101–106.

11. Herbert JM, Tissinier A, Defreyn G, Maffrand JP: Inhibitory effect of clopidogrel on platelet adhesion and intimal proliferation after arterial injury in rabbits. *Arterioscler Thromb* 1993;13:1171–1179.

12. Waksman R, Pakala R, Roy P, et al: Effect of clopidogrel on neointimal formation and inflammation in balloon-denuded and radiated hypercholesterolemic rabbit iliac arteries. *J Interv Cardiol* 2008;21:122–128.

13. Goncu T, Tiryakioglu O, Ozcan A, et al: Inhibitory effects of ticlopidine and clopidogrel on the intimal hyperplastic response after arterial injury. *Anadolu Kardiyol Derg* 2010;10:11-

14. Becquemin JP: Effect of ticlopidine on the long-term patency of saphenous-vein bypass grafts in the legs. Etude de la Ticlopidine apres Pontage Femoro-Poplite and the Association Universitaire de Recherche en Chirurgie. *N Engl J Med* 1997;337:1726–1731.

15. Belch JJ, Dormandy J, Biasi GM, et al: Results of the randomized, placebo-controlled clopidogrel and acetylsalicylic acid in bypass surgery for peripheral arterial disease (CASPAR) trial. *J Vasc Surg* 2010;52:825–33, 833.

16. Pepine CJ, Hirshfeld JW, Macdonald RG, et al: A controlled trial of corticosteroids to prevent restenosis after coronary angioplasty. M-HEART Group. *Circulation* 1990;81:1753–1761.

17. Colburn MD, Moore WS, Gelabert HA, Quinones-Baldrich WJ: Dose responsive suppression of myointimal hyperplasia by dexamethasone. *J Vasc Surg* 1992;15:510–518.

18. Schepers A, Pires NM, Eefting D, de Vries MR, van Bockel JH, Quax PH: Short-term dexamethasone treatment inhibits vein graft thickening in hypercholesterolemic ApoE3Leiden transgenic mice. *J Vasc Surg* 2006;43:809–815.

19. Jonasson L, Holm J, Hansson GK: Cyclosporin A inhibits smooth muscle proliferation in the vascular response to injury. *Proc Natl Acad Sci U S A* 1988;85:2303–2306.

20. Arruda JA, Costa MA, Brito FSJ, et al: Effect of systemic immunosuppression on coronary in-stent intimal hyperplasia in renal transplant patients. *Am J Cardiol* 2003;91:1363–1365.

21. McArthur CS, Sheahan MG, Pomposelli FBJ, et al: Infrainguinal revascularization after renal transplantation. *J Vasc Surg* 2003;37:1181–1185.

22. Grisafi JL, Dadachanji C, Rahbar R, Detschelt E, Benckart DH, Muluk SC: The effect of immunosuppression on lower extremity arterial bypass outcomes. *Ann Vasc Surg* 2011;25:165–168.

23. Marx SO, Jayaraman T, Go LO, Marks AR: Rapamycin-FKBP inhibits cell cycle regulators of proliferation in vascular smooth muscle cells. *Circ Res* 1995;76:412–417.

24. Morice MC, Serruys PW, Sousa JE, et al: A randomized comparison of a sirolimus-eluting stent with a standard stent for coronary revascularization. *N Engl J Med* 2002;346:1773–1780.

25. Duda SH, Bosiers M, Lammer J, et al: Drug-eluting and bare nitinol stents for the treatment of atherosclerotic lesions in the superficial femoral artery: long-term results from the SIROCCO trial. *J Endovasc Ther* 2006;13:701–710.

26. Sessa A, Esposito A, Giliberti A, et al: Immunosuppressive agents and metabolic factors of cardiovascular risk in renal transplant recipients. *Transplant Proc* 2009;41:1178–1182.

27. Muluk SC, Steed DL, Makaroun MS, et al: Aortic aneurysm in heart transplant recipients. *J Vasc Surg* 1995;22:689–694.

28. Kubota Y, Kichikawa K, Uchida H, et al: Pharmacologic treatment of intimal hyperplasia after metallic stent placement in the peripheral arteries. An experimental study. *Invest Radiol* 1995;30:532–537.

29. Douglas JSJ, Holmes DRJ, Kereiakes DJ, et al: Coronary stent restenosis in patients treated with cilostazol. *Circulation* 2005;112:2826–2832.

30. Morishita R: A scientific rationale for the CREST trial results: evidence for the mechanism of action of cilostazol in restenosis. *Atheroscler Suppl* 2005;6:41–46.

14

Deciding between Major Amputation and Attempts at Limb Salvage

Neal R. Barshes, MD, MPH and Michael Belkin, MD

INTRODUCTION

For most vascular surgeons, major amputation is considered a failure, and the merits of limb salvage require little discussion. The literature describing surgical bypass and endovascular revascularization is rich with details of the technique and results. Although the techniques of major amputation are well-described, few series describe the functional outcomes or examine the issue of patient selection. Indeed, the fundamental decision of whether to even pursue revascularization and limb salvage attempts at all or to perform a primary amputation instead is rarely discussed. With so little pertinent data, it is a decision-making process that vascular surgeons enter into frequently but with relatively little guidance.

It merits stating that one must begin the decision-making process with the end in mind: if the patient will derive little or no benefit from attempts at limb salvage, then revascularization accumulates costs, leads to prolonged hospitalization, and poses risk of adverse events with little reward. Simply put, the goal in this decision-making process is to optimize the patient's ability to ambulate and live independently in a manner that is safe, effective, and durable while being considerate of costs. Yet, as will be discussed in this chapter, although many factors may influence the likelihood of success of revascularization (and therefore the ultimate fate of the leg), there are few strong contraindications to undertaking limb salvage attempts in the motivated patient who is an acceptable candidate and interested in such efforts.

The focus of the vascular surgeon has predominately been on the vascular aspects of limb salvage. Adequate arterial perfusion is vital, but alone does not suffice for limb salvage: the bones and soft tissues of the foot also influence the ultimate viability of the weight-bearing surface of the foot, while limb- and patient-level factors determine whether this limb will be viable and functional. Herein we discuss the issues relevant to the vascular surgeon involved in limb salvage efforts, beginning with a focus on the foot and leg and expanding to incorporate other issues important to the decision between primary amputation and limb salvage efforts.

THE LEG AND FOOT

Amputation versus Limb Salvage in the Setting of Sepsis

Together, the extent of foot sepsis and/or necrosis and the clinical condition of the patient (viz. the degree of systemic signs of sepsis) are the two most important determinants of whether attempts at limb salvage are safe and worthwhile in the patient with lower extremity arterial occlusive disease presenting with wet gangrene of the foot. At some centers, the presence of systemic signs of sepsis (fever, tachycardia, hypotension, uncontrolled hyperglycemia or any other signs of organ failure) in the setting of foot gangrene or localized sepsis often serves as a clear indication for major amputation. This may offer a safe alternative but comes at the obvious price of limb loss. The alternative to this would be an aggressive debridement of the foot with planned re-debridement and a low threshold for proceeding to major amputation should the clinical condition of the patient worsen. The initial debridement should drain areas of localized sepsis, remove frankly necrotic soft tissue, and debride bone concerning for osteomyelitis. Any suspicious compartments of the foot should be opened to identify deep space abscesses. A planned second-look in the operating room within 24–48 hours of the initial debridement may be helpful if marginal areas were left at the initial operation in an attempt to spare tissue. This timeline should be shortened for patients who continue displaying clinical signs of sepsis or whose clinical condition is worsening, and attempts at limb-sparing management should be aborted if it appears that foot sepsis is jeopardizing the survival of the patient. A major amputation is in this situation can be life-sparing.

There is no single set of parameters that can be used with all patients to determine when the extent of foot sepsis mandates a primary amputation. This threshold should be tailored to each individual patient and should strongly consider the consequences of failure of attempts at limb salvage. An independently-functioning 55-year old man with diabetes but few other comorbidities, for example, would likely have better physiologic reserves than a homebound 88-year old man with chronic obstructive pulmonary disease and a mechanical heart valve. Whereas the former patient may be able to recover from a brief period of bacteremia or overt sepsis (until an operation can be performed), the latter may not. There are no mathematical models or decision trees that one can reliably turn to for this decision, however; experience and mature clinical judgment must serve as one's guide.

Identifying Arterial Insufficiency that Warrants Revascularization

Perfusion of the foot (the amount of oxygen and nutrient delivery per volume of tissue) by means of the arterial circulation is obviously among the most important determinants of the ultimate success of healing a foot wound or a minor amputation site. Thus a thorough vascular exam should be performed on every patient presenting with foot wounds, infections or rest pain to identify patients with inadequate foot perfusion. The combination of a thorough history and physical remains the best means to identify patients with lower extremity arterial occlusive disease. Yet perfusion can be thought of as a continuous variable, and in many patients an examination alone may not clearly distinguish those patients with perfusion that is marginal but adequate for wound healing from those in which it is marginal but inadequate. For such patients, quantifying perfusion may help in determining the need for revascularization. Transcutaneous oximetry may be the best surrogate measure available but is subject to measurement inaccuracies and is not widely available. Segmental Doppler pressures at the level of the ankle and the toe are more commonly used instead. At the level of the ankle, a pressure of 50 mmHg has been used as the upper limit that defines "adequate" perfusion. Ankle pressures below 30 mmHg clearly warrant revascularization, as wound healing would not be likely to occur. Ankle pressures that fall within the 30 to 50 mmHg range denote ischemia, and the need for revascularization depends on the individual patient's clinical situation. Toe pressures may also be useful, especially in diabetics with non-compressible vessels (i.e. falsely-elevated readings) at the ankle, as the vessels in the toe are much less likely to be non-compressible. A pressure of 30 mmHg at the toe is generally used as the threshold to indicate severe ischemia. Limitations to toe pressure measurements exist as well, the primary being the fact that measurements must be done on the first toe, which is not always present in patients who have had previous foot wounds or amputations[1,2].

Finally, it should be mentioned that primary amputation need not be done immediately in the event that perfusion is inadequate and the patient is not a candidate for revascularization. As will be discussed, there are few patients that truly cannot be revascularized in some fashion, but some patients do occasionally have truly nonreconstructable arterial disease or simply refuse an attempt at revascularization. A retrospective review by Marston and colleagues studied eighty-six Rutherford 5 CLI patients (viz. patients with chronic ulcers and a toe pressure of <40mmHG or an ankle pressure of <70mmHg) that were felt to be poor candidates for a variety of reasons. Ulcer healing was noted in approximately 50% by one year after the initiation of wound care, but the ulcer recurrence rate was high and the major amputation rate was 38.4%[3]. Thus the likelihood of escaping the need for a major amputation is low but not hopeless. Even though it may ultimately delay efforts at rehabilitation, this suggests that the decision to proceed with major amputation in this setting of limited dry gangrene or recalcitrant rest pain need not be made hastily.

Soft Tissue Considerations in the Setting of Dry Necrosis or Non-Healing Wounds

Once sepsis is controlled and the need for revascularization is identified, the decision must be made between revascularization and ultimate definitive foot reconstruction in an effort to achieve limb salvage or a primary major (transtibial or transfemoral) amputation (see Figure 14–1). Traditionally, most vascular surgeons have performed debridements and minor amputations (including single/multiple ray amputations or transmetatarsal amputations) in the forefoot but only limited debridements when a foot wound includes the midfoot or hindfoot. Some centers have reported moderate success in performing midfoot amputations (such as the Lisfranc and Chopart amputations) and hindfoot amputations (such as the Symes amputation) in diabetic populations, but the clinical success at many centers has been poor and attributed to the poor pedal circulation in diabetics. Furthermore, prosthetists can have difficulty fitting a prosthetic for even a successfully healed midfoot or hindfoot. As a result, extensive wounds extending into the midfoot and hindfoot have led many surgeons to pass over these amputation options and instead perform a transtibial (below-knee) amputation for extensive midfoot and hindfoot wounds. Ultimately, the

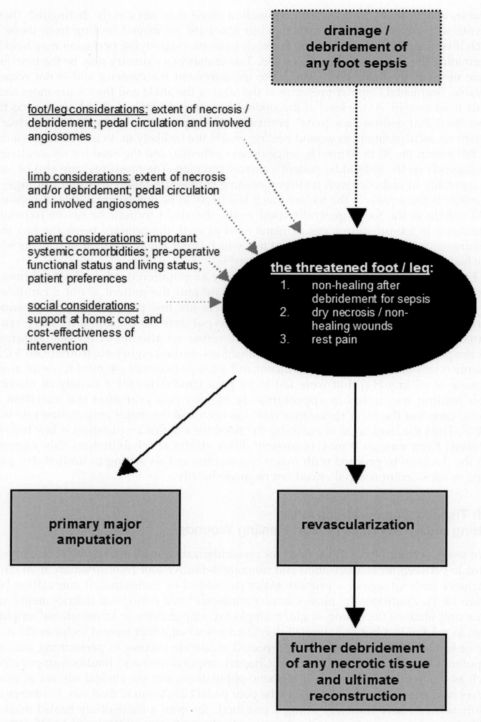

foot/leg considerations: extent of necrosis /
debridement; pedal circulation and involved
angiosomes

limb considerations: extent of necrosis
and/or debridement; pedal circulation
and involved angiosomes

patient considerations: important
systemic comorbidities; pre-operative
functional status and living status;
patient preferences

social considerations:
support at home; cost and
cost-effectiveness of
intervention

**drainage /
debridement of
any foot sepsis**

the threatened foot / leg:
1.   non-healing after
     debridement for sepsis
2.   dry necrosis / non-
     healing wounds
3.   rest pain

**primary major
amputation**

revascularization

**further debridement
of any necrotic tissue
and ultimate
reconstruction**

Figure 14–1. Schematic overview of the management and decision-making algorithm for patients with
critical limb ischemia.

question to consider is whether the remaining soft tissue will be a sufficient weight-bearing surface for ambulation. This is a difficult question to answer with a singular response. The ability to close foot wounds and reconstruct a foot may depend heavily on the availability and collaboration with orthopedic surgeons, plastic surgeons and/or podiatrists, and the ability of a patient to ultimately walk on the foot depends heavily on collaboration with a prosthetist and physical therapist. Thus the answer is in large part determined by the availability of resources within a given health care system. Whereas many vascular surgeons take sole responsibility for limb salvage efforts, more recently the focus has been on working within a multidisciplinary team of providers to manage these challenging, labor-intensive clinical problems.

Bone and Osteomyelitis

Osteomyelitis is common in the foot of diabetic patients with arterial insufficiency and structural foot deformities. Similar to soft tissue, active osteomyelitis should be at least controlled if it appears to be causing any local or systemic sequelae such as surrounding soft tissue infection or systemic sepsis. This is generally done with surgical debridement. Once the local and systemic problems are controlled, however, the definitive management of osteomyelitis should be reserved for after revascularization has occurred. Unlike the management of soft tissue infection or necrosis, however, the best management of foot osteomyelitis in not clear, and recommendations run the gamut of antibiotics alone, to antibiotics and selective debridements as needed, to aggressive debridements for all patients. While a detailed discussion of this topic cannot be covered here, it suffices to say that debridement can generally avoid major amputation in most cases of foot osteomyelitis in the sufficiently-revascularized limb. If done in conjunction with an experienced prosthetist and an orthopedic surgeon and/or podiatrist, surgical debridement can typically be achieved with ray amputations, midfoot osteotomies, and partial calcanectomies.

THE VASCULATURE

The Availability and Quality of Inflow and Outflow Sources

The availability of an inflow source is occasionally a problem in patients with critical limb ischemia. Those with inadequate inflow should undergo aortoiliac angioplasty and stenting, aortobifemoral bypass or other intervention to supply sufficient inflow below the level of the inguinal ligament. Those with inflow that seems marginal or in question should be aggressively investigated, evaluated and managed in accordance with general vascular surgical principles. Once sufficient inflow below the inguinal ligament is established, the site of the proximal anastomosis for infrainguinal surgical revascularization is typically selected as the distal-most arterial segment that is sufficiently non-calcified and provides in-line flow from the distal aorta. In many centers there is a strong preference for the common femoral artery as the origination of all infrainguinal bypass grafts, but this need not be the case: distal origin grafts are as durable and decrease the length of conduit required for limb salvage[4]. The distal target is typically the proximal-most vessel which is also sufficiently non-calcified and provides in-line flow to the foot. The majority of patients in need of revascularization have a tibial or pedal vessel available to serve as the distal target for bypass. Indeed, even among diabetic patients with critical limb ischemia and tissue loss and complete occlusion of all tibial vessels, angiography will demonstrate reconstitution of the dorsalis pedis in nearly 90%[5]. Several options exist in the event that high-quality digital subtraction angiography fails to demonstrate what would appear to be an adequate distal target. The use of magnetic resonance angiography (MRA) of the foot with dedicated foot coils may also demonstrate distal targets in the foot[6], but may not demonstrate more than high-quality digital subtraction angiography alone. Likewise, feet with dorsalis pedis or plantar artery Doppler signals but which cannot be visualized on digital subtraction angiography can be explored to determine their quality and usefulness as a distal target[7]. Finally, a distal anastomosis to an isolated tibial segment (defined as crural artery segments that are not in continuity with either the popliteal above or pedal vessels caudal to the malleoli of the ankle) should be considered. Even if it does not provide in-line flow to the foot, an isolated tibial segment of sufficient length (generally five centimeters or more) often provides enough outflow to maintain patency and also increases perfusion to the foot enough to achieve limb salvage. Indeed, the vascular surgeon that is aggressive about seeking out and utilizing distal targets for bypass operations will likely find that surprisingly few patients have truly "non-reconstructible" arterial disease.

The Quality of the Pedal and Tibial Arterial Circulation

The quality of outflow (i.e. arterial circulation distal to the graft or segment of endovascular intervention) impacts the success of revascularization and thus is worthy of consideration. The Bollinger score and the Society for Vascular Surgery Runoff score are two grading scales that can be used to assess crural and pedal vessel outflow. Both generate scores based on the number of vessels that are either stenotic or occluded, and higher scores in both scales indicate fewer patent outflow vessels. In practice, however, the assessment of outflow is typically more qualitative and focused on the degree of atherosclerotic disease in the outflow tract, the craniocaudal (proximal – distal) location, and the relation of the outflow tract to the area of concern in the foot.

O'Mara and colleagues demonstrated that the patients with an intact primary or secondary pedal arch had significantly higher graft patency rates at six months than patients with absence of a pedal arch[8], and Biancari and colleagues have demonstrated that poor tibial vessel outflow quality negatively impacts graft patency for surgical revascularizations[9]. In a similar fashion, Davies and colleagues have also demonstrated that poor quality tibial outflow can negatively impact the patency of endovascular superficial femoral artery interventions in the setting of critical limb ischemia[10]. Yet while such outflow characteristics do appear to negatively impact patency, these series and our own institution's experience with bypasses to isolated tibial segments[11] clearly demonstrate that reasonable success may be achieved with revascularization even in the setting of disadvantaged outflow tracts.

The concept of angiosomes is also worth consideration for both pre-operative planning and for prognosticating the ultimate fate of the foot. First described by British plastic surgeon G. Ian Taylor, angiosomes refer to the volume of tissue perfused by a particular source artery, and the angiosomes of the foot and leg in particular have been superbly detailed by Dr. Attinger and colleagues. In the foot, the dorsalis pedis angiosome is comprised of the forefoot and the dorsal midfoot; the posterior tibial angiosome is comprised of the plantar aspect of the midfoot and hindfoot; and posterior tibial and tarsal branch of the peroneal artery angiosomes are comprised of the medial and lateral aspects of the heel and ankle, respectively. In a situation in which multiple distal targets are available for bypass, choosing the source artery of the problematic territory (a so-called "direct revascularization") would be most consistent with the concept of angiosomes: for example, the anterior tibial or dorsalis pedis for a non-healing toe ulcer or the posterior tibial for a heel ulcer. In a retrospective study of patients undergoing surgical bypass for tissue loss of the foot, direct revascularizations resulted in a 91% healing rate and 9% major amputation rate, whereas bypasses done to non-source vessel distal targets resulted in a 62% healing rate and a 38% major amputation rate[12]. So, like many other factors, the ability to perform a direct revascularization is preferable, but the inability to do so should not preclude limb salvage attempts.

Conduit Availability and Quality

The availability of adequate conduit for infrainguinal bypass is among the most important factors to consider in pondering attempts at revascularization or bypass. Vascular surgeons seeking to optimize the outcomes of their infrainguinal bypasses in the setting of critical limb ischemia would do well to display a strong preference for the use of autogenous vein graft as a conduit. The published outcomes for bypasses to the above-knee popliteal suggest that prosthetic might be used here with patency results approaching that of greater saphenous vein. Bypasses to the below-knee popliteal and tibioperoneal trunk should be done preferentially with vein graft. Prosthetic conduits, especially when used together with a vein patch on the below-knee popliteal or tibioperoneal trunk, may provide outcomes that are acceptable. The long-term patency of bypasses to tibial vessels with prosthetic grafts is poor. These grafts may be used to augment arterial perfusion for the brief period of time needed to heel minor foot wounds, but their durability is insufficient for the relief of rest pain and claudication. Likewise, the long-term patency of cryopreserved saphenous vein and arterial allografts is low enough to preclude frequent use, but they may be considered in rare situation of a patient who needs augmented arterial flow for a limited period of time for the purposes of wound healing, has no available autogenous vein conduit, and otherwise appears to be a good candidate for attempts at limb salvage.

Saphenous vein from the ipsilateral leg is preferred, but vein should be taken from the contralateral side in the context of a threatened limb if it appears adequate for use in bypass. A vein graft that has a diameter of 3.5mm or larger is associated with better patency than a vein graft with a smaller conduit. Because of the frequent underestimation of vein diameter on pre-operative ultrasound vein mapping, greater saphenous vein segments that are 2.5mm or larger on pre-operative ultrasound vein mapping should not be excluded as usable conduits until they are exposed, harvested and gently distended with saline to avoid an underestimation of their full diameter. In the event that sufficient single segment of greater saphenous vein is not available or not usable, alternative vein conduits should be sought. These include composite saphenous vein grafts, arm vein grafts, lesser saphenous vein grafts, and (rarely) deep femoral vein grafts. Arm vein should probably not be used in patients with end-stage renal disease or advanced chronic kidney disease.

THE EXTREMITY & ITS FUNCTION

Infrainguinal revascularization appears quite effective in maintaining a patient's ability to walk, but is much less likely to improve the walking capacity of patients who are non-ambulatory at their pre-operative baseline. In their review of functional outcomes after infrainguinal bypass, Abou Zam-Zam and colleagues found that 97% of patients who were ambulatory at baseline and underwent infrainguinal bypass for critical limb ischemia remained ambulatory six months after the operation. This was no different for the subset of elderly patients: 98.3% of patients older than 80 years of age remained ambulatory post-operatively. Additionally, 99% of patients who lived independently in the community were able to remain so after the operation[13]. In contrast, only approximately half of patients undergoing major amputation for critical limb ischemia are able to maintain their ability to ambulate post-operatively, and 17% of patients previously living independently in the community remain in a nursing home at follow-up 10 months after major amputation[14].

Special consideration should be given to limb salvage in patients with a previous contralateral major amputation. Even among unilateral amputees who can tolerate the increased energy expenditures required for walking on a prosthesis after major amputation, fewer are capable of the further increase associated with bilateral major amputations. Even if not ambulatory with a prosthesis, the remaining limb is often of critical importance because it is of use in transfers from bed to a wheelchair, etc. Loss of the remaining limb will often forfeit any remaining functional independence the patient has, forcing them to be dependent on others in the home for activities of daily living or confining them to a nursing home.

THE PATIENT

The Presence of Diabetes and/or End-Stage Renal Disease

Diabetes mellitus is clearly the single most important etiologic factor that leads to foot loss. Of particular importance is the development of lower extremity arterial occlusive disease (especially tibial-level occlusions) that leads to critical limb ischemia. The motor, sensory and autonomic neuropathies that lead to foot deformity, impaired proprioception and nociception, and a compromised skin barrier, respectively, also play an important role. Glycosylation of the basement membrane of capillaries may affect the microcirculation of the foot to some degree, but the myth of "small vessel disease" in diabetics representing a contraindication to revascularization attempts has been laid to rest, as numerous large contemporary studies have demonstrated that outcomes of limb revascularization are identical for diabetics and non-diabetics (see, for example Taylor and Monahan[15,16]).

End-stage renal disease, on the other hand, does have both an etiologic role and a clear negative impact on the ultimate fate of the foot. In particular, limb loss in spite of a patent bypass graft occurs more frequently among patients with end-stage renal disease than those without. Although the outcomes are worse, limb salvage can be achieved with reasonable frequency, so the presence of end-stage renal disease should not represent a contraindication to limb salvage attempts. Meticulous wound debridements and local wound care may the key to achieving successful limb salvage in these challenging patients[17,18].

Other Systemic Comorbidities

The pre-operative evaluation of patients with critical limb ischemia is not unlike that of other patients. The presence of cardiac disease, especially severe arrhythmias, heart failure, heart valve problems, and significant coronary artery disease should be identified and used along with other patient factors to determine the need for non-invasive cardiac evaluation or intervention according to the American Heart Association/American College of

Cardiology guidelines[19]. At many centers the mere presence of major systemic comorbidities weighs heavily in the decision between amputation and revascularization attempts, and patients with multiple significant comorbidities may not be offered infrainguinal bypass because they are thought to represent an "excessive surgical risk" for revascularization and limb salvage attempts[20]. This rationale seems to be based on the premise that major amputation represents less of a physiologic disturbance than infrainguinal bypass. Although an infrainguinal bypass is typically much longer than a major amputation (median operative time of 265 minutes vs. 65 minutes, respectively), the relationship between operative duration and perioperative mortality is poor and not clearly causal. Other aspects of anesthetic care are the similar, and either revascularization or major amputation can be done under either regional/spinal/epidural anesthesia or general anesthesia.

Our group has studied the outcomes of major amputation and infrainguinal bypasses in the United States in an attempt to clarify the contribution of systemic comorbidities to the perioperative morbidity and mortality of these procedures. We first identified a subset of high-risk patients, defined as patients that were either: (1) American Society of Anesthesiologists (ASA) class[21] 4 or 5; or (2) ASA class 3 along with renal failure, dyspnea at rest, ventilator dependence, recent congestive heart failure, or recent myocardial infarct. Patients with systemic sepsis or a surgical site classified as contaminated, infected or dirty were excluded, as these were patients who may have had strong indications for major amputation. Propensity score matching was then used to balance the amputation and bypass groups. Among these high-risk patients, the 30-day post-operative mortality rate was significantly lower for patients undergoing infrainguinal bypass than for those undergoing major amputation (6.5% vs. 10.0%, respectively). The overall rate of major complications was similar, but the distribution was different: return to the operating room and post-operative transfusions were more common among bypass patients, while pulmonary emboli and urinary tract infections were more common among major amputation patients. While no non-randomized study is capable of completely eliminating differences between groups such as these, this study provides the best available risk-adjusted comparison of morbidity and mortality among these groups and challenges the presumption that a major amputation is safer than an infrainguinal bypass operation.

Perceptions or assumptions about a patient's lifespan are often included into the decision-making process when considering primary amputation or revascularization and sometimes cited as a reason to not be aggressive in limb salvage efforts. Indeed, with the annual mortality of these patients – mostly due to acute coronary and cerebrovascular events – on the order of 10-12% per year for patients with critical limb ischemia, some may perceive this practice to be warranted. With few exceptions, however, such attempts at forecasting should be discourage. The number of events occurring in a population of patients may be relatively predictable, but the accuracy of predictions degrade significantly at the level of individual patients and is thus unhelpful in informing individual-level decision-making in any meaningful way. The natural history of very few disease processes is so predictable as to allow the clinician to predict a patient's lifespan with any degree of certainty. Even in the case of aggressive metastatic cancers, the patient's eventual demise from the disease may be certain, but the time course is not.

Patient Compliance and Motivation

The vast majority of patients are interested in limb salvage, yet this interest should not be assumed. A general sense of a patient's overall interest in limb salvage, motivation for rehabilitation, compliance with medial therapy, and participation self care should be assessed. Full recovery for many patients presenting with critical limb ischemia and tissue loss may require many tedious months of clinic visits, physical therapy, and foot debridements, and a patient who is not fully engaged in this process may allow non-compliance to compromise outcomes. This being said, it would be difficult (if not unethical) to deny an interested patient the opportunity for revascularization based solely or predominately on a history of poor compliance with medical therapy.

Patient Peferences and Patient Autonomy

The psychological and emotional impact of a major amputation cannot be underestimated by those of us who remain bipedal. Others have demonstrated that of all the complications of diabetes, amputation has the highest negative impact on quality of life – even higher than dialysis[22]. Patients who undergo amputation have a higher incidence of anxiety and depression than the general population, something that appears to correlate with the degree of body image disturbance[23]. Most patients would choose to endure repeated hospitalizations, operations, and prolonged immobilization for the chance to avoid a major amputation. Occasionally, however, some patients – including those who have failed attempts to heal a chronic foot wound and have come to associate their leg with prolonged disability – are not uncomfortable considering an elective major amputation. The willingness to endure prolonged efforts at limb salvage and an acceptance of the inherent uncertainty surrounding the outcome of these efforts should be determined through repeated conversations with the patient with good amounts of listening on the part of the physician(s) involved.

Additional concepts that should be mentioned are patient autonomy and the idea of "futility" in health care. First, the clinician must always remember his or her primary role: to "exclusively and unequivocally promote the interests of his patient"[24]. We are charged with informing patients of the options and risks, and we often make explicit recommendations. Much of the discussion and recommendations are based on estimates of the probabilities of certain outcomes. Patients certainly should have such estimates – inherently subjective as they are – as a tool to aid decision making. Occasionally, however, an option that is perceived by a clinician as having a low likelihood of success and significant attendant risks is perceived as "futile" and not even offered to a patient. This serves as a *de facto* decision on the part of the physician and should be avoided. Options are deemed "futile" *not* if the likelihood of achieving a stated objective (such as limb salvage) is *low* but rather only if achieving such an objective is *impossible*. An example of this would be aggressive medical treatment in the setting of established brain death. Furthermore, the decision of whether a course of treatment is futile is *not* dependent on the costs or risks associated with it. Rather, these are additional factors that should be weighted by the patient in the decision making process along with the potential benefits[25]. Indeed, perhaps the single most important service that can be provided to a patient with a threatened limb is a detailed, realistic discussion of primary amputation and revascularization for limb salvage, including likelihood of success, risks, post-operative/rehabilitation expectations, and costs. This discussion should be lead by an experienced vascular surgeon and aided by any other providers that may be involved in the management (including the prosthetist and physical therapist). Recommendations should be given, but if a physician does not feel comfortable offering a non-futile option that the patient wants to pursue, he or she should refer the patient to a provider that is capable of providing that option[25]. As stated by Royall, the "role of the physician is to advise and propose, not to impose his judgments … the right to decide what is truly in the patient's best interests belong to the patient"[24].

THE PATIENT'S ENVIRONMENT

The support available for activities of daily living, dressing changes, weight transfers or otherwise functioning in the home should be considered. The physical structure of the patient's home is also pertinent and may require some modification post-operatively to facilitate movement around the home and maintain the ability to live independently. Perhaps the two most important environmental characteristics include the presence of stairs inside or outside the home and the patient's predominant form of transportation out-side of the home. The functional status of the patient can only be completely considered when viewed in the context of his or her home and family environment.

Currently there are few if any strict limits placed on the monetary costs of limb sal-vage efforts in the United States. This may soon change, however, as both patients and payors (especially governmental payors) are increasingly demanding "value" – that is, optimal benefit or effectiveness for the amount of healthcare dollars spent. Vascular surgeons will be challenged to find ways to maintain or improve the clinical effective-ness of their interventions while minimizing costs. We do not currently have enough cost-effectiveness or cost-utility analysis data to inform clinical decision-making, but vascular surgeons can act in a few ways to help improve cost-effectiveness and decrease charges to patients. Surgeons can begin the process by trying to understand their local "cost environment" by investigating the costs and charges of services within in his or her practice environment. Understanding the local and national coverage deci-sions of the payor for a given patient can also help avoid unnecessary or avoidable charges to patients. Finally, the decision-making discussion that takes place with patients should include at least some discussion of the relative costs (in monetary terms or in terms of "resource utilization" such as number of inpatient hospital days) and the relative effectiveness of various treatment options offered.

CASE EXAMPLES

Discussing options and making recommendations for limb salvage or primary major amputation can often be difficult, and the decision-making process is complex. Some exam-ples are provided to further review the issues presented above.

Case #1:   A 74 year-old man with diabetes and history of a right below-knee amputa-tion presents with a non-healing heal ulcer of this left foot, first noted one month ago. It was thought by the patient to be related to friction / repetitive trauma when using the heel to push himself up stair in their family's home. No improvement has been noticed with local wound care. In addition to diabetes, he has a history of hyperten-sion and hyperlipidemia, both poorly controlled. He is a former smoker. The right below-knee amputation was performed outside the country for what started as dry gangrene of the toes. He had been given a prescription for prosthesis fitting but said he could not afford the prosthetic. Even without a prosthesis, he says he transfers out of his wheelchair by standing and moves around within his home using his left leg. He lives in a multistory home with his wife and multiple adult children. His exam is notable for palpable left femoral and popliteal pulses and a biphasic Doppler signal over the dorsalis pedis. The heel ulcer is approximately 1cm in diameter and without any signs of soft tissue infection. Plain film demonstrates no signs of osteomyelitis. Vein mapping demonstrates 3.0+ mm greater saphenous vein in the ipsilateral thigh.

A diagnostic angiogram demonstrates complete occlusion of the tibial vessels with reconstitution of the dorsalis pedis, and this vessel is in continuity with the lateral plantar artery. Discussion of management options with the patient includes surgical bypass, local wound care alone, and primary amputation. Because of his good functional status, reliance on his left leg for movement, surgical bypass was strongly recommended to optimize the likelihood of limb salvage. He underwent a bypass from his below-knee popliteal to his dorsalis pedis artery using nonreversed greater saphenous vein. He was discharged to a rehabilitation facility but returns several weeks later for a brief hospitalization for debridement and local wound care of his leg incisions. He otherwise does well and remains functional his home.

Case #2: A 58 year-old man presents with his daughter after referral from a podiatrist for evaluation of a left heel ulcer. About three months ago he was discharged to a nursing home after hospitalization for a severe pneumonia that required prolonged intubation and mechanical ventilation. During that hospital stay he developed the above-mentioned heel ulcer. Prior to hospitalization he ambulated only within his home and with some difficulty. Due to severe debilitation during the recent hospitalization, he has remained confined to bed. He has end-stage renal disease and received hemodialysis three times per week. He also has a history of diabetes, hypertension, hyperlipidemia, history of right femorotibial bypass for rest pain, coronary artery bypass grafting. Exam demonstrates a cachectic, debilitated appearing man. His left femoral pulse is palpable. The left heel ulcer is approximately 4cm in diameter and probes to bone and necrotic edges surrounding the wound but no evidence of soft tissue infection. The right foot is warm and without ulcers or necrosis. Sensory neuropathy of both feet is noted, as are well-healed bilateral leg and calf incisions consistent with previous saphenous vein harvests. Noninvasive vascular studies demonstrate an ankle-brachial pressure of 0.22 on the left with a toe pressure of 20 mmHg. He undergoes angiography to entertain the possibility of endovascular intervention; this demonstrates occlusions of the distal superficial femoral artery, the popliteal artery and all tibial vessels with reconstitution of the dorsalis pedis artery. Given the inability to ambulate and the lack of available vein conduit for bypass, it is recommended that the patient undergo primary amputation. A bypass with prosthetic conduit is discussed but not recommended, and the rationale for not recommending this is also discussed. The patient and his daughter acknowledge understanding of this rationale; the patient declines and offer for referral to another vascular surgeon to further discuss the possibility of bypass surgery, and consents to primary amputation. It is performed without complication, and he eventually returns to his nursing home for convalescence.

CONCLUSIONS AND ADDITIONAL CONSIDERATIONS

Choosing between attempts at limb salvage and major amputation is a difficult decision, yet it is a decision that surgeons make frequently. It is a decision that must be individualized to the patient and must be made with the patient and his or her family as active participants in the decision-making process. As one might note from the detailed discussion above, there are very few factors that would absolutely prohibit attempts at limb salvage. The presence and extent of foot sepsis, baseline non-ambulatory status and the lack of available autogenous vein conduit are the three most influential factors that favor of primary amputation. However, in the sufficiently-motivated ambulatory patient with controlled sepsis or dry necrosis, adequate vein conduit available, many anatomic or patient-related factors might affect the outcome of revascularization and limb salvage attempts, but few would be prohibitive. All the factors reviewed above should be considered and discussed with the patient, and the decision between the options should be made between the patient and his physician or team of physicians.

REFERENCES

1. Faglia E, Clerici G, Caminiti M, et al. Predictive values of transcutaneous oxygen tension for above-the-ankle amputation in diabetic patients with critical limb ischemia. *Eur J Vasc Endovasc Surg* 2007;33(6):731–6.
2. Norgren L, Hiatt WR, Dormandy JA, et al. Inter-Society Consensus for the Management of Peripheral Arterial Disease (TASC II). *J Vasc Surg* 2007;45 Suppl S:S5–67.
3. Marston WA, Davies SW, Armstrong B, et al. Natural history of limbs with arterial insufficiency and chronic ulceration treated without revascularization. *J Vasc Surg* 2006;44(1): 108–114.
4. Reed AB, Conte MS, Belkin M, et al. Usefulness of autogenous bypass grafts originating distal to the groin. *J Vasc Surg* 2002;35(1):48–54; discussion, 54–5.
5. Graziani L, Silvestro A, Bertone V, et al. Vascular involvement in diabetic subjects with ischemic foot ulcer: a new morphologic categorization of disease severity. *Eur J Vasc Endovasc Surg* 2007;33(4):453–60.
6. Langer S, Kramer N, Mommertz G, et al. Unmasking pedal arteries in patients with critical ischemia using time-resolved contrast-enhanced 3D MRA. *J Vasc Surg* 2009; 49(5):1196–202.
7. Pomposelli FB, Kansal N, Hamdan AD, et al. A decade of experience with dorsalis pedis artery bypass: analysis of outcome in more than 1000 cases. *J Vasc Surg* 2003;37(2): 307–15.
8. O'Mara CS, Flinn WR, Neiman HL, et al. Correlation of foot arterial anatomy with early tibial bypass patency. *Surgery* 1981;89(6):743–52.
9. Biancari F, Alback A, Ihlberg L, et al. Angiographic runoff score as a predictor of outcome following femorocrural bypass surgery. *Eur J Vasc Endovasc Surg* 1999;17(6):480–5.
10. Davies MG, Saad WE, Peden EK, et al. Impact of runoff on superficial femoral artery endoluminal interventions for rest pain and tissue loss. *J Vasc Surg* 2008; 48(3):619–25; discussion 625–6.
11. Belkin M, Welch HJ, Mackey WC, et al. Clinical and hemodynamic results of bypass to isolated tibial artery segments for ischemic ulceration of the foot. *Am J Surg* 1992;164(3):281–4; discussion 284–5.
12. Neville R, Steinberg J, Babrowicz J, et al. A Comparison of Endovascular Revascularization and Bypass in Regards to Healing Rates of Ischemic Wounds. *J Vasc Surg* 2010;51(11S):11S-12S.
13. Abou-Zamzam AM, Jr., Lee RW, Moneta GL, et al. Functional outcome after infrainguinal bypass for limb salvage. *J Vasc Surg* 1997;25(2):287–95; discussion 295–7.
14. Nehler MR, Coll JR, Hiatt WR, et al. Functional outcome in a contemporary series of major lower extremity amputations. *J Vasc Surg* 2003;38(1):7–14.
15. Taylor SM, Kalbaugh CA, Blackhurst DW, et al. Determinants of functional outcome after revascularization for critical limb ischemia: an analysis of 1000 consecutive vascular interventions. *J Vasc Surg* 2006;44(4):747–55; discussion 755–6.
16. Monahan TS, Owens CD. Risk factors for lower-extremity vein graft failure. *Semin Vasc Surg* 2009;22(4):216–26.
17. Carsten CG, 3rd, Taylor SM, Langan EM, 3rd, et al. Factors associated with limb loss despite a patent infrainguinal bypass graft. *Am Surg* 1998;64(1):33–7; discussion 37–8.

18. Lantis JC, 2nd, Conte MS, Belkin M, et al. Infrainguinal bypass grafting in patients with end-stage renal disease: improving outcomes? *J Vasc Surg* 2001;33(6):1171–8.

19. Eagle KA, Berger PB, Calkins H, et al. ACC/AHA guideline update for perioperative cardiovascular evaluation for noncardiac surgery—executive summary a report of the American College of Cardiology/American Heart Association Task Force on Practice Guidelines (Committee to Update the 1996 Guidelines on Perioperative Cardiovascular Evaluation for Noncardiac Surgery). *Circulation* 2002;105(10):1257–67.

20. Abou-Zamzam AM, Jr., Teruya TH, Killeen JD, et al. Major lower extremity amputation in an academic vascular center. *Ann Vasc Surg* 2003;17(1):86–90.

21. Anesthesiologists ASo. ASA Physical Status Classification System. Available at: *http://www.asahq.org/clinical/physicalstatus.htm*. Accessed December 21st, 2009.

22. Clarke P, Gray A, Holman R. Estimating utility values for health states of type 2 diabetic patients using the EQ-5D (UKPDS 62). *Med Decis Making* 2002;22(4):340–9.

23. Coffey L, Gallagher P, Horgan O, et al. Psychosocial adjustment to diabetes-related lower limb amputation. *Diabet Med* 2009;26(10):1063–7.

24. Royall RM, Bartlett RH, Cornell RG, et al. Ethics and statistics in randomized clinical trials. *Stat Sci* 1991;6(1):52–88.

25. Wilson BE. Futility and the obligations of physicians. *Bioethics* 1996;10(1):43–55.

Lower Extremity II

15

Progress in SFA Interventions, Stents, and Stent Grafts

Timur P. Sarac, MD

Fifty percent of all peripheral vascular disease involves the superficial femoral artery (SFA). The first superficial femoral artery minimally invasive interventions for angioplasty or atherectomy were by Dotter,[1] Grunztig,[2] and Zarins.[3] Their success rates at one year were in the range of 60%. Since that time there has been a groundswell of new and exciting technology, which has attracted significant interest from not only clinicians, but also industry. In the United States it is estimated that the SFA market alone is close to 500 million dollars. The following review will discuss some of the existing SFA technologies. Particular attention should be paid to reporting standards for the devices as there is no one agreed upon method of reporting data. For example, several of the reporting metrics include primary, primary assisted, and secondary patency (based on Rutherford definition or based on velocity ratios), binary restenosis based on duplex, target limb revascularization (TLR), target vessel revascularization (TVR), freedom from TLR or TVR, freedom from clinically relevant TLR or TVR.

ATHERECTOMY

Atherectomy is the minimally invasive "coring out" or rechanneling the lumen of blood vessels. There are three types of atherectomy, laser, directional, and rotational. The first report on laser atherectomy was reported in 1986.[4] However, long-term results were unimpressive and the procedure fell into disuse. Recently there has been a resurgence in the procedure with the change to an excimer laser, which is touted as superior to other lasers because it is in the ultraviolet region at 308 nm. The largest known study reporting use of the excimer laser to treat SFA lesions is called the "LACI" trial.[5] This trial reported the results of 155 patients treated with laser atherectomy, and reported a 92% limb salvage rate at 6 months. Eight percent of the patients underwent amputation, and there was

45% bail out stenting. The result are discouraging, and has not lead to widespread adoption of this therapy.

Directional atherectomy involves blades that "shave" the plaque out of the vessel. Much like laser atherectomy, early results of directional atherectomy devices were unimpressive. Vroegindewig et al reported a two year primary patency of 34%,[6] and Tielbeek reported a 2 year primary patency of 44%.[7] However, this technology saw a reappearance with improvement of the device called the Silverhawk®. Excitement built up with the initial report of the results called the Talon registry.[8] However, after significant scrutiny of the results, the utility of the new improvements have come in to question. Sarac et al reported one year primary patency rates of 43% with a 25% one year amputation rate.[9] Since then, there has yet been a change to evaluating a different method of atherectomy, called rotational, where the plaque is drilled or bored. However, objective results of these devices have not yet been reported.

PLAIN OLD BALLOON ANGIOPLASTY (POBA)

Prior to development of stents, early results of angioplasty alone were not promising, despite a new legitimate, inexpensive minimally invasive solution to SFA occlusive disease. In a more contemporary analysis, The SCVIR Transluminal Angioplasty and Revascularization (STAR) registry is a database of patients who underwent conventional angioplasty or other percutaneous intervention for lower extremity occlusive disease performed at 7 hospitals over a 3 year period, and patients were followed for 5 years.[10] 219 limbs in 205 patients were treated in patients with both stenoses (78.5%) and occlusions (11%), with six percent of patients having chronic total occlusion (CTO). Mean lesion length was 3.8cm for stenotic lesions and 4.7cm for occlusions. Primary patency rates at 12, 24, and 36 months were 87%, 80%, and 69%. These patency results are higher than previously published rates, but the lesions were short in length.

A more recent meta-analysis including 19 studies from 1993-2000 included 923 balloon dilations.[11] The patients were divided into 4 categories by combinations of their lesion type (stenosis vs occlusion) and symptoms (claudication vs critical limb ischemia), and lesion length was <10cm in all but one study. Combined 3-year primary patency rates were 61% for patients with stenosis and claudication, 48% for those with occlusions and claudication, 43% in patients with stenosis and CLI, and 30% for occlusion plus CLI. These rates were found to be statistically similar to those for primary stenting with regard to patients with claudication and stenosis, but inferior with respect to stenting for occlusion or critical limb ischemia.

Comparison of balloon to stent is discussed below. However, there have been two new developments in balloon angioplasty which mention discussion. The first is the "cryoplasty". This is a balloon catheter, inflated with liquid nitrogen which works by freezing the tissue, theoretically leading to apoptosis of media cells which cause intimal hyperplasia. The first reported results of this were the "Big Chill Registry".[12] This was a registry of 104 patients treated with the Polar Cath®, and the results reported were "clinical patency" of 83% success at one year. The results had no objective duplex or angiographic data, and have never been reproduced. Subsequently, Sampsom et all reported on a reappraisal of the Polar Cath® and found a 53% restenosis rate at one year and 63% at 2 years.[13]

The most recent excitement has been from a new drug coated balloon.[14] The balloon is lined with paclitaxel, which is a mitotic inhibitor and works by stabilizing microtubules. The result is it interferes with the normal breakdown of microtubules during cell division. The reported results were the "Thunder Trial", which was a randomized prospective trial of 154 patients randomized to SFA treatment with POBA vs balloon coated with paclitaxel vs paclitaxel in the contrast media. The results were encouraging in that binary restenosis was 17% for the drug coated balloon vs 44% for POBA. However, results were only reported to 6 months, and in almost all other studies restenosis only begins to occur at 6 months.

BALLOON ANGIOPLASTY AND STENTING

The first reported stent in the SFA was by Katzen.[15] Initial treatment involved use of first generation balloon expandable and single wire mesh stainless steel stents.[16] Failure rates were 32-34% and were no different between PTA and stent vs POBA. However, the next generation of stents, which were self expanding stents made of titanium and nitinol offered better promise. The self-expanding stents recoil after compression, while balloon expandable stents do not. This was supported by a report from Mewissen et al. who reported patients treated with a SMART® stent for SFA occlusive disease had 76% primary patency at one year, and 60% at two years.[17]

All the self expanding stents used at that time were used "off label", and approved for use of bile duct strictures for cancer. Nevertheless, the use of the self expanding biliary stents initially was advanced to improve long-term patency rates from suboptimal balloon angioplasty by reducing vessel elastic recoil, and providing a scaffold to compress intimal dissections. What followed was reintroducing the question as to whether primary instead of optional stenting would lead to better outcomes. Three major randomized trials comparing primary nitinol stent placement with stent assisted angioplasty have recently been reported. The Femoral Artery Stenting Trial (FAST) studied outcomes with stand alone percutaneous transluminal angioplasty (PTA) versus primary stenting with a single self-expanding nitinol stent.[18] Only single, short segment lesions (<10cm) were included in the study with a mean lesion length of 45mm for both groups. One hundred and twenty one patients were randomized to PTA alone and 123 to primary stenting. Technical success was achieved in 79% in the PTA group and 95% in the stenting group. At one year restenosis rates determined by ultrasound were not statistically different between the two groups (38.6% in PTA, 31.7% in stent). Clinically, maximal walking distance was slightly improved in the stenting group but there was no difference in resting ABI or change in Rutherford class of symptoms. Stent fractures were also assessed, as concern exists regarding nitinol stent fracture risk and possible repercussions of an increase in restenosis. Stent fractures were found in 12% of patients with no statistically significant increase in restenosis associated with the presence of fracture.

Stent fractures soon became a widespread concern after Biamino et al. reported results of the FESTO trial.[19] They did plain film x-rays of 261 limbs following SFA angioplasty and stenting. The overall stent fracture rate was 25.4%. More importantly, not all self expanding stents performed the same, and 67% of all fractures lead to occlusions. The fractures were distributed to all areas of the SFA and were dependent on length of vessel treated and number of stents used. Restenosis clearly occurred at stent fracture sites.

However, engineering seems to have solved the stent fracture problem, as reported below in two randomized prospective trials which compared POBA to angioplasty and stenting. The first trial reported was the Vienna Trial.[20] In this trial the ABSOLUTE® stent was compared to POBA for treating symptomatic SFA stenosis. The overall primary patency rate at one year was 63% for stenting and 37% for POBA, with sustained walking improvement. The stent fracture rate was a low 2.2%. Subsequently, Schillinger et al. reported longer term outcomes in their patients 2 years post-procedure to determine if the benefit initially seen with stenting was sustained.[21] At 12 months primary stenting had shown a morphological and clinical benefit with respect to restenosis rates, walking capacity on the treadmill, and resting ABIs. Two-year follow-up was performed in 98 of the patients. Restenosis rates were found to be significantly lower in the primary stenting group at 2 years (45.7% vs 69.2%). There was no difference between the 2 groups with respect to Rutherford class, but there was a trend toward improved walking capacity and resting ABI in the stent group. Overall reintervention rates were lower in the primary stent group, but higher than anticipated.

In the RESILIENT trial, 234 limbs were treated in 206 patients over a year and a half in 24 centers throughout the United States and Europe.[22] Patients were randomized to primary stenting (134) or PTA alone (72). Mean lesion length in the stent group was 70.5+/−44mm and 64.4+/−40.7mm in the PTA group. Of note, 40% of the patients in the PTA group underwent bailout stent placement because of residual stenosis > 30% or flow-limiting dissection after PTA. These patients were kept with the PTA group for analysis purposes but were considered to have had a target lesion revascularization (TLR) event and loss of primary patency at day zero. Freedom from TLR (defined as any reintervention upon the target lesion) was significantly better in the stent group than the PTA group at 6 and 12 months (98.5% and 87.3% vs 52.6% and 45.1%). Primary patency at 6 and 12 months in the stent group were 94.2% and 81.3% which was significantly better than the PTA group which were 47.4% and 36.7% respectively. Stent fracture rate was 3% at 12 months and was not associated with any adverse clinical sequelae. The down side of the study was the close to 20% of patients were lost to follow, which presumably could have lead to diminished success, and the failure of several investigators to declare conflicts.

COVERED STENTS AND DRUG ELUTING STENTS

The first commercially viable stent approved for use in the United States in the SFA was the Viabahn®, which is a stent graft coated inside with expanded polyterafluroethylene (ePTFE). The published results n the PMA demonstrated similar efficacy as POBA with one year patency rates of 50%.[23] However, since that time Viabahn has been improved with the ePTFE now laced with heparin. A second randomized trial, called the VIBRANT trial, randomized patients with long segment stenosis (>8 cm) to be treated with the Viabahn or bare metal stents.[24] Treatment with the Viabahn resulted in a one year primary patency rate of 53% compared to 58% for bare metal stents, which was not significantly different. Interestingly, the freedom from TLR was better than patency, but not different between the two groups at 69% for Viabahn and 73% for bare metal stents. One new and exciting technology is the use of bovine peritoneal tissue lined stent grafts. This work is still investigational, with further trials in progress.[25]

Future directions currently being studied for treatment of femoro-popliteal artery occlusive disease are the use of drug-eluting stents. The initial study investigating drug eluting stents in SFA occlusive disease involved coating the SMART® stent with

Sirolimus, called the Scirroco trial.[26] The metric reported in this study was binary restenosis, and the investigators found that at 6 months, there was no difference in binary restenosis between the bare metal and the drug coated stent. The Scirroco II trial used a longer eluting time for drug on the stent, which pushed the restenosis out further, but again by 18 months there was no difference in binary restenosis between the drug coated stent and the bare metal stent.[27] The next trial was called the Strides trial, which evaluated everolimus on the Dynalink® self expanding stent for SFA occlusive disease.[28] By one year, there was no difference in outcomes between the drug eluting stent and the bare metal stent. Finally, one last drug coated stent trial was Zilver® stent coated with paclitaxel, but published results regarding this device are limited. It is likely that medicated stents and tissue lined stents, or a combination of the two, will add some benefit in treatment of these lesion. Medicated balloons have also shown some promise in reducing restenosis rates, but the application and method for these devices and the types of lesions these will work best for remains to be determined.

CONCLUSIONS

In conclusion, there are many different tools available to treat the superficial femoral artery, and to date none have stood out as superior to the other. In addition, randomized controlled trials comparing different therapies are lacking. Therefore, each patient's treatment should be tailored using a specific or combination of modalities to achieve the optimal short and long term results. This will vary for different TASC classifications, patient co-morbidities, and patient's life expectancy.

REFERENCES

1. Dotter CT, Rösch J, Judkins MP. Transluminal dilatation of atherosclerotic stenosis. *Surg Gynecol Obstet* 1968 Oct;127(4):794–804.
2. Grüntzig A, Schneider HJ. The percutaneous dilatation of chronic coronary stenoses—experiments and morphology. *Schweiz Med Wochenschr* 1977 Nov 5;107(44):1588.
3. Zarins CK, Lu CT, McDonnell AE, Whitehouse WM Jr. Limb salvage by percutaneous transluminal recanalization of the occluded superficial femoral artery. *Surgery* 1980 Jun;87(6):701–8.
4. Cumberland DC, Sanborn TA, Tayler DI, Moore DJ, Welsh CL, Greenfield AJ, et al. Percutaneous laser thermal angioplasty: initial clinical results with a laser probe in total peripheral artery occlusions. *Lancet* 1986;1:1457–9M.
5. Laird JR, Zeller T, Gray BH, Scheinert D, Vranic M, Reiser C, Biamino G; LACI Investigators. Limb salvage following laser-assisted angioplasty for critical limb ischemia: results of the LACI multicenter trial. *J Endovasc Ther* 2006 Feb;13(1):1–11.
6. Vroegindeweij D, Tielbeek AV, Buth J, Schol FP, Hop WC, Landman GH. Directional atherectomy versus balloon angioplasty in segmental femoropopliteal artery disease: two-year follow-up with color-flow duplex scanning. *J Vasc Surg* 1995 Feb;21(2):255–68; discussion 268–9.
7. Tielbeek AV, Vroegindeweij D, Buth J, Landman GH. Comparison of balloon angioplasty and Simpson atherectomy for lesions in the femoropopliteal artery: angiographic and clinical results of a prospective randomized trial. *J Vasc Interv Radiol* 1996 Nov-Dec;7(6):837–44.

8. Ramaiah V, Gammon R, Kiesz S, Cardenas J, Runyon JP, Fail P, Walker C, Allie DE, Chamberlin J, Solis M, Garcia L, Kandzari D; TALON Registry. Midterm outcomes from the TALON Registry: treating peripherals with SilverHawk: outcomes collection. *J Endovasc Ther* 2006 Oct;13(5):592–602.

9. Sarac TP, Altinel O, Bannazadeh M, Kashyap VS, Lyden S, Ouriel K, and Clair DG. Midterm outcome predictors for lower extremity atherectomy procedures. *J Vasc Surg* 2008;48:885–90.

10. Clark, T.W., J.L. Groffsky, and M.C. Soulen, Predictors of long-term patency after femoropopliteal angioplasty: results from the STAR registry. *J Vasc Interv Radiol* 2001. 12(8): p. 923–33.

11. Muradin, G.S., et al., Balloon dilation and stent implantation for treatment of femoropopliteal arterial disease: meta-analysis. *Radiology*, 2001. 221(1): p. 137–45

12. Laird J, Jaff MR, Biamino G, McNamara T, Scheinert D, Zetterlund P, Moen E, Joye JD. Cryoplasty for the treatment of femoropopliteal arterial disease: results of a prospective, multicenter registry. *J Vasc Interv Radiol* 2005 Aug;16(8):1067–73

13. Sampson RH, Showalter DP, Lepore M, Nair DG, Meriglano K. Cryoplasty therapy of the superficial femoral and popliteal arteries: A reappraisal after 44 months clinical experience. *J Vasc Surg* 2008;48:634–637

14. Tepe G, Zeller T, Albrecht T, Heller S, Schwarzwälder U, Beregi JP, Claussen CD, Oldenburg A, Scheller B, Speck U.. Local delivery of paclitaxel to inhibit restenosis during angioplasty of the leg. *New Engl J Med* 2008;358:689–99.

15. Katzen BT. Refinements widen utility of interventional devices. *Diagn Imaging* (San Franc). 1991 May;13(5):100–7. Review.

16. Becquemin JP, Favre JP, Marzelle J, Nemoz C, Corsin C, Leizorovicz A. "Systematic versus selective stent placement after superficial femoral artery balloon angioplasty: a multicenter prospective randomized study." *J Vasc Surg* 2003; 37(3):487–494.

17. Mewissen MW. Self-expanding nitinol stents in the femoral popliteal segment: technique and midterm results. *Tech Vasc Interv Radiol* 2004;7:2–5.

18. Krankenberg, H., et al., Nitinol stent implantation versus percutaneous transluminal angioplasty in superficial femoral artery lesions up to 10 cm in length: the femoral artery stenting trial (FAST). *Circulation* 2007;116(3): p. 285–92

19. Scheinert D, Scheinert S, Sax J, Piorkowski C, Bräunlich S, Ulrich M, Biamino G, Schmidt A. Prevalence and clinical impact of stent fractures after femoropopliteal stenting. *J Am Coll Cardiol* 2005 Jan 18;45(2):312–5.

20. Schillinger M, Sabeti S, Loewe C, Dick P, Amighi J, Mlekusch W, Schlager O, Cejna M, Lammer J, Minar E. Balloon angioplasty versus implantation of nitinol stents in the superficial femoral artery. *N Engl J Med* 2006 May 4;354(18):1879–88.

21. Schillinger, M., et al., Sustained benefit at 2 years of primary femoropopliteal stenting compared with balloon angioplasty with optional stenting. *Circulation* 2007; 115(21): p. 2745–9.

22. Laird, J.R., et al., Nitinol stent implantation versus balloon angioplasty for lesions in the superficial femoral artery and proximal popliteal artery: twelve-month results from the RESILIENT randomized trial. *Circ Cardiovasc Interv* 2010. 3(3): p. 267–76.

23. W.L Gore Inc. Gore Viabahn Endoprosthesis PMA: Summary of Safety and Effectiveness. 2005; http://www.accessdata.fda.gov/cdrh_docs/pdf4/P040037S007b.pdf

24. Ansel GM, Geraghty, PJ, Mewissen M, and Jaff MR. The VIBRANT Trial: Comparing bare-nitinol stents to stent grafts in long superficial femoral artery lesions. *Endovasc Today* 2010: March; 64–65.

25. Carnevale K, Ouriel K, Gabriel Y, Clair D, Bena JF, Silva MB, Sarac TP. Biological coating for arterial stents: the next evolutionary change in stents. *J Endovasc Ther* 2006 Apr;13(2): 164–74.

26. Duda SH, Pusich B, Richter G, Landwehr P, Oliva VL, Tielbeek A, Wiesinger B, Hak BH, Tielemans H, Ziemer G, Cristea E, Lansky A, Beregi JP. "Sirolimus-eluting stents for the treatment of obstructive superficial femoral artery disease," *Circulation* 2002b; 106: 1505–1509.

27. Duda SH, Bosiers M, Lammer J, et al. Sirolimus-eluting versus bare nitinol stent for obstructive superficial femoral artery disease: The SIROCCO II trial. *J Vasc Interv Radiol* 2005;16:331–338

28. Lammer L. Setback for drug eluting stents in the periphery as STRIDES follows SIROCCO. *Interventional News* 2009:14:43.

16

Atherectomy

Yazan Duwayri, MD and Brian G. Rubin, MD

DEFINITION

Atherectomy is defined as the endovascular intervention in which arterial occlusions and stenoses are treated by debulking the atherosclerotic plaque to reestablish an adequate arterial lumen.

HISTORY

Atherectomy was introduced clinically for the treatment of coronary artery disease in the mid 1980's. This technology was conceived initially to overcome the limitations of coronary balloon angioplasty, namely restenosis and acute dissections. However, despite initial encouraging results from single center studies, the combined experience from randomized trials suggested that coronary atherectomy failed to achieve improvements in periprocedure cardiac events, restenosis rates, and lesion revascularization.[1-3] Therefore, coronary atherectomy has largely fallen out of favor among coronary interventionalists, although it still exists as a niche lesion-specific technique.

Early clinical series of successful peripheral atherectomy were published towards the end of the 1980's[4,5] using first generation devices such as the Kensey rotational system and the Simpson directional atherectomy catheter. In spite of the early enthusiasm for this technology and the introduction of multiple atherectomy catheters, peripheral atherectomy did not gain wide acceptance among peripheral interventionalists largely due to the lack of success with early coronary atherectomy and because of disparate published early and midterm results of available peripheral atherectomy catheters. In their 1994 review article, Ahn and Concepcion critically analyzed the published early and midterm results of the Simpson AtheroCath, Transluminal Extraction Catheter (TEC), Trac-Wright Catheter, and Auth Rotablator atherectomy systems. They concluded that atherectomy devices have failed to reduce the restenosis and reocclusion rates from those reported for balloon angioplasty alone.[6]

149

CURRENT ATHERECTOMY DEVICES AVAILABLE IN THE UNITED STATES

The SilverHawk® and TurboHawk™
Plaque Excision Systems (ev3 Inc, Plymouth, MN)

This directional atherectomy device received FDA approval in 2003. It consists of two components: a catheter excision system and the cutter driver which powers the device. The target lesion should be crossed using 0.014" guide wire, over which the device is advanced as a monorail rapid exchange system. The cutting assembly is present at the distal portion of the catheter and is comprised of a tubular hinged nosecone that carries a rotating inner blade. The cutting blade is forced against the targeted site of the lesion when the nosecone is deflected, providing support at the opposite wall of the lumen, hence the term "directional atherectomy". To activate the cutting mechanism, the catheter is connected to the cutter driver and the positioning lever is pulled. This simultaneously spins the cutting blade and causes the distal portion of the cutter housing to deflect. With the blade spinning, the catheter is slowly advanced across the lesion, shaving the atherosclerotic plaque, which in turn is captured and stored in the tip of the device. This cutting sequence can be repeated. As the nosecone fills, the device is withdrawn to empty the collecting chamber. The number of lesion cuts per insertion depends on the length of the treated segment. SilverHawk® can treat vessels ranging from 1.5 to 7 mm in diameter, and requires sheath sizes 6, 7, or 8 Fr. TurboHawk™, which has an improved cutter blade for calcified lesions, can accommodate 2.0 to 7 mm vessels and requires 6, 7, or 8 Fr sheaths. (Figure 16–1a, Figure 16–1b)

The Diamondback and Predator 360°
Systems (Cardiovascular Systems Inc, St. Paul, MN)

This is an orbital atherectomy device that received FDA approval in 2007. It consists of a catheter with an eccentrically mounted diamond-coated crown on its shaft. The lesion needs to be crossed with the supplied guide wire, ViperWire Advance™, over which the catheter is advanced. The drive shaft is connected to a controller which powers the device. The centrifugal force, generated by rotation of the catheter at a range of speeds from 80,000 to 200,000 RPM, allows for sanding the plaque on the arterial wall as the catheter is advanced through the lesion. By virtue of its orbital mechanism, the crossing profile of the system increases as the crown rotates at higher speeds. The particles generated from this

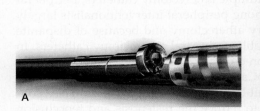
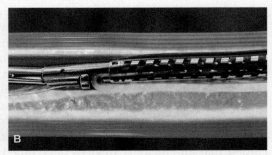

Figure 16–1. The SilverHawk® and TurboHawk™ Plaque Excision Systems (ev3 Inc, Plymouth, MN): **A.** rotating cutting blade and nosecone. **B.** the catheter advancing across the lesion, shaving the atherosclerotic plaque, which is captured in the nosecone. *Reproduced with permission from ev3 Inc, Plymouth, MN.*

sanding action are generally small and therefore carry no embolic risk. In contrast to the directional atherectomy devices, the particles are not collected. The Predator system is the newer generation and has a Tungsten coated crown with increased eccentricity that provides a wider orbital force despite lower rotating speeds. The crossing profile of the Diamondback is 1.8-2.0 mms, while the Predator's crossing profile is 1.8-2.25mms. The device requires 6 and 7Fr sheaths.

Jetstream Navitus™ and Jetstream G3® SF (Pathway Medical Technologies, Kirkland, WA)

This rotational atherectomy device initially received FDA approval, as Jetstream G2, in 2008. This device features a front-cutting, high-speed rotational catheter which has an active aspiration port that allows for continuous aspiration of debris. The lesion has to be crossed with 0.014 wire, over which the catheter is advanced. The catheter is connected to a console that generates a rotational speed of up to 73,000 rpm for the cutting tip. The Jetstream Navitus has a variable 2.1mm cutting tip in the "blades down" mode, and can be adjusted to a 3.0 mm cutting tip in the "blades up" mode (Figure 16–2a, Figure 16–2b). The Jetstream G3 SF features a smaller, fixed cutter. It therefore has enhanced performance in tortuosity and the infrageniculate arteries. There are two sizes of the Jetstream G3 SF available (1.6mm & 1.85mm). All three systems are compatible with a 7-F sheath (Figure 16–2c). Due to the infusion/ aspiration port, this is the only atherectomy device that also carries a thrombectomy indication.

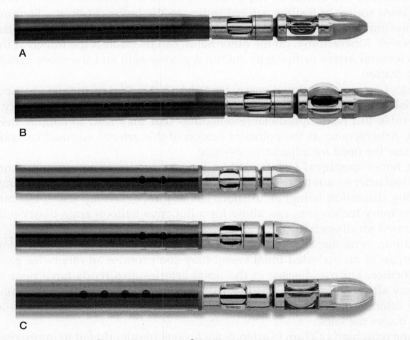

Figure 16–2. Jetstream Navitus™ and Jetstream G3® SF (Pathway Medical Technologies, Kirkland, WA): **A.** variable tip of Jetstream Navitus in the blade-down position (2.1mm) **B.** variable tip of Jetstream Navitus in the blade-up position (3.0 mm) **c.** Jetstream G3 SF fixed cutting tips (1.6mm and 1.85mm) compared to the Jetstream Navitus variable tip. *Reproduced with permission from Pathway Medical Technologies, Kirkland, WA.*

Turbo Elite® Excimer Laser Atheroablation (Spectranetics, Colorado Springs, CO)

The atheroablative laser technology that is currently available uses flexible multifiber fiber-optic catheters that transmit ultraviolet energy at 308 nm. The ultraviolet energy is delivered to the tip of the laser catheter to photoablate fibrous, calcific, and atheromatous lesions. The catheters have a lubricious coating to ease their trackability through arteries. The Turbo Elite catheter can be used in conjunction with a guide catheter, Turbo-Booster, to enhance the navigation of the system. The catheters are compatible with 0.014 wire, and range in diameter from 0.9 to 2.5 mm. The required sheath sizes range from 4 to 8 French. Cold saline flush should be used during laser atherectomy since laser does not work very well in a field that is filled with blood, which absorbs the laser energy and reduces its effectiveness. Laser atherectomy establishes a channel lumen which should almost always be treated with balloon angioplasty.

ADVANTAGES OF ATHERECTOMY

Atherectomy can extend the role of peripheral endovascular interventions to those lesions in which balloon angioplasty, with or without adjunctive stenting, has a limited role or is potentially harmful. Such situations include the following:

1. Osteal stenosis or flush occlusions of the superficial femoral artery: In this frequently encountered lesion, balloon angioplasty not uncommonly results in plaque shift towards the orifice of the profunda femoris, potentially compromising an important source of healthy arterial inflow to the lower extremity. Stenting in this location similarly results in jailing the origin of the profunda and potential loss of the vessel. Atherectomy, on the other hand, can reestablish the lumen at the superficial femoral artery orifice with minimal plaque spill and therefore avoids such a complication.
2. Popliteal artery occlusive disease: Stenting in this highly mobile location carries the risk of stent deformation, kinking, and fracture. Balloon angioplasty alone is preferable but has unpredictable outcomes that may lead to bailout stent placement. Atherectomy at the points of flexion of this arterial segment can potentially decrease the need for adjunctive stenting.
3. Long femoropopliteal lesions: When long segments of superficial femoral and popliteal arteries are treated with balloon angioplasty, the risk of creating a flow-limiting dissection is higher. A more stable lumen, created using the mentioned atherectomy techniques, can allow for adjunctive balloon angioplasty with lower likelihood for dissections.
4. Tibial interventions: Similar to orificial stenosis of the SFA, balloon angioplasty at the origin of an occluded tibial vessel may compromise an otherwise patent adjacent orifice. Diffuse disease in the tibial arteries also tends have poor midterm patency after angioplasty alone due to the intimal hyperplasia and the small size of these arteries. Therefore, atherectomy can be conceptually attractive in interventions below the knee.
5. Lesions with high calcium burden: Such lesions frequently fail to improve with balloon angioplasty, which also carries the risk of creating flow limiting dissections. The recoil of the calcified wall frequently results in significant residual stenosis despite adjunctive stenting. Debulking these lesions by atherectomy results in a patent regular lumen and is a good solution for this problem.

DRAWBACKS

1. Higher cost: The cost of atherectomy devices along with the increased time spent per intervention can significantly add to the cost of the endovascular intervention when compared to balloon angioplasty. In this era of increased cost of healthcare worldwide, the financial cost of every intervention should be taken into consideration.

2. Longer intervention duration: Overall, the use of atherectomy devices tends to be time consuming. This is largely due to device setup and the need for multiple slower passes to achieve the desired luminal recanalization. The radiation dose associated with atherectomy is therefore also higher than other peripheral interventions.[7]

3. Risk of embolization: All endovascular procedures of the femoropopliteal arterial segment carry the potential of embolization of atheromatous emboli. This largely depends on the plaque burden in the artery being treated. The significance of such an event depends largely on the particulate size and the quality of the patient's runoff vessels. The risk of distal embolization after atherectomy has been reported to range from 1% to 22%.[8] Embolic protection filters can be used to decrease this risk, but can also add to the time and cost of the procedure.

4. Vessel perforation and pseudoaneurysm formation: The risk of this complication is higher particularly if the atherectomy device is passed in a subintimal location inadvertently.

OUTCOME DATA FOR CONTEMPORARY ATHERECTOMY SYSTEMS

Due to its earlier availability, more outcome data are available for directional atherectomy than for any other atheroablative technology. Single center prospective registry data have been published by Zeller et al who reported midterm and long term results with Silver Hawk atherectomy. In a series of 131 femoropopliteal lesions, 45 lesions were de novo lesions (group 1; 34%), 43 were native vessel restenoses (group 2; 33%), and 43 were in-stent restenoses (group 3; 33%). Technical success rate was 86% for atherectomy only and 100% after additional balloon angioplasty with or without stenting. Primary patency, defined as freedom of a >50% restenosis detected by duplex, was 84%, 54%, and 54% at 12 months and 73%, 42%, and 49%, at 18 months; secondary patency rates were 100%, 93%, and 91% at 12 months and 89%, 67%, and 79% at 18 months, respectively. Target lesion revascularization (TLR) rate was 22%, 56%, and 49% at 18 months for group 1, group 2, and group 3, respectively. Ankle-brachial index was significantly improved after 12 months and 18 months in all groups.[9]

In a shorter series of 49 lesions below the knee, Zeller et al reported a 98% technical success rate. In 19 (39%) lesions, additional balloon angioplasty was performed, and 2 (4%) lesions required stent implantation as a result of dissection. Primary and secondary patency rates were 67% and 91% after 1 year and 60% and 80% after 24 months.[10]

These results were similar to those reported from 1258 lesions in 601 patients enrolled in the observational, nonrandomized, multicenter US TALON registry for directional atherectomy. Procedural success was 97.6%. 73.3% of the lesions did not require adjunctive therapy, and stent placement occurred in only 6.3% of lesions. The 6- and 12-month rates of survival free of TLR were 90% and 80%, respectively.[11]

Data supporting the use of orbital atherectomy are even more limited. The OASIS trial was a prospective non-randomized multicenter registry of 124 patients with severe infrapopliteal disease (201 lesions). The technical success rate was 90%, with stand-alone atherectomy performed in 57.4% of lesions. Six- month major adverse event rate (MAE) was 10.4% and included death, amputation, or target vessel revascularization. Improvement in Rutherford ordinal scale was observed in 78.2% of patients.[12]

A published series from a single center experience with infrainguinal disease treated with orbital atherectomy also demonstrated a similar efficacy profile. The authors evaluated 200 consecutive lesions among which 117 (58.5%) lesions were femoral, 31 (15.5%) were popliteal, and 52 (26.0%) were tibial. The procedural success (residual stenosis ≤30%) for femoral, popliteal and tibial lesions was 86.3%, 64.7%, and 92.5% respectively. MAE at 30-days occurred in 3 (2.2%) procedures. There were 31 (15.5%) dissections, 2 (1.0%) distal embolizations, 6 (3.0%) arterial spasms, and no perforations. Laboratory evidence of hemolysis was noted in 33.8% of cases.[13]

The COMPLIANCE 360° trial is a 50-patient pilot multicenter, prospective, randomized study comparing balloon angioplasty to the Diamondback 360° system in treating calcium-containing, de novo femoropopliteal lesions. The results of this trial have not been published to date. A calcium scoring system, to reflect the calcium distribution in this vascular territory, has been devised for this study. Low-pressure adjunctive balloon angioplasty (< 4 atm) was used in the Diamondback 360° arm (when required) to achieve a final residual stenosis < 30%. Bailout stenting was used in either arm where a residual stenosis of < 30% could not otherwise be achieved and will count as a target lesion revascularization (TLR) event for both arms. The primary endpoint is TLR or restenosis at 6 months with a secondary endpoint at 12 months. Clinical variables such as Rutherford class were obtained at baseline, 1, 6, and 12 months along with ankle brachial index measurement and duplex ultrasound examination.

Good results were also reported with Excimer Laser Atheroablation. The Laser Angioplasty for Critical Limb Ischemia (LACI) trial was a multicenter prospective registry of 155 critically ischemic limbs (423 lesions) treated at 15 sites in the United States and Germany. All patients were poor candidates for surgical revascularization. Lesions were located in the superficial femoral (41%), popliteal (15%), and infrapopliteal (41%) arteries. Procedural success, defined as <50% residual stenosis in all treated lesions, was seen in 86% of limbs. A limb-salvage rate of 93% was achieved at 6 months, despite the fact that mean treatment length was 16cm. Stents were implanted in 45% of limbs.[14]

The CliRpath Excimer Laser System to Enlarge Lumen Openings (CELLO) study was a single-arm, multicenter prospective registry. Sixty-five patients with stenotic lesions >70% underwent laser-assisted recanalization. 88% of patients received post laser adjunctive therapy (balloon angioplasty with or without stenting). Patency rates were 59% and 54% at 6 and 12 months, respectively. Target lesion revascularization was not required in 76.9% of CELLO participants within the 1-year follow-up.[15]

Pathway's rotational atherectomy and aspiration device, Jetstream, was the most recent addition to the available atheroablative catheters. Results from a multicenter prospective registry showed promising results. 172 patients (210 lesions) with femoropopliteal or infrapopliteal lesions were enrolled. Device success was 99%. MAE at 30 days was 1% (2 preplanned amputations). Clinically driven TLR rates at 6 and 12 months were 15% and 26%, respectively. The 1-year restenosis rate was 38.2% based on duplex imaging. The ankle-brachial index, mean Rutherford categories, and walking impairment questionnaire increased significantly at 12 months.[16,17]

Overall, the available prospective registry and retrospective data show promising results. However, public criticism of conflicts of interest cast doubt on the reported results of such registries, like the TALON directional atherectomy study.[18] Definitive prospective multicenter trials are lacking for the available atherectomy devices. Similar to other endovascular therapies, design and execution of comparative clinical trials have been challenging, in part because of the lack of consensus on relevant endpoints or definitions. Objective performance goals, set recently by the Society of Vascular Surgery, can facilitate such studies in the critical limb ischemia (CLI) arena. Using surgical bypass with autogenous vein as the standard for comparison, freedom from perioperative death or major adverse limb events was determined to be 76.9% at 1 year and should serve as the primary efficacy endpoint for a single-arm trial design in CLI.[19] Standardization of definitions and other endpoints should also allow for comparisons between atherectomy devices and contemporary endovascular therapies in different patient populations such as claudicants undergoing peripheral interventions.

CONCLUSION

Atherectomy can expand the endovascular options for vascular interventionalists. It is important, however, to mention that the literature lacks evidence of objective comparison between atherectomy and the simpler balloon angioplasty (with or without selective stenting). In addition, we lack a similar comparison between open bypass surgery and atherectomy. Such lack of evidence makes it difficult to provide conclusive statements regarding the use of these devices. If comparative studies are conducted, atherectomy devices will likely have a helpful role in select lesions.

REFERENCES

1. Bittl JA, Chew DP, Topol EJ, Kong DF, Califf RM. Meta-analysis of randomized trials of percutaneous transluminal coronary angioplasty versus atherectomy, cutting balloon atherotomy, or laser angioplasty. *J Am Coll Cardiol* Mar 17 2004;43(6):936–942.
2. vom Dahl J, Dietz U, Haager PK, et al. Rotational atherectomy does not reduce recurrent in-stent restenosis: results of the angioplasty versus rotational atherectomy for treatment of diffuse in-stent restenosis trial (ARTIST). *Circulation* Feb 5 2002;105(5):583–588.
3. Mauri L, Reisman M, Buchbinder M, et al. Comparison of rotational atherectomy with conventional balloon angioplasty in the prevention of restenosis of small coronary arteries: results of the Dilatation vs Ablation Revascularization Trial Targeting Restenosis (DART). *Am Heart J* May 2003;145(5):847–854.
4. Simpson JB, Selmon MR, Robertson GC, et al. Transluminal atherectomy for occlusive peripheral vascular disease. *Am J Cardiol* May 9 1988;61(14):96G–101G.
5. Snyder SO, Jr., Wheeler JR, Gregory RT, Gayle RG, Mariner DR. The Kensey catheter: preliminary results with a transluminal atherectomy tool. *J Vasc Surg* Oct 1988;8(4):541–543.
6. Ahn SS, Concepcion B. Current status of atherectomy for peripheral arterial occlusive disease. *World J Surg* Jul-Aug 1996;20(6):635–643.
7. Ketteler ER, Brown KR. Radiation exposure in endovascular procedures. *J Vasc Surg* Jan 2011;53(1 Suppl):35S-38S.
8. Shrikhande GV, Khan SZ, Hussain HG, Dayal R, McKinsey JF, Morrissey N. Lesion types and device characteristics that predict distal embolization during percutaneous lower extremity interventions. *J Vasc Surg* Feb 2011;53(2):347–352.
9. Zeller T, Rastan A, Sixt S, et al. Long-term results after directional atherectomy of femoropopliteal lesions. *J Am Coll Cardiol* Oct 17 2006;48(8):1573–1578.

10. Zeller T, Sixt S, Schwarzwalder U, et al. Two-year results after directional atherectomy of infrapopliteal arteries with the SilverHawk device. *J Endovasc Ther* Apr 2007;14(2):232–240.

11. Ramaiah V, Gammon R, Kiesz S, et al. Midterm outcomes from the TALON Registry: treating peripherals with SilverHawk: outcomes collection. *J Endovasc Ther* Oct 2006;13(5): 592–602.

12. Safian RD, Niazi K, Runyon JP, et al. Orbital atherectomy for infrapopliteal disease: device concept and outcome data for the OASIS trial. *Catheter Cardiovasc Interv* Feb 15 2009; 73(3):406–412.

13. Korabathina R, Mody KP, Yu J, Han SY, Patel R, Staniloae CS. Orbital atherectomy for symptomatic lower extremity disease. *Catheter Cardiovasc Interv* Sep 1 2010;76(3):326–332.

14. Laird JR, Zeller T, Gray BH, et al. Limb salvage following laser-assisted angioplasty for critical limb ischemia: results of the LACI multicenter trial. *J Endovasc Ther* Feb 2006;13(1):1–11.

15. Dave RM, Patlola R, Kollmeyer K, et al. Excimer laser recanalization of femoropopliteal lesions and 1-year patency: results of the CELLO registry. *J Endovasc Ther* Dec 2009;16(6): 665–675.

16. Sixt S, Rastan A, Scheinert D, et al. The 1-Year Clinical Impact of Rotational Aspiration Atherectomy of Infrainguinal Lesions. *Angiology* May 8 2011.

17. Zeller T, Krankenberg H, Steinkamp H, et al. One-year outcome of percutaneous rotational atherectomy with aspiration in infrainguinal peripheral arterial occlusive disease: the multicenter pathway PVD trial. *J Endovasc Ther* Dec 2009;16(6):653–662.

18. Reekers J. Challenging a myth: directional atherectomy. *Cardiovasc Intervent Radiol* Mar 2009;32(2):203–204.

19. Conte MS, Geraghty PJ, Bradbury AW, et al. Suggested objective performance goals and clinical trial design for evaluating catheter-based treatment of critical limb ischemia. *J Vasc Surg* Dec 2009;50(6):1462–1473 e1461–1463.

17

Gene and Cell-Based Therapies for Critical Limb Ischemia

Cheong J. Lee, MD, Jason A. Chin, BS and Melina R. Kibbe, MD

INTRODUCTION

Critical limb ischemia (CLI) represents the end stage of peripheral artery disease (PAD) and the diagnosis portends a high rate of limb loss and substantial mortality. Leg amputation due to atherosclerotic PAD gives rise to an acute mortality rate of approximately 30% and a 5-year survival rate of less than 30%.[1,2] Revascularization remains the cornerstone of limb salvage in the CLI patient, and surgical bypass is the established standard. Endovascular therapies, such as angioplasty, atherectomy, and stenting offer a less invasive option, but evidence of efficacy is lacking. Moreover, approximately 20% to 30% of patients with CLI are not considered candidates for open or endovascular revascularization with amputation often being the only option.[3] Further complicating this condition is the lack of effective pharmacologic treatments to alter the natural history of CLI. Over the past decade, investigative efforts in understanding the biologic mechanisms behind angiogenesis have led to clinically promising means of inducing neo-vascularization in ischemic tissue via gene and stem cell therapy. Thus, this chapter reviews emerging evidence from the fields of gene and cell-based therapies for the management of patients with CLI.

NEO-VASCULARIZATION: ANGIOGENESIS AND ARTERIOGENESIS

In patients with obstructive arterial disease, two different forms of compensatory vessel growth occur, angiogenesis and arteriogenesis. Angiogenesis is the formation of a capillary network, through the activation and proliferation of endothelial cells in ischemic tissue. It is mediated by hypoxia-induced release of cytokines, such as vascular endothelial growth factor (VEGF) and related growth factors.[4] The resulting capillaries are small, with a diameter of about 10 to 20 μm, and may not sufficiently compensate or substitute for a large occluded transport artery. Current gene-based therapies target upregulation of local angiogenic factors to augment compensatory angiogenesis.

Arteriogenesis, also called collateral growth, is the increase in the caliber of pre-existent collateral arterioles capable of compensating for the loss of function of occluded arteries.[4] The original diameter of a small, initially non-perfused arteriole may increase up to 20 times during the process of arteriogenesis.[5] It is initiated when elevated pressures and subsequent radial wall shear stresses increase in the collateral arterioles as stenosis or occlusion develops in a main artery. The increased shear stress leads to an upregulation of cell adhesion molecules for circulating monocytes, which subsequently accumulate around the proliferating arteries and provide the required cytokines and growth factors.[6] These circulating monocytes are bone marrow derived cells (BMC) and adhere to and invade the collateral vessel wall to induce arteriogenesis by paracrine or direct mechanisms to physically support the assembly of endothelial cells.[7–11] Current cell-based therapies and trials study the effectiveness of BMC administration to ischemic limbs in promoting neo-vascularization.

GENE THERAPY

With gene therapy, foreign pro-angiogenic nucleic acids are introduced into ischemic tissue by a variety of vectors and routes in order to increase the local expression of selected genes beyond native levels. Numerous angiogenic factors and their genes have been evaluated for therapeutic effect in CLI including VEGF, hepatocyte growth factor (HGF), fibroblast growth factor (FGF), hypoxia inducible factor-1 (HIF-1), and stromal cell derived factor-1 (SDF-1).

Gene Delivery

The transfer of genes into target cells to augment angiogenesis is accomplished by a number of mechanisms that can be broadly divided into non-viral (via plasmids) and viral means. Each method has advantages and disadvantages that must be considered in the design of an appropriate therapy. In addition to selecting a delivery vector for an angiogenic gene, an appropriate route of administration for the gene vector must be chosen. The more commonly studied modes of administration are via intravascular catheter delivery, intramuscular injection, and *ex vivo* gene transfer. Isner's initial trial of VEGF165 human plasmid used a hydrogel catheter involving balloon inflation for direct delivery of plasmid to the vascular endothelium.[12] Further work has demonstrated limitations in this approach by systemic dilution of the gene product and atherosclerotic disease of target vessels thus limiting transfer to ischemic cells and risking iatrogenic damage to calcified vessels.[13,14]

Both plasmid DNA and viral carriers of angiogenic genes can be transferred effectively to diseased tissues by direct intramuscular injection. In addition to the advantage of introducing the genes directly to the targeted tissue as opposed to being limited to patent vessels in the intravascular approach, this route of delivery is less invasive for the patient and easier to perform for the clinician. Animal models have also demonstrated augmented transfer efficiency with injection into ischemic muscle compared to non-ischemic muscle.[13] Other factors such as pre-injection with hypertonic sucrose have effected more uniform distribution and less variability in gene expression with intramuscular injection.[13]

Beyond these traditional gene therapy methods, more recent work has been undertaken in *ex vivo* gene transfer, wherein cells from the host organism are harvested, transfected with selected genes *in vitro*, and then re-introduced for gene expression. While this is a more involved process, it offers the opportunity to ensure introduction of only selected genetic material into specifically targeted cells in contrast to the relatively blind approach of intravascular and intramuscular routes. A limited number of studies have also examined the novel approach of using bacteria, specifically *Eschericia coli* containing VEGF and HIF-1 alpha genes, for angiogenesis.[12] This method suggests the possibility of regulated gene expression with the concurrent administration of antibiotics and other agents; however, this has only been carried out in rat models of intestinal ischemia with inconsistent results.[12]

Vascular Endothelial Growth Factor

VEGF is one of the primary growth factors currently being investigated to induce angiogenesis in ischemic tissues. In fact, injured tissue normally releases VEGF to stimulate endothelial progenitor cell (EPC) recruitment and differentiation to enhance blood vessel formation. Four isoforms of VEGF are derived from a single gene by mRNA splicing to yield molecules of 121, 165, 189, or 206 amino acids. The 165 isoform is the predominant isoform; however, all isoforms are mitogens for vascular endothelial cells and increase vascular permeability.[15] These properties have been seen to induce improved endothelial function, flow reserve, collateral vessel development, healing of ischemic ulcers, and limb salvage.[12]

In 1996, Isner et al reported a ground-breaking trial of angiogenic therapy using human plasmid VEGF165 via an intra-arterial hydrogel polymer-coated angioplasty balloon in the popliteal artery of a patient with CLI.[12] Angiography at 4 and 12 weeks showed an increase in collateral vessels at the knee and infra-popliteal levels along with unilateral edema and spider angiomata in the leg. The same laboratory later investigated intramuscular administration of plasmid VEGF165 in a small, uncontrolled trial of CLI and showed similar improvements in collateral formation, ulcer healing, and rest pain, and also demonstrated tolerability of injections.[15] It should be noted that 6 out of 9 subjects in the study experienced moderate to severe but transient edema associated with VEGF165 injections. Further Phase I studies of intramuscular VEGF165 administration in patients with CLI and chronic ischemic neuropathy supported benefits to ulcer healing, the ankle-brachial index (ABI), rest pain, neurologic disability, and electrophysiologic measures in ischemic limbs.[15]

Later and larger studies of VEGF have also investigated the use of adenoviral vectors in the delivery of VEGF to ischemic tissue. A Phase II double-blind, randomized, controlled trial by Makinen et al investigated the use of intra-arterial delivery of adenoviral VEGF165 after percutaneous transluminal angioplasty (PTA) in 40 intermittent claudication patients and 14 CLI patients.[16] It was previously noted that adenoviral vectors could prompt an immunologic and inflammatory response in patients. This study, however, showed that despite an increase in anti-adenovirus antibodies in the 61% of patients, no increased risk in other major gene transfer-related side effects were detected compared with placebo groups. Digital subtraction arteriography after 3 months showed significantly increased vascularization with VEGF treatment. Yet, secondary endpoints of improvement in Rutherford class and ABI showed no significant improvement compared to placebo. Another double-blind, randomized control Phase II trial examined the effects of intramuscular human plasmid VEGF165 in 54 diabetic patients with CLI. Although this trial did show evidence of improved ulcer healing, reduced pain, and improved ABI; the primary endpoint of a decreased amputation rate in the treatment group was not achieved.[12]

In summary, while VEGF is a well-studied angiogenic growth factor and has demonstrated increases in the vasculature of animal and human ischemic tissue, valuable clinical endpoints such as reduction in amputation rates in CLI remain to be proven.

Fibroblast Growth Factor

Fibroblast growth factor (FGF) represents a group of growth factors with 23 members that control the proliferation and migration of multiple cell types including endothelial, smooth muscle, and fibroblasts. Of these members, acidic FGF (FGF-1) is known to be a mitogen for vascular cells and has been shown to induce the formation of mature blood vessels.[15] Multiple trials have been and are being carried out in CLI patients with promising clinical results.

A Phase I trial of intramuscular human plasmid FGF-1 (NV1FGF) in 51 patients with CLI demonstrated an acceptable safety profile. Furthermore, the studied showed significant reductions in pain and ulcer size, and significant increases in the transcutaneous oxygen pressure (TcPO$_2$) and ABI. Additionally, 33% of patients showed new blood vessel formation in angiograms at the end of the study.[15] The TALISMAN study, a follow up Phase II, randomized control trial of NV1FGF was also conducted in 125 CLI patients found not to be candidates for surgical revascularization. The treatment group received a course of 8 injections over 2 months. After following groups to 52 weeks, a significant reduction in amputations was noted in the NV1FGF-treated group and a non-significant trend was also noted toward decreased mortality. The study had a primary endpoint of improved ulcer healing, which was not achieved; however, this was attributed to the heterogeneity and severity of lesions at the outset of the study in addition to sample size.[12]

The results of the phase III trial "therapeutic angiogenesis for the management of arteriosclerosis in a randomized international study" (TAMARIS) of NV1FGF was recently published with disappointing conclusions.[17] In this well-conducted multi-center, randomized trial, 525 patients unsuitable for revascularization were randomly allocated to intramuscular injections of NV1FGF or placebo. After 1 year follow-up, the primary endpoint of time to major amputation or death did not differ between the groups (hazard ratio 1.11, 95% CI 0.83–1.49, P=0.48). Endpoint rates were inconsistent between the placebo groups of the phase II and phase III trials, suggesting possible differences in patients' characteristics affecting response to treatment. Because the sample size for the phase III study was based on the 44% reduction in the endpoint shown in the phase II trial, rather than a smaller clinically meaningful reduction, the phase III study was possibly underpowered.

Hepatocyte Growth Factor

Hepatocyte growth factor (HGF) is a multifunctional cytokine that was first recognized as a potent hepatocyte mitogen but was also subsequently found to have dose-dependent stimulatory effects to endothelial cell proliferation without affecting vascular smooth muscle cell proliferation. Later studies into its angiogenic potential found that HGF could achieve therapeutic angiogenesis in animal models with introduction as either a recombinant protein or as naked plasmid DNA.[15] It has also been found to upregulate VEGF expression and function as a neurotrophic factor promoting the growth of sympathetic neurons. Since then, multiple clinical trials in PAD and CLI have been undertaken.

An initial Phase I/II randomized control trial (HGF-STAT) was carried out in 104 patients with CLI who were designated to receive either placebo or 1 of 3 different doses of HGF plasmid injections in ischemic leg muscle.[12] 80% of the high dose group exhibited higher $TcPO_2$ compared to the placebo group; however, no differences were found in the outcomes of ABI, wound healing, limb salvage, and survival. Of note, HGF gene transfer was not associated with limb edema as had been previously found in with VEGF.[12] A follow up Phase II randomized control trial of 27 Rutherford 5 and 6 CLI patients (HGF-0205 Trial) further assessed the safety and clinical efficacy of HGF.[18] This study showed HGF injections were associated with significant improvements in the toe-brachial index (TBI) and rest pain as assessed by a visual analogue scale with a non-significant trend toward complete ulcer healing in the HGF group at 6 months. Still, no differences in major amputation or mortality could be detected at 12 months.[18]

Another recent Phase II double-blind, randomized control trial was conducted in 41 Japanese patients with Rutherford 4 and 5 CLI who were randomized to either intramuscular HGF plasmid injection or placebo. After injections at 0 and 4 weeks and follow up to 12 weeks, the HGF group demonstrated significantly improved rest pain in Rutherford 4 patients and significantly reduced ulcer size in Rutherford 5 patients compared to the placebo group with no major safety problems. Improvement was also shown in quality of life; however, no differences could be observed in ABI or limb salvage rates.[19]

Additional studies are also ongoing in the United States, South Korea, and China for intramuscular injections of VM202, a non-viral plasmid DNA expressing two isoforms of HGF by differential splicing. A Phase I dose-escalation study demonstrated safety and tolerability as well as significantly improved ABI, TBI, and rest pain for this novel HGF plasmid design.[20] Given that this form of HGF therapy provides two isoforms, it is possible that this therapy may display greater potency and efficacy.

Despite the limitations of initial trials, HGF demonstrates another opportunity for angiogenic gene therapy in CLI without perhaps the adverse effects associated with VEGF such as edema. While most trials have been too small to show effects on more recognized clinical endpoints such as major amputation free survival, they warrant study with a larger multicenter trial.

Hypoxia Inducible Factor-1

Hypoxia inducible factor-1 (HIF-1) is a more recently investigated target for gene therapy in CLI. More than just an endothelial growth factor, it is a transcriptional activator and serves as a master regulator of oxygen homeostasis. HIF-1 is a heterodimeric protein composed of alpha and beta subunits. HIF-1alpha is regulated by oxygenation levels—increasing when oxygen levels decrease. The HIF-1beta subunit is constitutively expressed. The induction of HIF-1 in ischemic tissue has been shown to be involved in the activation of multiple vascular growth pathways including VEGF, SDF-1/CXCR4, and erythropoietin (EPO) expression. Previous animal models have demonstrated the recovery of blood flow in animal models of hind limb ischemia after injection of plasmid DNA coding for constitutively active HIF-1alpha (HIF1alpha-VP16).[15]

A Phase I dose-escalation trial has also been carried out including a double-blind, randomized control trial in 34 CLI patients who were not candidates for revascularization.[12] Patients were given escalation doses of intramuscular injections of adenoviral HIF1alpha-VP16. Safety and tolerability were shown for all doses; however, no improvement in any clinical endpoints could be demonstrated. Additionally, adverse events including peripheral edema were seen.[12]

HIF-1 is a novel approach to gene therapy in CLI with its transcriptional activation of multiple angiogenic pathways. This is attractive in possibly stimulating a more physiologic response to the hypoxia and ischemia of CLI. Conversely, this may present difficulties in the isolation of the effects of each pathway and could open the door to a wider range of adverse effects including those associated with VEGF such as peripheral edema.

Stromal Cell Derived Factor-1

Stromal cell derived factor-1 (SDF-1) is another newly emerging avenue of gene therapy for PAD and CLI, which could offer a bridge between classic growth factor administration, gene therapy, and cell-based therapies. Similar to VEGF, SDF-1 is also released from injured tissue in the same way to promote similar angiogenic processes; and HIF-1 may be a common factor unifying these pathways as noted previously.[15] In contrast to VEGF and FGF, SDF-1 is a chemokine that induces angiogenesis by binding CXCR4 and CXCR7 receptors to promote chemotaxis of EPCs. This lack of mitogenic function for SDF-1 may help prevent the uncontrolled proliferation of endothelial cells that can produce enlarged tortuous vessels like those seen with VEGF therapy. Thus, side effects like peripheral edema due to hyperpermeable vessels could be reduced with SDF-1 therapy.[21]

With respect to its possibility as a bridge between gene therapy and cell therapy for CLI, SDF-1 has been shown to increase blood flow in animal models of hind limb ischemia when overexpressed using gene therapy or in combination with cell therapy.[21] An experimental study in rat hind limb ischemia showed that ultrasound-mediated destruction of intravenous microbubbles carrying SDF-1 plasmid DNA resulted in targeted transfection of vascular endothelium in ischemic muscle and enhanced local engraftment of intravenously administered EPC. This combined treatment yields greater microvascular density compared to no treatment or treatment with either gene or cell monotherapy.

While SDF-1 remains in very early experimental animal studies, the possibilities for its use as a recombinant protein, gene therapy, or augmentation to cell therapy are promising. Moving forward, a more extensive understanding of SDF-1 physiologic mechanisms will be needed as well as evaluation of its safety and efficacy in human subjects.

CELL-BASED THERAPIES

BMC contain a population of EPC, which play an integral role in initiating neo-vascularization.[10] This discovery by Asahara et al is the basis for the use of autologous BMC in PAD to stimulate arteriogenesis by repopulating the ischemic tissue with needed EPC. The means by which EPC augment neo-vascularization are thought to be by direct incorporation into existing blood vessels, facilitating the sprouting of new capillaries, and through paracrine effects by stimulating resident endothelial cells with growth factors to induce proliferation.[7-9,11]

EPC are isolated based upon differential cell surface antigen expression. The cell surface antigen CD34 is lost as hematopoetic cells differentiate.[23] Consequently, derivation of BMC and peripherally circulating monocytes containing undifferentiated EPC populations were initially purified based upon CD34 expression (CD34+).[10] These CD34+ cells are seen to possess the capacity to differentiate into endothelial lineages, thus demonstrating an integral property of a putative stem cell. Since the initial observation, investigators have been able to isolate EPC populations from bone marrow-derived and circulating monocytes using cell surface markers CD133, and more recently an intracellular marker aldehyde dehydrogenase (ALDH)[24] Thus, identification of the putative endothelial stem cell remains a moving target as no consensus has been reached on which markers best isolate the EPC populations.

Methods of Delivery

Thus far, over 30 clinical studies have reported on the use of bone marrow-derived or peripheral blood-derived stem cells in patients with PAD and CLI, most of them reporting improvements in clinical parameters such as rest pain, pain free walking distance, ABI, and $TcPO_2$. Intramuscular injection of cells, intra-arterial injection, or a combination of both, have been reported as effective ways to administer cell-based therapies.[25] With intramuscular injection, local deposits of stem cells are created directly in the ischemic muscle, stimulating neo-vascularization by facilitating cell-to-cell contact, cell differentiation, and initiation of paracrine mechanisms; but survival of the stem cell may be reduced by implantation in an ischemic environment. With intra-arterial administration, stem cells travel to the border zone of ischemia in the nutrient- and oxygen-rich circulation which provides a more favorable environment for survival and engraftment. On the other hand, cell uptake from the circulation to the ischemic tissue may be limited. A review of clinical trials to date suggest that the intramuscular route of administration and the use of bone marrow cells maybe more effective than intra-arterial administration and the use of mobilized peripheral blood cells.[25] Clinical studies comparing different routes of administration have not yet been reported but will help to identify the most efficacious mode of delivering stem cell therapy in the critically ischemic patient. It should also be pointed out that autologous BMC or autologous peripheral blood cells were used in all of the above mentioned studies. Therapies with allogenous cells from another donor or pooled from several donors as in a placental cell concentrate are solely in animal trials or phase I trials with no publications on their effect in humans so far.

Cell Types

The first large report on the use of BMC for limb ischemia was published in the Therapeutic Angiogenesis by Cell Transplantation (TACT) study by Tateishi-Yuyama et al.[26] After establishing the feasibility and safety of autologous implantation of BMC intramuscularly, a randomized protocol comparing the efficacy of 40 intramuscular injections of BMC vs. peripheral blood monocytes (PBMC) as the control was carried out. Twenty two patients with bilateral leg ischemia were injected in the gastrocnemius muscle with control or treatment cells ($0.8-2.8 \times 10^9$ total cells) to each limb. At 4 weeks, the ABI was significantly improved in legs injected with BMC compared with those injected with PBMC. Similar improvements were seen for the $TcPO_2$, rest pain, and pain-free walking time.[26] Legs injected with PBMC showed much smaller increases in the ABI and $TcPO_2$. Overall, the effects observed with both treatment groups were sustained out to 24 weeks following therapy.[26] The authors concluded that the higher efficacy of implantation of BMC as compared to PBMC was due to the supply of CD34+ EPC. The study also proposed that the non-EPC populations (CD34- cells) release multiple angiogenic factors that aid in stabilizing the incorporation of EPC into ischemic tissue, an important consideration taken into account in subsequent clinical studies.

Since this first study, trials have used two modes of isolating stem cells: (1) bone marrow aspiration and (2) apheresis of peripheral blood after stimulation with granulocyte-macrophage colony-stimulating factor (GM-CSF).[25] In two cases of peripheral blood and in one case of bone marrow usage, CD34+ cells were selectively enriched and used for cell therapy. In all other cases unselected mononuclear cells were used.[25] The mean number of mononuclear cells implanted or infused was $3.56 \pm 2.81 \times 10^9$, while the mean number of CD34+ cells was $5.0 \pm 1.48 \times 10^7$, indicating that about 1.4% of transplanted cells were CD34+. The most common protocol was daily 5 µg/kg of GM-CSF for 4–5 consecutive days. The route of cell administration was intramuscular in 33 trials, intra-arterial in 4 trials and combined intra-arterial plus intramuscular in 1 trial; 1 trial compared intramuscular versus intramuscular plus intra-arterial cell administration.[25] The procedures appeared to be generally safe and well tolerated, with most adverse reactions occurring in patients treated with GM-CSF (in monotherapy or for stem cell mobilization).

In 2010, Fadini et al published a comprehensive review and meta-analysis of the clinical studies implementing cell-based therapy for CLI.[25] The analysis showed that autologous cell therapy was effective in improving clinical indexes of ischemia including ischemic rest pain, and hard endpoints of ulcer healing and limb salvage. On the contrary, GM-CSF monotherapy was not associated with significant improvement in the same endpoints. Patients with thromboangiitis obliterans showed some benefits over patients with atherosclerotic PAD. However, thromboangiitis obliterans patients and atherosclerotic PAD patients differed significantly in terms of cardiovascular risk profile. Thus, differences in outcomes cannot be interpreted such that thromboangiitis obliterans patients are more amenable to cell therapy.

Cell therapy for treatment of CLI using either whole BMC or GM-CSF-mobilized whole PBMC seemed to show more efficacy than use of subfractionated cell preparations (e.g., highly purified CD34+ or 133+ cells) from peripheral blood after GM-CSF mobilization.[27] Furthermore, some studies propose improved efficacy of GM-CSF induced PBMC compared to BMC. In a study by Huang et al, comparative analysis of thromboangiitis obliterans patients receiving BMC treatment versus PBMC treatment revealed that at 12 weeks after cell implantation, improvement of the ABI, skin temperature, and rest pain was significantly better for patients receiving GM-CSF mobilized PBMC than for those receiving BMC.[28] There was, however, no significant difference between the two groups for pain-free walking distance, $TcPO_2$, ulcers, and rate of lower limb amputation.[28] Other reports inclusive of atherosclerosis- related PAD patients showed slight but insignificant improvements in the ABI, $TcPO_2$, and pain free walking distance with GM-CSF derived PBMC therapy over BMC therapy. Pain-scale reduction was significantly better with mobilized PB-MNC than with BM-MNC ($P = 0.006$).[25] Bone marrow derived cell therapy, however, significantly improved hard end points such as ulcer healing (OR 7.23; $P = 0.038$) while PBMC treatments failed to show significance (OR 2.24; $P = 0.13$).[25] This may be explained by the observation that mobilized cells are transiently dysfunctional due to cleavage of the chemokine receptor CXCR4, which is directly involved in stem cell homing.[29]

Identification of the most effective bone marrow derived isolate for clinical application continues to remain a moving target as purification of BMC based on markers other than CD34 may deliver subpopulations with more effective pluripotent capacity. Perin et al recently published a randomized clinical trial using bone marrow derived cells with aldehyde dehydrogenase (ALDH) expression. ALDH is an intracellular marker which has been shown to confer "stemness" in multiple tissue types.[30] A population of bone marrow stem and progenitor cells that expresses high levels of ALDH makes up about 1% of bone marrow mononuclear cells and contains potent stem and progenitor cells of all cell types thought to be needed for ischemic repair, including hematopoietic, endothelial, and mesenchymal progenitor cells.[31] In a preclinical study, ALDH+ cells derived from human bone marrow were highly angiogenic and restored blood flow to ischemic hindlimbs in immunodeficient mice.[32] In the study, the safety and efficacy of ALDH+ cell injections were compared to non-purified autologous BMC injections. Clinical endpoints were measured by assessment of Rutherford category, ABI, $TcPO_2$, quality of life, and pain. No therapy-related serious adverse events occurred in the study. Patients treated with ALDH+ cells ($n = 11$) showed significant improvements in Rutherford category from baseline to 12 weeks and in ABI at 6 and 12 weeks compared with baseline.[32] Patients receiving non-purified autologus BMC ($n = 10$) showed no significant improvements at 6 or 12 weeks in Rutherford category but did show improvement in ABI from baseline to 12 weeks. No significant changes from baseline were noted in ischemic ulcer grade or $TcPO_2$ in either group. The results of the study show promise for ALDH+ derived stem cells and highlight the need for studies that best characterize EPC populations in bone marrow as a clear and physiologically relevant definition of endothelial stem cells still remains elusive.

Cell Therapy Limitations

Regenerative repair mechanisms of arteriogenesis by recruitment of BMC fail to work adequately in patients with advanced peripheral ischemia and, ultimately results in limb loss.[22] Coincidentally, low levels of circulating EPC are seen in patient populations with risk factors observed for advanced ischemia including diabetes, smoking, hyperlipidemia, and advanced age.[33–35] This observation has been heralded as a novel pathogenic mechanism of advanced PAD and further heightens the impetus for advancements in cell-based therapies. Moreover, recent findings suggest that a number of these risk factors not only reduce the number of circulating EPC but also cause an innate dysfunction in these cells which may potentially limit the success of autologous cell therapy.[25,34] Regardless of these limitations, evidence continues to amass reporting the benefits of treating PAD patients with direct injection of autologous BMC. Further research on the influence of patient characteristics on the effects of stem cell therapy will help to determine patient suitability for stem cell therapy.

Multiple randomized trials involving stem cell therapy for treatment of CLI are currently underway with two in phase III; Autologous Bone Marrow Stem Cell Transplantation for Critical, Limb-threatening Ischemia (BONMOT-CLI), and Bone Marrow Aspirate Concentrate for Treatment of Critical Limb Ischemia (BMAC-CLI). Table 17–1 lists a summary of these trials. Results of these trials will provide more data on the effectiveness of cell therapy and will further elucidate the mechanisms of neovascularization leading to critical advancements in the treatment of CLI.

TABLE 17-1. RECENT STEM CELL THERAPY TRIALS

National Clinical Trial No.	Phase	Inclusion Criteria	Treatment	No. Subjects	Outcome measure	End date
NCT00523731	I	PAD, CLI	ACPs or Vescell	6	Attenuation of CLI, reduction of amputation rate, ulcer size	03/07
NCT-00377897	I	CLI	BM-MNC	20	ABI, TcPO$_2$	12/09
NCT00955669	I	Diabetic Foot	BM-MNC and BM-MSC	40	Safety, MRA, TcPO$_2$, ABI, amputation rate, ulcer healing rate, pain	08/10
NCT00951210	I	PAD, PVD, CLI	PLX-PAD	12	AE, amputation rate, incidence of death	12/10
NCT00919958	I	PAD, PVD, CLI	PLX-PAD IM injection	15	AE, SLV, tumorigenesis	05/12
NCT00913900	I	CLI, AOD, VD	Autologous CD133+ cells	24	Death or amputation, vascular hemodynamics and function	09/12
NCT00392509	I/II	CLI, PAD, PVD	ALDH+ BM cells vs MN-BMC	20	ABI, TcPO$_2$, QoL, LPR	12/08
NCT00616980	I/II	PAD, PVD, CLI	ASC (CD34+)	75	Ulcer healing, functional improvement, limb salvage	10/09
NCT00595257	I/II	AOD	SmartPReP2 BMAC system	60	Avoid amputation, measurement of HR	04/10
NCT00956332	I/II	PAD, CLI	MultiGeneAngio	18	AE, improvement of CLI symptoms	01/26
NCT01065337	II	Diabetic foot	TRC, BMC	30	ABI, TcPO$_2$, amputation status, ulcer healing	02/09
NCT00468000	II	PAD	Autologous BMC, electrolyte solution (-C)	150	Safety of TRCs in CLI patients, amputation rate, ABI, QoL, TcPO$_2$	03/11
NCT00434616	II/III	CLI	ABMC vs placebo	90	Reduction of amputation, induce wound healing, ABI, QoL, TcPO$_2$	03/10
NCT01232673	II	CLI	BMC (CD34+)	40	Major limb amputation, ABI, TcPO$_2$, QoL	12/11
NCT01245335	III	CLI due to PAD	BMC vs placebo	210	Change in Rutherford classification, pain	06/14

ABMC, Autologous bone marrow cell concentrate; ABI, ankle-brachial index; AE, adverse events; AOD, arterial occlusive disease; ASC, autologous stem cells; BMCs, bone marrow stem cells; BM-MNCs, bone marrow mononuclear cells; -C, without cells; BM-MSC, bone marrow mesenchymal stem cells; CLI, critical limb ischemia; HR, hemodynamic response; i.m., intramuscular; LPR, level of pain at rest; MRA, magnetic resonance angiography; PAD, peripheral arterial disease; PVD, peripheral vascular disease; QoL, quality of life (as determined by questionnaire form); SLV, safety laboratory values; TcPO$_2$, transcutaneous partial oxygen tension; TRC, tissue repair cells; VD, vascular disease.

CONCLUSION

Gene and cell-based therapy appear to be promising strategies to augment neo-vascularization in CLI patients. The long-term clinical benefit of any of these regimens remains to be elucidated in upcoming clinical trials. Ongoing trials may also shed light upon the open issue still remaining to be resolved, such as selection of an optimal gene and cell type, isolation method of cells, method for delivery for genes and cells, routes of administration, need for targeted delivery based on anatomy, number and dose of injections, and determination of critical paracrine stimulation mechanisms in ischemic environments. A logical direction for future research may be to combine growth factor and cell-based therapy; intramuscular gene therapy could be administered in the ischemic tissue as pretreatment of the target tissue to augment homing of implanted stem cells. In summary, gene and cell-based revascularization techniques offer hopeful alternatives for the treatment of CLI.

REFERENCES

1. Norgren L, Hiatt WR, Dormandy JA, Nehler MR, Harris KA, Fowkes FG. Inter-Society Consensus for the Management of Peripheral Arterial Disease (TASC II). *J Vasc Surg* 2007;45 Suppl S:S5–67.
2. Feinglass J, Pearce WH, Martin GJ, et al. Postoperative and late survival outcomes after major amputation: findings from the Department of Veterans Affairs National Surgical Quality Improvement Program. *Surgery* 2001;130:21–9.
3. Norgren L, Hiatt WR, Dormandy JA, et al. Inter-Society Consensus for the Management of Peripheral Arterial Disease (TASC II). *Eur J Vasc Endovasc Surg* 2007;33 Suppl 1:S1–75.
4. Voskuil M, van Royen N, Hoefer I, Buschmann I, Schaper W, Piek JJ. [Angiogenesis and arteriogenesis; the long road from concept to clinical application]. *Ned Tijdschr Geneeskd* 2001;145:670–5.
5. Buschmann I, Schaper W. The pathophysiology of the collateral circulation (arteriogenesis). *J Pathol* 2000;190:338–42.
6. Hoefer IE, van Royen N, Rectenwald JE, et al. Arteriogenesis proceeds via ICAM-1/Mac-1-mediated mechanisms. *Circ Res* 2004;94:1179–85.
7. Kinnaird T, Stabile E, Burnett MS, et al. Marrow-derived stromal cells express genes encoding a broad spectrum of arteriogenic cytokines and promote in vitro and in vivo arteriogenesis through paracrine mechanisms. *Circ Res* 2004;94:678–85.
8. Jin DK, Shido K, Kopp HG, et al. Cytokine-mediated deployment of SDF-1 induces revascularization through recruitment of CXCR4+ hemangiocytes. Nat Med 2006;12:557–67.
9. Asahara T. Cell therapy and gene therapy using endothelial progenitor cells for vascular regeneration. *Handb Exp Pharmacol* 2007:181–94.
10. Asahara T, Murohara T, Sullivan A, et al. Isolation of putative progenitor endothelial cells for angiogenesis. *Science* 1997;275:964–7.
11. Rehman J, Li J, Orschell CM, March KL. Peripheral blood "endothelial progenitor cells" are derived from monocyte/macrophages and secrete angiogenic growth factors. *Circulation* 2003;107:1164–9.
12. Attanasio S, Snell J. Therapeutic angiogenesis in the management of critical limb ischemia: current concepts and review. *Cardiol Rev* 2009;17:115–20.
13. Bobek V, Taltynov O, Pinterova D, Kolostova K. Gene therapy of the ischemic lower limb—Therapeutic angiogenesis. *Vasc Pharmacol* 2006;44:395–405.
14. Emmerich J. Current state and perspective on medical treatment of critical leg ischemia: gene and cell therapy. The international journal of lower extremity wounds 2005;4:234–41.
15. Germani A, Di Campli C, Pompilio G, Biglioli P, Capogrossi MC. Regenerative therapy in peripheral artery disease. *Cardiovasc Ther* 2009;27:289–304.

16. Makinen K, Manninen H, Hedman M, et al. Increased vascularity detected by digital sub-traction angiography after VEGF gene transfer to human lower limb artery: a randomized, placebo-controlled, double-blinded phase II study. Molecular therapy: *J Am Society of Gene Ther* 2002;6:127–33.

17. Fowkes FG, Price JF. Gene therapy for critical limb ischaemia: the TAMARIS trial. *Lancet* 2011;377:1894–6.

18. Powell RJ, Goodney P, Mendelsohn FO, Moen EK, Annex BH. Safety and efficacy of patient specific intramuscular injection of HGF plasmid gene therapy on limb perfusion and wound healing in patients with ischemic lower extremity ulceration: results of the HGF-0205 trial. *J Vasc Surg* 2010;52:1525–30.

19. Shigematsu H, Yasuda K, Iwai T, et al. Randomized, double-blind, placebo-controlled clini-cal trial of hepatocyte growth factor plasmid for critical limb ischemia. *Gene Ther* 2010;17: 1152–61.

20. Henry TD, Hirsch AT, Goldman J, et al. Safety of a non-viral plasmid-encoding dual iso-forms of heypatocyte growth factor in critical limb ischemia patients: a phase I study. *Gene Ther* 2011.

21. Frangogiannis NG. Stromal cell-derived factor-1-mediated angiogenesis for peripheral arte-rial disease: ready for prime time? *Circulation* 2011;123:1267–9.

22. Kuliszewski MA, Kobulnik J, Lindner JR, Stewart DJ, Leong-Poi H. Vascular Gene Transfer of SDF-1 Promotes Endothelial Progenitor Cell Engraftment and Enhances Angiogenesis in Ischemic Muscle. Molecular therapy: *J Amer Society Gene Ther* 2011;19:895–902.

23. Civin CI, Strauss LC, Brovall C, Fackler MJ, Schwartz JF, Shaper JH. Antigenic analysis of hematopoiesis. III. A hematopoietic progenitor cell surface antigen defined by a monoclonal antibody raised against KG-1a cells. *J Immunol* 1984;133:157–65.

24. Hess DA, Wirthlin L, Craft TP, et al. Selection based on CD133 and high aldehyde dehydro-genase activity isolates long-term reconstituting human hematopoietic stem cells. *Blood* 2006;107:2162–9.

25. Fadini GP, Sartore S, Albiero M, et al. Number and function of endothelial progenitor cells as a marker of severity for diabetic vasculopathy. *Arterioscler Thromb Vasc Biol* 2006;26: 2140–6.

26. Tateishi-Yuyama E, Matsubara H, Murohara T, et al. Therapeutic angiogenesis for patients with limb ischaemia by autologous transplantation of bone-marrow cells: a pilot study and a randomised controlled trial. *Lancet* 2002;360:427–35.

27. Canizo MC, Lozano F, Gonzalez-Porras JR, et al. Peripheral endothelial progenitor cells (CD133 +) for therapeutic vasculogenesis in a patient with critical limb ischemia. One year follow-up. *Cytotherapy* 2007;9:99–102.

28. Huang PP, Yang XF, Li SZ, Wen JC, Zhang Y, Han ZC. Randomised comparison of G-CSF-mobilized peripheral blood mononuclear cells versus bone marrow-mononuclear cells for the treatment of patients with lower limb arteriosclerosis obliterans. *Thromb Haemost* 2007; 98:1335–42.

29. Honold J, Lehmann R, Heeschen C, et al. Effects of granulocyte colony simulating factor on functional activities of endothelial progenitor cells in patients with chronic ischemic heart disease. *Arterioscler Thromb Vasc Biol* 2006;26:2238–43.

30. Moreb JS. Aldehyde dehydrogenase as a marker for stem cells. *Curr Stem Cell Res Ther* 2008;3:237–46.

31. Gentry T, Deibert E, Foster SJ, Haley R, Kurtzberg J, Balber AE. Isolation of early hematopoietic cells, including megakaryocyte progenitors, in the ALDH-bright cell popula-tion of cryopreserved, banked UC blood. *Cytotherapy* 2007;9:569–76.

32. Perin EC, Silva G, Gahremanpour A, et al. A randomized, controlled study of autologous therapy with bone marrow-derived aldehyde dehydrogenase bright cells in patients with critical limb ischemia. *Catheter Cardiovasc Interv* 2011.

33. Kondo T, Hayashi M, Takeshita K, et al. Smoking cessation rapidly increases circulating progenitor cells in peripheral blood in chronic smokers. *Arterioscler Thromb Vasc Biol* 2004;24:1442–7.

34. Loomans CJ, de Koning EJ, Staal FJ, et al. Endothelial progenitor cell dysfunction: a novel concept in the pathogenesis of vascular complications of type 1 diabetes. *Diabetes* 2004;53:195–9.

35. Zhu S, Liu X, Li Y, Goldschmidt-Clermont PJ, Dong C. Aging in the atherosclerosis milieu may accelerate the consumption of bone marrow endothelial progenitor cells. *Arterioscler Thromb Vasc Biol* 2007;27:113–9.

18

Open Surgery for Critical Limb Ischemia (CLI)

John Byrne, MCh, FRCSI(Gen), Benjamin B. Chang, MD and R. Clement Darling III, MD

In 2008, a little-cited paper was published in the *Annals of Vascular Surgery* from the University of Cincinnati[1]. The premise was simple. A vascular nurse carried out a telephone survey of 78 amputees. All patients were recent 'vascular' amputees. All had undergone multiple attempts at limb salvage (a median of 1 percutaneous procedure and 3 bypasses) before they finally consented to a major leg amputation. The question asked was a simple one: if you had to do it all again, knowing the outcome would likely be an amputation, would you do it? Eighty-five percent of those surveyed stated they would do everything to save the leg if faced with a similar scenario, regardless of the number of procedures needed. These patients were already experiencing life as a vascular amputee. This study was also skewed. The rehabilitation teams were excellent: Fifty-four percent of these patients were actively using a prosthesis and 91% were living at home. In most studies, only 20% of vascular amputees walk with an artificial limb.

In the past, physicians were accused of having a paternalistic attitude to their patients. In the twenty-first century we feel that we have moved beyond that and will only provide treatment based on evidence and good clinical practices. Patients with critical leg ischemia already know they are facing a life-changing event. Their goal is to maintain their leg and their ability to walk at any cost. The patients in the Cincinnati study were not asked about (but made no mention of) the cosmetic result of their procedure, their in-patient length of stay or how impressed they were with the technology used. As vascular physicians, we should bear in mind that angiograms or arterial reconstructions that impress our colleagues may not mean much to amputees.

In this chapter, we will address the best choice for patients with critical limb ischemia. We will not discuss "quality of life" issues such as intermittent claudication. We will review the evidence supporting open surgery and our algorithm at Albany Medical Center for management. We will also look at what patients in the United States in 2011 can expect after a technically perfect procedure. At the outset, it is clear that most controversy attends the best therapy for femoropopliteal and tibioperoneal disease. For most patients with aortoiliac occlusive disease, an endovascular approach will be the preferred one, especially for TASC A and B lesions. It is also apparent that CLI is a broad church. Patients with rest pain due to a TASC A superficial femoral artery lesion may fall under the definition. The other end of the spectrum is a patient with extensive forefoot gangrene and no obvious target vessel in the affected foot. Not quite the same thing.

DEFINITIONS

Critical Limb ischemia was defined by the International Vascular Symposium Working Party Committee as "severe rest pain requiring opiate analgesia for at least four weeks and either an ankle pressure of less than 40 mmHg or tissue necrosis or digital gangrene[2]." The Second European Consensus Document produced a remarkably similar definition: "persistently recurring ischemic pain requiring analgesia for more than two weeks and an ankle systolic pressure of less than 50 mmHg and/or toe systolic pressure of less than 30 mmHg or ulceration and gangrene of the foot or toes with an ankle pressure of less than 50 mmHg or toe pressure of less than 50 mmHg[3]". Regardless of the precise wording, these are patients who require urgent revascularization.

EXTENT OF THE PROBLEM

In developing management strategies for any disease, it is important to have an idea of the magnitude of the problem faced. There has been only one large, prospective population study on the incidence of CLI. This showed its prevalence in the Norwegian population was 0.24% or 2,400 per million population[4]. The prevalence in of CLI in the United States is estimated to be higher (0.5–1%) and the TASC II document[5] suggested an incidence of 500–1000 new cases every year in a North American population of one million. The single largest risk factor for CLI (as opposed to intermittent claudication) is diabetes followed by cigarette smoking. Many of us wonder how many patients with claudication will ultimately require limb salvage surgery. One of the largest natural history studies was by Acquino[6] who followed up 1,244 male patients over 45 months. After 10 years, 30% progressed to rest pain. The risk of developing an ulcer was 23%. The annual rate of progression from claudication to CLI was 5.3%. Most vascular surgeons have an aggressive approach to CLI. In many centers, intervention rates approach 90% for CLI. For those who do not or cannot undergo intervention, the prognosis is dreadful: approximately 40% will lose their leg within 6 months and 30% will die. (Figure 18–1)

THE ROLE OF MEDICAL THERAPY

Unlike patients with intermittent claudication, patients with CLI do not have an effective conservative or medical option. Medical therapies have been tried but have proven harmless at best and useless at worst. Intravenous Prostanoids (Iloprost™) are licensed for use in Europe but not the United States. Theoretically, prostanoids prevent platelet adherence

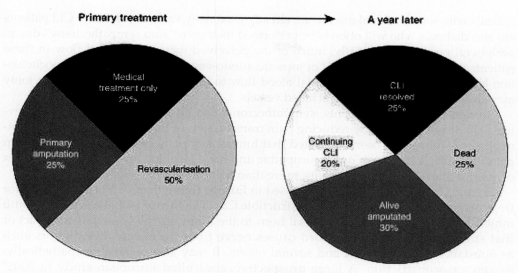

Figure 18–1. Fate of Patients Presenting with CLI (After TASCII)[5]. *Reproduced with permission from the Journal of Vascular Surgery.*

and leukocyte activation and protect the vascular endothelium. They are administered over several weeks and frequently as an in-patient due to possible side effects including hypotension. According to the TASC II document[5], nine double blind randomized control trials have been published. Three showed a benefit in reducing ulcer size but no other benefits. The other studies showed marginal benefit at best. Prostanoids have not proven to be any kind of "silver bullet" for CLI. Vasoactive drugs such as naftidrofuryl and pentoxifylline are worthless for CLI. Vasodilators are also ineffective in CLI as they improve perfusion to healthy tissue only. Hyperbaric physicians are familiar with requests from their vascular colleagues to treat patients with CLI who are not enticing surgical or interventional candidates. However, hyperbaric oxygen therapy works by delivering supersaturated plasma (or "oxygen loaded" plasma) to unhealthy tissues. If patients have severe tibial occlusive disease, for example, the fallacy of subjecting them to HBOT can be seen. Interestingly, the TASC II authors[5] suggest it may have a role in selected patients with CLI. They are wrong.

THE ROLE OF NEUROVASCULAR INTERVENTIONS

Lumbar sympathectomy has been around for a long time. Jaboulay first described it in 1896. Prior to 1948 and the first operation for arterial occlusive disease, the mainstays of vascular surgery were heparin, amputation and lumbar sympathectomy. In theory, it works by abolishing basal and reflex control of arterioles and pre-capillary sphincters and experimentally, this can increase flow by 20–100%[7]. However, as far back as 1921, Leriche observed that the results for CLI were disappointing. The initial hyperemia associated with successful open lumbar sympathectomy often dissipates within a few weeks and resting vasomotor tone returns in 2–6 months. There are several explanations for its lack of benefit.

Patients with severe arterial disease are already maximally vasodilated. Many CLI patients are also diabetics who will often have performed their own "auto-sympathectomy" due to peripheral neuropathy. Finally, much of the perceived increase in blood flow in these patients will actually be the result of increase arterio-venous shunting at the microcirculation level with little added nutritional blood flow to the tissues. Lumbar sympathectomy may also increase flow in collateral blood vessels.

In non-neuropathic patients, sympathectomy can be an effective means of relieving pain. It relieves pain by reducing pain transmission or by decreasing tissue norepinephrine levels. It has been suggested that lumbar sympathectomy may have a role in patients with CLI who are non-neuropathic and have an ankle brachial pressure index of greater than 0.3. In these patients, more than half can expect relief of rest pain.

Spinal cord stimulation has been used in Europe (more than in North America) for treatment of patients with non-reconstructible CLI. The theory is that electrical stimuli inhibit pain signaling from the dorsal horn to the brain via the spinothalamic tract or that stimulation of the spinal cord causes nerve fibers to release vasodilators such as Substance P, prostacyclin and several others. It may also reverse sympathetically-driven vasoconstriction. A large prospective, controlled European study in 2003[8] reported that SCS was significantly better than conservative management of patients with non-reconstructible arterial disease. A Cochrane Collaborative Database study also concluded benefit in patients with no surgical option[9].

THE ROLE OF WOUND CARE

We are all familiar with the rare patient who refuses intervention for a foot ulcer only to be healed when next seen, despite known arterial disease. So, is there a cohort of patients with critical limb ischemia who do not require intervention and who can be managed conservatively? Recently, two studies addressed this question. The first, from Loma Linda in California[10], was published last year. The authors reviewed the outcomes for 49 patients with arterial ulcers deemed unfit for surgical or endovascular intervention. After a mean of 14 months follow-up, 67% of wounds had healed with aggressive local wound care. Significant predictors of wound healing were a transcutaneous oxygen value of >30mmHg and ankle pressures >70mmHg. This confirmed the findings of the University of North Carolina at Chapel Hill[11] who reviewed outcomes in 142 patients with arterial insufficiency undergoing wound care only. Complete wound closure was achieved in 52% of patients by 12 months. Patients with an ABI of less than 0.5 were less likely to heal and more likely to undergo an amputation. Of course, the catch here is than the patients most likely to heal in these studies did not, strictly speaking, conform to our accepted definitions of CLI. They also required a lot of input and healing times were long. There were also a lot of patients who did not heal. However, they undoubtedly are representative of a large group of patients who undergo revascularization in many North American vascular centers.

WHAT WORKS FOR PATIENTS WITH CLI?

So far, we have seen what, by and large, doesn't work or works only in carefully-selected patients with CLI. So, what works? In the last decade, there has been an exponential increase (Figure 18–2) in the number of endovascular procedures performed in the United

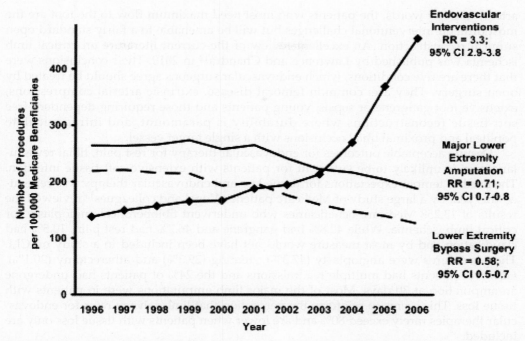

Figure 18–2. Trends in endovascular interventions, major amputation and leg bypass surgery 1996–2006. *Reproduced with permission from the Journal of Vascular Surgery.*

States. There has also been a corresponding, but less dramatic, decrease both in the number of open vascular procedures and the amputation rate. Our goal for CLI patients is not patency. It is limb salvage and survival, which is why amputation-free survival is such a good composite outcome measure for these patients. Resolution of rest pain, healing of ulcers and maintenance of independence are more subjective terms but have also been studied in this context.

THE EVIDENCE FOR ENDOVASCULAR PROCEDURES

The mantra at all vascular meetings in the last few years has been "an endovascular-first approach". A dwindling minority advocates "an open-first approach." There is also an equally fatuous term: "one size fits all". Endovascular therapy has been a boon to many patients with intermittent claudication, saving them the trauma and complications of open surgery with improvement of symptoms. But, in patients with CLI, the therapeutic goals require qualification and there is room for a more nuanced approach.

Critical limb ischemia covers a wide spectrum from rest pain to extensive gangrene. Conventional wisdom is that correcting a single level of occlusive disease is sufficient to cure rest pain. It will clearly not be enough to heal a transmetatarsal amputation performed for forefoot sepsis. For patients with tissue loss, straight line, pulsatile blood flow to the foot is needed. This often means recannulating tibial occlusions with their unique challenges. These vessels are often extremely calcified with multiple occlusions. Occasionally there may be no radiographically obvious outflow artery. In other words, the patients who most need maximum flow to the foot are the most difficult interventional challenges but will be amenable to a fairly standard open surgical reconstruction. An excellent review of the current literature on critical limb ischemia was published by Lawrence and Chandra[12] in 2010. Their conclusions were that there are five conditions, which endovascular surgeons agree should be treated by open surgery. They are: common femoral disease, extrinsic arterial compressions, extensive foot gangrene or sepsis, young patients and those requiring dependent-free soft-tissue reconstructions where durability is paramount, and infrageniculate popliteal and proximal tibial occlusions with a single target vessel.

Despite acceptable outcomes for endovascular therapy for rest pain, tibial revascularization is unlikely to be sufficient for patients with extensive soft tissue infection. The need to temper expectations for tissue loss and endovascular therapy was reiterated this year by a large study of Medicare patients. Vogel and colleagues[13] reviewed the results of 13,258 Medicare beneficiaries who underwent tibioperoneal angioplasty for critical limb ischemia. While 42.8% had gangrene and 46.7% had rest pain, 10.5% had claudication and by most measure would not have been included in a study on CLI. The procedures were angioplasty (47.3%), stenting (29.3%) and atherectomy (20.1%). However patients had multiple readmissions and the 24% of patients had undergone an amputation at 30 days. Most of the major limb amputations were in patients with tissue loss. This seems to reinforce the perception that limb salvage rates for endovascular therapies rarely exceed 80% and are lower when patients with tissue loss only are included.

Of course, no discussion of this area is complete without mention of the Bypass versus Angioplasty in Severe Ischemia of the Leg (BASIL) trial's tribulations[14]. To date, it is the only substantive trial comparing outcomes for surgery and endovascular therapy. The authors looked at outcomes in 452 patients with severe leg ischemia which was defined as rest pain or tissue loss (but not necessarily CLI, by definition) undergoing an 'endovascular-first' versus an 'open-first' approach. The primary outcome measure was amputation-free survival. Secondary outcome measures included all-cause mortality, morbidity, re-intervention, quality of life and hospital costs. The 30-day mortality was low in both groups, at 5% for surgery and 3% for angioplasty. Surgery was associated with a significantly higher morbidity (57% vs. 41%), mainly due to myocardial infarction and wound infection. The surgical patients also stayed in the hospital longer, and this contributed to the cost of surgery being one-third higher than angioplasty at one year. By three years, however, the difference in costs was no longer significant because angioplasty patients had a significantly higher failure rate (20% vs. 3% within 12 months) resulting in a higher re-intervention rate (28% vs. 17%). There was no difference in quality of life, amputation-free survival, or all-cause mortality at any time interval out to two years; and by five years, 36% of patients had died. The conclusions were fairly clear-cut: For patients living at least 2 years, bypass was better, preferably with vein (Figure 18–3). For those unlikely to live two years, and those in whom vein is not available, they are better served by balloon angioplasty. Criticisms of the trial were that it was a multi-center trial with differing definitions of what constituted a best-first option for patients. At each center, the majority of patients evaluated were not considered study patients for reasons that were not made clear. It was also criticized for its combined end point, the high mortality that accounted for 75% of the end points, the failure to address the secondary risk factors, and the absence of data on diabetic control. However, at the least, the BASIL trial was a good starting point for discussion.

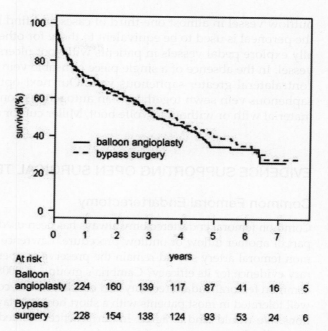

Figure 18–3. Amputation-free survival in BASIL trial patients randomized to a bypass-first or balloon-first revascularization strategy[14]. *Reproduced with permission from the Journal of Vascular Surgery.*

At risk	years						
	0	1	2	3	4	5	6	7
Balloon angioplasty	224	160	139	117	87	41	16	5
Bypass surgery	228	154	138	124	93	53	24	6

OPEN SURGERY ALGORITHMS FOR CLI

As stated at the outset, there appears to be general agreement about the best approach to aortoiliac occlusive disease. The TASC II document[5] summarizes it nicely: Endovascular therapy is the treatment of choice for type A lesions and surgery is the treatment of choice for type D lesions. For TASC B and C lesions: Endovascular treatment is the preferred treatment for type B lesions and surgery is the preferred treatment for good-risk patients with type C lesions. The real controversies are at the infrainguinal level. Therefore, this will be the focus of this section.

The Albany Medical Center Algorithm for Open Infrainguinal Revascularization for CLI

Our approach to open reconstruction in patients with CLI is based on over three decades of experience. Some may argue with our choice of techniques (and some may indeed seem idiosyncratic), but our limb salvage rate is consistently over 90%, suggesting that something is working.

For isolated femoropopliteal disease, we perform a common femoral to below-knee popliteal in situ bypass, as we believe the patency rates for an autologous in situ reconstruction to the infrageniculate popliteal artery is superior to that for a reversed common femoral to above-knee popliteal bypass. This has been our practice for the last twenty years. In fact, we rarely perform a common femoral to above knee popliteal bypass using reversed greater saphenous vein (GSV) unless acceptable conduit is limited.

For tibial disease, we perform in situ bypass in the majority of patients. In 60–70% of patients, we employ our so-called 'closed' technique using the 3mm Leather cutter, supplemented by a modified Mills' valvulotome. We use the peroneal artery as our outflow vessel in almost one-third of cases and find healing rates for foot ulcers when the peroneal is used to be equivalent to those for other tibial vessels. We will also liberally explore pedal vessels in patients with foot ulcers or rest pain for a usable outflow vessel. In the absence of a single piece of usable vein from the affected leg, we will use contralateral greater saphenous vein. Our next option is spliced arm vein or lesser saphenous vein sewn together as an autogenous conduit. Our last option is prosthetic material with or without a Wolfe boot, Miller cuff or arteriovenous fistula.

EVIDENCE SUPPORTING OPEN SURGICAL TECHNIQUES FOR CLI

Common Femoral Endarterectomy

Common femoral endarterectomy always has been used extensively, either in isolation or as part of another inflow or outflow procedure. Lawrence and Chandra[12] stated that the common femoral artery should remain the preserve of open surgery. So, what's the contemporary evidence for its efficacy? Cambria's group[15] in 2008 reviewed contemporary results for common femoral endarterectomy and concluded that common femoral endarterectomy was well tolerated in most patients with a short hospital stay (mean 3.2 days) and few complications. We would tend to agree. In our practice, isolated common femoral disease is treated surgically. Endarterectomy of vessels below the common femoral should be done sparingly, if at all. Superficial femoral artery lesions that would do well with endarterectomy (limited in length and stenosis) are better treated by endovascular techniques. Endarterectomy of infrageniculate arteries only rarely works despite an initial pleasing cosmetic outcome.

Profundaplasty

Profundaplasty has always been an important tool in any vascular surgeon's toolbox. In latter years, isolated profundaplasty has been disregarded in favor of more extensive bypass operations. However, it has not been totally discarded. In 2010 Koscielny and colleagues[16] from Bonn reviewed their experience 28 matched patient pairs who underwent supragenicular bypass or profundaplasty. The authors reinforce our previous argument that tissue loss and rest pain ought to be considered as opposite ends of the CLI spectrum: The outcomes for claudication and rest pain in these patients were identical. However, profundaplasty patients did less well if they had ulcers or gangrene or a single tibial artery runoff.

Femoropopliteal Bypass

Although the first procedure was performed in 1949, there are still controversies. Our preferences and prejudices regarding vein bypass have been described above. Yet, there are contemporary data that contradict some of our and Veith's practices[17]. In 2007 the Project of Ex-vivo Vein graft Engineering via Transfection III (PREVENT III) trial was published[18]. Shah and colleagues[19] commented that although the agent under investigation (edifoglide) was ineffective, the study provided high-quality prospective data on leg bypasses with vein. Some of the findings were predictable: Single-segment GSV is better than arm vein or lesser saphenous vein, with spliced vein performing worst (64% Vs 52% vs. 42% one-year patency). GSV grafts less than 3 mm did worse that GSV veins greater than 3.5 mm (68% Vs 42% one-year patency). Length of bypass appeared important: bypasses less than 40 cm in length had a one-year patency of 69% Vs 54% for those over 60 cm. Contradicting our practices, in-situ graft were found to be equal to reversed and site of inflow and outflow had no bearing on patency.

Tibial and Pedal Bypass

Our techniques of tibial artery and pedal artery bypasses have been described in previously (Figure 18–4). Our own preference is for in situ vein bypass to the tibial and pedal vessels for rest pain and gangrene. We have also published our outcomes for claudicants undergoing this procedure, although such patients comprise fewer than 10% of our total vein tibial bypass patients. The durability of tibial and pedal bypass is surprisingly good with limb salvage rates in our center approaching 80% at five years.

However, our patients are living longer. As a result, they have often already had either a coronary or peripheral artery bypass by the time they present. In the late 1980's, in our practice, 80% of patients had an intact ipsilateral greater saphenous vein. Now, fewer than 50% of our patients have this option left. As a result, many of our reconstructions are orthograde single vein or spliced vein reconstructions. Spliced arm vein has been used extensively by us and others[20,21]. The results from our center in 2002 showed similar primary patency rates: 44% for arm vein at two years and 49% for prosthetic grafts) but better secondary patency rates for arm vein (87% versus 59%) although arm vein bypasses required a lot of secondary interventions to maintain patency[21]. More recent data from Helsinki, in 2010, confirmed the superiority of spliced arm vein over prosthetic for infrapopliteal bypass[22]. In a review of 290 consecutive

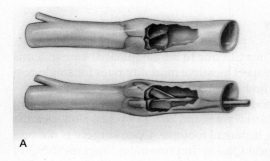

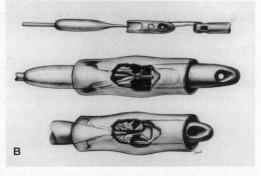

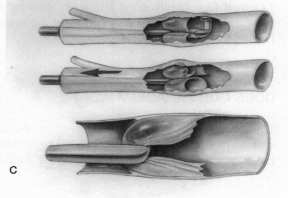

Figure 18–4. The technique of **a.** proximal valve lysis under direct vision, **b.** use of the Leather cutter for the 'closed' part of the in situ bypass and **c.** finally, lysis of the remaining valves using a modified Mills valvulotome from the inaugural edition of the Journal of Vascular Surgery in 1984. *Reproduced with permission from the Journal of Vascular Surgery.*

bypasses, spliced arm vein had a secondary patency at three years of 57% versus 11% for prosthetic grafts with a better limb salvage rate also (75% versus 57%).

In some cases, there is little choice but to pursue a prosthetic option. The initial results for direct anastomosis of synthetic graft to tibial arteries were poor. In part it was thought that the reason was the difference in compliance between the synthetic graft and the native artery. The addition of ancillary techniques such as the Miller cuff, Taylor patch and Wolfe boot seemed to improve patency rates as, it was thought, it mitigated "compliance mismatch". Work by Harris and his group[23] subsequently suggested that the benefits were due to the unique geometry of these reconstructions rather than any compliance issues. This led to the development of preformed cuffed grafts (the DistaFlo® and Dynaflo® grafts). Warfarinization is an essential adjunct to treatment.

The latest advance has been the Heparin-bonded graft (Propaten™) with reported[24] patency rates approaching those of greater saphenous vein (and without the need for adjuncts such as cuffs or patches), which seems almost too good to be true.

Some subgroups of CLI patients bear special mention. Chronic renal failure patients are notoriously difficult to affect limb salvage, even with the performance of a successful bypass. They are poor candidates for open surgery due to their often profound comorbidities. In addition, tibial angioplasty in these frequently heavily-calcified arteries is less efficacious compared to non-renal failure patients.Their autogenous conduit is usually limited to the legs, as arm veins are usually needed, or have been used, for dialysis access. In this group, a less optimistic approach is warranted, but we still advocate an aggressive effort toward limb salvage, particularly if patient physiology and enthusiasm permit.

COMPLICATIONS OF OPEN SURGERY

Open revascularization is the "gold standard" for CLI due to infrainguinal disease in terms of durability, relief of symptoms and limb salvage. Operative mortality rates for single centers are reported as less than 2% range and limb salvage rates at 5 years approach 90%. Even in "real life" situations, outcomes are good. A 2009 report[25] on 28,128 Californian leg bypass patients reported limb salvage was 82% at 5 years and 76% at 9 years. However, the 'gold standard' (in its original sense) is now a historical footnote. Open surgery is not perfect. A 2009 study[26] using the National Surgical Quality Improvement Program (NSQIP) database reviewed contemporary outcomes in 2404 patients. Operative (30 day) mortality was 2.7%. Major complications occurred in 18.7%. There were graft thromboses in 7.4% and 9.4% had wound infections. Ironically, healing the surgical incision is the Achilles heel of these operations, taking an average of 4.2 months in one frequently quoted study from Portland, Oregon.[27]

DOES OUR PARADIGM WORK?

The priority for our patients is retention of a functioning healthy limb. For them, terms such as patency rates and target lesion restenosis are of passing interest. Relief of rest pain can be predicted by successful surgical (or endovascular) revascularization in patients with

CLI. What we know less about, however, is how patients with ulcers or tissue loss fare after they leave the OR or the hospital. As vascular surgeons, we tend, naturally, to be procedure-oriented. Although we tend to follow our patients afterwards, our appreciation of successful healing is less than perfect. Pure interventionalists are probably even less aware of long term outcomes, explaining some of the more optimistic expectations of endovascular interventions. What we all have in common, however, is the assumption that once a limb is revascularized, and the graft or stent remains patent, the wound will heal.

There is a growing body of literature that suggests this is not the case. In 2011, Taylor and colleagues[28] presented a very honest appraisal of their success in treating ischemic and neuropathic diabetic foot ulcers (DFU's). Their 5-year limb salvage for revascularized DFU's was 61%, amputation-free survival was 37% and maintenance of ambulation was 55%. While this was striking, the equivalent outcome measures for non-revascularized ischemic DFU's were 51%, 17% and 55%. Their conclusions (as vascular surgeons) were that although revascularization is an effective treatment for ischemia, it is probably overvalued when compared with the potential improvement afforded by better medical foot wound management (control of foot wound sepsis, liberal ulcer debridement, plantar offloading). They further suggested ulcer healing should be the goal of treatment rather than procedure patency. The need for a multidisciplinary approach to foot ulcers was also mentioned in the TASC II report[5]. Others have coined the term "toe and flow" to emphasize the need for co-operation between specialists from vascular surgery (flow) to plastics, orthopedics, infectious disease and finally podiatry ("toe") to achieve ulcer healing.

So, are there any hemodynamic reasons why our interventions don't work? Part of the reason may lie in angiosomes. The foot can be divided into six separate anatomic segments or angiosomes fed by distinct 'source arteries'. Three angiosomes are fed by the posterior tibial artery, two by the peroneal (surprisingly!) and one by the anterior tibial artery (Figure 18–5). Neville and colleagues[29] from Georgetown University looked at whether this had any bearing on wound healing outcomes in 48 patients undergoing tibial bypass. When they directly revascularized the angiosome containing a wound,

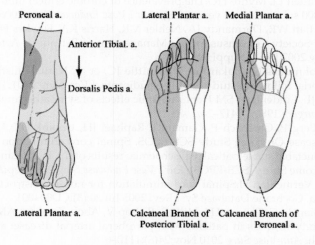

Figure 18–5. Angiosomes of the foot and ankle. *Reproduced with permission from Endovascular Today.*

healing rates were 91%. In those patients in whom the angiosome was not directly revascularized, e.g. a bypass to the peroneal artery was performed when the wound was in the anterior tibial distribution, wound healing was only 62%. Obviously, it is not always possible to perform direct revascularization on all patients. Some patients may have only one patent artery supplying their foot. In some the appropriate artery may be so diseased that it will clearly not support a bypass graft. In still others, there may be no angiographically visible vessels at all. This idea, however, is gaining acceptance with some endovascular specialists beginning to report their results in terms of angiosome specific interventions[30].

CONCLUSIONS

Critical limb ischemia is not a single entity. Therefore, it requires a tailored approach. Tissue loss is the more technically challenging end of the spectrum. Revascularization for these patients is best achieved by open surgery, if they are to have a chance of healing. However, restoring flow is only part of the answer. Graft patency must be supplemented by good wound healing practices. Endovascular procedures cannot always provide in-line, pulsatile flow. Endovascular specialists should recognize these limitations. The only request our patients have is that we preserve their limb.

REFERENCES

1. Reed AB, Delvecchio C, Giglia JS. Major lower extremity amputation after multiple revascularizations:was it worth it? *Ann Vasc Surg* 2008;22(3)335–40.
2. Bell PRF, Charlesworth D, DePalma PG. The definition of critical ischemia of the limb.: Working Party of the International Vascular Symposiu. *Br J Surg* 1982;69:S2
3. Second European Consensus document on chronic critical limb ischemia. *Circulation* 1991;84(4 Suppl):IV1–IV26.
4. Jensen SA, Vatten LJ, Myhre HO The prevalence of chronic critical limb iscaemia in a population of 20,000 subjects 40–69 years of age *Eur J Vasc Endovasc Surg* 2006;32(1):60–65.
5. Norgren L, Hiatt WR, Dormandy JA, Nehler MR, Harris KA, Fowkes FG; TASC II Working Group. Inter-Society Consensus for the Management of Peripheral Arterial Disease (TASC II).*J Vasc Surg* 2007 Jan;45 Suppl S:S5–67
6. Aquino R, Johnnides C, Makaroun M, Whittle JC, et al. Natural history of claudication: Long term serial follow-up study of 1244 claudicants. *J Vasc Surg* 2001;34:962–970
7. Cronenwett JL, Lindenauer SM Hemodynamic effects of sympathectomy in ischemic canine hindlimbs. *Surgery* 1980;87:417–24.
8. Amann W, Berg P, Gersbach P, Gamain J, Raphael JH, Ubbink DT; European Peripheral Vascular Disease Outcome Study SCS-EPOS. Spinal cord stimulation in the treatment of non-reconstructable stable critical leg ischaemia: results of the European Peripheral Vascular Disease Outcome Study (SCS-EPOS). *Eur J Vasc Endovasc Surg* 2003 Sep;26(3):280–6.
9. Ubbink DT, Vermeulen H.Spinal cord stimulation for non-reconstructable chronic critical leg ischaemia. Cochrane Database Syst Rev. 2005 Jul 20;(3):CD004001
10. Chiriano J, Bianchi C, Teruya TH, Mills B, Bishop V, Abou-Zamzam AM Jr. Management of lower extremity wounds in patients with peripheral arterial disease: a stratified conservative approach. *Ann Vasc Surg* 2010 Nov;24(8):1110–6

11. Marston WA, Davies SW, Armstrong B, Farber MA, Mendes RC, Fulton JJ, Keagy BA. Natural history of limbs with arterial insufficiency and chronic ulceration treated without revascularization. *J Vasc Surg* 2006 Jul;44(1):108–114

12. Lawrence PF, Chandra A. When should open surgery be the initial option for critical limb ischemia? *Eur J Vasc Endovasc Surg* 2010 Mar;39 Suppl 1:S32–7

13. Vogel TR, Dombrovskiy VY, Carson JL, Graham AM. In-hospital and 30-day outcomes after tibioperoneal interventions in the US Medicare population with critical limb ischemia. *J Vasc Surg* 2011 Mar 10. [Epub ahead of print]

14. Adam DJ, Beard JD, Cleveland T, Bell J, Bradbury AW, Forbes JF, Fowkes FG, Gillepsie I, Ruckley CV, Raab G, Storkey H; BASIL trial participants. Bypass versus angioplasty in severe ischaemia of the leg (BASIL): multicentre, randomised controlled trial. *Lancet* 2005 Dec 3;366(9501):1925–34.

15. Kang JL, Patel VI, Conrad MF, Lamuraglia GM, Chung TK, Cambria RP.Common femoral artery occlusive disease: contemporary results following surgical endarterectomy. *J Vasc Surg* 2008 Oct;48(4):872–7.

16. Koscielny A, Pütz U, Willinek W, Hirner A, Mommertz G. Case-control comparison of pro-fundaplasty and femoropopliteal supragenicular bypass for peripheral arterial disease. *Br J Surg* 2010 Mar;97(3):344–8

17. Veith FJ, Gupta SK, Ascer E, White-Flores S, Samson RH, Scher LA, Towne JB, Bernhard VM, Bonier P, Flinn WR, et al. Six-year prospective multicenter randomized comparison of autologous saphenous vein and expanded polytetrafluoroethylene grafts in infrainguinal arterial reconstructions. *J Vasc Surg* 1986 Jan;3(1):104–14

18. Schanzer A, Hevelone N, Owens CD, Belkin M, Bandyk DF, Clowes AW, Moneta GL, Conte MS. Technical factors affecting autogenous vein graft failure: observations from a large multicenter trial. *J Vasc Surg* 2007 Dec;46(6):1180–90

19. Shah SK, Baxi KH, Clair DG Critical limb ischemia:surgical perspectives and options Vascular Disease Management 2010;7:214–218.

20. Varcoe RL, Chee W, Subramaniam P, Roach DM, Benveniste GL, Fitridge RA. Arm vein as a last autogenous option for infrainguinal bypass surgery: it is worth the effort. *Eur J Vasc Endovasc Surg* 2007 Jun;33(6):737–41

21. Kreienberg PB, Darling RC 3rd, Chang BB, Champagne BJ, Paty PS, Roddy SP, Lloyd WE, Ozsvath KJ, Shah DM Early results of a prospective randomized trial of spliced vein versus polytetrafluoroethylene graft with a distal vein cuff for limb-threatening ischemia. *J Vasc Surg* 2002 Feb;35(2):299–306

22. Arvela E, Söderström M, Albäck A, Aho PS, Venermo M, Lepäntalo M.Arm vein conduit vs prosthetic graft in infrainguinal revascularization for critical leg ischemia. *J Vasc Surg* 2010 Sep;52(3):616–23

23. Harnessing haemodynamic forces for the suppression of anastomotic intimal hyperplasia: the rational for precuffed grafts. Fisher RK, How TV, Toonder IM, Hoedt MT, Brennan JA, Gilling-Smith GL, Harris PL. *Eur J Vasc Endovasc Surg* 2001 Jun;21(6):520–8

24. Lindholt JS, Gottschalksen B, Johannesen N, Dueholm D, Ravn H, Christensen ED, Viddal B, Flørenes T, Pedersen G, Rasmussen M, Carstensen M, Grøndal N, Fasting H. The Scandinavian Propaten(®) Trial - 1-Year Patency of PTFE Vascular Prostheses with Heparin-Bonded Luminal Surfaces Compared to Ordinary Pure PTFE Vascular Prostheses - A Randomised Clinical Controlled Multi-centre Trial. *Eur J Vasc Endovasc Surg* 2011 May;41(5): 668–73.

25. Feinglass J, Sohn MW, Rodriguez H, Martin GJ, Pearce WH. Perioperative outcomes and amputation-free survival after lower extremity bypass surgery in California hospitals, 1996–1999, with follow-up through 2004. *J Vasc Surg* 2009 Oct;50(4):776–783.

26. LaMuraglia GM, Conrad MF, Chung T, Hutter M, Watkins MT, Cambria RP. Significant perioperative morbidity accompanies contemporary infrainguinal bypass surgery: an NSQIP report. *J Vasc Surg* 2009 Aug;50(2):299–304.

27. Nicoloff AD, Taylor LM Jr, McLafferty RB, Moneta GL, Porter JM.Patient recovery after infrainguinal bypass grafting for limb salvage. *J Vasc Surg* 1998 Feb;27(2):256–63

28. Taylor SM, Johnson BL, Samies NL, Rawlinson RD, Williamson LE, Davis SA, Kotrady JA, York JW, Langan EM 3rd, Cull DL. Contemporary management of diabetic neuropathic foot ulceration: a study of 917 consecutively treated limbs. *J Am Coll Surg* 2011 Apr;212(4): 532–45

29. Neville RF, Attinger CE, Bulan EJ, Ducic I, Thomassen M, Sidawy AN. Revascularization of a specific angiosome for limb salvage: does the target artery matter? *Ann Vasc Surg* 2009 May-Jun;23(3):367–73.

SECTION V

EVAR

19

Using Duplex Ultrasound for Surveillance after EVAR

*Shardul B. Nagre, MBBS, MS, MPH and
William D. Jordan, Jr., MD*

INTRODUCTION

Since its FDA approval in 1999, endovascular repair for abdominal aortic aneurysm (EVAR) is now an accepted modality of treatment as an alternative to open repair. Studies and clinical experience have led clinicians to maintain vigorous imaging standards after EVAR to insure a durable outcome with fixation of the endograft and exclusion of the aneurysm from rupture. One concern after EVAR includes endoleak i.e. continuing blood flow around the graft into the aneurysm sac with a potential risk of aneurysm rupture. Regular surveillance after EVAR is required to identify patients with increasing aneurysm diameter or presence of endoleaks. Computed tomographic angiography (CTA) has been used as preferred modality for surveillance in majority of the clinical trial protocols. CTA provides detailed information about anatomy of aneurysm sac, and can identify endoleaks by demonstrating flow of contrast into the sac. However, exposures to radiation, contrast-related nephrotoxicity, and its costs have raised concern about the suitability of EVAR. Due to its relatively novel nature, EVAR requires more intense imaging than open AAA but this increased surveillance need may inappropriately increase the total treatment cost creating a problem in the cost-conscious age of health care reform. Instead clinicians have sought alternative imaging means to avoid some of these detrimental aspects of CTA. Specifically, duplex ultrasound (DUS) has been advocated to supplement and potentially replace CTA for post-operative surveillance after EVAR. We present a case for increase utilization of DUS for post-EVAR surveillance to limit the deleterious aspects of CTA and maintain a reliable monitor to assure endograft durability and freedom from rupture.

BACKGROUND STUDIES

Ultrasound is commonly used as a screening tool to evaluate the abdominal aorta in patients who have an abnormal exam or in whom there is a suspicion for AAA. This modality can accurately identify aneurysms that reach a large enough diameter that there is concern for rupture. After EVAR, aneurysm diameter as measured by DUS correlates well with diameter on CTA as shown by Wolf et al.[1] When adding the duplex portion to an ultrasound examination, one can assess the flow through the iliac limbs and endoleaks. Some studies have shown that DUS is insensitive in endoleak detection.[2,3,4] More recent studies show that DUS is comparable to and sometimes superior to CTA in detecting endoleaks and can also predict need for re-intervention.[5,6,7,8] A recent study suggested a protocol demonstrating exclusive and early use of DUS in patients with shrinking or stable aneurysms as a safe method of surveillance.[9]

CT Angiography

CT angiography has been used as the standard after EVAR to assess endograft stability and exclusion of the aneurysm to avoid rupture. Multiple clinical trials have been completed with careful clinical surveillance to satisfy a critical community of vascular surgeons who had doubt about the durability of EVAR and to satisfy the regulatory agencies before approval for the general medical community. It has been accepted that patients who undergo EVAR require continued surveillance and increased re-intervention rate compared to open AAA to maintain clinical success after EVAR. CTA can accurately demonstrate the patients who have endoleaks or graft migration that might require re-intervention. However, there has been concern that the CTA sometimes shows minor findings that have little clinical significance. Instead, we suppose that DUS, while not as sensitive, can identify those patients who have a clinically significant endoleak or an increase in aneurysm diameter that necessitates further intervention.

UAB Experience

We reviewed our experience at UAB to determine the suitability of DUS compared to CTA to identify endoleaks and then to predict the need for re-intervention after EVAR.[10] Over a 10-year period (1999–2009), we identified 1062 EVARs in 992 patients. After EVAR, our initial imaging included CTA and DUS at the first visit to evaluate the correlation between the two modalities. We compared the ability of the imaging techniques to identify an endoleak and the correlation of the maximum diameter size. Ultimately our goal was to use DUS as the primary imaging tool and our surveillance pattern reflected that goal by a continuous shift to DUS with an abdominal x-ray. DUS imaging and CTA were evaluated with attention towards maximum aneurysm diameter, patency of graft and presence of an endoleak. A change in size by more than 5 mm from the first post-op follow-up CTA or DUS was termed significant and was investigated more thoroughly for possible re-intervention. Our study evaluated patients with EVAR who had discrepancies in endoleak detection between CTA and DUS and to determine whether these discrepancies played a role in the long term outcome after EVAR. We sought to determine that CTA might be overly sensitive in identifying endoleaks and the DUS might be a better tool for identifying endoleaks and predicting the need for re-intervention based upon other markers in spite missing endoleaks.

Imaging: All color duplex ultrasounds was done using a Sequoia 512 Acuson Sonography System (Siemens Medical Solutions, Mountain View, CA, USA) by a registered vascular technician in our accredited vascular laboratory. Using 4C1 transducers, the abdominal aorta and iliac arteries were investigated in transverse and anterior-posterior images were obtained. Maximum diameter of the sac was determined using these images. Color Doppler was used to identify any endoleak, graft patency, and limb flow abnormalities. The DUS exam was done on a limited basis without a time-intense study to identify a small endoleak particularly considering the CTA was done during the same visit. Computed tomographic angiography was performed using GE LightSpeed 16 CT scanner (General Electric Medical Systems, Milwaukee, WI). Both contrast and non-contrast images were obtained by performing helical scans from the diaphragm to upper thigh using a thin section CT angiography protocol. Nonionic intravenous contrast material was administered. The scan delay was determined by bolus tracking. In patients with abnormal renal function (Creatinine > 1.4 mg/dl) CT without contrast along with DUS was obtained.

Statistical Analysis: Patients with both CTA and DUS studies recorded at the same visit or within 7 days of each other were selected. Endoleaks that were identified within 30 days of follow-up were classified as early endoleaks while those detected after 30 days were classified as late endoleaks.

Statistical analysis included demographics, operative and clinical characteristics. Chi-square test was used for categorical data while mean +/– standard deviation was used for continuous variables. P value less than 0.05 was considered significant.

UAB Experience - *Results*

There were a total of 3120 post-operative imaging encounters recorded via the surveillance protocol. Of these 3120 encounters, 1729 were DUS encounters (1.9 per patient) while 2001 were CTA scans (2.2 per patient) with 610 of these encounters recording a CTA and DUS at the same visit. Contrast was not used in 49 CT scans, leaving 561 encounters, in 455 patients, for comparing CTA imaging with DUS findings.

In this matched group of 561 encounters, 173 (31%) had a documented endoleak either on CTA or DUS. CTA scan recorded 14 Type I, 135 Type II and 5 Type III endoleaks, while DUS recorded 9 Type I, 62 Type II, 2 Type III endoleaks. Table 19–1 shows the distribution of the type of endoleaks for CTA and DUS. CTA and DUS findings correlated in 442 encounters (78.8%). Discrepancies occurred in 119 encounters (21.2%) as follows: CTA scan only endoleak in 17.8% (N=100; Type I=6, Type II=91; Type III=3) (Figure 19–1) and DUS only endoleak in 3.4% (N=19; Type II=19) encounters.

Most (99) of these 119 encounters did not require secondary interventions suggesting that the CT might be very sensitive for finding endoleaks but it may be finding endoleaks that are small and have little clinical significance. Only 15 patients required

TABLE 19–1. COMPARING CT ANGIOGRAPHY AND DUPLEX ULTRASOUND FINDINGS AFTER 561 SIMULTANEOUS IMAGING ENCOUNTERS (N=561)

Endoleak detected	Type I	Type II	Type III	No Endoleak	Total (%)
CTA (+), DUS (+)	8	44	2	–	54 (9.6)
CTA (+), DUS (–)	6	91	3	–	100 (17.8)
CTA (–), DUS (+)	0	19	0	–	19 (3.4)
CTA (–), DUS (–)	–	–	–	388	388 (69.2)
Total	14	154	5	388	

CTA – CT angiography; DUS – Duplex ultrasound.

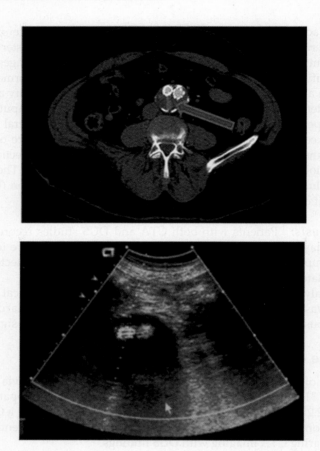

Figure 19–1. CT angiography identifies a type II endoleak that is not visible on an ultrasound exam.

19 re-interventions after 20 discrepant encounters (3.6%). Eleven patients continued with the surveillance protocol via CTA or DUS imaging, while 4 were followed by CTA imaging due to the absence of endoleak on DUS and the usually large patient size that made DUS imaging so difficult. Rarely, had a Type II endoleak that was missed by CTA and detected on DUS on subsequent follow-up. Of these 15 patients, 12 were diagnosed with an early endoleak, while the remaining 3 were diagnosed with a late endoleak. There was no rupture, graft migration, limb occlusion, or structural failure in any of these 15 patients who maintained the surveillance protocol.

ENDOLEAKS MISSED BY DUS

Type I Endoleak

Interventions: Of the 6 patients where DUS missed a Type I endoleak, 5 required re-interventions. Three patients required iliac extenders to resolve a Type Ib endoleak, of which one patient required two interventions. One patient required a proximal cuff while the fifth required a complete relining of the graft due to the greater clinical concern of endotension as a contributing factor to the aneurysm expansion. The sixth patient had an endoleak visible on the first follow-up visit that resolved in his subsequent visits.

Other indicators by DUS: Considering these 5 patients who required intervention, DUS was able to use other surrogates to determine the need for re-intervention. Specifically, DUS demonstrated an increase in size of the aneurysm sac in 2 other patients while DUS identified the endoleak in one patient on a subsequent scan even though it was not seen on the first scan. The difference in a later DUS could also be related to a different DUS operator or additional time that was taken on later examinations to interrogate for an endoleak. The 2 remaining patients were followed with CTA (due to the identified inability of DUS to adequately follow the EL) only after the first visit until subsequent intervention was required.

Type II Endoleak

Interventions: Most patients (76) with type II endoleaks did not require intervention. Only 9 patients underwent re-intervention for an increase in aneurysm size even though DUS missed the Type II endoleak. These interventions included embolizations (6), explants (2), and relining (1). The relining was done due to the judged minor type II endoleak and the concern about endotension.

Other indicators by DUS: DUS identified the endoleak during a subsequent follow-up in 3 patients. Two patients were followed with CTA only due to the clinician's judgment after the first visit until they underwent intervention; one with embolization and the other with endograft explant. DUS demonstrated an increase in size of the aneurysm sac in 2 other patients who later underwent embolization, one of which also had a Type III endoleak treated with distal extender. DUS failed to demonstrate an endoleak and did not show a significant increase in size in only 2 patients during the entire follow-up period. Both these patients underwent embolization due to CT findings that raised clinical concern about the aneurysm.

Type III Endoleak

Interventions: There were 3 patients with type III endoleaks that were missed by DUS, of which only one patient required re-intervention with distal iliac extender. The first patient who was treated with an extender limb graft underwent an angiogram intra-operatively that CT had demonstrated a type III endoleak. The same patient also had 2 embolization procedures as previously mentioned. That is, DUS saw the type II but had missed the type III. The second patient was previously treated for a type III endoleak. At the first visit after this re-intervention, CTA showed a minor residual endoleak that subsequently resolved, while DUS did not visualize the endoleak. In the third patient, DUS missed an endoleak that CTA detected as type III endoleak that was not seen on the subsequent angiogram. Instead it was a type II that was not treated at the time. He has remained asymptomatic with stable aneurysm size 3 years into follow-up and has not required subsequent intervention. These "type III" interventions that were done suggest that the CT may be overly sensitive in identifying clinically relevant problems considering the subsequent angiogram and treatment was not needed for a type III endoleak.

One patient had a type II endoleak that was detected on DUS but missed on CTA on multiple visits. This patient eventually underwent complete relining of the endograft due to the clinical suspicion of endotension. In retrospect, the DUS showed the increase in aneurysm diameter but not the endoleak. If both parameters (diameter and endoleak) are considered then the patient can often be identified as needing further intervention to stabilize the aneurysm.

REVIEW OF CONCEPT

Surveillance after EVAR is necessary and is recognized to improve outcome of the primary repair. The primary goal is to identify potential complications and determine the need for intervention. Possible complications include different types of endoleaks, increase in aneurysm size, migration of graft, graft limb failure or occlusion, structural failure and risk of potential rupture. Lifelong surveillance is important after any vascular procedure due to the recurring nature of the disease. There is no standard protocol for surveillance after EVAR and usually a varying combination of CTA, DUS and angiography is utilized. Many surgeons employ CTA as the exclusive method in surveillance. It provides very reliable and reproducible information on complications after EVAR. But CTA carries the risk of repeated radiation exposure and contrast use. Side effects include contrast allergy, renal function impairment due to iodinated contrast, and increased risk of malignancy.[11] Annual CT scans do not provide additional benefit in majority of EVAR patients thus reducing the frequency of CTA may simplify surveillance with an improved safety profile.[12] In addition, the high costs associated with CTA are concerning in long-term follow-up. It is estimated that CTA alone accounts for 65% of the total cost of EVAR,[13] thus justifying limiting its use while promoting other modalities that offer equivalent results when used alone or combined with CTA.

DUS is being increasingly used in surveillance after EVAR and is effective as demonstrated in many studies. Even though it has not been established for exclusive surveillance, it does offer many advantages. It is safe, non-invasive, easily available, less costly and associated with no known side effects. However, it is operator dependent, it can be difficult to perform in large body habitus or with excess bowel gas, requires a long time for complete assessment and may miss some subtle complications after EVAR. Graft limb occlusion and aneurysm size can be assessed reliably with DUS. It correlates well with CTA for detecting aneurysm size during follow-up.[14,15,16] Wolf et al studied 100 patients who had undergone EVAR and followed them up with both CTA and DUS at regular intervals. They found that maximal aneurysm diameter correlated very well ($r = 0.93$; $P < 0.001$) without a significant difference in paired analysis.[17] Endoleak assessment with DUS has conflicting reports as to sensitivity, specificity, positive predictive value, and negative predictive value. Some studies have reported high values,[18,19,20] while others have mixed results in these tests.[21,22,23] The UAB study results demonstrate a low sensitivity (35%), high specificity (95%), 74% positive predictive value and 79% negative predictive value. Our current technique involves a focused scan that is done relatively quickly as opposed to doing a more thorough interrogation of the aneurysm; hence we might be missing small endoleaks. With newer equipment, continued experience and improvement of technique for a focused scan, these results may be able to demonstrate the endoleaks that are clinically important. Taking into account these findings, we decided to focus our attention on analyzing the long-term outcome following EVAR in patients that had both CTA and DUS done at the same time. We identified discrepancies in the two that were further analyzed to assess the need for re-intervention. We hypothesized that DUS could provide better indicators for re-intervention even if it failed to identify a small endoleak and that majority of the endoleaks missed by DUS either resolved over time or were not clinically significant.

The suggested DUS protocol emphasizes that the need for both modalities recorded at the same time at the first post-implant visit, and at the first visit after re-intervention. Then depending upon clinical findings, aneurysm size and presence of endoleak, CTA or DUS can be used at intervals of 6 months or 1 year. The treating clinician can then judge when to change to DUS only after a correlating CT scan ensures safety. While 3 ruptures occurred in our entire EVAR treatment experience, no rupture occurred in patients who maintained the prescribed surveillance protocol. The total re-intervention rate in the UAB cohort of 561 patients was 11.9%; patients in whom both modalities ruled out endoleak, it was 8.2%, while patients in whom both modalities identified an endoleak, it was 29.6%.

No major complication occurred in our study cohort when DUS missed an endoleak. DUS detected the endoleak on subsequent visits, or detected a significant increase in size in all patients that underwent intervention. Conclusions cannot be drawn on those 4 patients who were followed with CTA only after the first visit but one should consider the importance of clinical judgment in choosing the best surveillance modality. Endoleaks may be missed initially if they are small or due to patient factors like body habitus, or bowel gas. However, these small endoleaks may not have real clinical significance. Aneurysm size increase can be reliably detected even if endoleak is missed, as a persistent endoleak may pressurize the sac and lead to enlargement.[24]

Many of these studies, including our own, are retrospective in nature and face those usual limitations. However, as the collective clinical experience has grown throughout the world, more data is available to show the value and efficacy of DUS as the major surveillance tool after EVAR. But practical constraints in clinical practice do not allow for both investigations to be done at each visit and thus is difficult to implement. An extensive DUS was not obtained in our patients, which resulted in the low sensitivity that we observed. The number of endoleaks that were missed with DUS and were detected on CTA was more than those missed by CTA scan and detected on DUS. While DUS has lower sensitivity in detecting endoleaks, comparison with CTA findings can identify the appropriate patients for US surveillance only. Even considering the discrepancies between the two modalities, repeat US surveillance may identify an unstable aneurysm (i.e., increase in diameter) that requires further intervention.

As the frequency of CT scanning as increased across multiple areas of medicine, there has been an increasing concern about the deleterious effects of this imaging modality, Instead, MRI and DUS have been increasingly used for surveillance after EVAR. More recently, contrasted DUS has gained attention as an even more sensitive modality for imaging the abdominal aorta without nephrotoxic agents or ionizing radiation.[25] However, these new methods of contrast-enhanced duplex ultrasound,[26] magnetic resonance angiography[27,28] carry more cost and are not readily available. These new modalities are sensitive but remain some limited in their widespread use. Additionally, these may reflect the same sensitivity as CT imaging and thus may be better used for the unusual post-EVAR situation that requires more intensive monitoring. Instead, DUS, while less sensitive, may represent the appropriate balance between adequate imaging at relatively low cost with wide applicability. DUS is available in most centers treating aneurysms and can continue as a valuable tool in this regard.

CONCLUSION

EVAR requires long term surveillance to prevent potential complications associated with EVAR and to identify patients for possible re-intervention. An ideal surveillance protocol will not only reduce the costs and risks associated with CTA scan, but also provide comparable sensitivity and specificity. With EVAR procedures gaining in popularity, it is important to develop a protocol that is both economically viable and reliable. Although DUS has not been established as an exclusive surveillance tool, it can be used to effectively monitor most patients after EVAR with reduced need for CT imaging.

REFERENCES

1. Wolf YG, Johnson BL, Hill BB, et al. Duplex ultrasound scanning versus computed tomographic angiography for postoperative evaluation of endovascular abdominal aortic aneurysm repair. *J Vasc Surg* 2000; 32(6):1142–48.
2. AbuRahma AF, Welch CA, Mullins BB, et al. Computed Tomography versus Color Duplex Ultrasound for Surveillance of Abdominal Aortic Stent-Grafts. *J Endovasc Ther* 2005; 12: 568–73.
3. Roy A, Brown LC, Rodway A, et al. Color Duplex Ultrasonography Is Insensitive for the Detection of Endoleak After Aortic Endografting: A Systematic Review. *J Endovasc Ther* 2005;12:297–305.
4. Raman KG, Missig-Carroll N, Richardson T, et al. Color-flow duplex ultrasound scan versus computed tomographic scan in the surveillance of endovascular aneurysm repair. *J Vasc Surg* 2003; 38(4):645–51.
5. Schmieder GC, Stout CL, Stokes GK, et al. Endoleak after endovascular aneurysm repair: Duplex ultrasound imaging is better than computed tomography at determining the need for intervention. *J Vasc Surg* 2009; 50(5):1012–18.
6. Manning BJ, O'Neill SM, Haider SN, et al. Duplex ultrasound in aneurysm surveillance following endovascular aneurysm repair: a comparison with computed tomography aortography. *J Vasc Surg* 2009; 49(1):60–5.
7. Collins JT, Boros MJ, Combs K. Ultrasound Surveillance of Endovascular Aneurysm Repair: A Safe Modality versus Computed Tomography. *Ann Vasc Surg* 2007; 21(6):671–5.
8. Nagre SB, Taylor SM, Passman MA, Patterson MA, Combs BR, Lowman BG, Jordan WD Jr. Evaluating outcomes of endoleak discrepancies between computed tomography scan and ultrasound imaging after endovascular abdominal aneurysm repair. *Ann Vasc Surg* 2011 Jan;25(1):94–100.
9. Chaer RA, Gushchin A, Rhee R, et al. Duplex ultrasound as the sole long-term surveillance method post-endovascular aneurysm repair: A safe alternative for stable aneurysms. *J Vasc Surg* 2009; 49(4):845–9.
10. Nagre SB, Taylor SM, Passman MA, Patterson MA, Combs BR, Lowman BG, Jordan WD Jr. Evaluating outcomes of endoleak discrepancies between computed tomography scan and ultrasound imaging after endovascular abdominal aneurysm repair. *Ann Vasc Surg* 2011 Jan;25(1):94–100.
11. Brenner DJ, Hall EJ. Computed Tomography – An Increasing Source of Radiation Exposure. *N Engl J Med* 2007; 357(22):2277–84.
12. Dias NV, Riva L, Ivancev K, et al. Is There a Benefit of Frequent CT Follow-up After EVAR? *Eur J Vasc Endovasc Surg* 2009; 37(4):425–30.
13. Prinssen M, Wixon CL, Buskens E, et al. Surveillance after Endovascular Aneurysm Repair: Diagnostics, Complications, and Associated Costs. *Ann Vasc Surg* 2004; 18(4):421–7.
14. Wolf YG, Johnson BL, Hill BB, et al. Duplex ultrasound scanning versus computed tomographic angiography for postoperative evaluation of endovascular abdominal aortic aneurysm repair. *J Vasc Surg* 2000; 32(6):1142–48.

15. Raman KG, Missig-Carroll N, Richardson T, et al. Color-flow duplex ultrasound scan versus computed tomographic scan in the surveillance of endovascular aneurysm repair. *J Vasc Surg* 2003; 38(4):645–51.
16. Beeman BR, Doctor LM, Doerr K, et al. Duplex ultrasound imaging alone is sufficient for midterm endovascular aneurysm repair surveillance: A cost analysis study and prospective comparison with computed tomography scan. *J Vasc Surg* 2009; 50(5):1019–24.
17. Wolf YG, Johnson BL, Hill BB, et al. Duplex ultrasound scanning versus computed tomographic angiography for postoperative evaluation of endovascular abdominal aortic aneurysm repair. *J Vasc Surg* 2000; 32(6):1142–48.
18. Wolf YG, Johnson BL, Hill BB, et al. Duplex ultrasound scanning versus computed tomographic angiography for postoperative evaluation of endovascular abdominal aortic aneurysm repair. *J Vasc Surg* 2000; 32(6):1142–48.
19. Schmieder GC, Stout CL, Stokes GK, et al. Endoleak after endovascular aneurysm repair: Duplex ultrasound imaging is better than computed tomography at determining the need for intervention. *J Vasc Surg* 2009; 50(5):1012–18
20. Manning BJ, O'Neill SM, Haider SN, et al. Duplex ultrasound in aneurysm surveillance following endovascular aneurysm repair: a comparison with computed tomography aortography. *J Vasc Surg* 2009; 49(1):60–5.
21. AbuRahma AF, Welch CA, Mullins BB, et al. Computed Tomography Versus Color Duplex Ultrasound for Surveillance of Abdominal Aortic Stent-Grafts. *J Endovasc Ther* 2005; 12: 568–73.
22. Roy A, Brown LC, Rodway A, et al. Color Duplex Ultrasonography Is Insensitive for the Detection of Endoleak after Aortic Endografting: A Systematic Review. *J Endovasc Ther* 2005; 12:297–305.
23. AbuRahma AF. Fate of Endoleaks Detected by CT Angiography and Missed by Color Duplex Ultrasound in Endovascular Grafts for Abdominal Aortic Aneurysms. *J Endovasc Ther* 2006; 13:490–5.
24. Veith FJ, Baum RA, Ohki T, et al. Nature and significance of endoleaks and endotension: Summary of opinions expressed at an international conference. *J Vasc Surg* 2002; 35(5): 1029–35.
25. Cantisani V, Ricci P, Grazhdani H, Napoli A, Fanelli F, Catalano C, Galati G, D'Andrea V, Biancari F, Passariello R. Prospective comparative analysis of colour-Doppler ultrasound, contrast-enhanced ultrasound, computed tomography and magnetic resonance in detecting endoleak after endovascular abdominal aortic aneurysm repair. *Eur J Vasc Endovasc Surg* 2011 Feb;41(2):186–92. Epub 2010 Nov 20.
26. Iezzi R, Basilico R, Giancristofaro D, et al. Contrast-enhanced ultrasound versus color duplex ultrasound imaging in the follow-up of patients after endovascular abdominal aortic aneurysm repair. *J Vasc Surg* 2009; 49(3):552–60.
27. van der Laan MJ, Bartels LW, Viergever MA, et al. Computed Tomography versus Magnetic Resonance Imaging of Endoleaks after EVAR. *Eur J Vasc Endovasc Surg* 2006; 32(4):361–5.
28. Stavropoulos SW, Baum RA. Imaging modalities for the detection and management of endoleaks. *Semin Vasc Surg* 2004; 17(2):154–60.

20

Aneurysmal Extension to the Iliac Bifurcation in Patients Undergoing EVAR

Peter A. Naughton, MD, M. Park, MD,
E. A. Kheirelseid, MD, A. Moriarty, MD,
M. P. Colgan, MD, D. J. Moore, MD, S. M. O'Neill, MD,
H. E. Rodriguez, MD, Mark D. Morasch, MD,
P. Madhavan, MD and Mark K. Eskandari, MD

INTRODUCTION

Endovascular abdominal aortic aneurysm repair (EVAR) has evolved as a feasible, less-invasive alternative to open repair[1]. Increased experience and improved understanding of EVAR has enabled refinement of this technique. However, treating aneurysms by endovascular intervention with unfavorable anatomy or outside the manufacturers IFU (instructions for use) may predispose to treatment failure. Limiting the long-term complications specific to EVAR is a challenge.

Poor patient or stent-graft selection undermines the effectiveness of EVAR[2]. Various pre-, intra- and post-operative factors may compromise repair and must be considered at the time of pre-operative planning, intervention and follow-up. To date most studies report the outcome of EVAR in patients with adverse morphological features at the proximal seal, including neck angulation, diameter and thrombus[3,4]. Post-operatively aortic remodeling following successful sac exclusion and late progression of aneurysmal degeneration may predispose to late endoleaks[5,6].

The common iliac artery serves as the distal stent-graft implantation site. Like the proximal landing zone a durable distal seal is essential. Aneurysmal involvement at the common iliac artery aneursym (CIAA) may limit full exclusion of the aneurysm and increase the complexity of EVAR[7-9]. In this review we examine the clinical significance of aneurysmal extension into the common iliac artery and outline the surgical options available to attenuate the risk of early and late complications.

CLINICAL SIGNIFICANCE OF CIAA IN EVAR

Concomitant CIA aneurysms are present in 15–40% of patients with AAA[10]. These CIA aneurysms may challenge the long-term benefits of EVAR if a robust distal seal is not achieved. Alternatively, the risks of deploying additional stent-grafts into external iliac arteries may also compromise long-term stent-graft patency[7]. There is also evidence that patients with a challenging CIA have additional unfavourable anatomical factors and more extensive medical co-morbidities[8].

Three contemporary large single-center studies examine re-intervention following EVAR and highlight the importance of achieving good distal stent-graft apposition and iliac limb patency[9–11]. Mehta et al report the largest single-center experience of 1768 patients who underwent EVAR with a mean follow-up of 34 months[12]. 19.2 % of patients underwent re-intervention for aneurysm-related complications. Progressive iliac artery aneurysm formation was the third most common indication (11.5%) for reintervention and an additional 7.4% of reinterventions were for iliac limb thrombosis. Iliac limb occlusion was the second most common indication for re-intervention in a series of 832 EVAR patients[10]. Becquemin et al in a series of 250 patients report that type 1b endoleaks were the second most common indication for re-intervention[11]. In all three studies problems related to the distal landing zone were a more common indication for re-intervention than proximal seal compromise. Indeed in our series of patients who underwent endovascular re-intervention following EVAR in Northwestern Memorial hospital type 1b endoleak was the most common indication for re-intervention[2].

Clearly distal limb seal and patency are of paramount importance but few studies focus on outcome of patients with concomitant CIAA during EVAR[7,12–14]. Results are conflicting. Three studies report that concomitant CIAA is associated with increased complexity of procedure, AAA-related complications and re-interventions[7,12–14]. Hobo et al using data from the Eurostar Registry (n-6668) compared outcomes after EVAR in patients with and without concomitant CIAA[7]. Those with concomitant CIAA had a higher incidence of type 1b endoleaks, iliac limb occlusion, re-interventions and aneurysm rupture. Albertini et al had similar results in patients with or without concomitant CIAA extending to the distal third of the CIA[12]. All cases of graft limb thrombosis were associated with stent-graft deployment into the external iliac artery. Parlani et al demonstrated that the presence of CIAA rendered EVAR more complex with significantly longer operative and fluoroscopic time and more contrast used[14].

In contrast, data from the Cook Zenith trial (n=736) failed to show any significant difference in technical success, AAA-related complications or re-intervention in patients with concomitant CIAA[13]. This study involved the use of more contemporary stent-graft technology and a higher proportion of patients received flared limbs rather than endograft extension to the external iliac artery compared to the previous studies. Importantly approximately 30% of all EVAR patients developed CIA expansion and stent-graft oversizing was the only identified risk factor for expansion.

SURGICAL OPTIONS FOR CONCOMITANT CIAA DURING EVAR

A variety of open and endovascular techniques are available to treat patients with concomitant CIAA during EVAR. In the absence of any randomized controlled studies and only two comparative studies evidence standardization of treatment is poor[15,16].

Mainstays of treatment include achieving successful distal exclusion of aneurysm and maintaining limb perfusion. Secondly a decision on preserving or sacrificing the internal iliac artery needs to be made.

Options on how to effectively treat this cohort of patients include:

1. Internal iliac embolization/occlusion with extension of stent-graft to the external iliac extension (IIE+EE)
2. Flared limb or Bell-Bottom technique to the CIA (BBT)
3. Iliac Side Branch Device (IBD)
4. Open advancement of the CIA bifurcation by internal iliac artery bypass/transposition.
5. Aorto-uniiliac stent-graft with femoral-femoral bypass (AUI) with a retrograde EIA-IIA endograft

Approach adopted may be influenced by patient anatomy, operator preference, availability of appropriate stent-graft and financial constraints. Detailed pre-operative imaging using computed tomographic angiography with 3-D reconstruction is essential in case planning to anticipate access difficulties, facilitate wire and catheter choice and optimise positioning of the C-arm. At this time evaluation of the contra-lateral landing zone and patency of the contralateral IIA is also of great importance and is discussed later.

Internal Iliac Embolization/Occlusion with Extension of Stent-Graft to the External Iliac Extension (IIE+EE) (Figure 20–1)

IIE+EE is generally favoured when aneurysmal disease extends to or beyond the bifurcation of the CIA and in the presence of significant thrombus in the distal CIAA[15]. IIE is required prior to stent-graft deployment to obviate the risk of type II endoleaks. Occasionally, when the orifice of the internal iliac artery (IIA) is very stenotic, in cases of chronic renal failure when use of contrast volume needs to be minimised or in emergency cases the origin may be covered by the graft limb without embolization[17].

In most cases access to the internal iliac artery is from a contra-lateral groin approach. Access may be complicated by contra-lateral external iliac tortuosity, unfavourable angulation of the aortic bifurcation and a large ipsilateral CIAA. Alternative access sites include an ipsilateral or brachial approach.

Once stable access is achieved embolization of the IIA can be achieved using coils (MR Eye Coils, Cook Inc) or an Amplatzer vascular plug (AVP, AGA Medical, Golden Valley, MN). Coils or AVP are placed at the origin of the IIA . The presence of an IIA aneurysm may preclude flush occlusion and proximal embolization. In these circumstances the primary branches of the IIA are embolized. The relative benefits of embolizing with coils is that they can be delivered via a standard 5 French 0.038 catheter making them particularly suitable in patients with extreme tortuosity, reverse taper, severe IIA stenosis and/ or a short IIA main trunk[18]. The main pitfalls associated with coil embolization are coil prolapse into the external iliac artery or coil migration beyond the IIA main trunk. Alternatively, the AVP device is a self-expanding nitinol cylindrical wire mesh plug deployed through an appropriately sized guiding sheath or guiding catheter, while the newest AVP, the AVP 4 can be delivered via a 0.038 diagnostic catheter. Attributes of this system include the ability to accurately position the AVP at the target site while preserving flow of the IIA bifurcation and the ability to reconstrain and reposition the device as needed following deployment but prior to release[18]. This precision of positioning at the origin of the IIA prevents the risks

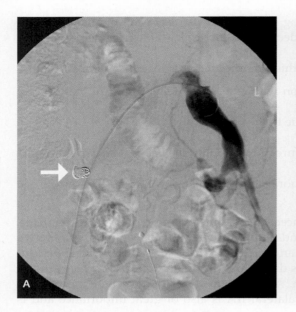

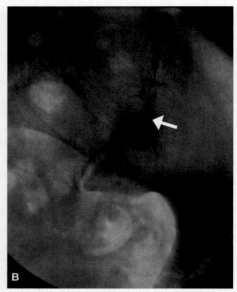

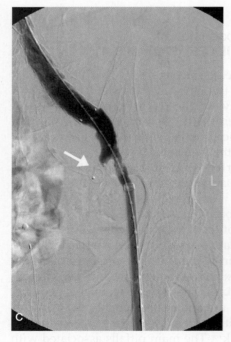

Figure 20–1a. Digital subtraction angiogram demonstrates an aneurysmal left common iliac artery extending to the bifurcation. Note the coil pack in the contralateral internal iliac (arrow) placed on a separate occasion for a staged bilateral iliac embolization. **b.** Fluoroscopic unsubtracted obliqued image shows the amplatazer vascular plug (AVP) II (arrow) following deployment in the left internal iliac artery. Note the characteristic dumbbell shape of the deployed device (arrow). **c.** Check angiography demonstrates no flow into the embolized left internal iliac artery.

inherent with inadvertent coil malpositioning and the use of a single device assists with cost reduction[19]. The main limitation of AVP use is difficulty in delivering the guiding sheath to the target site.

The risk of ischemic complications limits the appeal of IIE. Ischemia may be caused by coils misplacement and is most commonly associated with pelvic malperfusion. Ipsilateral buttock claudication and sexual dysfunction is reported in 40% and 20% of patients respectively[20–22]. In addition there are documented cases of bowel infarction, paraplegia and gluteal compartment syndrome[23]. There is contrasting evidence that buttock claudication may dissipate with time due to the development of a collateral blood supply[24].

The severity of symptoms following sacrifice of one or both IIA is unpredictable. Symptoms may be affected by demand of the end organs in the territory of the IIA and by the presence of a collateral blood supply. Younger, more active patients and patients with a reduced cardiac output are at highest risk of ischemic symptoms[25]. Collateral blood supply is provided from the contralateral IIA, profunda femoris and external iliac branches[26]. Intuitively, strategies to preserve this collateral network may assuage ischemic complications. This may be achieved by interrupting the IIA as proximally as possible thereby preserving the IIA bifurcation[20]. Some advocate timing (staging) of IIE prior to EVAR facilitates development of pelvic collaterals[20]. However there is also no evidence for the benefit of sequential rather than simultaneous bilateral IIE[27]. A systematic literature review failed to demonstrate a higher incidence of pelvic ischemia in patients undergoing bilateral IIE prior to EVAR compared to unilateral IIE[28]. In view of the unpredictability of complications techniques to preserving IIA flow should always be considered.

Following IIE, extension of the stent-graft to the external iliac artery (EE) completes EVAR. Use of additional iliac stent-graft limbs are associated with increased risks of limb occlusion[7,10]. Velazques et al used centerline software-assisted measurements to significantly reduce the need for iliac extensions[29]. Cochennec et al reviewed 33 patients with graft thrombosis and found that kinking was the most frequent predictor of thrombosis[30]. To diminish this risk, Conrad et al advocate removing the stiff wire at the timing of completion angiogram and if a kink is identified treating it with deployment of an additional stent[10].

Flared Limb or Bell-Bottom Technique to the CIA (BBT) (Figure 20–2)

The distal attachment zone of the stent-graft must be completely sealed to ensure exclusion of the aneurysm. Initially the BBT involved deploying an aortic extension cuff or a reverse-mounted iliac limb stent-graft in the distal CIA landing zone[31-33]. This strategy has the benefit of preserving antegrade flow into the IIA. This technique has now been superseded by the introduction of commercially available large diameter iliac extension limbs of up to 28mm diameter (Endurant stent-graft, Medtronic Cardiovascular, Santa Rosa, California).

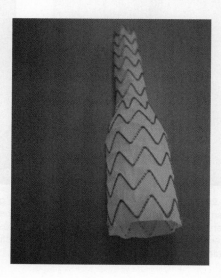

Figure 20–2. Photograph of a flared iliac limb (Medtronic Endurant, CA, USA) used in the bell bottom technique.

Concerns exist about the long-term durability of deploying large diameter iliac extension limbs into a CIAA thereby predisposing to future aneurysmal degeneration after EVAR and development of a distal type 1b endoleak. Data on the progression of CIA diameter after open AAA repair show that growth is directly proportional to baseline diameter[34]. Ballotta et al found that CIAs 19-22mm in diameter expanded at twice the growth rate of non-aneurysmal CIAs[34]. While long-term follow-up is lacking for patients with concomitant CIA undergoing EVAR with flared limbs, Kirkwood et al reported that patients treated with flared limbs were not predisposed to future CIA growth but care needs to be taken to avoid stent-graft oversizing[13].

Iliac Side Branch Device (IBD) (Figure 20–3)

IBD extend distally from the main-body of the conventional stent-graft to the EIA and preserves flow into the IIA via a side-branch. A variety of clinical and morphological indications for IBD deployed are reported[35]. Tielliu et al excluded IBD in patients with limited levels of activity[36]. IBD is particularly preferred in patients with contralateral IIA occlusion. Anatomical requirements for successful treatment with IBD include; suitable 15mm length of EIA for distal fixation; absence of excessive iliac tortuosity; patent lumen of CIA of at least 20mm in diameter and 40mm in length; a landing zone of at least 10mm in the main internal iliac trunk and a normal diameter IIA[15,35].

There are two IBD systems commercially available; the Helical Iliac Side Branch (HBIS) (Cook Inc., Bloomington, IN, USA) and the Zenith Bifurcated Side Branch device (ZBIS) (Cook Inc., Bloomington, IN, USA). Both devices involve using a pre-loaded wire from the side branch that is snared from the contra-lateral common femoral artery thereby enabling a through-and-through access into the IIA[15,37]. The HBIS consists of a 6- or 8-mm branch emerging in a helical fashion from the 12-mm main body and has a left and right model. This branch assumes a helical path around the external portion of

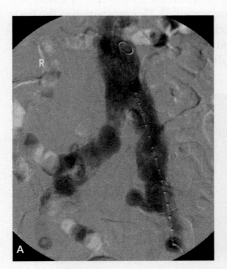 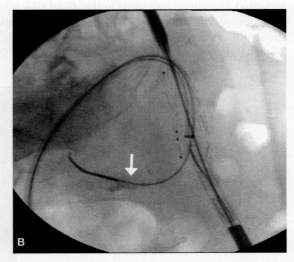

Figure 20–3a. Digital subtraction angiogram with a graduated pigtail catheter in the aorta demonstrates an aneurysmal abdominal aorta extending into both common iliac arteries. **b.** Fluoroscopic unsubstracted obliqued image shows the left iliac limb partially deployed across the orifice of the left internal iliac artery. The left internal iliac artery has been canulated via the iliac limb fenestration with a Kumpe catheter (arrow) via an up and over contralateral approach. *(continued)*

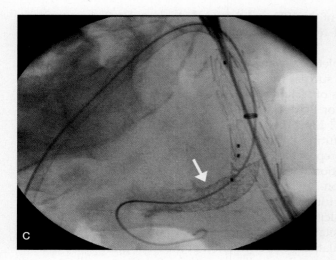

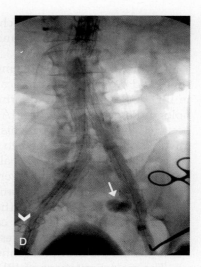

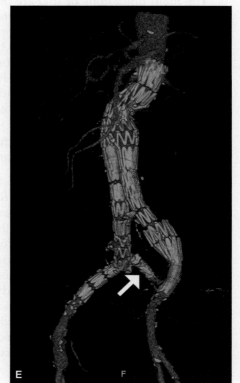

Figure 20–3c. *(continued)* A V12 (Advanta, Atrium Medical Corporation, New Hampshire, USA) stentgraft (arrow) has been deployed within the left internal iliac artery through the iliac limb fenestration. **d.** Completion angiography following entire branched stentgraft deployment demonstrates preserved patency of left internal iliac artery via the iliac limb fenestration and V12 stentgraft (arrow). Note the contralateral coils within the right internal iliac artery (arrowhead). **e.** Volume rendered view of a CT angiogram demonstrating patency of the left internal iliac artery (arrow) following EVAR with a branched stentgraft technique.

the main body to optimise flow dynamics into the IIA[37]. The ZBIS is similar to the Zenith AAA modular stent-graft main body and the same model can be used on the left or right side. The ZBIS is introduced over a stiff-wire and orientated under fluoroscopic guidance. After the iliac branch is deployed a covered stent (Advanta V12; Atrium Medical, Hudson, NH or Fluency; C.R Bard Inc, Murray Hill, NJ) is deployed to fill the gap between the side branch of the IBD and the IIA[19]. A more detailed comparison between these two devices and techniques of deployment is reported by Ferreira et al[38].

Karthikesalingam et al completed a systemic review of IBD[35]. This included nine series and 196 patients. Technical success was 85–100%. A learning curve was identified in IBD deployment both in terms of technical expertise and improved stent-graft technology. Re-occlusion of the IIA or EIA occurred in 12% of patients and claudication occurred in half of these patients[35]. Most IBD occlusions of the IIA were treated conservatively and did not portend to future endoleaks. Only one type 1b and two type III endoleaks occurred. Verzini et al report the only comparative study of IBD to IIE + EE[15]. Technical success and reintervention rates are similar but IIE + EE had higher rates of endoleaks and buttock claudication.

A variety of technical difficulties can be encountered during IBD deployment. Negotiation of tortousity and calcification in the iliac arteries or sharp angulation of the aortic bifurcation may necessitate a brachial approach. Caution must also be taken not to dissect the IIA upon cannulation or over-dilation of the stent-graft in the IIA.

The main limitations of IBD are only small proportion of patients with concomitant CIAA are anatomically suitable for these devices and the additional cost to the procedure. IIA embolization costs approximately $470, whereas a ZBIS device costs $6000 with an addition cost for the bridging stent[39]. Cautious patient selection is appropriate, some advocate this approach in younger, active patients with the highest risk of symptomatic pelvic ischemia if the IIA flow is sacrificed[15]. Improvements in experience, stent-graft technology and standardization of patients at highest risk of pelvis ischemia will expand the applicability of this technique in the future.

Open Advancement of the CIA Bifurcation by Internal Iliac Artery Bypass/Transposition

This procedure involves advancing the CIA bifurcation by re-siting the origin of the IIA thereby preserving flow. Access to the IIA and EIA may be achieved by a retroperitoneal approach[16]. Unlike conventional bypass procedures the distal anastomosis to the IIA should be performed first to simplify the procedure in view of the deep location of the IIA[40]. The proximal anastomosis is performed to the underside of the EIA by rotating the vessel with the vascular clamps. The oversown proximal IIA should be marked with a large clip to assist identification of the distal landing zone at stent-graft deployment.

Lee et al report a comparative study of IIE+EE to IIA bypass[16]. Procedure time and blood loss was significantly greater in the bypass group. Bypass patients experienced less buttock ischemia than IIE+EE and had a 36 month graft patency of 91%. Patient obesity and patients with very calcified IIA and EIA are relative contra-indication for this procedure. Patient preference very often is for a completely endovascular option if possible[16].

Aorto-Uniiliac Stent-Graft with Femoral-Femoral Bypass (AUI) with a Retrograde EIA-IIA Endograft

This hybrid repair involves ipsilateral IIE, deployment of an aorto-uniiliac stent-graft to the ipsilateral EIA, femoral-femoral bypass and contralateral EIA to IIA stent-graft to maintain pelvic perfusion. This technique is reported in only a small series of patients[41]. While an attempt is made to maintain IIA perfusion, long-term durability may be undermined by the use of an extra-anatomical bypass and the unproven long-term patency of an EIA to IIA endograft[42]. Improvements in endovascular technology and technique mean that this approach is rarely employed.

CONCLUSION

Concomitant CIAA is present in a significant proportion of patients undergoing EVAR. A number of surgical approaches are available and should be carefully considered at pre-operative planning. We advocate preservation of pelvic perfusion when feasible due to the unpredictable nature of ischemic complications encountered in IIE. Further improvements in stent-graft technology may improve results and assist in the preservation of pelvic perfusion.

REFERENCES

1. Greenhalgh RM, Brown LC, Kwong GP, et al. Comparison of endovascular aneurysm repair with open repair in patients with abdominal aortic aneurysm (EVAR trial 1), 30-day operative mortality results: randomised controlled trial. *Lancet* 2004 Sep 4;364(9437):843–8.
2. Naughton PA, Garcia-Toca M, Rodriguez HE, et al. Endovascular Treatment of Delayed Type 1 and 3 Endoleaks. *Cardiovasc Intervent Radiol* 2010 Nov 25.
3. Zayed HA, Attia R, Modarai B, et al. Predictors of reintervention after endovascular repair of isolated iliac artery aneurysm. *Cardiovasc Intervent Radiol* 2011 Feb;34(1):61–6.
4. Sampaio SM, Panneton JM, Mozes GI, et al. Proximal type I endoleak after endovascular abdominal aortic aneurysm repair: predictive factors. *Ann Vasc Surg* 2004 Nov;18(6):621–8.
5. Matsumura JS, Pearce WH, McCarthy WJ, et al. Reduction in aortic aneurysm size: early results after endovascular graft placement. EVT Investigators. *J Vasc Surg* 1997 Jan;25(1):113–23.
6. Harris P, Brennan J, Martin J, et al. Longitudinal aneurysm shrinkage following endovascular aortic aneurysm repair: a source of intermediate and late complications. *J Endovasc Surg* 1999 Feb;6(1):11–6.
7. Hobo R, Laheij RJ, Buth J. The influence of aortic cuffs and iliac limb extensions on the outcome of endovascular abdominal aortic aneurysm repair. *J Vasc Surg* 2007 Jan;45(1):79–85.
8. Hobo R, Sybrandy JE, Harris PL, et al. Endovascular repair of abdominal aortic aneurysms with concomitant common iliac artery aneurysm: outcome analysis of the EUROSTAR Experience. *J Endovasc Ther* 2008 Feb;15(1):12–22.
9. Mehta M, Sternbach Y, Taggert JB, et al. Long-term outcomes of secondary procedures after endovascular aneurysm repair. *J Vasc Surg* 2010 Dec;52(6):1442–9.
10. Conrad MF, Adams AB, Guest JM, et al. Secondary intervention after endovascular abdominal aortic aneurysm repair. *Ann Surg* 2009 Sep;250(3):383–9.
11. Becquemin JP, Kelley L, Zubilewicz T, et al. Outcomes of secondary interventions after abdominal aortic aneurysm endovascular repair. *J Vasc Surg* 2004 Feb;39(2):298–305.
12. Albertini JN, Favre JP, Bouziane Z, et al. Aneurysmal extension to the iliac bifurcation increases the risk of complications and secondary procedures after endovascular repair of abdominal aortic aneurysms. *Ann Vasc Surg* 2010 Jul;24(5):663–9.
13. Kirkwood ML, Saunders A, Jackson BM, et al. Aneurysmal iliac arteries do not portend future iliac aneurysmal enlargement after endovascular aneurysm repair for abdominal aortic aneurysm. *J Vasc Surg* 2011 Feb;53(2):269–73.
14. Parlani G, Zannetti S, Verzini F, et al. Does the presence of an iliac aneurysm affect outcome of endoluminal AAA repair? An analysis of 336 cases. *Eur J Vasc Endovasc Surg* 2002 Aug;24(2):134–8.

15. Verzini F, Parlani G, Romano L, et al. Endovascular treatment of iliac aneurysm: Concurrent comparison of side branch endograft versus hypogastric exclusion. *J Vasc Surg* 2009 May;49(5):1154–61.

16. Lee WA, Nelson PR, Berceli SA, et al. Outcome after hypogastric artery bypass and embolization during endovascular aneurysm repair. *J Vasc Surg* 2006 Dec;44(6):1162–8.

17. Rhee RY, Muluk SC, Tzeng E, et al. Can the internal iliac artery be safely covered during endovascular repair of abdominal aortic and iliac artery aneurysms? *Ann Vasc Surg* 2002 Jan;16(1):29–36.

18. Resnick SA, Eskandari MK. Outcomes of Amplatzer vascular plugs for occlusion of internal iliacs during aortoiliac aneurysm stent grafting. *Ann Vasc Surg* 2008 Sep;22(5):613–7.

19. Ha CD, Calcagno D. Amplatzer Vascular Plug to occlude the internal iliac arteries in patients undergoing aortoiliac aneurysm repair. *J Vasc Surg* 2005 Dec;42(6):1058–62.

20. Mehta M, Veith FJ, Ohki T, et al. Unilateral and bilateral hypogastric artery interruption during aortoiliac aneurysm repair in 154 patients: a relatively innocuous procedure. *J Vasc Surg* 2001 Feb;33(2 Suppl):S27–S32.

21. Lin PH, Bush RL, Chaikof EL, et al. A prospective evaluation of hypogastric artery embolization in endovascular aortoiliac aneurysm repair. *J Vasc Surg* 2002 Sep;36(3):500–6.

22. Karch LA, Hodgson KJ, Mattos MA, et al. Adverse consequences of internal iliac artery occlusion during endovascular repair of abdominal aortic aneurysms. *J Vasc Surg* 2000 Oct;32(4):676–83.

23. Kritpracha B, Comerota AJ. Unilateral lower extremity paralysis after coil embolization of an internal iliac artery aneurysm. *J Vasc Surg* 2004 Oct;40(4):819–21.

24. Farahmand P, Becquemin JP, Desgranges P, et al. Is hypogastric artery embolization during endovascular aortoiliac aneurysm repair (EVAR) innocuous and useful? *Eur J Vasc Endovasc Surg* 2008 Apr;35(4):429–35.

25. Wyers MC, Schermerhorn ML, Fillinger MF, et al. Internal iliac occlusion without coil embolization during endovascular abdominal aortic aneurysm repair. *J Vasc Surg* 2002 Dec;36(6):1138–45.

26. Iliopoulos JI, Hermreck AS, Thomas JH, et al. Hemodynamics of the hypogastric arterial circulation. *J Vasc Surg* 1989 May;9(5):637–41.

27. Bratby MJ, Munneke GM, Belli AM, et al. How safe is bilateral internal iliac artery embolization prior to EVAR? *Cardiovasc Intervent Radiol* 2008 Mar;31(2):246–53.

28. Rayt HS, Bown MJ, Lambert KV, et al. Buttock claudication and erectile dysfunction after internal iliac artery embolization in patients prior to endovascular aortic aneurysm repair. *Cardiovasc Intervent Radiol* 2008 Jul;31(4):728–34.

29. Velazquez OC, Woo EY, Carpenter JP, et al. Decreased use of iliac extensions and reduced graft junctions with software-assisted centerline measurements in selection of endograft components for endovascular aneurysm repair. *J Vasc Surg* 2004 Aug;40(2):222–7.

30. Cochennec F, Becquemin JP, Desgranges P, et al. Limb graft occlusion following EVAR: clinical pattern, outcomes and predictive factors of occurrence. *Eur J Vasc Endovasc Surg* 2007 Jul;34(1):59–65.

31. Torsello G, Schonefeld E, Osada N, et al. Endovascular treatment of common iliac artery aneurysms using the bell-bottom technique: long-term results. *J Endovasc Ther* 2010 Aug; 17(4):504–9.

32. Kritpracha B, Pigott JP, Russell TE, et al. Bell-bottom aortoiliac endografts: an alternative that preserves pelvic blood flow. *J Vasc Surg* 2002 May;35(5):874–81.

33. Karch LA, Hodgson KJ, Mattos MA, et al. Management of ectatic, nonaneurysmal iliac arteries during endoluminal aortic aneurysm repair. *J Vasc Surg* 2001 Feb;33(2 Suppl): S33–S38.

34. Ballotta E, Da Giau G, Gruppo M, et al. Natural history of common iliac arteries after aorto-aortic graft insertion during elective open abdominal aortic aneurysm repair: a prospective study. *Surgery* 2008 Nov;144(5):822–6.

35. Karthikesalingam A, Hinchliffe RJ, Holt PJ, et al. Endovascular aneurysm repair with preservation of the internal iliac artery using the iliac branch graft device. *Eur J Vasc Endovasc Surg* 2010 Mar;39(3):285–94.

36. Tielliu IF, Bos WT, Zeebregts CJ, et al. The role of branched endografts in preserving internal iliac arteries. *J Cardiovasc Surg (Torino)* 2009 Apr;50(2):213–8.
37. Greenberg RK, West K, Pfaff K, et al. Beyond the aortic bifurcation: branched endovascular grafts for thoracoabdominal and aortoiliac aneurysms. *J Vasc Surg* 2006 May;43(5):879–86.
38. Ferreira M, Monteiro M, Lanziotti L. Technical aspects and midterm patency of iliac branched devices. *J Vasc Surg* 2010 Mar;51(3):545–50.
39. Vandy F, Criado E, Upchurch GR, Jr., et al. Transluminal hypogastric artery occlusion with an Amplatzer vascular plug during endovascular aortic aneurysm repair. *J Vasc Surg* 2008 Nov;48(5):1121–4.
40. Faries PL, Morrissey N, Burks JA, et al. Internal iliac artery revascularization as an adjunct to endovascular repair of aortoiliac aneurysms. *J Vasc Surg* 2001 Nov;34(5):892–9.
41. Bergamini TM, Rachel ES, Kinney EV, et al. External iliac artery-to-internal iliac artery endograft: a novel approach to preserve pelvic inflow in aortoiliac stent grafting. *J Vasc Surg* 2002 Jan;35(1):120–4.
42. Tsang JS, Naughton PA, Wang TT, et al. Endovascular repair of para-anastomotic aortoiliac aneurysms. *Cardiovasc Intervent Radiol* 2009 Nov;32(6):1165–70.

21

Long-term Results of Palmaz Stenting

Samir K. Shah, MD and Daniel G. Clair, MD

Since its inception roughly 20 years ago endovascular aneurysm repair (EVAR) has revolutionized the treatment of infrarenal abdominal aortic aneurysms. Although device modifications have ameliorated a number of problems that hampered early use – device migration, stent fatigue and fracture, maldeployment, and others – they remain present to varying degrees even today. Indeed, type I endoleak was a crucial problem in Parodi's original experience and remains at present a formidable obstacle to achieving the principal goal of EVAR, namely complete and durable exclusion of the aneurysm[1].

Proximal attachment site endoleaks (type Ia) have been reported to occur intraoperatively in 6–7% of contemporary EVAR cases[2,3]. Type Ia endoleaks have been associated with unfavorable proximal anatomy: short neck length, large neck diameter, excessive neck angulation, the presence of attachment-site mural thrombus or calcification, and a reverse taper neck morphology[4–6]. Proximal endoleaks discovered intraoperatively are not expected to resolve spontaneously and, given the risk of sac pressurization and consequent rupture, mandate prompt intervention. Furthermore, intraoperative proximal endoleaks are likely to become more frequent despite ongoing device improvements due to the increasingly common use of EVAR in patients whose anatomy falls outside the instructions for use for currently approved devices. These two facts taken together clearly demonstrate the critical importance of elucidating appropriate endoleak management and its long-term implications.

There are numerous options for treatment, including placement of periaortic sutures[7], external banding[8], and coil and glue embolization[9], but the mainstay of current treatment of immediate proximal endoleaks first involves molding balloon angioplasty to improve graft-aorta apposition. If the endoleak persists, distance to the lowest renal artery should be examined. It has previously been demonstrated that this distance should be minimized to reduce the risk of migration[10], but in case of suboptimal deployment there may be adequate distance for the placement of an extension cuff. If cuff placement risks coverage of the renal artery ostia, giant Palmaz stent (Cordis Endovascular, Warren, NJ) placement is appropriate.

Despite universal acceptance of the use of Palmaz stents for treatment of proximal endoleaks with self-expanding stent grafts, data regarding long-term outcomes, including delayed endoleak, mortality, graft migration, and aneurysm growth, are sparse. Chung et al. provided intermediate-term data in late 2010[11]. The study retrospectively examined 56 patients who received one of four commercially available self-expanding stent grafts: 7 required balloon angioplasty only, 22 received extension cuffs, 15 received Palmaz stents, while 12 required both extension cuffs and Palmaz stent placement to achieve endoleak resolution. The indication for adjunctive therapy was proximal endoleak in 87.5% of patients, with stent graft migration accounting for the balance. Patients who received adjunctive neck therapy were not statistically different from 118 EVAR patients who did not require such treatment with respect to age, gender, medical comorbidities, and neck morphology (angulation, length, diameter, presence of >50% thrombus, reverse taper configuration). Thirty-day rates of death, reintervention, and endoleak were similar between the two groups. Palmaz stent use was associated with an overall decreased freedom from a graft-related event, defined as survival without aneurysm-related intervention (e.g. repeat adjunctive neck procedure risk, conversion to open repair) and aneurysm-related morbidity (migration, recurrent type I endoleak, limb thrombosis, aneurysm enlargement, rupture). This was significant on univariate analysis but not multivariate analysis, in which only increasing age and elevated preoperative serum creatinine remained significant. Although lending support to the safety and effectiveness of Palmaz stent use, this study, which provided the longest-term results at the time of its publication, was severely limited by the loss to follow-up of 50% of the cohort by 12 months and a mean follow-up of 15.2 +/– 12.2 months. Additionally, as the authors noted, the small study size poses a significant risk of type II error.

Nevertheless, Chung's conclusions are broadly supported by two recent studies from Cleveland Clinic that had more extensive follow-up and data. Rajani et al. provide stronger evidence of freedom from recurrent endoleak with Palmaz use[3]. They studied 72 self-expanding stent graft recipients from 2001 to 2009, who received 48 extension cuffs and 24 Palmaz stents after intraoperative discovery of proximal endoleak. All patients treated exclusively with Palmaz stents had immediate endoleak resolution; 3 cuff patients additionally required Palmaz placement and were subsequently analyzed as part of the Palmaz group. There was no recurrent endoleak in the latter group, while three patients who had received extension cuffs developed recurrent proximal endoleak at 3, 12, and 60 months. Mean CT follow-up was 25.2 and 34.9 months in the cuff and Palmaz stent groups, respectively. However, only 65% of the entire cohort had a CT beyond 3 months. Admittedly, the sample size, although slightly larger than Chung's, was still small.

The most detailed study with the lengthiest follow-up is provided by Arthurs et al. in a report on 31 patients with immediate type Ia endoleak after placement of a Zenith stent graft (Cook Medical, Bloomington, IN)[2]. All patients had a single Palmaz stent placed; 6 patients had a Zenith extender placed before Palmaz stenting at the surgeon's discretion to guard against tearing of the graft fabric. All patients had resolution of endoleak with placement. No patient had recurrent endoleak during the follow-up period, 58 +/– 49 months. Significant percentages of patients experienced aortic degeneration immediately below the superior mesenteric artery (36%), infrarenal neck (34%), and 15 mm below the lowest renal artery (63%). Average increase in diameter was 1.9 mm, 2.8 mm, and 3.2 mm, respectively. Aneurysm sac growth of at least 10% aneurysm diameter was seen in 25% of patients. Although statistically insignificant, at last follow-up the stent graft was caudally displaced 1.3 mm (p=0.53) along with a mean aortic neck length loss of 2.1 mm (p=0.45), resulting in a proximal seal zone loss of 3.3 mm (p=0.06). No graft, however, had migrated more than 10 mm. It is important to note that patients experiencing loss of neck length had statistically longer follow-up than those without: 98 vs. 44 months (p<0.05). Likewise, patients with proximal seal zone loss had greater follow-up: 81 vs. 46 months (p<0.05). Clearly, the fraction of patients experiencing these phenomena may be higher with more extensive follow-up.

These studies collectively suggest that Palmaz stent placement is a highly effective treatment for proximal endoleak both immediately and in the long-term, and that placement does not seem to increase risk of perioperative reintervention or mortality. Maldeployment (secondary to "watermelon seeding"), graft fabric perforation, and aortic rupture were not seen and risks of these events may be overstated. There are, however, two significant concerns regarding the use of a balloon-expandable Palmaz stent with a self-expanding stent graft. The first of these is the gradual aortic neck degeneration observed in numerous studies[12–15]. Arthurs et al. also noted a similar phenomenon at both the suprarenal and infrarenal segments[2]. Indeed, they report that 3/31 patients demonstrated complete separation of the Palmaz stent and stent graft. Although none of these 3 patients required additional intervention, this is problematic. Continued incremental aortic degeneration coupled with a fixed, non-expanding Palmaz could lead to loss of Palmaz-aorta apposition superiorly and stent-graft-aorta apposition inferiorly. Frank endoleak would not be observed because of thrombus interposed between these surfaces, leading instead to an occult type Ia from trans-thrombus pressure transmission, which has been previously documented[16]. This theoretical risk requires detailed investigation and may indeed clarify the durability and appropriateness of Palmaz use.

The second concern is the continued aneurysm expansion noted in patients who had initial success achieving a proximal seal after Palmaz stent placement. While none of these patients experienced rupture or graft migration, the fact that at least one quarter of patients had some aneurysm expansion, implies that either Palmaz stent/graft separation may pose a risk in terms of continued proximal seal, or that a graft treated with a Palmaz may be inherently unstable when followed for a long period of time[2].

It is evident that Palmaz stents are acutely helpful in treating proximal seal issues. Nonetheless, long-term use of these devices warrants further evaluation to assure that aneurysm expansion and Palmaz/graft separation will not jeopardize outcomes for patients.

REFERENCES

1. Parodi J, Palmaz J, Barone H. Transfemoral Intraluminal Graft Implantation for Abdominal Aortic Aneurysms. *Ann Vasc Surg* 1991;5(6):491–499.
2. Arthurs ZM, Lyden SP, Rajani RR, Eagleton MJ, Clair DG. Long-Term Outcomes of Palmaz Stent Placement for Intraoperative Type Ia Endoleak During Endovascular Aneurysm Repair. *Ann Vasc Surg* 2011;25(1):120–126.
3. Rajani RR, Arthurs ZM, Srivastava SD, Lyden SP, Clair DG, Eagleton MJ. Repairing immediate proximal endoleaks during abdominal aortic aneurysm repair. *J Vasc Surg* 2011.
4. Cao P, De Rango P, Verzini F, Parlani G. Endoleak after endovascular aortic repair: classification, diagnosis and management following endovascular thoracic and abdominal aortic repair. *J Cardiovasc Surg (Torino)* Feb 2010;51(1):53–69.

5. Stanley BM, Semmens JB, Mai Q, et al. Evaluation of patient selection guidelines for endoluminal AAA repair with the Zenith Stent-Graft: the Australasian experience. *J Endovasc Ther* Oct 2001;8(5):457–464.

6. Sternbergh Iii WC, Carter G, York JW, Yoselevitz M, Money SR. Aortic neck angulation predicts adverse outcome with endovascular abdominal aortic aneurysm repair. *J Vasc Surg* 2002;35(3):482–486.

7. Tzortzis E, Hinchliffe RJ, Hopkinson BR. Adjunctive procedures for the treatment of proximal type I endoleak: the role of peri-aortic ligatures and Palmaz stenting. *J Endovasc Ther* Apr 2003;10(2):233–239.

8. Younis G, Messner G, Gregoric I, Krajcer Z. Aortic wrap as a novel technique of type I endoleak repair. *Ann Vasc Surg* Sep 2006;20(5):690–695.

9. Maldonado TS, Rosen RJ, Rockman CB, et al. Initial successful management of type I endoleak after endovascular aortic aneurysm repair with n-butyl cyanoacrylate adhesive. *J Vasc Surg* Oct 2003;38(4):664–670.

10. Zarins CK, Bloch DA, Crabtree T, Matsumoto AH, White RA, Fogarty TJ. Stent graft migration after endovascular aneurysm repair: importance of proximal fixation. *J Vasc Surg* Dec 2003;38(6):1264–1272; discussion 1272.

11. Chung J, Corriere MA, Milner R, et al. Midterm results of adjunctive neck therapies performed during elective infrarenal aortic aneurysm repair. *J Vasc Surg* 2010;52(6):1435–1441.

12. Badran M, Gould D, Raza I, et al. Aneurysm Neck Diameter after Endovascular Repair of Abdominal Aortic Aneurysms. *JVIR* 2002;13(9):887–892.

13. Cao P. Predictive factors and clinical consequences of proximal aortic neck dilatation in 230 patients undergoing abdominal aorta aneurysm repair with self-expandable stent-grafts. *J Vasc Surg* 2003;37(6):1200–1205.

14. Maldonado TS, Rosen RJ, Rockman CB, et al. Initial successful management of type I endoleak after endovascular aortic aneurysm repair with n-butyl cyanoacrylate adhesive. *J Vasc Surg* 2003;38(4):664–670.

15. Napoli V, Sardella SG, Bargellini I, et al. Evaluation of the proximal aortic neck enlargement following endovascular repair of abdominal aortic aneurysm: 3-years experience. *EJR* 2003;13(8):1962–1971.

16. Schurink GW, van Baalen JM, Visser MJ, van Bockel JH. Thrombus within an aortic aneurysm does not reduce pressure on the aneurysmal wall. *J Vasc Surg* Mar 2000;31(3): 501–506.

22

Endoleaks after Endovascular Repair of Ruptured AAA: Do They Matter?

Nam T. Tran, MD and Benjamin W. Starnes, MD

INTRODUCTION

It is estimated that approximately 4,500 to 5,000 patients present each year with ruptured abdominal aortic aneurysm (rAAA).[1] Despite advances in peri-operative management and critical care, outcomes of open repair of rAAA have not changed significantly over the last two decades. A recent population analysis showed operative mortality at 40–50% with a 30 days mortality approaching 70%.[2]

In the last 20 years, the surgical management of abdominal aortic aneurysm has undergone a complete metamorphosis from open surgical repair to endovascular repair. With endovascular repair, lifelong follow up is required to prevent aneurysm related morbidity and mortality. Stent graft failure, migration, infection, and aneurysm sac enlargement from endoleak and endotension have all been reported. As the indication for endovascular aneurysm repair (EVAR) has expanded to rAAA, the natural history and management strategy of endoleak become even more relevance.

BACKGROUNDS

In 1990, Juan Parodi and colleagues performed the 1st endovascular abdominal aortic aneurysm repair.[3] Since that time, the surgical treatment of abdominal aortic aneurysm (AAA) has undergone a revolutionary change as a direct result of the endovascular evolution. In the beginning, only a small number of patients would qualify for endovascular repair while many would not due to anatomic factors such as short infrarenal neck, significant neck angulation, and iliac tortuosity. Since then, substantial advances have been made in both endograft technology and the endovascular management of patients with

213

AAA. Smaller delivery system, trans renal fixation, advanced image processing with 3-D reconstruction, and branched/fenestrated endograft technology have made it possible for virtually all aneurysms to be approached with endovascular techniques. Today, EVAR is considered relatively safe and effective for the treatment of AAA. Furthermore, it is often offered as the first line therapy for patients with aneurismal disease. Recent analysis of the Medicare population shows that up to 78% of patients with AAA are repaired with endovascular techniques as compared to only 35% in 2001.[4]

Similarly, the endovascular evolution has carried over to the emergent setting where patients present with rupture aneurysm. Ohki and Veith first reported on using endograft and endovascular technology to manage rAAA in 2000.[5] At that time, their institutional series included only 12 patients who were treated with a custom-made aortouni-iliac stent graft and femoral to femoral crossover bypass. The overall mortality was only 12%, a drastic improvement over open repair. Subsequently, familiarity and expertise with endovascular repair of elective AAA have translated into the management of rAAA. Ruptured endovascular repair of aneurysm, or rEVAR, has became much more common and is available in virtually all metropolitan areas in the United Stated. More and more centers have transition to endovascular techniques as the preferred method of treatment for rAAA. In 2008, over 30% of rAAA underwent endovascular repair as compared to 0% in 1995.[4]

ENDOVASCULAR REPAIR OF RUPTURED AAA (REVAR)

Endovascular management of ruptured AAA requires a system wide approach involving pre hospital personnel such as paramedics and EMT unit, emergency department support, and a surgical team well versed with endovascular procedures. Peri-operative anesthetic care is especially important due to the inherent hemodynamic instability of the ruptured patient. In our institution as well as reported by others, most rEVAR are performed with the patient awaked with only conscious sedation.[6] We find this to be advantageous as it avoids the "sympathectomy" and hypotension associated with a general anesthetic. Lastly, a successful rEVAR outcome is inherently linked to the availability of a large endograft inventory to deal with a wide range and often unexpected anatomic variation in the urgent/emergent setting.

Mehta and his group has been leaders in this field and has published a standardized algorithm for the management of rAAA (Figure 22–1)[7]. This has been adopted elsewhere including our own institution and has been shown to significantly reduced the mortality associated with the unstable rAAA patients[6]. A recent meta analysis by Ricotta and colleagues showed endovascular repair of rAAA has a mortality of 32% as compared to 44% for open repair (Table 22–1).[8]

EVAR AND ENDOLEAK

The introduction of endovascular aneurysm repair (EVAR) has resulted in post-procedure morbidity that is entirely unique and has not occurred with open surgical repair. The term endoleak was first used in 1996 to define persistent perfusion and pressurization of the aneurysm sac after endovascular repair due to incomplete sealing or exclusion of the aneurysm sac or vessel segment.[9] In brief, the presence of an endoleak implies lack of complete aneurysm sac exclusion and thus the patient is at continued risk of aneurysm rupture.

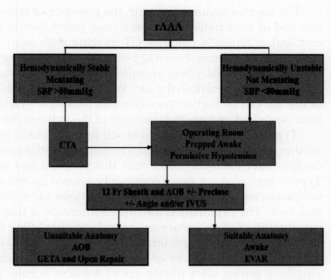

Figure 22–1. Algorithm for management of patients presenting with ruptured AAA.

Mehta et al JVS 2006;44:1–8

TABLE 22–1. SUMMARY OF ALL RECENT PUBLISHED SERIES COMPARING OPEN REPAIR VERSUS ENDOVASCULAR REPAIR FOR MANAGEMENT OF rAAA.

Study	n	EBM level	Data source	Operative Mortality	
				OR % (n)	rEVAR % (n)
Hinchliffe et al.	32	I	Single institution	53 (9/17)	53 (8/15)
Peppelenbosch et al.	100	II-1	Multicenter trial	39 (20/51)	35 (17/49)
Visser et al.	55	II-2	Single institution	31 (9/29)	31 (8/26)
Arya et al.	51	II-2	Single institution	24 (4/17)	47 (16/34)
Vaddineni et al.	24	II-2	Single institution	26 (4/15)	22 (2/9)
Lesperance et al.	9,931	II-3	National data set	42 (3772/8982)	31 (294/949)*
Greco et al.	5,798	II-3	Regional data set	48 (2,627/5,508)	39 (114/290)*
Starnes et al.	51	II-3	Single institution	54 (13/24)	19 (5/27)*
Leon et al.	894	II-3	Regional data set	42 (874/2,059)	36 (20/55)
Sharif et al.	126	II-3	Single institution	51 (38/74)	33 (17/52)
Acosta et al.	162	II-3	Single institution	45 (48/106)	34 (19/56)
Verhoeven et al.	125	II-3	Multicenter, institution	28 (25/89)	14 (5/36)
Coppi et al.	124	II-3	Single institution	46 (42/91)	30 (10/33)*
Ockert et al.	58	II-3	Single institution	31 (9/29)	31 (9/29)
Wibmer et al.	47	II-3	Single institution	13 (4/31)	0 (0/16)
Castelli et al.	46	II-3	Single institution	47 (10/21)	20 (5/25)*
Larzon et al.	41	II-3	Single institution	46 (12/26)	13 (2/15)*
Anain et al.	40	II-3	Multicenter, institution	40 (4/10)	17 (5/30)
Brandt et al.	39	II-3	Single institution	53 (8/15)	8 (2/24)*
Alsac et al.	37	II-3	Single institution	50 (10/20)	24 (4/17)
Lee et al.	37	II-3	Single institution	75 (15/20)	35 (6/17)*
Dalainas et al.	28	II-3	Single institution	63 (5/8)	40 (8/20)
TOT	17,874	–	–	44 (7,562/17,242)	32 (576/1,824)*

*$p < 0.05$
EBM – Evidence Based Medicine level of evidence

For elective aneurysm repair, the presence of endoleak has been reported in nearly one out of four patients at some time point during follow-up.[10,11] The diagnosis of endoleak is typically made by CT imaging with delayed views, although duplex ultra-sonography has been shown to be an effective imaging modality as well.[12,13,14] The typical endoleak usually has an inflow source and an outflow vessel thus resulting in elevated pressure within the sac. When there is no outflow vessel, the diastolic pressure in the sac can be higher than systemic pressure.[15] Overall, five kinds of endoleak have been described and are independent of the make of the endograft.

Type IV endoleak represents self-limiting blood seepage through the graft materials due to porosity. While common with the initial generation of endograft, newer graft designs have essentially eliminate this problem and usually treatment is not required. Type V endoleak, or more commonly known as endotension, denotes continual pressurization and enlargement of the aneurysm sac without radiographic evidence of an endoleak. The explanation for this endotension is that it is from persistent or recurrent pressurization of an aneurysm sac include blood flow that is below the sensitivity limits for detection with current imaging technology. Also, systemic aortic pressure can transmit through thrombus or endograft fabric thus causing the aneurysm sac to growth. Finally, a serous ultra filtrate across a micro porous fabric can fill the aneurysm and increase pressure. Both type IV and type V endoleak require individualized treatment which may include serial observation, endograft "relining", to graft explants and open aneurysm repair.

Unlike these less common endoleaks, type I through III endoleak comprise of the majority of the observed endoleaks and are ones which management guidelines have been established. Currently, the SVS published guidelines suggest conservative treatment of type II endoleak unless aneurysm sac is enlarging. Type I and III endoleak should be treated although the timing of the intervention does not necessary have to be at the index operation.[15]

ENDOLEAK AND RUPTURED ENDOVASCULAR ANEURYSM REPAIR

Adequate neck seal is critical to a successful endovascular aneurysm repair. In the elective setting, short or angulated infrarenal neck is the most common contraindication that disqualifies a patient from an endovascular repair. In recent years, shorter and more angulated aneurysm neck are approached with endovascular techniques due to increase in overall experience with the procedure as well as advances in endograft technology. As such, the incidence of endoleak, especially type I, has correspondingly increased and techniques have been described to address this problem. A recent report from the Cleveland Clinic demonstrates the feasibility of using Palmaz stent and aortic cuff placement for repairing of type Ia endoleak.[16]

Endovascular repair of the ruptured AAA is essentially a "damage control" operation where the main goal is to arrest hemorrhage and stabilize the hemodynamically unstable patient. Furthermore, one does not have the luxury of detailed imaging or 3-D reconstruction that is available during elective aneurysm repair. Patients with less than ideal anatomy are accepted for repair when they present with rupture. While it is ideal to implant the best "fit" endograft for each individual patient, this may not be possible in an emergent setting due to graft inventory, etc.... Taking all these factors together, one would theorize that rEVAR should result in higher endoleak rate than that of elective repair.

Lastly, unlike elective aneurysm repair, the ruptured aortic aneurysm is inherently different. The ruptured aneurysm sac has a defect, an "opening", that is essentially in communication with the retroperitoneal space. For endoleak such as that of type I, the blood flow will continue to pressurize the ruptured aneurysm sac directly. Correspondingly, that blood will continues to leak out of the ruptured sac. This can lead to catastrophic bleeding as the aneurysm sac is not fully excluded. Similarly, type II endoleak from either lumbar vessels or the IMA will continue to bleed into the retroperitoneal hematoma. This is similar to a back bleeding lumbar or IMA encountered during open aneurysm repair where the sac is opened. The patient will continue to bleed unless the vessel is oversewn. In the endovascular setting, the type II endoleak would then need to be embolized or bleeding will continued.

PRIMARY ENDOLEAK (EARLY)

While much as been written regarding the outcomes of rEVAR, there are only few reports detailing the incidence as well as management of endoleak encountered during repair of the ruptured AAA. The first report of endoleak associated with endovascular repair of a ruptured AAA was presented in 2001. That particular patient had stable rAAA and underwent repair with an aorto-uniiliac endograft, contralateral iliac Excluder plug placement, and femoral to femoral crossover graft. The completion arteriogram showed both type Ia endoleak from the proximal graft as well as a distal type Ib endoleak from the excluder plug. The patient did well and was discharged to home shortly after hospital admission. On follow up exam at 3 months, a CT scan was performed and both type Ia and Ib endoleaks were detected. Most surprisingly, the aneurysm sac had shrunk even with the presence of these endoleaks. On review of the intraoperative imaging, the endoleaks were present but unfortunately were not diagnosed at that time. This was attributed to poor image resolution on the OR monitor. Re-intervention was undertaken where a proximal aortic cuff was placed. Another Excluder plug was placed. On further follow up, the endoleaks had resolved and the patient had no adverse outcome.[17]

In another case report by Hartung et al., a 62 years old male underwent unremarkable rEVAR with a Zenith Cook aorto-uniiliac graft, contralateral iliac Excluder plug placement, and a femoral to femoral crossover graft.[18] Several hours after the procedure, the patient experienced continual hemodynamic instability with an associated drop in his blood count. An urgent CT scan was performed which demonstrated a type II endoleak from the IMA. This was successfully treated with coil embolization. The patient recovered, maintained a stable hematocrit, and was shortly discharged to home.

Frank Veith and colleagues were the first to report on their experience with endovascular treatment of rAAA using a custom made an aorto-uniiliac graft. Unlike the previous two case reports, they reported no endoleak in their case series of 25 patients.[5] However, it was unclear what was the exact protocol of follow up as well as what type of imaging was performed. Furthermore, it was also unclear the time interval from the operation until the first imaging study. If the CT scan was done early versus later at 30 day, would it detect type II endoleak that eventually went on to thrombosis? Was there truly no endoleak, or is this just a function of a low number of cases done so far?

In our institution at Harborview Medical Center, an established protocol for the management of ruptured AAA was established in July of 2007 with preference of approaching all rAAA with endovascular techniques regardless of the patient's hemo-dynamic status. Since that time, a total of 43 patients have been treated with endovas-cular techniques, with the majority of patients undergoing bifurcated endograft placement. We noted a total of 6 endoleaks out of 43 cases, or 14%. Of these, four were type II endoleak and the remaining two were type I.

In the first case of type I endoleak, the patient left the OR with completion arteri-ogram demonstrating the presence of no endoleak and complete aneurysm sac exclu-sion without contrast extravasations. Postoperatively, she continued to show evidence of bleeding and was taken back to the OR where a repeated arteriogram still could not demonstrate any abnormality. Laparotomy was performed and the aneurysm sac was found to be pulsatile. A posterior jet was observed at the proximal neck when the aneurysm sac was opened. This was treated successfully by local plication of the native aortic tissue to the endograft. In the second case, the patient was found with the type I endoleak on a post-op day #1 on CT scan after a normal completion arteriogram. At that time, he was hemodynamically stable. Even so, we took the patient to the angio suite where the endoleak was detected and was confirmed to be type Ia. A prox-imal aortic cuff was placed and successfully sealed the leak. The patient has since done well on follow up with CT scan imaging of aneurysm sac regression. At his 2-year fol-low up, his aneurysm sac has essentially disappeared.

As for the 4 patients with type II endoleak, they were managed conservatively as the patients were stable after their endovascular procedure. In two patients, the endoleak resolved on subsequent CT imaging at one month. The remaining two patients still have endoleak at twelve and eighteen month follow up respectively. Both have aneurysm sac size regression.

A review of the literature showed that the incidence of endoleak after rEVAR is somewhat lower than that of elective endovascular aneurysm repair. However, one would think that rEVAR should have a higher endoleak rate when compared to elec-tive aneurysm repair due to less than ideal circumstances where there is just not enough time to fully reconstruct the patient's CT scan on a workstation to analyze the anatomy or plan the procedure. Furthermore, one may not have the exact size endo-graft for implantation due to limited inventory. Lastly, as rEVAR is a "damaged con-trol" procedure, one may accept a patient with less than ideal anatomy such as that of a short or angulated infrarenal neck.

So, why is the reported rate of endoleak after rEVAR lower than that of its elective counterpart? First, most of these procedures are done in an operating room with a portable C-arm unit. As such, image quality will be suboptimal as compared to a fixed fluoroscopy unit. This can contribute to an under detection of endoleak at the time of the operation. With a tortuous and angulated infrarenal neck, one can miss a posterior type Ia endoleak unless dedicated views in multiple obliquity are performed. Type II endoleak can be missed if not enough contrast was used for the completion arteri-ogram or if the filming was not carried out far enough. Postoperative CT scans are done at different intervals as there is no standardized protocol or guideline to follow for these ruptured patients. Thus, detection and reporting rate can vary and may not truly represent the actual incidence or prevalence of endoleak. When one reviewed the body of literature on endovascular repair of aneurysm, reports of endoleak are few and scattered. Primary endoleaks, or those that occurred within the first 30 days, range from 0 to 25% (Table 22–2).[19,20,21,22,23] Overall, the incidence is slightly lower than that reported for elective aneurysm repair. However, it is difficult to tease out what actual-ly happened to these patients when one reviewed the published data. Did they all

TABLE 22–2. REPORTED INCIDENCE OF PRIMARY (< 30 D) ENDOLEAK AFTER ENDOVASCULAR REPAIR OF RUPTURED AAA.

	Incidence		
	Range	Average	Number of Citations
Primary endoleak[a]			
Type I	2–16%	9% (38/421)	10
Type Ia	2–6%	3% (10/323)	8
Type II	0–25%	11% (40/375)	9
Type III	0–3%	1% (3/318)	8
Overall endoleak	7–42%	20% (86/423)	12

[a]Primary (early) endoleak defined as postoperative endoleak < 30 d

require re-intervention for type I endoleak like those in our series? Or, were they able to be managed conservatively as reported by Hechelhammer and his group for 6 of out of 17 type I endoleak?[21]

SECONDARY ENDOLEAK (LATE)

In elective aneurysm repair, established guidelines have been set forth to follow EVAR over time. This is critical as endovascular repaired aneurysm can have delayed complications and require much more re-intervention than that of its open counterpart.[24] Furthermore, delayed ruptured after EVAR is a real entity with reported rate as high as 1.5%.[25] The majority of ruptured AAA after endograft placement demonstrates aneurysm sac enlargement when one reviewed previous serial imaging. Furthermore, most of these cases demonstrated either type I or type III endoleak.

Late endoleaks after rEVAR have been reported from multiple centers. Similar to early endoleaks, they appear to be less as compared to elective EVAR (Table 22–3). Likely, the low number is the result of loss to follow-up as most of these patients are not part of a registry or clinical trial. As such, postoperative imaging is infrequent and unreliable. In fact, Mehta and his group reported that up to 74% of their patients are lost to follow up at > 1 year.[25]

It is comforting to know that an analysis of long-term follow-up (> 30 d) of rEVAR showed that the aneurysm sac remains stable or regresses over time in the majority of

TABLE 22–3. REPORTED INCIDENCE OF SECONDARY (> 30D) ENDOLEAK AFTER ENDOVASCULAR REPAIR OF RUPTURED AAA

	Incidence		
	Range	Average	Number of Citations
Secondary endoleak[b]			
Type I	0–12%	4% (10/236)	8
Type Ia	0–15%	3% (7/217)	6
Type II	0–13%	7% (11/154)	5
Type III	0–10%	2% (5/219)	6

[b]Secondary (late) endoleak defined as postoperative endoleak >30 d

TABLE 22–4. BEHAVIOR OF RUPTURED ANEURYSM SAC AFTER ENDOVASCULAR REPAIR

	Incidence		
	Range	Average (n)	Number of Citations
Sac shrinkage	28–80%	51% (72/142)	5
Stable AAA sac	12–72%	42% (60/142)	5
Sac enlargement	0–24%	7% (10/142)	5

cases. In these patients, all types of endoleak were detected and most were followed conservatively and not treated. Unfortunately, there are also reports of aneurysm sac enlargement over time after rEVAR (Table 22–4). Even though the incidence is low, this can lead to a re-rupture. In fact, we have recently treated a gentleman who is 2 years s/p a rEVAR at another facility. He presented with a contained ruptured and large retroperitoneal hematoma. Review of his previous CT scans showed a type Ia endoleak and gradual aneurysm sac expansion. Intervention was not carried out as the patient did not return to see his surgeon.

DISCUSSION

All data so far indicates that endoleaks in ruptured AAA do not behave in the same way as those of open aneurysm repair. Furthermore, the incidence and prevalence of endoleak are also different for rEVAR as compared to elective endovascular aneurysm repair. As multiple investigators have shown, most endoleak including type I will not result in continual hemorrhage in the acute ruptured setting. In fact, the majority of acute (< 30 days) type I endoleak after rEVAR were managed conservatively and do not require intervention. Similarly, the majority of type II and III endoleak was also managed successfully without the need for surgical treatment.

What is it about the ruptured abdominal aortic aneurysm that allows acute endoleak to be managed in this fashion? Likely, the initial hemorrhage with its associated retroperitoneal hematoma plays a significant role. It could tamponade bleeding from endoleak by exerting pressure in the retroperitoneal space surrounding the defect in the aneurysm sac. The limited use of systemic heparinization in rEVAR and the patient's own up regulated coagulation profile could also contribute to the natural history of endoleak, especially type II, in the ruptured setting. This, of course, can change as uncontrolled bleeding continues and the patient becomes coagulopathic from uncontrolled hemorrhage.

In the end, the overall literature and our knowledge of endoleak in the setting of rEVAR is quite limited. This is likely due to differences in the follow up protocol of different centers. The timing of the initial post-operative CT scan varied from postoperative day #1 to 30 days after the operation. Furthermore, some centers will perform duplex imaging prior to sending the patient home but not get the CT scan until the follow up appointment. Data from our center suggests that duplex ultrasonography is unable to reliably pick up flow within the aneurysm sac and endoleak when performed in the post-operative setting (pending publication). This is likely secondary to the significant retroperitoneal hematoma which can impede full visualization of the aneurysm sac.

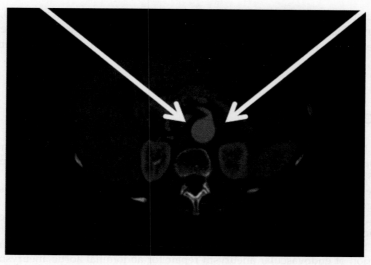

Figure 22–2 Imaging of the aneurysm neck to include both RAO and LAO projection to ensure that there is no type Ia endoleak.

So, how does one manage endoleaks in the setting of endovascular repair of rAAA? In our opinion, type I and III endoleak is equivalent to bleeding at the anastomotic line in an open repair. Without intervention, they can be rapidly fatal. As such, the patient should not leave the operating room unless type I and III endoleaks are definitely excluded. In centers with dedicated fixed imaging, a focused and magnified view of the aneurysm neck, especially in cases where the anatomy is tortuous, should be sufficient to rule out a type Ia endoleak (Figure 22–2). In those centers where portable C-arm imaging is used, one may need to perform not only dedicated views of the proximal seal zone but also views in multiple obliquity such as that of LAO and RAO. This will enable one to adequately rule out most type Ia endoleaks.

As for type II endoleak, all data so far would suggest that these can be managed conservatively. However, one should have a low threshold of investigational imaging study if the ruptured patient demonstrates signs of continual hemorrhage. This can indicate continual bleed into the retroperitoneal space through the ruptured aneurysm sac. In these cases, a return trip to the interventional suite and coil embolization of the offending vessel should be performed.

CONCLUSION

The surgical management of ruptured abdominal aortic aneurysm has undergone an evolutionary change within the last decade. A disease which was once thought to be lethal with mortality approaching 70% now can be managed with the majority of the patients surviving their rupture and being discharged from the hospital to their home within several days of admission. Endoleak in the ruptured AAA is clearly different than its elective counterpart. Until evidence suggests otherwise, type I and III endoleak should be investigated and managed aggressively in the acute setting. On the other hand, type II endoleak can be managed expectantly unless the patient exhibits signs of continual bleeding. At that time, aggressive management should be sought.

As more ruptured AAAs are managed with endovascular techniques, the natural history of endoleak will be better defined. Over time, it is hoped that enough data will be collected so firm recommendations regarding endoleak management can be put forth.

REFERENCES

1. Egorova N, Giacovelli J, Greco G, et al. National outcomes for the treatment of ruptured abdominal aortic aneurysm: comparison of open versus endovascular repairs. *J Vasc Surg* 2008;48(5):1092–100, 1100.e1–2.
2. Heikkinen M, Salenius J, Auvinen O. Ruptured abdominal aortic aneurysm in a well-defined geographic area. *J Vasc Surg* 2002;36(2):291–296.
3. Parodi JC, Palmaz JC, Barone HD. Transfemoral intraluminal graft implantation for abdominal aortic aneurysms. *Ann Vasc Surg* 1991;5(6):491–499.
4. Sachs T, Schermerhorn M, Pomposelli F, et al. Resident and fellow experiences after the introduction of endovascular aneurysm repair for abdominal aortic aneurysm. *J Vasc Surg* 2011.
5. Ohki T, Veith FJ. Endovascular grafts and other image-guided catheter-based adjuncts to improve the treatment of ruptured aortoiliac aneurysms. *Ann Surg* 2000;232(4):466–479.
6. Starnes BW, Quiroga E, Hutter C, et al. Management of ruptured abdominal aortic aneurysm in the endovascular era. *J Vasc Surg* 2010;51(1):9–17; discussion 17–8.
7. Mehta M, Kreienberg PB, Roddy SP, et al. Ruptured abdominal aortic aneurysm: endovascular program development and results. *Sem in Vasc Surg* 2010;23(4):206–214.
8. Ricotta JJ, Malgor RD, Oderich GS. Ruptured endovascular abdominal aortic aneurysm repair: part II. *Ann Vasc Surg* 2010;24(2):269–277.
9. White GH, Yu W, May J. Endoleak–a proposed new terminology to describe incomplete aneurysm exclusion by an endoluminal graft. *J Endovasc Surg* 1996;3(1):124–125.
10. Sheehan MK, Ouriel K, Greenberg R, et al. Are type II endoleaks after endovascular aneurysm repair endograft dependent? *J Vasc Surg* 2006;43(4):657–661.
11. Ouriel K, Clair DG, Greenberg RK, et al. Endovascular repair of abdominal aortic aneurysms: device-specific outcome. *J Vasc Surg* 2003;37(5):991–998.
12. Manning B, O'Neill S, Haider S, et al. Duplex ultrasound in aneurysm surveillance following endovascular aneurysm repair: a comparison with computed tomography aortography. *J Vasc Surg* 2009;49(1):60–65.
13. Schmieder GC, Stout CL, Stokes GK, Parent FN, Panneton JM. Endoleak after endovascular aneurysm repair: duplex ultrasound imaging is better than computed tomography at determining the need for intervention. *J Vasc Surg* 2009;50(5):1012–7; discussion 1017–8.
14. Bakken AM, Illig KA. Long-term follow-up after endovascular aneurysm repair: is ultrasound alone enough? *Perspet Vasc Surg Endovas Ther* 2010;22(3):145–151.
15. Chaikof EL, Brewster DC, Dalman RL, et al. The care of patients with an abdominal aortic aneurysm: the Society for Vascular Surgery practice guidelines. *J Vasc Surg* 2009;50 (4 Suppl):S2–49.
16. Rajani RR, Arthurs ZM, Srivastava SD, et al. Repairing immediate proximal endoleaks during abdominal aortic aneurysm repair. *J Vasc Surg* 2011;53(5):1174–1177.
17. Verhagen HJM, Prinssen M, Milner R, Blankensteijn JD. Endoleak after endovascular repair of ruptured abdominal aortic aneurysm: is it a problem? *J Endovasc Ther* 2003;10(4):766–771.
18. Hartung O, Vidal V, Marani I, et al. Treatment of an early type II endoleak causing hemorrhage after endovascular aneurysm repair for ruptured abdominal aortic aneurysm. *J Vasc Surg* 2007;45(5):1062–1065.
19. Alsac J, Desgranges P, Kobeiter H, Becquemin J. Emergency endovascular repair for ruptured abdominal aortic aneurysms: feasibility and comparison of early results with conventional open repair. *Eur J Vasc Endovasc Surg* 2005;30(6):632–639.

20. Coppi G, Silingardi R, Gennai S, Saitta G, Ciardullo AV. A single-center experience in open and endovascular treatment of hemodynamically unstable and stable patients with ruptured abdominal aortic aneurysms. *J Vasc Surg* 2006;44(6):1140–1147.
21. Hechelhammer L, Lachat ML, Wildermuth S, et al. Midterm outcome of endovascular repair of ruptured abdominal aortic aneurysms. *J Vasc Surg* 2005;41(5):752–757.
22. Mayer D, Pfammatter T, Rancic Z, et al. 10 years of emergency endovascular aneurysm repair for ruptured abdominal aortoiliac aneurysms: lessons learned. *Ann Surg* 2009; 249(3):510–515.
23. Scharrer-Pamler R, Kotsis T, Kapfer X. Endovascular stent-graft repair of ruptured aortic aneurysms. *J Endovasc Ther* 2003;10:447–452.
24. de Bruin J, Baas A, Buth J. Long-term outcome of open or endovascular repair of abdominal aortic aneurysm. *N Engl J Med* 2010;362(20):1881–9.
25. Mehta M, Paty P, Roddy S, Taggert J. Treatment options for delayed AAA rupture following endovascular repair. *J Vasc Surg* 2011;53:14–20.

SECTION **VI**

TAAA I

23

Management of Adult Aortic Coarctation

Hyde M. Russell, MD and S. Chris Malaisrie, MD

INTRODUCTION

Aortic coarctation is a narrowing of the aorta that occurs in 0.4 out of every 1000 live births. The location of this narrowing is almost always just distal to the left subclavian artery at the aortic isthmus. (Figure 23–1). Prior classifications of coarctation into infantile or "pre-ductal" versus adult or "post-ductal" subgroups have been fallen out of favor because nearly all coarctations are, in fact, juxta-ductal and involve the tissue of the ductus arteriosus.[1] In adults with aortic coarctation, the aortic isthmus is not hypoplastic and the coarctation occurs at the level of a closed ductus arteriosus (ligamentum arteriosum).

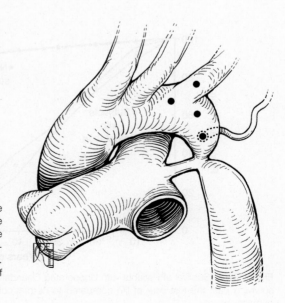

Figure 23–1. Juxtaductal or "Adult" Coarctation. The area of aortic narrowing is at the same level as the ligamentum arteriosum. A prominent posterior ridge protrudes into the aorta. Abbott's artery is an anomalous artery arising from the posterior aortic isthmus. Black circles show other possible sites of origin of Abbott's artery. Reproduced with permission.

PATHOPHYSIOLOGY

There is a bi-modal distribution of presentation of patients with coarctation of the aorta. Infants with ductal-dependent flow (where the majority of the descending aorta blood flow is provided by an open ductus arteriosus downstream from the critical coarctation) may present with shock following natural ductus closure in the first week of life. With the advent of prostaglandin E1 (PGE1) which relaxes the ductal smooth musculature allowing reopening of the ductus, these infants can be resuscitated and subsequently taken for surgical repair after stabilization. The second group of patients is those with an asymptomatic coarctation that present late in childhood or even adulthood. These patients often have developed significant collaterals around the coarctation, and rib notching from enlarged intercostal arteries. Femoral pulses may be weak or absent and there is often a delay between radial and femoral pulsations. A gradient between right arm and leg using blood pressure cuff measurement is diagnostic. The presentation of a third group of patients, those with recurrent coarctation, deserves mention. These patients are generally identified by arm-leg blood pressure gradients, but unexplained hypertension may be the initial clue to the clinician.

NATURAL HISTORY

The natural history of unrepaired coarctation is notable for hypertension, aneurysm, and early death (Figure 23–2). Berry aneurysms occur in 10% of patients with coarctation, even after repair. Bicuspid aortic valve disease is indentified in over 50% of patients with coarctation. Before the advent of surgical repair, fatal aortic dissection was the cause of death in 19% of patients with coarctation, and 50% of patients with combined coarctation and bicuspid aortic valve disease.[2] The high incidence of aneurysm and dissection supports the theory that aortic coarctation is but one manifestation of a diffuse aortopathy rather than a

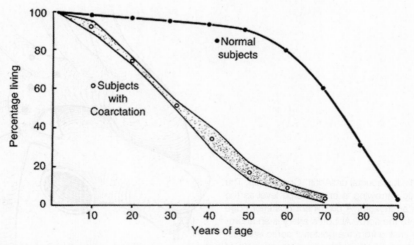

Figure 23–2. Survival of Patients with Unoperated Coarctation. Survival curve of patients with aortic coarctation surviving past the first year of life compared to normal cohort of patients from the 1970's. Reproduced with permission.

localized disease. The "unnatural" or operative history of patients with repaired coarctation varies depending on the type of repair employed. The next section will describe the various techniques used to repair aortic coarctation and their long term results.

SURGICAL REPAIR

Class I indications for operation in adults with coarctation include a peak-to-peak gradient of 20mmHg between right arm and leg, and a peak-to-peak gradient less than 20mmHg in the presence of significant coarctation and collaterals.[3] Systemic hypertension, leg claudication, and aneurysm formation are additional factors to be considered in deciding to intervene. Intended pregnancy should also prompt strong consideration of repair as left sided obstruction represents one of the highest risk cardiac conditions in pregnancy. The population of adults with aortic coarctation includes both patients with unoperated lesions and patients who have undergone previous repair and have developed recoarctation. Because their original repair technique is germane to their care, a brief description of the various operations performed in children over the past 5 decades is presented.

The following variations of surgical repairs are performed through a left posterolateral thoracotomy entering the third or fourth interspace. Operations performed on infants and small children are generally performed with a "clamp and sew" technique. Upper body blood pressure measured in the right arm is allowed to stay elevated to aid lower body perfusion via collaterals. Left heart bypass is utilized in older children and adults in whom a lower extremity blood pressure fails to maintain a level of 45 mmHg during test clamping due to insufficient collateralization. All patients are allowed to passively cool to 35 degrees to lower the metabolic demands of the kidneys and spinal cord during the ischemic interval.

Resection and End to End anastomosis: The first attempts at repair of aortic coarctation were reported by Crafoord and Nylin in 1945. This technique excises the ductal tissue distal to the left subclavian and utilizes a direct end-to-end anastomosis with mobilization of the aorta (Figure23-3). Because no attempt is made to address the arch, patients with a hypoplastic distal arch may have residual obstruction. The recurrence rate of series using this technique published in the 1980's is reported between 20–80%.[4-6]

Patch Aortoplasty: Prosthetic patch aortoplasty was first reported in 1957 as an alternative to resection and end-to-end anastomosis secondary to the high rate of recoarctation observed in those early patients. This technique utilizes a longitudinal incision on the aorta with an oval patch to enlarge the luminal area (Figure 23–4). The main late complication of this technique is aneurysm formation opposite the patch which occurs in 5–13% of patients.[7-9] Aneurysm formation is higher when the posterior ductal shelf is excised at the time of surgery, thus such excision is no longer recommended. Patch aortoplasty has a favorable rate of recoarctation of less than 10%[9,10] and is useful in the older child who is too large for an extended end-to-end anastomosis but too small for an interposition graft.

Subclavian Flap Aortoplasty: In this repair, the left subclavian artery is ligated distally. Following aortic cross clamp, the subclavian artery is divided and opened longitudinally along its inferior aspect. The arteriotomy continues down onto the aorta

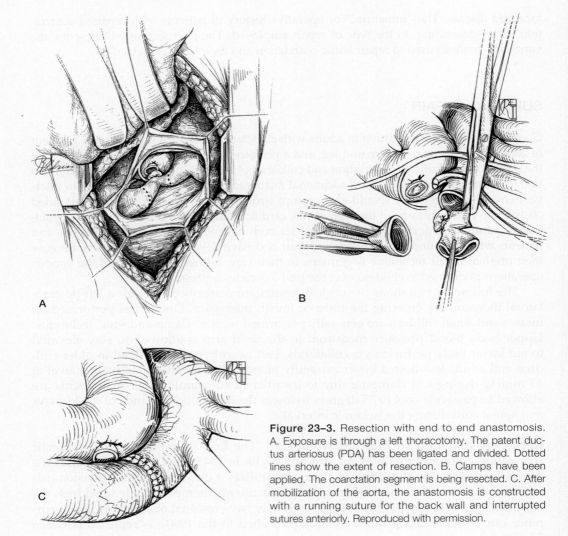

Figure 23–3. Resection with end to end anastomosis. A. Exposure is through a left thoracotomy. The patent ductus arteriosus (PDA) has been ligated and divided. Dotted lines show the extent of resection. B. Clamps have been applied. The coarctation segment is being resected. C. After mobilization of the aorta, the anastomosis is constructed with a running suture for the back wall and interrupted sutures anteriorly. Reproduced with permission.

and across the coarctation site. The opened subclavian artery is then "flapped" down onto the opened aorta as a patch and a running suture line is used to close the aortotomy. (Figure 23–5). The lack of subclavian blood flow is tolerated quite well by young children due to collateral formation but concerns over limb growth and subclavian steal syndrome remain. The long-term results of subclavian flap aortoplasty are better in terms of recoarctation compared to direct end-to-end anastomosis with an overall rate of 12%.[1]

Extended End to End anastomosis: Extended end-to-end anastomosis which has now gained acceptance as the standard repair for coarctation in infants was first described by Amato in 1977.[11] This operation modified the original end-to-end anastomosis by spatulating the aorta to create a larger anastomotic area. In order to do this, the proximal clamp is placed across the transverse arch between the innominate and left carotid arteries leaving cerebral blood flow dependent on the right carotid and

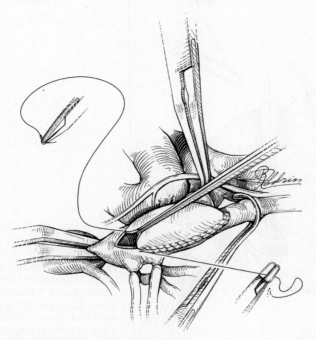

Figure 23–4. Patch Aortoplasty. An elliptical polytetrafluoroethylene (PTFE) patch is sutured into place so that the patch creates a roof over the coarctation ridge. Reproduced with permission.

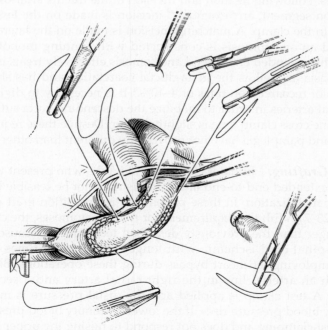

Figure 23–5. Sublclavian Flap Aortoplasty. The left subclavian artery (LSA) has been ligated distally and opened into the aorta creating a flap. The LSA is turned down over the coarctation site and carried as far distal as possible. Three polypropylene sutures are used to create the anastomosis. Reproduced with permission.

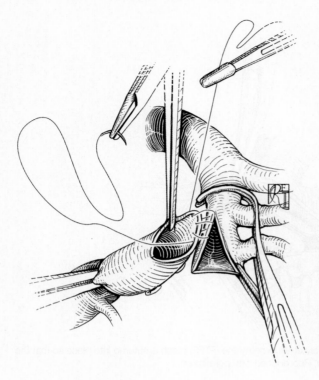

Figure 23–6. Extended end-to-end anastomosis. The proximal clamp occludes the left carotid and left subclavian arteries. Incisions have been made on the undersurface of the arch and lateral wall of the descending aorta. A running propylene suture is used to complete the extended anastomosis. Reproduced with permission.

vertebral arteries. Following ligation and division of the ductus arteriosus and excision of the coarctation segment, an "extended" incision is made on the lesser curve of the arch extending to the clamp. A matching incision is made on the lateral surface of the distal aorta and an anastomosis is constructed with running monofilament suture (Figure 23–6). This extended end-to-end anastomosis effectively treats isthmus and distal arch hypoplasia as well as the juxta-ductal coarctation and has shown improved results in terms of recoarctation rates of 4–10%.[1] It is necessary to divide two or three sets of intercostal arteries in order to mobilize the descending aorta sufficiently for this operation, and the cross clamp time is slightly longer. Despite these requirements, operative mortality and paraplegia have not proven any different than other techniques.

Interposition Grafting: In older children and adults who present with unrepaired coarctation, an extended end-to-end anastomosis may not be feasible because of limitations of aortic mobilization. In these patients an interposition graft may be the best option (Figure 23–7). With the requirement for two anastomoses, the cross clamp time is generally longer than the previously described techniques. Because of the concern for renal and spinal cord ischemia with longer cross clamp times we have a low threshold for employing left heart bypass during these operations. Blood pressure is monitored with an arterial line in the right radial artery and a second line in the femoral artery. A test clamp is applied and the distal pressure is monitored as the upper extremity blood pressure rises. If the lower extremity blood pressure falls below 45 mmHg on test clamping and does not respond to raising the upper extremity blood pressure to 180 mmHg with volume expanders, then a decision is made to use left-heart bypass. Patients with aberrant right subclavian arteries arising from the descending aorta are of particular concern because of the lack of collateral blood flow when

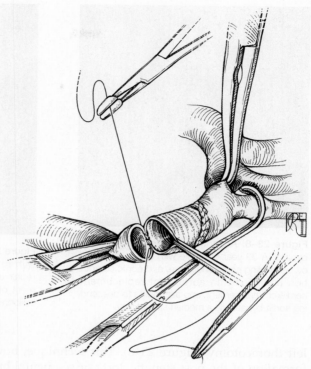

Figure 23–7. Interposition Grafting. The proximal anastomosis of the interposition graft has been completed. The distal anastomosis is similarly completed with a running polypropylene suture. Reproduced with permission.

both subclavian arteries are deprived of flow during the cross clamp period. We recommend left heart bypass for all of these patients.

We perform left heart bypass using systemic heparinization with a venous cannula in the left atrial appendage or inferior pulmonary vein and an aortic cannula in the descending aorta. We do not use an oxygenator in the circuit and ventilation must be continued. Flows of 50%–60% of calculated maximal flow (2.5 L/min/m2) are generally sufficient to achieve a distal mean blood pressure of 45 mmHg.[12]

The size of the interposition graft is important as patients can "outgrow" a small graft and produce functional recoarctation with a gradient across the graft following somatic growth. No smaller than a 16 mm tube graft should be used for the interposition graft. This technique, therefore, is generally reserved for older teenagers and adults in whom a larger graft can be accommodated.

Bypass Grafting: Surgery for coarctation can also be performed using a bypass graft rather than an interposition graft, leaving the native aorta unresected. In this scenario, the proximal end of the graft can be anastomosed to the left subclavian artery, the transverse arch, or the ascending aorta using a partial occlusion clamp. The graft can be routed parallel to the aorta in the left chest or can be routed to the right of and posterior to the heart if performing the operation through a sternotomy.[13] This repair is attractive as it maintains spinal cord and lower body perfusion as the aorta is partially clamped and avoids the need for left heart bypass. In addition, patients with concomitant cardiac disease such as bicuspid aortic valve or ascending aortic aneurysm can have all of their pathology addressed though a median sternotomy in a single operation rather than a two-staged operation involving median sternotomy followed by a

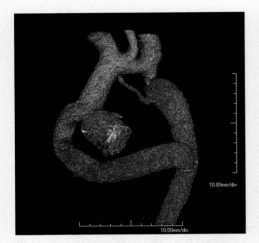

Figure 23–8. Ascending to descending aortic bypass. A 39 year-old male with aortic insufficiency, ascending aortic aneurysm, and aortic coarctation underwent an aortic root replacement, hemiarch replacement, and ascending to descending aortic bypass via a median sternotomy.

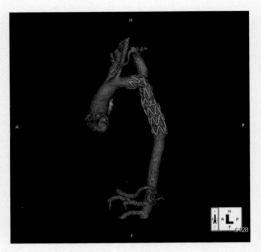

Figure 23–9. Endovascular Repair. 51 year old male with recurrent coarctation after previous surgical repair underwent endovascular repair using placement of a 26 mm x 10 cm stent-graft followed by balloon angioplasty.

left thoracotomy (Figure 23–8). This technique, however does not address aneurysm formation of the post-stenotic aorta or segmental branches which often occur in adult patients.

Endovascular Repair: Endovascular repair can be accomplished by balloon angioplasty with or without stent placement (Figure 23–9). The placement of an uncovered stent can prevent immediate recoil of the aorta but is associated with long-term intimal hyperplasia. The placement of a stent-graft protects against immediate rupture during aggressive balloon angioplasty and may prevent long-term aneurysm formation. Mortality and morbidity after endovascular repair is similar to surgery, however endovascular repair is associated greater rate of recoarctation (11–15%) and reintervention (10–14%) which differed significantly from surgical repair of adult aortic coarctation (less than 2%).[14] Despite lack of randomized clinical data, endovascular repair is a class I recommendation for patients with either recurrent coarctation or discrete coarctation as an acceptable alternative to surgery as a primary intervention.[3]

OUTCOMES

The mortality after surgical repair of adult aortic coarctation is 1% or less with reported rates of paralysis also less than 1%.[14] Laryngeal nerve injury and bleeding are the most common morbidities after surgery, compared to free rupture, acute dissection, and traumatic aneurysm formation after endovascular repair.

Although the benefit of repair of aortic coarctation is greatest amongst younger patients there does not appear to be an age over which repair fails to afford improvement in hypertension. The long term effects of coarctation repair in the adult have been described by several groups.[15–17] In a large series of adult patients undergoing surgical repair, 69% had resolution of their systemic hypertension and 42% did not require any antihypertensive medications.[16]

CONCLUSIONS

Options for surgical repair of adult aortic coarctation include resection with interposition grafting, bypass grafting without resection, and endovascular repair. Safety after interposition grafting for adult coarctation is excellent and is associated with greater than 60% rate of resolution of hypertension and less than 2% rate of recoarcation and reintervention. Endovascular repair is an acceptable alternative for patients who develop recurrent coarctation after previous coarctation repair and for patients with discrete narrowing; however is associated with higher rate of recoarctation and reintervention. Bypass grafting from the ascending aorta to the descending aorta is useful in patients who require concomitant cardiac surgery such as aortic valve surgery or ascending aortic repair, but does not address post-coarctation dilatation.

REFERENCES

1. Backer CL, Mavroudis C. Coarctation of the Aorta. In: Mavroudis C, Backer CL, editors. *Pediatric Cardiac Surgery*, 3rd Edition. Philadelphia: Mosby (An Affiliate of Elsevier); 2003. pp 251–272.
2. Abbott ME. Coarctation of the aorta of adult-type. *Am Heart J* 1928;3:574–628.
3. Warnes CA, Williams RG, Bashore TM, et al. ACC/AHA 2008 Guidelines for the Management of Adults with Congenital Heart Disease: a report of the American College of Cardiology/American Heart Association Task Force on Practice Guidelines (writing committee to develop guidelines on the management of adults with congenital heart disease). *Circulation* Dec 2 2008;118(23):e714–833.
4. Kappetein AP, Zwinderman AH, Bogers AJ, Rohmer J, Huysmans HA. More than thirty-five years of coarctation repair. An unexpected high relapse rate. *J Thorac Cardiovasc Surg* Jan 1994;107(1):87–95.
5. Williams WG, Shindo G, Trusler GA, Dische MR, Olley PM. Results of repair of coarctation of the aorta during infancy. *J Thorac Cardiovasc Surg* Apr 1980;79(4):603–608.
6. Ziemer G, Jonas RA, Perry SB, Freed MD, Castaneda AR. Surgery for coarctation of the aorta in the neonate. *Circulation* Sep 1986;74(3 Pt 2):I25–31.
7. Clarkson PM, Brandt PW, Barratt-Boyes BG, Rutherford JD, Kerr AR, Neutze JM. Prosthetic repair of coarctation of the aorta with particular reference to Dacron onlay patch grafts and late aneurysm formation. *Am J Cardiol* Aug 1 1985;56(4):342–346.
8. del Nido PJ, Williams WG, Wilson GJ, et al. Synthetic patch angioplasty for repair of coarctation of the aorta: experience with aneurysm formation. *Circulation* Sep 1986;74(3 Pt 2):I32–36.
9. Hehrlein FW, Mulch J, Rautenburg HW, Schlepper M, Scheld HH. Incidence and pathogenesis of late aneurysms after patch graft aortoplasty for coarctation. *J Thorac Cardiovasc Surg* Aug 1986;92(2):226–230.
10. Backer CL, Paape K, Zales VR, Weigel TJ, Mavroudis C. Coarctation of the aorta. Repair with polytetrafluoroethylene patch aortoplasty. *Circulation* Nov 1 1995;92(9 Suppl):II132–136.
11. Amato JJ, Rheinlander HF, Cleveland RJ. A method of enlarging the distal transverse arch in infants with hypoplasia and coarctation of the aorta. *Ann Thorac Surg* Mar 1977;23(3): 261–263.

12. Backer CL, Stewart RD, Kelle AM, Mavroudis C. Use of partial cardiopulmonary bypass for coarctation repair through a left thoracotomy in children without collaterals. *Ann Thorac Surg* Sep 2006;82(3):964–972.

13. Connolly HM, Schaff HV, Izhar U, Dearani JA, Warnes CA, Orszulak TA. Posterior pericardial ascending-to-descending aortic bypass: an alternative surgical approach for complex coarctation of the aorta. *Circulation* Sep 18 2001;104(12 Suppl 1):I133–137.

14. Carr JA. The results of catheter-based therapy compared with surgical repair of adult aortic coarctation. *J Am Coll Cardiol* Mar 21 2006;47(6):1101–1107.

15. Aris A, Subirana MT, Ferres P, Torner-Soler M. Repair of aortic coarctation in patients more than 50 years of age. *Ann Thorac Surg* May 1999;67(5):1376–1379.

16. Bhat MA, Neelakandhan KS, Unnikrishnan M, Rathore RS, Mohan Singh MP, Lone GN. Fate of hypertension after repair of coarctation of the aorta in adults. *Br J Surg* Apr 2001;88(4): 536–538.

17. Wells WJ, Prendergast TW, Berdjis F, et al. Repair of coarctation of the aorta in adults: the fate of systolic hypertension. *Ann Thorac Surg* Apr 1996;61(4):1168–1171.

24

Penetrating Aortic Ulcers
An Overview

Tanya R. Flohr, MD, Margaret C. Tracci, MD,
John A. Kern, MD, Irving L. Kron, MD,
Gorav Ailawadi, MD, Kenneth J. Cherry, MD and
Gilbert R. Upchurch, Jr., MD

INTRODUCTION

Penetrating aortic ulcers (PAUs) are one of three unique vascular pathologies included in acute aortic syndromes (AAS).This spectrum of vascular disorders also includes intramural hematomas (IMHs) and aortic dissections (ADs). According to a recent study, AAS affects 2.6% of the population.[1] Isolated PAUs, however, are rare with the true incidence yet to be determined. The prevalence of PAUs among patients with AAS is 2-8% with the majority of these lesions found in the descending thoracic aorta.[2, 3] In a study of 120 patients undergoing transesophageal echocardiograms for suspected aortic disease, only 2.5% patients had a PAU, whereas 37.5% patients were found to have classic aortic dissections.[4] Stanson et al. also reported an incidence of 2.3% of PAUs in 684 consecutive aortograms performed for suspected aortic dissection.[5] Other studies suggest the incidence is slightly higher. In a retrospective review of 198 patients with the initial diagnosis of aortic dissection, Coady et al. noted the incidence of PAUs to be 7.6%.[2] Symptoms associated with PAUs can be similar to IMH and AD. Moreover, the lesion can be found isolated in the absence of other AAS pathologies. Currently, whether a PAU is the inciting lesion leading to the progression of an IMH or AD or the PAU is an entirely distinct pathology is unknown. It is known that patients presenting with a PAU, especially if accompanied with symptoms or signs of hemodynamic instability, are at an increased risk for aortic rupture. Therefore, these lesions should be treated if discovered in a symptomatic patient.[2, 3, 6] This review discusses PAUs primarily in the descending thoracic aorta, their pathophysiology, diagnosis and treatment options.

PATHOPHYSIOLOGY

PAUs were first described by Shennan in 1934 and later distinguished from other aortic syndromes by Stanson in 1986.[5,7] A PAU is a focal ulcerative lesion that penetrates the internal elastic lamina of the vascular wall. PAUs may or may not have an associated hematoma within the medial layer of the aortic wall and can progress to form an AD. PAUs are generally not associated with traumatic injuries or genetic mutations associated with AD, such as Marfan's syndrome, cystic media necrosis or seronegative spondyloarthropathies. Whether or not local inflammation is the cause or the result is still uncertain; however, macrophages are frequently present in the vascular wall media of a PAU. PAUs can be circumferential or longitudinal lesions. In contrast to ADs or traumatic dissections, PAUs do not necessarily occur at points of maximal hydraulic stress, namely the right lateral wall of the ascending aorta or at the ligamentum arteriosum of the descending aorta.[8]

With the increasing use of medical or endovascular therapy to the exclusion of open surgery for PAUs, a true histologic diagnosis is not possible in most patients believed to be affected by these lesions. The diagnosis of a PAU therefore has become one of radiologic appearance. Imaging shows a localized, contrast material-filled, craterlike, outpouching of the endoluminal border with discontinuity of the internal elastic lamina into the aortic wall. Distinct from AD, there is an absence of an intimal flap or a double-barreled lumen. PAUs are found with or without subinitimal hemorrhage depending on the presence of an associated IMH. If an IMH is associated with the PAU, it is generally limited in location without much extension. Often PAUs occur in an area of significant atheroma, but not all PAUs are associated with atherosclerosis. Park et al. noted 53% of PAUs found on imaging are associated with atherosclerotic lesions.[9] Regardless of the etiology of the PAUs, the pathology resolves with treatment, as even after endovascular stenting, most PAUs are found to regress on follow-up imaging.

A PAU can be single or multiple in as many as 17% to 22% of cases.[10] They occur all along the length of the aorta with the most common location being the descending thoracic aorta. (Table 24–1) As such, most of the studies included in this review focused mostly on the descending thoracic aortic PAU. In a retrospective review of PAUs, 87% were found in the descending thoracic aorta, while 13% were isolated in the ascending aorta and arch.[2] PAUs found in the infrarenal aorta are exceptionally rare with less than 4% of patients with abdominal vascular pathologies being affected.[21, 24] PAUs in the ascending aorta and aortic arch are infrequent.[19, 29]

A PAU should not be confused with mycotic aneurysms, which are also rare. Mycotic aneurysms can also appear as ulcerations; however, their presence often is accompanied with a systemic response including fevers, leukocytosis, tachypnea, or tachycardia. Patients may also present with florid sepsis. Characteristic radiographic findings of a mycotic aneurysm include the appearance of surrounding infected fluid, which may contain air-fluid levels, an aortoenteric fistula or aortobronchial fistula. Patients presenting with such symptoms or radiographic findings should have blood cultures evaluated and treated with broad spectrum antibiotics prior to repair.[30]

CLINICAL PRESENTATION

PAUs can be associated with sudden onset of pain that is often intense tearing, throbbing and even migratory depending on the location. (Figure 24–1) If the ascending aorta is

TABLE 24–1. LOCATION OF PAUs IN STUDIES REVIEWED (UPCHURCH)

	n	Ascending (%)	Arch (%)	Descending Thoracic (%)	Abdominal (%)
Stanson AW, et al. 1986[5]	16	6		94	
Yucel EK, et al. 1990[11]	7			100	
Kazerooni EA, et al. 1992[12]	16		6	88	6
Harris JA, et al. 1994[13]	18		3	87	10
Coady MA, et al. 1998[2]	15	13		87	
Vilacosta I, et al. 1998[14]	12		13	87	
Murgo S, et al. 1998[15]	4			100	
Brittenden J, et al. 1999[16]	2			100	
Hayashi H, et al. 2000[17]	12			92	8
Quint LE, et al. 2001[18]	38	2	25	62	11
Cho KR, et al. 2004[19]	96		11	89	
Demers P, et al. 2004[20]	26		4	96	
Batt M, et al. 2005[21]	8				100
Brinster DR, et al. 2006[22]	21			100	
Eggebrech H, et al. 2006[23]	22			91	9
Piffaretti G, et al. 2007[24]	11			100	
Dalainas I, et al. 2007[25]	18			89	11
Geisbüsch P, et al. 2008[10]	48			73	27
Gottardi R, et al. 2008[26]	27		19	81	
Botta L, et al. 2008[27]	19			100	
Patel HJ, et al. 2009[28]	37			100	

involved, the affected patient can have anterior chest, neck and jaw pain. Upper back, mid-scapular and abdominal pain is frequently present if the arch or high descending aorta is involved. Descending thoracic PAUs present with chest, back and abdominal pain. Abdominal PAUs can also present with abdominal and lower back pain. Collectively, more than 75% of patients present with symptoms of acutely worsened pain for less than 14 days.[9, 22]

Alternatively, patients with a PAU can be asymptomatic on presentation. Coady et al. noted 20% of patients with a thoracic PAU were asymptomatic at presentation.[2] Piffaretti et al. found that 23% of the patients with an infrarenal aortic PAU treated with endovascular stent grafting had no complaints when being evaluated initially.[24]

Most patients affected by a PAU are elderly, ranging in age from 66 to 76 years.[2, 10, 22, 24-26, 28] Patients with PAUs are considerably older than those with other aortic pathologies, with the exception of patients with aortic aneurysms.[19, 24] There does not seem to be a gender disposition. However, Demers et al. noted interestingly that female gender was associated with negative outcomes for PAUs.[20]

Hypertension is a universal risk factor for the development of all AAS pathologies. It is therefore not unexpected that it is the most common comorbid disease associated with PAUs. The percentage of patients identified with a PAU and a history of hypertension ranges from 73 to 100%.[2, 10, 25, 28] In addition to hypertension, patients presenting with PAUs are likely to have a history of atherosclerosis, coronary artery disease, prior myocardial infarction, peripheral vascular disease and cerebrovascular accident history. Multiple other risk factors for a PAU include a smoking history, chronic obstructive pulmonary disease and diabetes.[10, 21, 22, 25, 26] Botta et al. only noted

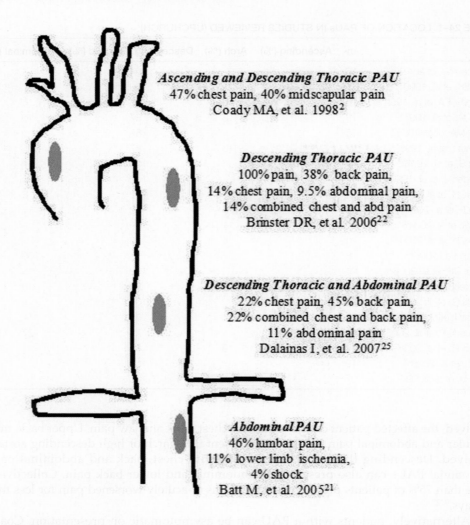

Ascending and Descending Thoracic PAU
47% chest pain, 40% midscapular pain
Coady MA, et al. 1998[2]

Descending Thoracic PAU
100% pain, 38% back pain,
14% chest pain, 9.5% abdominal pain,
14% combined chest and abd pain
Brinster DR, et al. 2006[22]

Descending Thoracic and Abdominal PAU
22% chest pain, 45% back pain,
22% combined chest and back pain,
11% abdominal pain
Dalainas I, et al. 2007[25]

Abdominal PAU
46% lumbar pain,
11% lower limb ischemia,
4% shock
Batt M, et al. 2005[21]

Figure 24–1. Symptoms associated with PAUs based on location along the aorta.

approximately 40% of patients affected by a PAU had a history of smoking or currently smoked, but most studies suggest the smoking incidence to be between 60% and 80%.[10, 19-22, 25, 27]

Distinct clinical presentations between patients with a PAU and an AD are focused on differences in pulse exam and associated neurologic deficits. Peripheral pulses are typically equivalent in bilateral upper and lower extremities in patients with PAUs, whereas pulses may not be equivalent in patients with AD, especially in those with lower extremity malperfusion. Patients with AD also present with neurologic deficits, which are not typically found in patients even with symptomatic PAUs. Moreover, patients with PAUs seldom have aortic valve regurgitation, which is frequently observed in patients with type A AD.

Generally, patients with PAUs have a larger aortic diameter at the time of diagnosis. Coady et al. found concomitant abdominal aortic aneurysms (AAA) in 6 of

15 patients (40%) with PAUs. The incidence of AAA associated with PAUs is significantly higher as compared to type A and B dissections (9% and 31%, respectively).[2] Stanson et al. and Kazerooni et al. found 38% and 75% of patients with a PAU to have an associated aortic aneurysm.[5, 12] Geisbusch et al. found the aortic diameter in 48 patients with PAUs to be a mean of 5.0±1.7cm (range 27-105).[10]

Pulmonary complications frequently occur in conjunction with PAUs, especially if other vascular pathologies (IMH, AD and rupture) are present. Pleural effusions are found in conjunction with PAUs 10% to 44% of the time.[12, 19, 22, 27] Brinster et al. noted 9.5% of the patients in their study presented with evidence of an increasing, bloody effusion in the left chest. These patients were included in the group of patients with an acute presentation of PAUs necessitating urgent endovascular treatment whether or not they presented with pain.[22]

PAUs may also present with embolization of atheromatous debris, which can result in ischemia or even infarction distal to the PAU, even though this is considered rare.[24] However, if there are no indications suggesting a cardiac origin for the source of a lower limb embolism, a search for an aortic cause, particularly a PAU, should be pursued with computed tomography angiography (CTA) of the chest, abdomen and pelvis. Abdominal PAUs are more likely than thoracic PAUs to cause embolization.[5, 31, 32]

OTHER AORTIC PATHOLOGIES ASSOCIATED WITH PAU

IMHs are not universally associated with PAUs; however, the incidence of IMHs in conjunction with PAUs is frequent. Multiple reports have determined that IMHs occurs with PAUs in 22% to 94% of cases.[2, 9, 12, 25, 28, 33] Initial studies have shown that the population presenting with both a PAU and an IMH versus those presenting with a solitary PAU are similar in age, prevalence of comorbidities, and frequency of associated rupture. However, a recent study by Patel et al. suggests patients with a PAU and an associated IMH require urgent or emergent intervention more frequently.[28] The mean longitudinal extension of an IMH found with a PAU is limited and was noted to be approximately 2.8cm.[25] The surrounding aortic wall is typically thickened and there is often an inward displacement of intimal calcification. It is speculated that chronic atherosclerosis in the affected area leads to fibrosis in the vascular media preventing hematoma propagation.

In the aforementioned study of the 11 patients with an IMH found to have a concurrent PAU, seven of these patients (64%) progressed to an atypical AD or a new intimal tear during their hospital stay. Thirty-six percent of the patients with an IMH and a PAU died during the follow up period, while only 8% of the patients with solitary IMH died.[33] This study implied that IMHs found in the presence of a coexisting PAU might be associated with worse outcomes and that PAU found in conjunction with an IMH might be the cause of newly developed dissections with intimal tear and rupture of the aorta. Patel et al. however found no difference in overall patient survival between those presenting with a PAU and an IMH compared to PAU alone.[28]

When ADs are found in conjunction with PAUs, they, like IMHs, are also typically shorter in length as compared to a classic AD. Hussain et al. studied PAU in association with AD of the thoracic aorta and found the frequency of PAUs in a group of 47 patients with ADs to be approximately 11%, while Park et al. found the number of patients with a PAU and concurrent AD to be 20%.[9, 34] Often a thicker calcified and static flap is affiliated with the tear.[14]

Pseudoaneurysms can result when PAUs erode into the adventitia. Previous studies have shown that pseudoaneurysms occur with a PAU in 19% to 44% of cases.[5, 12] Transmural rupture of the pseudoaneurysm occurs into the mediastinum or rupture can result in a hemithorax. While the rate of rupture is quite variable, rupture is almost immediately lethal. Rupture is more common in patients with a PAU compared to dissection. Nine to 44% percent of patients presenting with a symptomatic PAU were observed to have an aortic rupture in the studies evaluated for this summary.[3, 5, 10, 19, 20, 22, 24-28, 36] Patel et al. found that 41% of the patients evaluated with a PAU of the descending thoracic aorta presented emergently with rupture. Similarly, Stanson et al. recognized the rate of rupture associated with a PAU to be around 44%.[5] Unlike descending thoracic PAUs, abdominal PAUs are thought to be responsible for only 1% to 5% of all aortic ruptures.[24]

DIAGNOSTIC IMAGING

The once gold standard for the detection of PAUs, aortography, is now largely replaced by CTA. CTA accurately visualizes other vascular pathologies, including aortic wall enhancement, thrombosed IMH external to the calcified intima, contrast extravasation through the ulceration, the absence of a double lumen, a thrombosed pseudoaneurysm and transmural rupture.[34] The greatest disadvantage of CTA is the requirement for iodinated contrast and radiation exposure. Additionally, if intimal calcification is not present, CTA can have difficulty distinguishing between intraluminal thrombus and an IMH.[11] Imaging techniques used to identify PAUs generally demonstrate an outpouching of the aortic wall with the presence of jagged edges surrounded by extensive aortic atheroma (Figure 24–2). The imaging is quite unlike that of aortic dissections. The starting point for a PAU is distinct, whereas, the starting point for an AD is often difficult to determine.

Magnetic resonance angiography (MRA) reveals the PAU as craterlike ulcerations in the absence of an intimal flap or false lumen. As compared to aortography, Yucel et al. reported that MRA identified six of seven PAU.[11] The aortic wall was thickened and showed up as high intensity signals on T1 and T2 weighted images when the PAU

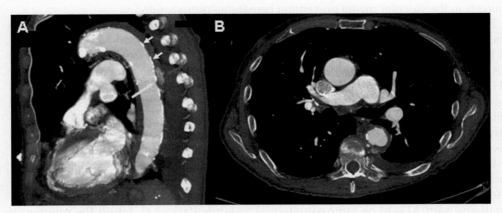

Figure 24–2. A. CTA patient #1, lateral view of descending thoracic PAU, yellow arrow indicates lesion, red arrow indicates associated IMH, white arrows indicate associated atherosclerosis, **B.** CTA patient #1, sagittal view of associated IMH.

was complicated by an acute IMH. MRA may be superior to aortography at identifying complications of aortic ulcerations. An advantage of MRA is that no iodinated contrast is required and images may be acquired using time of flight sequences. Additionally, images can be acquired in multiple planes unlike aortography. Unfortunately, the high cost of MRA, the long time needed for evaluation, the difficulty monitoring unstable patients and the inability for patients with metallic devices to be imaged still limits its use. Additionally, MRA is of little value in the identification of an IMH and aortic wall calcification.

On transesophageal echocardiography (TEE), PAUs appear as crater-like ulcers with ragged edges in the presence of extensive atheroma without an intimal flap or false lumen. If an IMH is present in conjunction with a PAU, they appear echolucent with mottled thickening of the aortic wall and inward displacement of intimal calcification. The greatest benefit of TEE is being able to evaluate cardiac function, as well as to identify regional cardiac wall motion abnormalities. The limitation of TEE is that the results are operator dependent based on the ability to obtain accurate images and the interpreter's read of the imaging acquired.

Since the diagnosis of PAU is often performed using imaging techniques, pre-intervention histologic confirmation is not possible. This is important as there is some concern that PAUs are actually re-entry tears associated with IMHs. Unfortunately, there are no reliable criteria at this point to distinguish between the two different pathologies by imaging alone. The presence of extensive calcification in the aortic wall surrounding the lesion favors the presence of a PAU over a bland tear associated with IMH. [28]

The presence of PAUs with other vascular arteriopathies indicates increased severity of the pathology and tends to correlate with worsened survival. When studied in conjunction with AD, patients with PAUs are more likely to suffer aortic rupture than patients with AD alone (AD + PAU, 40% versus type A AD alone 7.0% and type B AD alone 3.6%).[2] The survival trend of AD in association with a PAU is worse as compared to solitary AD because PAUs more often progress to rupture.[2]

APPROACH TO THERAPY

An understanding of PAU evolution, significance and need for treatment is warranted. Prognosis for the PAU is correlated with size with most believing that PAUs with larger diameters (>20mm) and longer depths (>10mm) require earlier intervention. Geisbusch et al. found a mean ulcer diameter of 2.2±0.9 cm.[10] In contrast, Dalainas et al. found a mean crater diameter of 1.2cm (range 0.5-2cm). [20]

In a study following patients with an IMH and PAU, there is a correlation between PAU size and progression of aortic pathology as defined by an enlarging IMH, development of dissection or rupture. According to Ganaha et al., the diameter and depth of a PAU found in patients with more severe worsening aortic disease during follow up was significantly larger than those patients who did not have disease progression. The mean diameter and depth of a PAU that progressed was 2.1±0.8cm and 1.4±0.4 cm, respectively. They concluded that patients with a PAU initially measuring 2.0 cm or more in maximum diameter or 1.0 cm or greater in maximum depth have a high risk of disease progression and therefore should be considered for early surgical or endovascular repair.[3]

There is also a correlation between PAUs and larger aortic diameter. Coady et al. noted that patients with PAUs tended to have larger aortic diameters at presentation as compared to patients with dissection and were significantly more likely to have AAA at the time of presentation. This might be a function of age since patients with PAUs are often older than patients with an AD. Tittle et al. found progression of aortic diameter to be 0.2cm/year in the presence of a PAU arguing for annual surveillance.[6] Demers et al. identified increased aortic diameter as a risk factor for treatment failure.[20]

Conservative management is preferred if patients presenting with a PAU have only descending aorta involvement and they have no associated symptoms or symptoms are well controlled with antihypertensive medications. Strict blood pressure control with beta blockade or vasodilators and pain control with morphine should be performed. In a study of conservative management of a PAU with blood pressure control and observation with repeat imaging over a one to seven year period, Harris et al. found that approximately one third of patients progressed to form a saccular or fusiform aneurysm.[13] Cho et al. presented a retrospective series of 105 patients with conservatively treated PAUs. Medical management in this study was associated with a significantly lower early mortality rate compared to open surgical repair, 4% and 21%, respectively.[19] Conservative treatment with antihypertensive therapy generally results in only one third of patients requiring intervention for progression of PAUs to aneurysms, dissection or perforation over a 25 year period.[19]

Contrary to the aforementioned studies, Hussain et al. found few if any patients treated with conservative management progressed to aneurysm formation or rupture. In this study, Hussain followed patients with PAUs for 30 months. None of the patients required surgical intervention. Within six months of diagnosis, all patients were symptom-free and imaging showed that 80% patients had a resolution of their PAU with no signs of progression to aneurysm or rupture.[34]

Obviously, a PAU located in the descending thoracic aorta should be repaired if there are signs of progression (accelerated growth) or impending vascular compromise. These signs include an expanding IMH, an evolving AD, distal embolization or hemodynamic instability. Failure of medical management to control pain or blood pressure is another indication for surgical repair. Ganaha et al. noted the patients presenting with PAUs and either symptoms that started acutely, uncontrolled pain or a pleural effusion were indicators for a more malignant form of PAU that was associated with a higher risk of progression to aortic rupture. These patients require urgent operative intervention.[3] Dalainas et al. found that the median time between admission and endovascular repair for patients who failed conservative management for their PAU was two days (range 1-4 days).[25] Geisbusch et al. advocated for PAU repair, specifically with endovascular intervention in their study, within 48 hours of symptom onset.[10]

OPERATIVE REPAIR

Historically, PAUs were treated with open aortic repair. In 1959, Shumacker and King described the first successful operative repair of a ruptured descending thoracic aorta directly caused by a PAU.[35] The open surgical repair of aortic pathologies, including those directly related to a PAU, has since improved greatly with decreased mortality and morbidity rates documented over time. Recent studies from specialized aortic surgery centers have demonstrated 30-day mortality rates as low as 6%.[36] Yet, operative mortality for patients undergoing open repair of PAU can be as high as 60% especially for patients with

TABLE 24–2. COMPARISON OF STUDIES REPORTING ENDOVASCULAR TREATMENT FOR PAUs

	n	Average Age	Average (months)	Follow-Technical Success (%)	30-Day Mortality (%)	Overall Mortality (%)	Endoleaks (%)
Demers P, et al.[20] 2004	26	70	51	92	12	30	4
Brinster DR, et al.[22] 2006	21	73	14	100	0	5	0
Eggebrech H, et al.[23] 2006	22	69	27	96	0	18	5
Piffaretti G, et al.[24] 2007	11	73	15	100	0	10	0
Geibüsch P, et al.[10] 2008	48	70	31	94	6	39	23
Gottardi R, et al.[26] 2008	27	66	42	100	11	15	7
Botta L, et al.[27] 2008	19	72	22	95	11	21	16
Patel HJ, et al.[28] 2009	37	72	37	100	5	38	24

significant comorbidities.[24] One of the few advantages of open surgical repair is that it allows for a histological diagnosis. However, open surgical repair requires clamping the aorta, often a large thoracotomy, cardiopulmonary bypass, and an extended hospital stay requiring an intensive care unit admission.

ENDOVASCULAR REPAIR

In general, patients affected by PAUs are often not ideal candidates for open repair because of advanced age and poor functional status. In addition, as the field has evolved towards treating more pathologies endovascularly, this approach is now the primary form of therapy. Importantly, endovascular repair of PAU has been demonstrated to be at least as effective as traditional open surgical repair or a hybrid procedure. Multiple groups have pursued endovascular repair of PAUs. (Table 24–2) For PAU treatment, the clinical success of endovascular stenting ranges from 76% to 100%.[10, 20, 22, 24, 26-28] The reported 30-day mortality for patients undergoing endovascular repair for PAUs is 0% to 26%.[10, 20, 22-24, 26-28] Geisbusch P et al. reported a slightly higher 30-day mortality (6.2%) and in-hospital mortality (14.6%); however, some of the patients included in this study had AD and/or aneurysms in addition to their PAU.[10] Moreover, the same study found that patients with a PAU whom were asymptomatic at presentation had a lower in hospital mortality rate than symptomatic patients, 0 vs. 23%, respectively.[10] By univariate analysis, Patel et al. found older age correlated with early mortality.[28]

There are many advantages to endovascular over open repair in the treatment of PAUs (Figure 24–3). For example, mean operative time with endovascular stent graft placement is decreased compared to open repair. [22-24] In addition, the number of hospital days post-procedure are minimized with endovascular stent placement for PAUs with multiple studies reporting a mean length of hospital stay after endovascular repair ranging from four to eight days.[22, 24, 28]

As endovascular repair continues to evolve, long term mortality associated with stent graft placement for aortic PAUs improves, even for complicated PAUs associated with other aortic pathologies. The median survival for the 37 patients with descending thoracic PAUs treated by Patel et al. was 90 months. The same study found overall late mortality (>30 days postoperative) after endovascular repair to be 38%. Mortality directly related to an aortic pathology was noted in 11%. PAUs presentation with IMH was associated with an increased risk for treatment failure defined as the need for

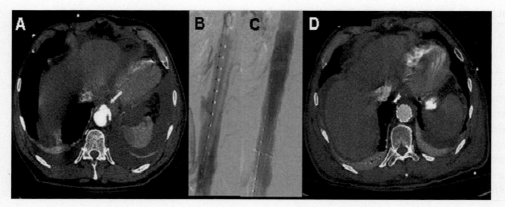

Figure 24–3. A. CTA patient #2, saggital view, yellow arrow indicates PAU, **B.** angiography of PAU, **C.** angiography of PAU after stent placement, **D.** CTA sagittal view, three months after PAU stent placement.

open or endovascular aortic re-intervention, aortic rupture or aortic related death. Not surprisingly, late mortality was found to be correlated with urgent or emergent endovascular repair.[28]

Limitations for endovascular repair include unfavorable anatomy, inadequate working length (insufficient landing zones) and aortic pathology that includes branch vessels. Sufficient landing zones remain important for successful a PAU exclusion and a minimum of 20 mm proximal and distal to the PAU seems mandatory. Hybrid approaches, including bypasses to brachiocephalic, mesenteric and renal vessels can be followed by endovascular repair of a PAU. Fenestrated endografts have been used for investigational purposes in patients with inadequate landing zones. Because PAUs are rare and the procedures used to intervene upon the PAU have evolved with time, it is difficult to say which stent grafts are best to use to treat lesions. Most studies evaluated agree that only a 5% to 10% maximum oversizing should be performed.[25, 28] D'Ancona and others agree that aggressive attempts to dilate the landing zones for stent grafts are usually not indicated.[37]

Post-procedural imaging usually with CTA typically demonstrates lesion regression or thrombosis. It is therefore not surprising that clinical symptoms associated with PAU in most cases resolved after endovascular treatment. One hundred percent of the patients treated for PAUs with preoperative pain had symptomatic relief after stent placement in a study by Brinster et al.[22]

Complications after stent-grafting for PAUs include endoleak, peripheral embolization, stent migration or fragmentation. Endoleaks are infrequently encountered during follow-up of patients with PAU treated endovascularly. Early endoleaks were observed in 19% of patients included in the study by Geisbusch et al. However, this study included PAUs found in conjunction with multiple other aortic pathologies including AD, associated aneurysms, and aortic fistulas.[10] Others describe a less frequent rate of endoleaks. Dalainas et al. demonstrated a 5.5% rate of endoleak after endovascular repair of PAUs. The only endoleak experienced in this study was associated with covering a pseudoaneurysm found in association with a PAU at the time of presentation.[25] Park et al. found endoleaks affecting approximately 13% of the 15 patients treated for a thoracic PAU.[9] These endoleaks were noted initially during post-procedural follow-up and all disappeared spontaneously. Piffaretti et al. showed no patients with infrarenal PAUs found to have endoleaks after endovascular stent placement during a mean 26 month follow-up period.[24]

Patel et al. identified endovascular repair that included the aortic arch might be protective against future rupture or new aneurysmal development for PAU. While the study lacked sufficient numbers of patients treated to yield statistical significance, the group theorized that the use of a short stent graft for a PAU occurring in the mid-descending aorta may leave the distal arch and proximal descending aorta untreated and susceptible to further dissection.[28] There is a subset of patients with a PAU with a history of peripheral vascular occlusive disease with femoral and iliac vessels not amenable to percutaneous access. This can be circumvented via multiple approaches including retroperitoneal access to the iliac vessels. Brinster et al. found that 10% of the patients with PAUs treated endovascularly required a retroperitoneal approach.[22] Dalainas et al. found that 12% of patients treated endovascularly for a PAU required a retroperitoneal approach or direct aortic access to perform the intervention.[25] In a study including only descending thoracic PAUs treated with endovascular repair, Patel et al. documented that 14% of patients required iliac artery access via a retroperitoneal approach with conduit.[28]

Neurologic complications, primarily spinal cord paraplegia and paraparesis, were initially encountered not infrequently, following endovascular therapy. However, increased use of lumbar drains has decreased these complications. Recent studies show the rate of transient paraplegia requiring lumbar drains to be approximately 5%. [9, 28] Other long term neurologic complications including stroke were encountered 0-5%.[9, 20, 28] It is implied that neurologic complications might be reduced with decreased aortic coverage.[9, 22]

SUMMARY

Despite being rare as compared to the other AAS pathologies, PAUs are important lesions of which vascular surgeons should be aware. With the aging population and improvements in vascular imaging, their observed frequency will likely increase. The presence of a bland PAU in an asymptomatic patient is not necessarily predictive of an evolving vascular pathology. However, those presenting with symptoms and other associated aortic pathologies in addition to a PAU are at increased risk for poor outcomes, even after intervention. The onset of endovascular stent-grafting has provided patients with PAU, whom would have not been eligible for open repair, an opportunity for therapeutic intervention. It is likely that endovascular repair will remain the gold standard for PAU treatment.

REFERENCES

1. Rothwell PM, Coull AJ, Silver LE, Fairhead JF, Giles MF, Lovelock CE, et al. Population-based study of event-rate, incidence, case fatality, and mortality for all acute vascular events in all arterial territories (Oxford Vascular Study). *Lancet* 2005;19:1773–83.
2. Coady MA, Rizzo JA, Hammond GL, Pierce JG, Kopf GS, Elefteriades JA. Penetrating ulcer of the thoracic aorta: what is it? How do we recognize it? How do we manage it? *J Vasc Surg* 1998;27:1006–15.

3. Ganaha F, Miller DC, Sugimoto K, Do YS, Minamiguchi H, Saito H, et al. Prognosis of aortic intramural hematoma with and without penetrating atherosclerotic ulcer: a clinical and radiological analysis. *Circulation* 2002;16:342–8.

4. Movsowitz HD, Lampert C, Jacobs LE, Kotler MN. Penetrating atherosclerotic aortic ulcers. *Am Heart J* 1994;128:1210–7.

5. Stanson AW, Kazmier FJ, Hollier LH, Edwards WD, Pairolero PC, Sheedy PF, et al. Penetrating atherosclerotic ulcers of the thoracic aorta: natural history and clinicopathologic correlations. *Ann Vasc Surg* 1986;1:15–23.

6. Tittle SL, Lynch RJ, Cole PE, Singh HS, Rizzo JA, Kopf GS, et al. Midterm follow-up of penetrating ulcer and intramural hematoma of the aorta. *J Thorac Cardiovasc Surg* 2002;123: 1051–9.

7. Sheenan T. Dissecting Aneurysms. Medical Research Council, Special Report Series no. 193. London: HMSO; 1934.

8. Coady MA, Rizzo JA, Elefteriades JA. Pathologic variants of thoracic dissections: penetrating atherosclerotic ulcers and intramural hematomas. *Cardiology Clinics* 1999;17:637–57.

9. Park JS, Lim SH, Shin JH. Unusual aortic dissection mimicking penetrating atherosclerotic ulcer after blunt chest trauma. *J Cardiovasc Ultrasound* 2009;17:110–11.

10. Geisbüsch P, Kotelis D, Weber TF, Hyhlik-Dürr A, Kauczor HU, Böckler D. Early and midterm results after endovascular stent graft repair of penetrating aortic ulcers. *J Vasc Surg* 2008;48:1361–8.

11. Yucel EK, Steinberg FL, Egglin TK, Geller SC, Waltman AC, Athanasoulis CA. Penetrating aortic ulcers: diagnosis with MR imaging. *Radiology* 1990;177:779–81.

12. Kazerooni EA, Bree RL, Williams DM. Penetrating atherosclerotic ulcers of the descending thoracic aorta: evaluation with CT and distinction from aortic dissection. *Radiology* 1992;183:759–65.

13. Harris JA, Bis KG, Glover JL, Bendick PJ, Shetty A, Brown OW. Penetrating atherosclerotic ulcers of the aorta. *J Vasc Surg* 1994;19:90–8.

14. Vilacosta I, San Román JA, Aragoncillo P, Ferreirós J, Mendez R, Graupner C. Penetrating atherosclerotic aortic ulcer: documentation by transesophageal echocardiography. *J Am Coll Cardiol* 1998;32:83–9.

15. Murgo S, Dussaussois L, Golzarian J, Cavenaile JC, Abada HT, Ferreira J, et al. Penetrating atherosclerotic ulcer of the descending aorta: treatment by endovascular stent graft. *Cardiovasc Intervent Radiol* 1998;21:454–8.

16. Brittenden J, McBride K, McInnes G, Gillespie IN, Bradbury AW. The use of endovascular stents in the treatment of penetrating ulcers of the thoracic aorta. *J Vasc Surg* 1999;30:946–9.

17. Hayashi H, Matsuoka Y, Sakamoto I, Sueyoshi E, Okimoto T, Hayashi K, et al. Penetrating atherosclerotic ulcer of the aorta: imaging features and disease concept. *Radiographics* 2000;20:995–1005.

18. Quint LE, Williams DM, Francis IR, Monaghan HM, Sonnad SS, Patel S, et al. Ulcerlike lesions of the aorta: imaging features and natural history. *Radiology* 2001;218:719–23.

19. Cho KR, Stanson AW, Potter DD, Cherry KJ, Schaff HV, Sundt TM. Penetrating atherosclerotic ulcer of the descending thoracic aorta and arch. *J Thorac Cardiovasc Surg* 2004;127: 1393–9.

20. Demers P, Miller DC, Mitchell RS, Kee ST, Chagonjian L, Dake MD. Stent-graft repair of penetrating atherosclerotic ulcers in the descending thoracic aorta: mid-term results. *Ann Thorac Surg* 2004;77:81–6.

21. Batt M, Haudebourg P, Planchard PF, Ferrari E, Hassen-Khodja R, Bouillanne PJ. Penetrating atherosclerotic ulcers of the infrarenal aorta: life-threatening lesions. *Eur J Vasc Endovasc Surg.* 2005;29:35–42.

22. Brinster DR, Wheatley GH, Williams J, Ramaiah VG, Diethrich EB, Rodriguez-Lopez JA. Are penetrating aortic ulcers best treated using an endovascular approach? *Ann Thorac Surg* 2006 Nov;82:1688–91.

23. Eggebrecht H, Herold U, Schmermund A, Lind AY, Kuhnt O, Martini S, et al. Endovascular stent-graft treatment of penetrating aortic ulcer: results over a median follow-up of 27 months. *Am Heart J* 2006; 151:530–6.

24. Piffaretti G, Tozzi M, Lomazzi C, Rivolta N, Riva F, Maida S, Caronno R, et al. Penetrating ulcers of the thoracic aorta: results from a single-centre experience. *Am J Surg* 2007;193: 443–7.
25. Dalainas I, Nano G, Medda M, Bianchi P, Casana R, Ramponi F, et al. Endovascular treatment of penetrating aortic ulcers: mid-term results. *Eur J Vasc Endovasc Surg* 2007;34:74–8.
26. Gottardi R, Zimpfer D, Funovics M, Schoder M, Lammer J, Wolner E, et al. Mid-term results after endovascular stent-graft placement due to penetrating atherosclerotic ulcers of the thoracic aorta. *Eur J Cardiothorac Surg* 2008;33:1019–24.
27. Botta L, Buttazzi K, Russo V, Parlapiano M, Gostoli V, Di Bartolomeo R, et al. Endovascular repair for penetrating atherosclerotic ulcers of the descending thoracic aorta: early and mid-term results. *Ann Thorac Surg* 2008;85:987–92.
28. Patel HJ, Williams DM, Upchurch GR Jr, Dasika NL, Deeb GM. The challenge of associated intramural hematoma with endovascular repair for penetrating ulcers of the descending thoracic aorta. *J Vasc Surg* 2010;51:829–35.
29. Troxler M, Mavor AI, Homer-Vanniasinkam S. Penetrating atherosclerotic ulcers of the aorta. *Br J Surg* 2001;88:1169–77.
30. Lew WK, Rowe VL, Cunningham MJ, Weaver FA. Endovascular management of mycotic aortic aneurysms and associated aortoaerodigestive fistulas. *Ann Vasc Surg* 2009;23:81–9.
31. Goldstein DJ, Flores RM, Todd GJ. Rupture of a nonaneurysmal atherosclerotic infrarenal aorta. *J Vasc Surg* 1997;26:700–3.
32. Farooq MM, Kling K, Yamini D, Gelabert HA, Baker JD, Freischlag JA. Penetrating ulceration of the infrarenal aorta: case reports of an embolic and an asymptomatic lesion. *Ann Vasc Surg* 2001;15:255–9.
33. Shimizu H, Yoshino H, Udagawa H, Watanuki A, Yano K, Ide H, et al. Prognosis of aortic intramural hemorrhage compared with classic aortic dissection. *Am J Cardiol* 2000;85:792–5.
34. Hussain S, Glover JL, Bree R, Bendick PJ. Penetrating atherosclerotic ulcers of the thoracic aorta. *J Vasc Surg* 1989;9:710–17.
35. Shumacker HB Jr, King H. Surgical management of rapidly expanding intrathoracic pulsating hematomas. *Surg Gynecol Obstet* 1959;109:155–64.
36. Coselli JS, Conklin LD, LeMaire SA. Thoracoabdominal aortic aneurysm repair: review and update of current strategies. *Ann Thorac Surg* 2002;74:S1881–4.
37. D'Ancona G, Bauset R, Normand JP, Turcotte R, Dagenais F. Endovascular stent-graft repair of a complicated penetrating ulcer of the descending thoracic aorta: a word of caution. *J Endovasc Ther* 2003;10:928–31.

25

Contemporary Management of Aortic Arch Aneurysms

B. Ramlawi, MD, M.J. Reardon, MD,
M.G. Davies, MD and A.B. Lumsden, MD

INTRODUCTION

Thoracic aortic aneurysm is a progressive, life threatening disease that occurs with an incidence of about 10/100,000.[1] Progressive expansion and subsequent rupture will lead to death in 45% to 85% of untreated patients by 5 years.[2] This dismal prognosis has led our surgical department to an early interest in the repair of thoracic aortic aneurysm that persists today.[3] The earliest repairs of aortic arch aneurysm required extra anatomic bypass to maintain cerebral blood flow, cardiopulmonary bypass with resection and reconstruction of the aortic arch aneurysm and subsequent take down of the previously created extra anatomic bypass. This was simplified by Griepp with the introduction of profound hypothermia and circulatory arrest to allow cerebral protection during aortic arch resection.[4] Despite continued improvement of surgical techniques, open aortic arch repair remains a challenge to the surgeon and the patient. Current results from the Mayo group in a series of 95 open aortic arch repairs revealed a mortality of 16.8% and a stroke rate of 9.5%.[5] The introduction of axillary cannulation and antegrade cerebral profusion did allow a decrease in mortality to 6% and stroke rate to 6% but still highlights the complexity of this disease. For our increasingly elderly and often frail patient population, open aortic arch repair continues to be associated with an in hospital mortality of up to 20% and stroke rate of up to 12%.[6,7] For patients with significant comorbidities such as severe chronic obstructive lung disease, dialysis dependent renal failure, heart failure, diabetes or previous stroke, open surgical repair may not be a viable option due to prohibitive estimated mortality and permanent morbidity. Hybrid repair of aortic arch aneurysm has been developed by our group and others to address this high risk patient cohort without the use of circulatory arrest and often cardiopulmonary bypass which can be poorly tolerated.[8–12]

RATIONALE FOR HYBRID APPROACH

Debranching is fundamentally performed for two reasons:

1. Provide an appropriate landing zone for thoracic stent graft.
2. Provide ongoing perfusion to the supra-aortic vessels.

It is clear from the previous discussion that traditional open repair of aortic arch aneurysms is possible but comes at a significant cost to the patient.[13–18] This cost is not only dependent on the magnitude of the incision and dissection needed for open repair but heavily influenced by the need for cardiopulmonary bypass, cardiac arrest and profound hypothermia with circulatory arrest. Hybrid procedures were developed to help minimize or eliminate these whenever possible in hopes of decreasing mortality and morbidity and allowing us to extend therapy to a group previously believed to have a prohibitive risk using standard repair techniques.[19–26]

The endovascular repair of infrarenal abdominal aortic aneurysm and descending thoracic aortic aneurysm with adequate landing zones has become common-place and well accepted as an alternative to traditional open repair in appropriate cases.[27–29] Thoracic aneurysms that would require coverage of the innominate artery or the left subclavian artery for proper graft fixation are not amenable to standard, isolated endovascular techniques. Aortic arch aneurysm can be isolated or involve the ascending and/or descending thoracic aorta. When isolated or involving the descending thoracic aorta, these aneurysms can be repaired by extra anatomic bypass of the cerebral vessels and the left subclavian when desired and antegrade or retrograde endografts deployment with cardiopulmonary bypass, cardiac arrest or circulatory arrest removing many of the technical risks factors. For arch aneurysm that also involves the ascending thoracic aorta, cardiopulmonary bypass and cardiac arrest is necessary for ascending aortic replacement but debranching and endografts repair will eliminate the need for profound hypothermia and circulatory arrest and can shorten the overall procedure. (Figure 25–1)

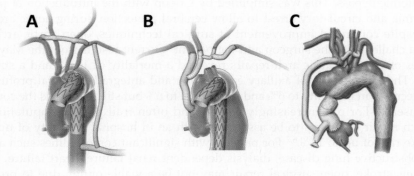

Figure 25–1. A Arch vessels debranching using 14-mm inflow conduit from ascending aorta followed by 10-mm bypass graft to the innominate, left common carotid and left subclavian arteries; **B** Arch vessels debranching using 10-mm Dacron graft with retrograde inflow through 10-mm graft. Endograft was delivered using 14-mm conduit; **C** Arch vessels showing a 10-mm limb being sutured to a 14-mm trunk. The 10-mm limb is tunneled superiorly to revascularize the supra-aortic trunks, whereas the 14-mm trunk is used as the conduit for antegrade stent-graft placement. The 14-mm stump is oversewn after completion of the stent-graft deployment.[10,11] Figures A and B reprinted with permission from Elsevier/Society for Vascular Surgery/Department of Cardiovascular Surgery, Methodist DeBakey Heart & Vascular Center. Figure C reprinted with permission from Elsevier/Society for Vascular Surgery.

TECHNICAL ISSUES WITH ARCH ANEURYSMS

Endograft repair of aneurysms requires anatomically appropriate necks or landing zones for the proper fixation and sealing of the aneurysm at its proximal and distal extent. It also requires that critically important arteries not be covered unless revascularized in some method as well as access to deliver the graft for deployment. Aortic arch aneurysms can provide challenges in each of these areas. The thoracic aorta has been divided into 4 zones. Zone 0 includes the ascending aorta to just beyond the take off of the innominate artery. Zone 1 begins at the end of zone 0 and extends to just beyond the take off of the left carotid artery. Zone 2 begins at the end of zone 1 and extends to just beyond the take off of the left subclavian artery. Zone 3 represents the proximal descending thoracic aorta from just beyond the left subclavian to the mid descending thoracic aorta and finally zone 4 comprises the rest of the descending thoracic aorta. (Figure 25–2) We will now consider specific technical aspects of a hybrid procedure for each zone.

Zone 0-Deployment Principles

This is the most complex debranching procedure to perform, necessitating revascularization of all 3 supra aortic trunks. There are numerous considerations:

1. Either a full sternotomy or a right anterior mini thoracotomy can be utilized. The intercostal space is selected based on correlation with the pre op CT scan to provide the optimal approach to the most proximal ascending aorta.
2. Quality of the ascending aorta. We have had one death from sutures tearing out of the ascending aorta on postoperative day #1. The aorta cannot be severely calcified or aneurysmal.

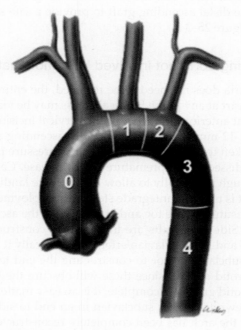

Figure 25–2. Ishimaru arch map depicting the different landing zones.[44]
Reprinted with permission from Elsevier.

3. The surgeon must consciously work to place the Dacron graft as far proximal as possible. The anastamosis always uses up a significant portion of the ascending aorta and it is imperative to preserve landing zone for the stent graft proximal to the aneurysm.

4. Patients with prior ascending grafts, although more difficult to expose, provide secure clamping of the aorta and we have approached these through a small right thoracotomy, using visible sternal wires to "tee-off" the intercostals space selection.

5. The left subclavian artery in most cases can be exposed through a median sternotomy. In this case it can be simply divided and bypassed.

6. We routinely utilize TCD for cerebral monitoring all thoracic endografting procedures

7. In most cases we perform the entire operation: debranching and stent grafting, in one setting. The stent graft is deployed through a 10mm side limb originating from the proximal end of the bypass grafts.

8. If a two-stage procedure is planned, make sure that the iliac arteries and distal aorta is adequate to permit stent graft insertion in the standard retrograde fashion.

Scenario 1: Ascending aortic involved

If the ascending aorta is involved and must be replaced, we use a standard median sternotomy for surgical access. Cardiopulmonary bypass with cardioplegic cardiac arrest and standard distal ascending aortic cross clamp technique is used for ascending aortic replacement. The arch aneurysm is left in place, thus avoiding the need for profound hypothermia and circulatory arrest. A 12-mm graft is attached to the proximal ascending graft and from this 12-mm graft separate side arms are constructed and attached end to end to the innominate artery, the left carotid artery and the left subclavian artery. This allows the proximal stent graft to land in the distal ascending graft to provide a safe seal of the proximal component of the repair. (Figure 25–3 A)

Scenario 2: Ascending aorta not involved but innominate artery involved

When the ascending aorta does not need to be replaced, the entire procedure can be done without stopping the heart at any point. Surgical access may be via a standard median sternotomy or via mini right anterior thoracotomy and cervical incisions.[30] Median sternotomy allows attachment of a 12-mm graft to the proximal ascending aorta using a side biting clamp. Care must be taken to lower the systemic blood pressure prior to applying the side biting clamp to avoid dissection or premature clamp release. Care must also be taken to attach this graft far enough proximally to allow an adequate landing zone in the ascending aorta. Because this graft is used for antegrade stent graft deployment we bolster the anastomosis with a pledgeted suture at the toe and at the heel of the ascending aortic attachment to prevent disruption. Side arm grafts are individually constructed and attached to the innominate, left carotid and left subclavian arteries. Technically it is easiest to attach a graft end to end to the left subclavian prior to constructing the end to end anastomoses to the innominate and left carotid arteries since these will obscure the left subclavian. After the innominate and left carotid grafts are complete, it is an easy matter to attach the left subclavian graft previously sewn to the left subclavian in an end to side manner to the existing left carotid graft. Once the arch has been completely reconstructed in this extra anatomic fashion the stent graft is deployed in an antegrade fashion through the 12-mm graft

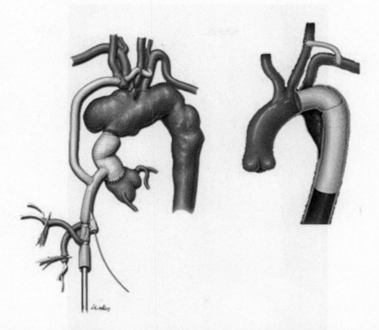

Figure 25–3. Extra-anatomic debranching of aortic arch vessels with replacement of ascending aorta and ante-grade TEVAR via Dacron side branch.[12] Reprinted with permission from Elsevier/Society for Vascular Surgery.

attached to the ascending aorta. The distal extent of the stent graft is dependent on the distal extent of the aneurysm and achieving an adequate distal landing zone. We have used this approach to debranch the entire aortic arch and the celiac and superior mesenteric arteries allowing a distal graft landing at just above the renal arteries. (Figure 25–3 B; Figure 25–4)

MINIMALLY-INVASIVE HYBRID ARCH REPAIR – TECHNICAL DETAILS

The alternative to a median sternotomy is a small anterior right thoracotomy and cervical incision.[31–34] Our group has used a small right anterior thoracotomy as access for aortic valve replacement and finds it provides good access to the ascending aorta.[30] A small incision at the lower sternocleidomastoid muscle on each side allows access for the right and left common carotid arteries. A small left supraclavicular incision allows exposure of the left subclavian artery. A 10-mm Dacron graft is pre sewn onto a 12-mm graft on the back table and tailored to fit the proximal ascending aorta. The 12-mm graft is attached to the proximal ascending aorta as described in the previous section. At the completion of this anastomosis, clamps are placed on the 12-mm and the 10-mm grafts and the side biting clamp is removed. Pledgeted sutures are again placed at the toe and heel of the ascending attachment and the anastomosis carefully inspected for any bleeding. At this point the 10-mm graft is within the chest and next to the ascending aorta and would not be an easy anastomosis if not already done. The 10-mm graft must then be passed through the sternal outlet into the right cervical incision for anastomosis to the right common carotid artery.

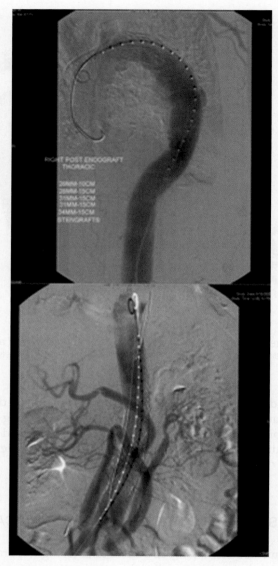

Figure 25–4. Completion angiography after stent grafting in a patient that underwent arch and abdominal debranching shows the patency of bypass grafts and the exclusion on the aneurysm.[10] Reprinted with permission from Elsevier/Society for Vascular Surgery.

Great care must be exercised at this point to exit the sternum in the midline and against the posterior table of the sternum to avoid injury to the innominate vein. An 8-mm graft is then attached to this 10-mm graft and passed anterior to the trachea and making a loop low behind the upper sternum and attached to the left common carotid artery. A low loop of this graft leaves the trachea uncovered by graft in case a future tracheostomy is ever needed. A standard left carotid subclavian bypass completes the arch debranching. The proximal left carotid and innominate arteries are ligated to prevent type II endoleaks. The left subclavian is closed proximally with a coil or plug via the left arm to prevent endoleak while preserving the vertebral artery. Antegrade deployment of the stent graft can then be

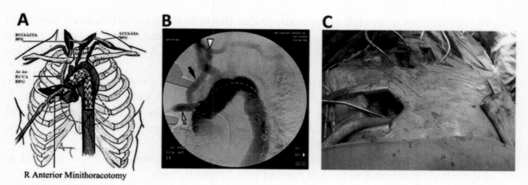

R Anterior Minithoracotomy

Figure 25–5. A Schematic drawing showing the procedure. Via a 5 cm incision at the 3rd- intercostal space to access the ascending arch, a 12-mm – 10-mm bifurcated hemashield Dacron graft is created. A partial occluding clamp is used on the ascending aorta to attach the 10-mm arm of the bifurcated 10/12-mm graft to the Right common carotid or Innominate artery. Remaining arch vessels are bypassed through carotid-carotid and left carotid-subclavian bypass. Antegrade stenting of the aortic arch is carried out through the RAM via the remaining 12-mm limb.[30] **B** Intraoperative angiogram showed the ascending aorta to R common carotid artery BPG (Black arrow), RCCA to LCCA BPG (White arrow) and the stent graft deployment via a 12-mm limb (hollow arrow) through the anterior minithoracotomy and complete exclusion of the aneurysmal sac.[30] **C** Intraoperative photograph.[10] Figures A and B reprinted with permission from Elsevier/The American Association for Thoracic Surgery. Figure C reprinted with permission from Elsevier/Society for Vascular Surgery.

carried out via the original 12-mm graft attached to the ascending aorta. We prefer to do all our aortic arch hybrid cases as a single stage, using antegrade deployment whenever possible in contrast to visceral debranching and stent grafting for thoracocabdominal aortic aneurysm which we prefer to do as a staged procedure with retrograde deployment.[35] (Figure 25–5)

Zone 1-Deployment Principles

This includes the origin of the left common carotid artery and is usually shorter than depicted in the illustration, consequently, simple bypass of the left carotid artery usually adds little additional landing zone. However, it is helpful in some patients, so the technique is well worth understanding.

1. Carotid to carotid bypass, our preference is a looped subcutaneous tunnel. We always combine this with carotid to left subclavian bypass.
2. Bovine origins are common and usually associated with a wide innominate origin. However, these origins are very variable in their anatomical configuration, which must be taken into consideration. When broad, with a left CCA arising from within the innominate, away from the aortic wall, it is reasonable to "cheat a little" and project the stent graft into the innominate orifice thereby proving a maximal landing zone length.

Zone 2-Deployment Principles

1. Left subclavian must be covered: selective revascularization is performed by most surgeons, BUT, the threshold for revascularization has been decreasing. Although the left subclavian artery can be covered without untoward effect in some patients, there is a growing belief that revascularization of the left subclavian in these circumstances may improve outcomes.[36]

2. We revascularize the left subclavian under the following circumstances: absent or atretic right vertebral, LIMA, known left PICA syndrome, thoracic stent grafting in presence of prior infrarenal open or endovascular AAA repair, type B aortic dissections.
3. There must be an adequate area between the distal margin of the left CCA origin and the proximal margin of the left subclavian orifice. Occasionally the origin of the left subclavian is so wide and funnel shaped that the endograft tends to displace up into the subclavian artery. This must be judged in advance with a low threshold for anticipatory left CCA bypass.
4. Cervical incisions are required for right carotid to left carotid bypass as well as supraclavicular incision for left carotid subclavian bypass.

ISSUES COMMON TO ALL ZONES

1. Regardless of zone deployment it is essential to consider arch angulation and tortuosity when selecting the proximal landing zone in order to prevent lack of apposition to the inner curve, or "bird beaking" of the graft.[37]
2. The final technical consideration is delivering the stent graft to the site of deployment. This can be done in an antegrade or a retrograde fashion. When deploying through the ascending aorta, care should be taken to minimize strain applied by insertion of the sheath to the suture line by angling the take off of the Dacron graft.

RESULTS

Hybrid arch procedures provide a safe and viable alternative to open traditional surgical repair. In general, hybrid approaches have a lower mortality and morbidity for high-risk older patients. Recently, such approaches have extended hybrid repair indications for complex arch pathology once thought to be prohibitively high risk for open arch surgical repair.

At The MDHVC, hybrid TAAA and arch repairs have become the preferred approach with open procedures performed only if hybrid approaches are not possible for technical reasons. We reviewed our experience with hybrid aortic repair in patients who were denied open surgery due to preoperative comorbidities and low physiologic reserve. Fifty-five percent of cases were symptomatic on presentation and 83% were done emergently. Seventy-six percent underwent debranching of the aortic arch, 17% of the visceral vessels, and 7% required both. Primary technical success was achieved in all cases and of these, 43% were staged. The 30-day mortality was 5%. Myocardial infarction developed in 6% and respiratory failure in 33%. (Table 25–1) These hybrid approaches, while initially performed mostly for very sick or emergent cases, proved the technical feasibility given the medical and anatomical complexity of these patients with encouraging results.[8,10–12]

Milewski and coworkers compared a hybrid arch repair cohort with an open aortic arch repair cohort and found a trend for lower incidence of neurologic deficit of 4% compared to 9% per group, while the short-term/in-hospital mortality rate was 11% and 16% respectively. The only statistically significant difference was the mortality rate between age groups and not among surgical approaches; the older patients[1] had a higher mortality rate of 36%.[38]

TABLE 25-1. COMPARISON OF THE OUTCOME OF ANEURYSM AND DISSECTION (%).[10]

Complication	Hybrid aneurysm (n = 33)	Hybrid dissection (n = 7)	P value
MI	6%	0%	1
Respiratory failure	33%	20%	.65
Renal failure	15%	20%	1
GI	24%	0%	.38
SCI	15%	0%	.56
CVA/TIA	18%	40%	.61
Death (30 days)	24%	0%	.31
Composite endpoint	13%	0%	.07

CVA, Cerebrovascular accident; *GI*, gastrointestinal; *MI*, myocardial infarction; *SCI*, spinal cord ischemia; *TIA*, transient ischemic attack. Composite endpoint is the combined death and permanent paraplegia rate at 30 days. Reprinted with permission from Elsevier/Society for Vascular Surgery.

In another series reported by Hughes and colleagues, 28 patients underwent hybrid arch repair with a thirty-day/in-hospital rates of death, stroke, and permanent paraplegia/paresis at 0%, 0%, and 3.6% respectively. At a mean follow-up of 14 +/− 11 months, there were no late aortic-related events. Two patients[39] required secondary endovascular reintervention for a type 1 endovascular leak. No patient has a type 1 or 3 endovascular leak at latest follow-up.[40–41] Similarly, Canaud reported a 6.8% risk of stroke with an actuarial survival of 70% at a mean follow up of 29.9 months.[42]

Regardless of the configuration used, hybrid approaches to arch repair are achieving similar or better short- and long-term outcomes compared the open arch replacement procedures in most reported series.

FUTURE DIRECTIONS

Every major endograft manufacturer currently has an active branched endograft program. Although this initially focused on the visceral segment, there will shortly be branch arch grafts. Basically these are single branch devices, designed to revascularize the left subclavian primarily. However, flow to at least one of the supra aortic trunks allows us to connect the other vessels with extra anatomical bypass. At the present time these devices are not available, however some physicians are using in situ fenestration techniques to perforate the device using a retrograde laser catheter passed from the left brachial artery. Once the fenestration is created the defect is widened with balloon angioplasty and a branch created by placing a self-expanding covered stent, also from the brachial approach.

CONCLUSION

In the future, branched endografts (Figure 25–6) may play a role in the management of aortic arch pathology.[43] The technology for this, however, remains in the development phase. In the meantime, open aortic arch repair for aortic arch aneurysm can be carried out at reasonable but not insignificant risk in appropriate patients. Hybrid endovascular stent graft

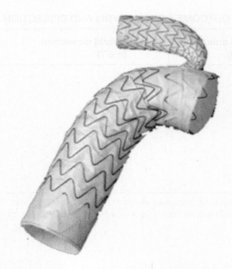

Figure 25–6. Prototype of branched aortic endograft.

approaches have been developed in an attempt to decrease the mortality and morbidity of open arch repair and to allow extension of life saving therapy to high risk patients who may not be reasonable candidates for open repair.

REFERENCES

1. Clouse WD, Hallett JW, Jr., Schaff HV, Gayari MM, Ilstrup DM, Melton LJ, 3rd. Improved prognosis of thoracic aortic aneurysms: a population-based study. *JAMA* 1998;280:1926–9.
2. Juvonen T, Ergin MA, Galla JD, Lansman SL, Nguyen KH, McCullough JN, Levy D, de Asla RA, Bodian CA, Griepp RB. Prospective study of the natural history of thoracic aortic aneurysms. *Ann Thorac Surg* 1997;63:1533–45.
3. de Bakey ME, McCollum CH, Graham JM. Surgical treatment of aneurysms of the descending thoracic aorta: long-term results in 500 patients. *J Cardiovasc Surg (Torino)* 1978;19:571–6.
4. Griepp RB, Stinson EB, Oyer PE, Copeland JG, Shumway NE. The superiority of aortic cross-clamping with profound local hypothermia for myocardial protection during aorta-coronary bypass grafting. *J Thorac Cardiovasc Surg* 1975;70:995–1009.
5. Sundt TM, 3rd, Orszulak TA, Cook DJ, Schaff HV. Improving results of open arch replacement. *Ann Thorac Surg* 2008;86:787–96; discussion 787–96.
6. Coselli JS, Buket S, Djukanovic B. Aortic arch operation: current treatment and results. *Ann Thorac Surg* 1995;59:19–26; discussion 26–7.
7. Svensson LG, Crawford ES, Hess KR, Coselli JS, Raskin S, Shenaq SA, Safi HJ. Deep hypothermia with circulatory arrest. Determinants of stroke and early mortality in 656 patients. *J Thorac Cardiovasc Surg* 1993;106:19–28; discussion 28–31.
8. Mussa FF, Walkes JC, Lumsden AB, Reardon MJ. Novel technique for arch and visceral artery debranching using ascending aortic inflow. *Vascular* 2008;16:275–8.
9. Smolock CJ, Chen G, Anaya-Ayala JE, Martinez K, Lumsden AB, Davies MG, Naoum JJ, Peden EK. Successful Endovascular Repair of Two Ruptured Thoracic Aortic Aneurysms in Nonagenarians. *Ann Vasc Surg* 2011;25:697.e9–12.
10. Younes HK, Davies MG, Bismuth J, Naoum JJ, Peden EK, Reardon MJ, Lumsden AB. Hybrid thoracic endovascular aortic repair: pushing the envelope. *J Vasc Surg* 2010;51:259–66.

11. Zhou W, Reardon M, Peden EK, Lin PH, Lumsden AB. Hybrid approach to complex thoracic aortic aneurysms in high-risk patients: surgical challenges and clinical outcomes. *J Vasc Surg* 2006;44:688–93.

12. Zhou W, Reardon ME, Peden EK, Lin PH, Bush RL, Lumsden AB. Endovascular repair of a proximal aortic arch aneurysm: a novel approach of supra-aortic debranching with antegrade endograft deployment via an anterior thoracotomy approach. *J Vasc Surg* 2006;43:1045–8.

13. Di Eusanio M, Schepens MA, Morshuis WJ, Dossche KM, Di Bartolomeo R, Pacini D, Pierangeli A, Kazui T, Ohkura K, Washiyama N. Brain protection using antegrade selective cerebral perfusion: a multicenter study. *Ann Thorac Surg* 2003;76:1181–8; discussion 1188–9.

14. Kazui T, Washiyama N, Muhammad BA, Terada H, Yamashita K, Takinami M. Improved results of atherosclerotic arch aneurysm operations with a refined technique. *J Thorac Cardiovasc Surg* 2001;121:491–9.

15. Keeling WB, Kerendi F, Chen EP. Total aortic arch replacement for the treatment of Kommerell's diverticulum in a Jehovah's Witness. *J Card Surg* 2010;25:333–5.

16. Ogino H, Ueda Y, Sugita T, Matsuyama K, Matsubayashi K, Nomoto T, Yoshioka T. Aortic arch repairs through three different approaches. *Eur J Cardiothorac Surg* 2001;19:25–9.

17. Spielvogel D, Halstead JC, Meier M, Kadir I, Lansman SL, Shahani R, Griepp RB. Aortic arch replacement using a trifurcated graft: simple, versatile, and safe. *Ann Thorac Surg* 2005;80:90–5; discussion 95.

18. Ueda Y. Retrograde cerebral perfusion with hypothermic circulatory arrest in aortic arch surgery: operative and long-term results. *Nagoya J Med Sci* 2001;64:93–102.

19. Akhyari P, Kamiya H, Heye T, Lichtenberg A, Karck M. Aortic dissection type A after supra-aortic debranching and implantation of an endovascular stent-graft for type B dissection: A word of caution. *J Thorac Cardiovasc Surg* 2009;137:1290–2.

20. Chiesa R, Tshomba Y, Melissano G, Marone EM, Bertoglio L, Setacci F, Calliari FM. Hybrid approach to thoracoabdominal aortic aneurysms in patients with prior aortic surgery. *J Vasc Surg* 2007;45:1128–35.

21. Donas KP, Lachat M, Rancic Z, Oberkofler C, Pfammatter T, Guber I, Veith FJ, Mayer D. Early and midterm outcome of a novel technique to simplify the hybrid procedures in the treatment of thoracoabdominal and pararenal aortic aneurysms. *J Vasc Surg* 2009;50:1280–4.

22. Esposito G, Marullo AG, Pennetta AR, Bichi S, Conte M, Cricco AM, Salcuni M. Hybrid treatment of thoracoabdominal aortic aneurysms with the use of a new prosthesis. *Ann Thorac Surg* 2008;85:1443–5.

23. Greenberg RK, Haddad F, Svensson L, O'Neill S, Walker E, Lyden SP, Clair D, Lytle B. Hybrid approaches to thoracic aortic aneurysms: the role of endovascular elephant trunk completion. *Circulation* 2005;112:2619–26.

24. Kawaharada N, Kurimoto Y, Ito T, Koyanagi T, Yamauchi A, Nakamura M, Takagi N, Higami T. Hybrid treatment for aortic arch and proximal descending thoracic aneurysm: experience with stent grafting for second-stage elephant trunk repair. *Eur J Cardiothorac Surg* 2009;36:956–61.

25. Rancic Z, Pfammatter T, Lachat M, Frauenfelder T, Veith FJ, Mayer D. Floating aortic arch thrombus involving the supraaortic trunks: successful treatment with supra-aortic debranching and antegrade endograft implantation. *J Vasc Surg* 2009;50:1177–80.

26. Szeto WY, Bavaria JE, Bowen FW, Woo EY, Fairman RM, Pochettino A. The hybrid total arch repair: brachiocephalic bypass and concomitant endovascular aortic arch stent graft placement. *J Card Surg* 2007;22:97–102; discussion 103–4.

27. Bavaria JE, Appoo JJ, Makaroun MS, Verter J, Yu ZF, Mitchell RS. Endovascular stent grafting versus open surgical repair of descending thoracic aortic aneurysms in low-risk patients: a multicenter comparative trial. *J Thorac Cardiovasc Surg* 2007;133:369–77.

28. Greenhalgh RM, Brown LC, Powell JT, Thompson SG, Epstein D, Sculpher MJ. Endovascular versus open repair of abdominal aortic aneurysm. *N Engl J Med* 2010;362:1863–71.

29. Makaroun MS, Dillavou ED, Wheatley GH, Cambria RP. Five-year results of endovascular treatment with the Gore TAG device compared with open repair of thoracic aortic aneurysms. *J Vasc Surg* 2008;47:912–8.

30. Anaya-Ayala JE, Cheema ZF, Davies MG, Bismuth J, Ramlawi B, Lumsden AB, Reardon MJ. Hybrid Thoracic Endovascular Aortic Repair via Right Anterior Minithoracotomy. *J Thorac Cardiovasc Surg* 2011;142(2):314–318.

31. Donas KP, Czerny M, Guber I, Teufelsbauer H, Nanobachvili J. Hybrid open-endovascular repair for thoracoabdominal aortic aneurysms: current status and level of evidence. *Eur J Vasc Endovasc Surg* 2007;34:528–33.

32. Saleh HM, Inglese L. Combined surgical and endovascular treatment of aortic arch aneurysms. *J Vasc Surg* 2006;44:460–466.

33. Shimamura K, Kuratani T, Matsumiya G, Kato M, Shirakawa Y, Takano H, Ohta N, Sawa Y. Long-term results of the open stent-grafting technique for extended aortic arch disease. *J Thorac Cardiovasc Surg* 2008;135:1261–9.

34. Zierer A, Sanchez LA, Moon MR. Combined open proximal and stent-graft distal repair for distal arch aneurysms: an alternative to total debranching. *Ann Thorac Surg* 2009;88:307–9.

35. Estrera AL, Miller CC, 3rd, Porat EE, Huynh TT, Winnerkvist A, Safi HJ. Staged repair of extensive aortic aneurysms. *Ann Thorac Surg* 2002;74:S1803–5; discussion S1825–32.

36. Holt PJ, Johnson C, Hinchliffe RJ, Morgan R, Jahingiri M, Loftus IM, Thompson MM. Outcomes of the endovascular management of aortic arch aneurysm: implications for management of the left subclavian artery. *J Vasc Surg* 2010;51(6):1329–38.

37. Wang S, Chang G, Li X, Hu Z, Li S, Yang J, Chen W, Li J. Endovascular treatment of arch and proximal thoracic aortic lesions. *J Vasc Surg* 2008;48:64–8.

38. Milewski RK, Szeto WY, Pochettino A, Moser GW, Moeller P, Bavaria JE. Have hybrid procedures replaced open aortic arch reconstruction in high-risk patients? A comparative study of elective open arch debranching with endovascular stent graft placement and conventional elective open total and distal aortic arch reconstruction. *J Thorac Cardiovasc Surg* 2010;140:590–7.

39. Hughes GC, Daneshmand MA, Balsara KR, Achneck HA, Sileshi B, Lee SM, McCann RL. "Hybrid" repair of aneurysms of the transverse aortic arch: midterm results. *Ann Thorac Surg* 2009;88:1882–7; discussion 1887–8.

40. Hughes GC, McCann RL. Hybrid thoracoabdominal aortic aneurysm repair: concomitant visceral revascularization and endovascular aneurysm exclusion. *Semin Thorac Cardiovasc Surg* 2009;21:355–62.

41. Hughes GC, Nienaber JJ, Bush EL, Daneshmand MA, McCann RL. Use of custom Dacron branch grafts for "hybrid" aortic debranching during endovascular repair of thoracic and thoracoabdominal aortic aneurysms. *J Thorac Cardiovasc Surg* 2008;136:21–8, 28 e1–6.

42. Canaud L, Hireche K, Berthet JP, Branchereau P, Marty-Ane C, Alric P. Endovascular repair of aortic arch lesions in high-risk patients or after previous aortic surgery: midterm results. *J Thorac Cardiovasc Surg* 2010;140:52–8.

43. Chuter TA, Hiramoto JS, Chang C, Wakil L, Schneider DB, Rapp JH, Reilly LM. Branched stent-grafts: will these become the new standard? *J Vasc Interv Radiol* 2008;19:S57–62.

44. Cronenwett JL, Johnston W. *Rutherford's Vascular Surgery*. 7th ed. Vol. 2. Philadelphia: Saunders; 2010. p. 1309.

26

Endovascular Reconstruction of the Aortic Arch

Jason N. MacTaggart, MD and G. Matthew Longo, MD

INTRODUCTION

It's difficult to catch up to over 50 years of experience and technical refinement of open aortic surgery. Yet in a relatively short span, endovascular aortic aneurysm repair has equaled or surpassed open repair in almost every key aspect, save for long-term durability.[1-3] For infrarenal aortic aneurysms, the use of stent grafts has dramatically reduced perioperative complications and death while significantly shortening hospital stays and recovery time.[4] For the aortic arch, open repair is still the gold standard, but it carries significantly more morbidity and mortality than open repair of the infrarenal aorta. The use of cardiopulmonary bypass and hypothermia with various cerebral perfusion strategies have made these operations safer,[5-7] but the extensive operative exposures, the susceptibility of the brain to emboli and ischemia, and the addition of dissection to the common pathophysiologic processes, continue to make arch repair particularly treacherous.

Many patients with arch disease are not open operative candidates due to their underlying medical conditions. Although many will have a limited life expectancy as a result of these comorbidities, a large majority will die from aneurysm rupture. Some of these patients could prolong their survival and maintain a satisfactory quality of life if less morbid operative solutions were available. These are the patients who have the most to gain from endovascular aortic arch reconstruction.

The benefits of stent graft technology as applied to the aortic arch are the same as those for other arterial locations. One major advantage is the ability to deliver the prosthesis from a remote location, minimizing collateral damage imparted by major operative exposures. Another is the elimination of significant periods of organ ischemia and reperfusion injury that accompany open surgery and vessel clamping. Despite these advantages however, stent graft repair of the arch remains one of the remaining frontiers of endovascular surgery for a number of reasons. First, arch curvature and the presence of critical branch vessels make it difficult to apply currently available devices without either some type of modification to the implant site or to the devices themselves. Larger aortic diameters in the arch require larger stent grafts and higher profile delivery systems that may not safely traverse the usual routes of access. In addition, the harsh physical conditions found within the arch are significantly more violent than those in encountered in the infrarenal aorta.[8] All of these problems, unique to the arch, require better delivery systems and more robust devices with different strategies for access,[9] fixation and sealing in order to produce safe and durable results.

PATIENT SELECTION AND EVALUATION

High quality imaging is required for diagnosis, patient selection and operative planning. Gated CT or MR angiography is best used to assess aneurysm size, implant site dimensions and the routes of access. For CT angiography, contrast injection through the right upper extremity minimizes innominate vein artifact and provides excellent visualization of the arch and proximal branch vessels. The use of three-dimensional post-processing software is highly desirable to obtain true axial diameters, accurate centerline lengths and realistic depictions of vessel angulations and morphology. Commonly cited aneurysm repair size thresholds should be balanced with the patients overall functional status and anatomic suitability for the various repair options.[10] All patients should be evaluated for the presence of cardiac disease, with particular attention paid to the coronary arteries and aortic valve structure and function. If a patient requires a transthoracic exposure, pulmonary function tests should be obtained. The presence of preexisting cerebrovascular disease should also be determined. Significant amounts of thrombus within the arch may increase the risk of stroke during endovascular manipulations and alternative techniques or specific methods of embolic protection, such as the embrella device, should be considered.[11] Last, the use of aortic stent grafts in patients with connective tissue diseases, such as Marfan's syndrome, is currently not advised.[10]

ENDOVASCULAR ARCH RECONSTRUCTION

Endovascular management of aortic arch pathology consists of two primary approaches: hybrid operations involving a combination of open bypasses and endovascular aortic stent grafting, and endovascular repair without open revascularization of the arch vessels prior to aortic stent graft deployment. The former incorporate anatomic or extra-anatomic bypasses to the supra aortic trunks and are designed to allow branch vessel coverage by the aortic stent graft while maintaining flow to the brain and upper extremities. The latter can be grouped into three basic techniques: 1) Retrograde branch stenting (double barrel/chimney/snorkel techniques) 2) Fenestrated stent grafts and 3) Branched stent grafts. Similar to hybrid repair, these three techniques also provide the opportunity to extend the landing zone of thoracic stent grafts to a more proximal location within the arch to improve endograft fixation and seal, but use additional devices or stent graft modifications to preserve critical branch flow.

HYBRID PROCEDURES

Hybrid procedures involve open reconstruction of the supra aortic trunks to "debranch" the aorta and provide more suitable landing zones for the placement of commercially available stent grafts within the arch.[12,13] These procedures can be broadly classified as those

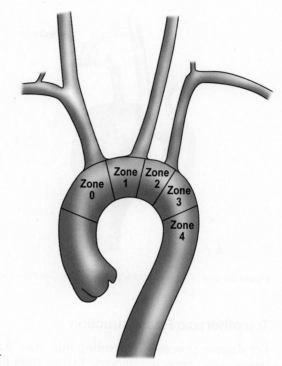

Figure 26–1. Attachment zones of the aortic arch.

that employ transcervical revascularization versus those that require transthoracic reconstruction.

Transcervical Reconstruction

Transcervical rerouting of blood flow through the supra-aortic trunks is applicable to patients with disease requiring placement of stent grafts into zones 1 and 2 of the arch (Figure 26–1). For zone 2 implantations, the importance of subclavian revascularization in conjunction with stent graft coverage has been increasingly recognized, and it's now recommended that most patients undergo carotid subclavian bypass or transposition to reduce the risk of neurologic complications.[14] (Figure 26–2) If coronary perfusion is dependent upon a left internal mammary graft, a carotid-subclavian bypass is preferable to a transposition. Origin of the left vertebral artery directly from the aortic arch is not uncommon and should prompt proximal ligation and reimplantation into the carotid artery or bypass graft. Endovascular embolization of the proximal left subclavian artery may be a safer alternative to dissecting down below the clavicle and ligating the subclavian artery to prevent type 2 endoleak.

For zone 1 implantation, a retropharyngeal end-to-side bypass from the right carotid artery to the left subclavian artery with an 8 mm ringed polytetrafluoroethylene (PTFE) graft is our preferred technique. The left common carotid artery can then be ligated proximally and reimplanted into the side of the bypass graft. Various other configurations are depicted in Figure 26–3. Large series of transcervical bypass operations demonstrate these techniques to be durable, with relatively low rates of perioperative complications.[15] These reconstructions can be performed simultaneously with aortic stent grafting, or in a staged fashion.

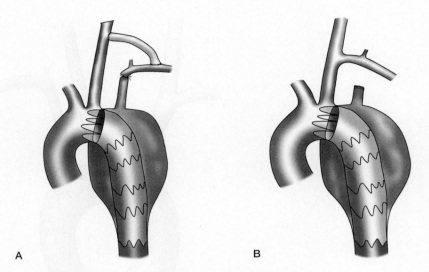

Figure 26–2. A. Carotid-subclavian bypass **B.** Carotid-subclavian transposition

Transthoracic Reconstruction

For disease processes extending into zone 0 and requiring stent graft coverage of the innominate artery, intrathoracic bypass from the ascending aorta is required. Though this does require a more invasive exposure with more morbidity and mortality than the transcervical approaches,[16] the safe application of a side-biting clamp to the ascending aorta

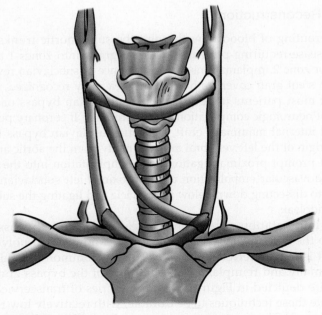

Figure 26–3. Configurations of a carotid-carotid bypass

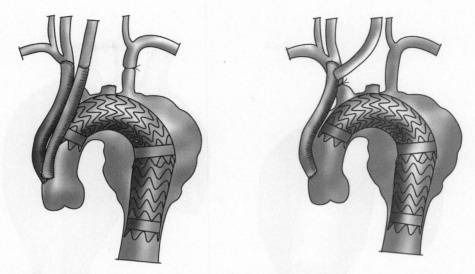

Figure 26–4. Configurations of an arch debranching with ascending aortic bypass to the supra-aortic trunks utilized for Zone 0 arch aneurysms.

and construction of the bypass still does eliminate the need for cardiopulmonary bypass and hypothermic circulatory arrest. (Figure 26–4) Careful review of preoperative imaging to assess for calcification and thrombus in the ascending aorta is mandatory when opting for this technique. An additional conduit limb attached to next to the origin of the bypass can facilitate antegrade delivery of the thoracic stent graft, eliminating the need to traverse potentially diseased and tortuous iliac arteries and distal aorta (Figure 26–5). The sutureless telescoping anastomotic technique initially described by Lachat may be of some utility

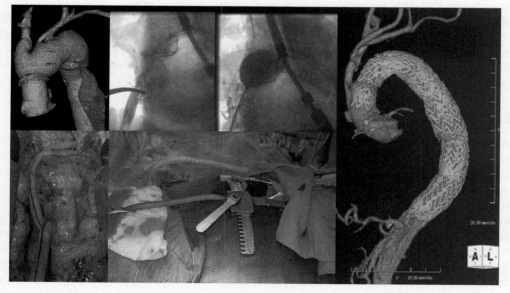

Figure 26–5. A Zone 0 arch debranching with an additional conduit placed for antegrade placement of a thoracic stent graft.

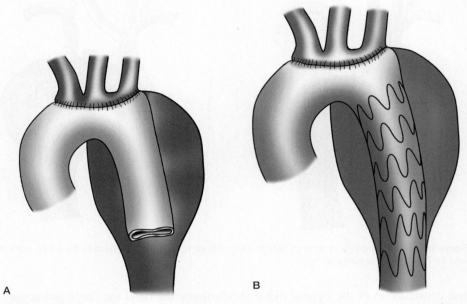

Figure 26–6. a. Depiction of elephant trunk placement for Zone 0 arch aneurysm **b.** Stent graft placement within the elephant trunk.

in these operations, reducing ischemic times and arterial dissection required for supra aortic trunk revascularization.[17]

Use of an elephant trunk technique is another method of dealing with Zone 0 aneurysms.[18,19] This operation can be performed in either one or two stages, and it allows for both antegrade access to the arch or femoral access at the time of endografting. Elephant trunk reconstruction avoids bypasses to the supra-aortic vessels, thus removing the potential of bypass failure, while maintaining normal arch anatomy. Furthermore, it allows construction of a specific diameter and length to the proximal landing zone. (Figure 26–6)

Endovascular Procedures

Advanced endovascular techniques may be used in lieu of hybrid debranching procedures to maintain arch branch vessel perfusion with aortic arch stent grafting. The utility of the following operations compared with the hybrid procedures described above is somewhat questionable, as they are much more complex and require significantly advanced endovascular skills and experience to perform safely. Nevertheless, these techniques are evolving and allow arch repair without entering the chest and placing a clamp on the ascending aorta. In some cases, they may even be done entirely percutaneously, permitting a greater number of individuals to undergo endovascular repair of aortic arch pathology in situations where open surgery and general anesthesia carry a prohibitive risk. Each of the interventions described below utilize equipment in a manner that has not been thoroughly tested or approved for these specific maneuvers or techniques and thus, the long-term durability are uncertain.

Aortic Branch Stenting

A variety of monikers have been used to describe the technique of retrograde stenting to preserve perfusion to the aortic arch vessels – double-barrel technique, chimney technique and snorkel technique.[20,21] In situations where the need to obtain an adequate proximal landing zone for stent graft fixation or seal encroaches on a critical arch branch, retrograde stenting is useful both as a planned or bail out procedure. If there is a high likelihood that a critical arch vessel will be threatened by stent graft placement, it's beneficial to gain access and position a rescue wire in the threatened vessel prior to stent graft deployment in case rapid restoration of flow becomes necessary.

In this technique (Figure 26–7), percutaneous or open transcervical access is obtained for the artery requiring coverage. Though we typically access these vessels using an open approach, the common carotid artery can be accessed percutaneously with ultrasound guidance, and the left subclavian artery may be accessed via a brachial artery puncture. A 6 to 8 Fr sheath is placed in the vessel using the Seldinger technique. From the chosen access site, a 0.035-inch wire is advanced into the aortic arch, and subsequently positioned in the ascending aorta. The thoracic stent graft is then positioned and deployed as usual. An arch arteriogram is performed to visualize the aortic arch branches. If there has been significant encroachment upon or coverage of the arch vessel, the introducer and sheath are advanced out of the respective artery alongside the thoracic stent graft. A balloon expandable or self expanding stent is then advanced through the sheath, and positioned with only a short segment of the stent protruding beyond the proximal margin of the aortic stent graft into the arch. The sheath is then withdrawn, leaving the stent in position, where it is deployed. The sheath allows more accurate placement of the stent, while simultaneously making it easier to pass the stent alongside the thoracic stent graft. Additional stents may be required within the initially placed branch stent to assure that the aortic stent graft does not crush it.

Sizing of the branch stent is based on the size of the arch vessel requiring salvage. If this technique is used to ensure patency of the left subclavian artery, the distal landing zone of the branch stent should be positioned proximal to the origin of the vertebral artery. If completion ballooning of the thoracic stent graft is undertaken, the arch vessel stents are simultaneously balloon dilated to optimize the apposition of the aortic stent and maintain expansion of the branch stent. Leakage through the gutters

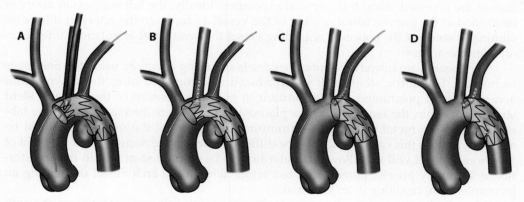

Figure 26–7. a. Sheath is advanced along the lateral edge of the thoracic graft. **b.** A balloon-expandable stent is placed to restore perfusion to the covered vessel. **c.** and **d.** Retrograde stenting of the left subclavian artery origin.

around the snorkel stent can be managed by coil remobilization or placement of a balloon expandable stent inside the aortic stent graft. This procedure is most applicable to disease that is focal and located on the inner curvature of the arch. Mastery of the concepts and techniques employed in this approach allow for endovascular salvage of an arch vessel if it is inadvertently covered, without having to resort to open operations to maintain perfusion.

Fenestrated Stent Grafts

A fenestration is a hole in the fabric of the stent graft that allows flow through to a branch vessel. There are three different varieties of fenestrated stent grafts. Prefabricated, custom designed fenestrated grafts are made to order, with reinforced fenestrations precisely placed and sized based on preoperative imaging. During implantation the fenestrations are aligned with the origins of the branch vessels and are typically held into place by an additional stent or stent graft placed through the fenestration out into the branch artery. Prefabricated fenestrated devices are only available outside the United States and require months to build. Homemade fenestrated grafts are constructed in the operating room at the time of surgery using commercially available stent grafts and components harvested from other endovascular instruments and devices.[22] These "back-table" fenestrated stent grafts must be deployed for modification and then replaced back into the delivery system. Extensive experience and knowledge of the selected stent graft and delivery system are required for the safe application of this technique, and even then it is fraught with potential difficulties. Both prefabricated and homemade fenestrated devices can be extremely difficult to properly align when delivered into the curvature of the arch through tortuous access vessels, and small errors either in fenestration placement, or graft implantation, can lead to occlusion of the branch vessel and catastrophic ischemic complications.

In situ fenestration theoretically appears to be a safer and more versatile approach than the other fenestration options and calls for initial placement of the stent graft into the arch with subsequent retrograde fenestration from the covered branch arteries. As with the other techniques, the decision to electively fenestrate a stent graft requires detailed pre-operative imaging to determine which vessels will be covered. If the both carotid arteries require coverage, a temporary shunt must be planned to maintain cerebral perfusion.[23] Access for the aortic stent graft is typically obtained via the common femoral artery or 10 mm iliac conduit, and each of the arch vessels requiring revascularization are accessed using transcervical exposures. Ideally, the left subclavian artery is controlled at the paravertebral portion of the vessel as access to the artery at this point eliminates some of the concerns regarding vessel tortuosity and angulation of its takeoff from the aorta.[24]

6 Fr sheaths are introduced into the vessels requiring coverage using the Seldinger technique. The aortic stent graft is introduced into the arch from the downstream access site and positioned. It is important to note the position of the thoracic stent struts. If possible, the fenestrations are placed at points where there are gaps in the fabric between the metal stents. At a minimum, the apices of the metal stent must be avoided, though this can occasionally be difficult to determine accurately. If the stent of the thoracic graft will not allow a circular hole to be cut, the stent within the fenestration will deploy poorly, potentially obstructing flow in the arch vessel or creating an incomplete seal resulting in an endoleak.

After deployment of the thoracic stent graft, the sheath originating from the arch vessel is advanced, abutting the fabric of the aortic graft. With the sheath now against the graft fabric, graft fenestration can be achieved using a variety of techniques. In the method initially described by McWilliams et al., the back end of a 0.014-inch or

0.018-inch guidewire is used to puncture the fabric.[25] If the wire buckles or has diffi-culty penetrating the fabric, a balloon sized for the arch vessel is positioned at the ostia of the artery and inflated. The stiff end of the wire is brought through the balloon lumen to puncture the graft, using the inflated balloon for support.

An alternative method for *in situ* fenestration involves advancement of a 20-gauge spinal needle over a wire through the sheath. The needle is positioned against the graft fabric and then used to puncture the fabric with subsequent advancement of a wire into the thoracic graft lumen. In an arch vessel with significant tortuosity, a TIPS sheath with an inner metal core can be pre-curved, allowing for safer introduction of the 20-gauge needle. The perforation is serially dilated first with a 2mm balloon fol-lowed by a 3 or 4mm cutting balloon. The sheath and introducer are the advanced into the lumen of the thoracic graft, allowing for exchange to a 0.035-inch wire. This wire is directed into the descending thoracic aorta where it can be snared and brought out through the groin, establishing through-and-through wire access. The fenestration is now enlarged, with either a 7 or 8mm cutting balloon. After dilation to the appropriate size, an additional stent graft can safely be deployed through the fenestration and may be flared proximally and distally to achieve a seal. In situations where the branch aris-es from a non-aneurysmal portion of the arch, a bare metal, balloon-expandable stent is preferred to a covered stent. (Figure 26–8)

A third method for graft fenestration was recently described using an endoluminal laser.[26] As before, a sheath is brought up against the endograft fabric for both support and prevention of injury. The laser is advanced through the sheath, positioned against the fabric and when activated, burns a hole through the stent graft fabric. With the fen-estration created, the wire and sheath are then advanced through the hole and into the thoracic graft lumen. The perforation is dilated and stenting proceeds as previously described. The long delivery system of the laser catheter allows for percutaneous access from the brachial artery rather than subclavian artery cutdown. Another advantage of

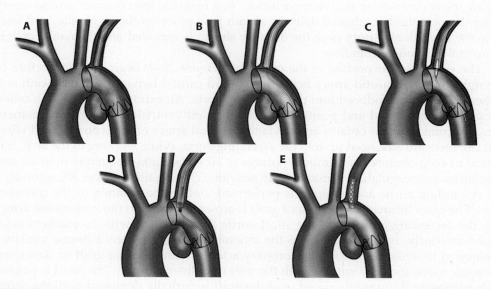

Figure 26–8. a. Stent graft is positioned, with needle and sheath against the graft, and the graft is punctured. **b.** The wire is advanced into the lumen of the graft. **c.** Balloons are passed into the fenestration and used to seri-ally dilate the puncture site. **d.** The 0.014-inch wire is exchanged for a stiff 0.035-inch wire and the sheath is advanced across the fenestration with the stent. **e.** The stent is deployed and flared proximally and distally.

this method is that it does not require the application of large amounts of mechanical force to penetrate the tough fabric of the stent graft, which may dislodge the graft from its position in the arch and potentially put previously constructed fenestrations and stents out of alignment. It should be noted that this technique has only been described with use of a polyester thoracic grafts and has not been attempted on PTFE grafts, and thus, the effect of the laser on this material is unknown. It is known that when PTFE is heated or burned at high temperatures hydrogen chloride, trifluoroacetate, and other toxic substances are released (26 PTFE chemicals with burning).

Branched Stent Grafts

Inoue was the first to report a catheter-based, total aortic arch repair in 1999 using a custom designed unibody multi-branched stent graft.[27] A more extensive series using the same basic design, but primarily using stent grafts with only a single side branch to the left subclavian artery demonstrated excellent perioperative results with good medium-term durability.[28] Though unibody designs may be more durable over time, they are less versatile and arguably more difficult to implant than modular stent graft systems.

The modular branched arch stent graft designed by Hartley and Chuter has been successfully implanted into a small series of patients.[29,30] Though stent grafts employing multiple branches to each of the supra aortic trunks are possible, a single side branch arch device, in combination with transcervical debranching, appears to be the safest and least complex method to accomplish extrathoracic repair of arch pathology extending well into zone 0.[30] When this approach is used, the right common carotid artery is the preferred route of access for stent graft delivery and the artery must be able to accommodate a large introducer sheath, otherwise a 10 mm conduit must be placed on the innominate artery. Prior to introduction of the stent graft delivery system, a left subclavian to carotid transposition is performed, followed by a carotid-carotid bypass. The debranching allows for virtually continuous cerebral perfusion during the endovascular arch reconstruction, first from the left common carotid artery when the potentially occlusive delivery sheath is in place on the right side, and later from the innominate artery once the delivery sheath is removed and the native arch is completely excluded from flow.

The endovascular portion of the operation (Figure 26–9) begins with puncture of the right common carotid artery below the carotid-carotid bypass. A short sheath and catheter are then introduced into the ascending aorta. An extra-stiff wire with a coiled floppy tip is advanced and positioned inside the left ventricle. During these maneuvers, a second operator obtains access via the femoral artery or iliac conduit, and wires and catheters are advanced up into the ascending aorta. While working in the arch, it is critical to keep clean wires, eliminate sources of air emboli and frequently monitor and administer anticoagulation to maintain an activated clotting time of over 300 seconds.

Ascending aortic angiography is performed, noting the position of the coronary ostia. The main bifurcated aortic stent graft is advanced through the innominate artery into the ascending aorta, until the short aortic limb opening with its markers positioned inferiorly, is just proximal to the innominate artery orifice. Extreme vigilance is required to avoid occluding the coronary arteries with the stent graft or damaging the aortic valve and left ventricle with the wire or delivery system. The heart is paused with adenosine,[32] or rapidly paced, and the graft is partially deployed until the short, wide aortic limb opens in the ascending aorta. Repeat angiography confirms patency of the coronary arteries before the remaining long limb of the bifurcated stent graft is

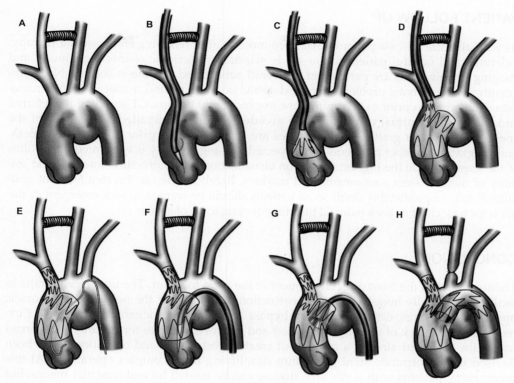

Figure 26–9. a. Carotid-Carotid bypass and subclavian-carotid reimplantation. **b.** Insertion of the first sheath. **c.** Deployment of the bifurcated proximal component, proximal stent **d.** Deployment of the bifurcated proximal component, short aortic limb. **e.** Catheterization of bifurcated proximal component. **f.** Insertion of the second sheath. **g.** Deployment of tubular distal component. **h.** Ligation of left common carotid artery. Reprinted with permission from Chuter TAM et al. *J Vasc Surg* 2003;38:859–63.

deployed into the innominate artery. Proper sizing of stent graft length should avoid coverage of the right subclavian artery.

The large diameter short aortic limb is then cannulated in the ascending aorta from the distal access site, and an extra-stiff wire is placed through the stent graft and out into the ascending aorta. The distal aortic component is advanced over the extra-stiff wire and positioned to achieve satisfactory overlap. It is then deployed, again with adenosine-induced asystole, creating a seal in the descending thoracic aorta excluding the arch from flow. Care must be taken not to dislodge the bifurcated main body of stent graft during passage and deployment of the distal aortic component. Magnified fluoroscopic views are useful to enhance visibility and facilitate cannulation and safe placement of the distal aortic stent graft. Completion angiography confirms patency and seal. If the long innominate limb portion of the stent graft, supplying the entirety of blood flow to the brain, does not appear without kinks or irregularities, it is lined with a braided self-expanding stent. Branched stent grafts are theoretically superior to both the retrograde stenting and fenestrated approaches because of more secure inter-component junctions and better sealing. Branched stent grafts also require less precise placement to preserve branch vessel flow and are capable treating a multitude of patient anatomies with a single off-the-shelf bifurcated device.

PATIENT FOLLOW UP

As with all aortic disease patients, and even more so after receiving endovascular therapy, indefinite and faithful patient follow-up is mandatory. Periodic counseling, clinical and imaging examinations are paramount to overall patient and prosthesis success. Not infrequently, asymptomatic problems can be detected on imaging and managed with percutaneous intervention prior to becoming catastrophic complications. CT scanning is preferred and the use of contrast can usually be avoided as long as detailed assessment of the aneurysm and stent graft sizes and shapes are compared with prior images. If endoleak, graft migration or other problems are suspected, CT angiography is warranted. Plain films of the chest provide the highest resolution visualization of the structural integrity and stability of metallic stent components and markers. Rarely, acute life-threatening stent graft failures may unpredictably occur so all patients should be warned to seek emergent evaluation for new chest or back pain, GI bleeding or symptoms of stroke.

CONCLUSION

The aortic arch is the most difficult segment of the aorta to repair. The use of stent grafts to facilitate minimally invasive arch reconstruction can eliminate the need for intrathoracic operative exposures, cardiopulmonary bypass and hypothermic circulatory arrest. Currently there is a lack of thoroughly studied and approved devices for routine, widespread use in the arch, but already a number of creative techniques and operations have been devised that incorporate stent grafts into simplifying these complex operations. At this point, many patients with aortic arch disease can be treated by endovascular means, but the question is whether or not they should be. Younger, healthier patients that can tolerate an open repair should get an open repair. For patients that cannot tolerate open repair these methods can improve short term survival and reduce perioperative morbidity, but have unknown long term outcomes. Devices currently exist outside of the United States for grafting of the aortic arch. Within the United States they are being used by select centers on an experimental basis. (Figure 26–10) With continued evolution of techniques and

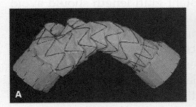
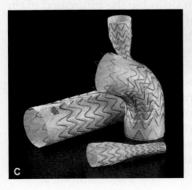
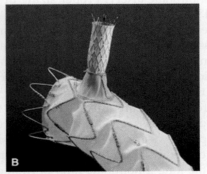

Figure 26–10. a. COOK arch branch device, with two branches for the innominate and left common carotid arteries. **b.** Medtronic arch branch device, with a single branch. **c.** Gore arch branch device, with a single branch. Reprinted with permission from Greenberg RK et al. *J Vasc Surg* 2010;52:15S–21S.

devices, soon the entire aorta from the valve to the bifurcation will be conquered by endovascular surgery.

REFERENCES

1. Parodi J, Palmaz J, Barone H. Transfemoral intraluminal graft implantation for abdominal aortic aneurysms. *Ann Vasc Surg* 1991;5(6):491–499.
2. Schermerhorn ML, O'Malley AJ, Jhaveri A, et al. Endovascular vs. open repair of abdominal aortic aneurysms in the Medicare population. *New Engl J Med* 2008;358(5):464–474.
3. Schanzer A, Greenberg RK, Hevelone N, et al. Predictors of abdominal aortic aneurysm sac enlargement after endovascular repair. *Circulation.* 2011;123(24):2848–2855.
4. Lederle FA, Freischlag JA, Kyriakides TC, et al. Outcomes following endovascular vs. open repair of abdominal aortic aneurysm. *JAMA* 2009;302(14):1535 -1542.
5. Griepp R, Stinson E, Hollingsworth J, Buehler D. Prosthetic replacement of the aortic arch. *J Thorac Cardiov Surg* 1975;70(6):1051–1063.
6. Sundt III TM, Orszulak TA, Cook DJ, Schaff HV. Improving results of open arch replacement. *Ann Thorac Surg* 2008;86(3):787–796.
7. Patel HJ, Nguyen C, Diener AC, et al. Open arch reconstruction in the endovascular era: Analysis of 721 patients over 17 years. *J Thorac Cardiov Surg* 2011;141(6):1417–1423.
8. Figueroa CA, Taylor CA, Chiou AJ, Yeh V, Zarins CK. Magnitude and direction of pulsatile displacement forces acting on thoracic aortic endografts. *J Endovasc Ther* 2009;16(3):350–358.
9. MacDonald S, Cheung A, Sidhu R, et al. Endovascular aortic aneurysm repair via the left ventricular apex of a beating heart. *J Vasc Surg* 2009;49(3):759–762.
10. WRITING GROUP MEMBERS, Hiratzka LF, Bakris GL, et al. 2010 ACCF/AHA/AATS/ ACR/ASA/SCA/SCAI/SIR/STS/SVM Guidelines for the diagnosis and management of patients with thoracic aortic disease: A Report of the American College of Cardiology Foundation/American Heart Association Task Force on Practice Guidelines, American Association for Thoracic Surgery, American College of Radiology, American Stroke Association, Society of Cardiovascular Anesthesiologists, Society for Cardiovascular Angiography and Interventions, Society of Interventional Radiology, Society of Thoracic Surgeons, and Society for Vascular Medicine. *Circulation.* 2010;121(13):e266–e369.
11. Carpenter JP, Carpenter JT, Tellez A, et al. A percutaneous aortic device for cerebral embolic protection during cardiovascular intervention. *J Vasc Surg* 2011. Available at: http://www.jvascsurg.org/article/S0741-5214(10)02866-1/abstract. Accessed July 3, 2011.
12. Melissano G, Civilini E, Bertoglio L, et al. Results of endografting of the aortic arch in different landing zones. *Eur J Vasc Endovasc* 2007;33(5):561–566.
13. Lee WA, Daniels MJ, Beaver TM, et al. Late outcomes of a single-center experience of 400 consecutive thoracic endovascular aortic repairs. *Circulation.* 2011;123(25):2938–2945.
14. Matsumura JS, Lee WA, Mitchell RS, et al. The Society for Vascular Surgery Practice Guidelines: Management of the left subclavian artery with thoracic endovascular aortic repair. *J Vasc Surg* 2009;50(5):1155–1158.
15. Byrne J, Darling RC, Roddy S, et al. Long term outcome for extra-anatomic arch reconstruction. An analysis of 143 procedures. *Eur J Vasc Endovasc* 2007;34(4):444–450.
16. Berguer R, Morasch MD, Kline RA. Transthoracic repair of innominate and common carotid artery disease: immediate and long-term outcome for 100 consecutive surgical reconstructions. *J Vasc Surg* 1998;27(1):34–42.
17. Rancic Z, Mayer D, Pfammatter T, et al. A new sutureless telescoping anastomotic technique for major aortic branch revascularization with minimal dissection and ischemia. *Ann Surg* 2010;252(5):884–889.
18. Greenberg RK, Haddad F, Svensson L, et al. Hybrid approaches to thoracic aortic aneurysms: the role of endovascular elephant trunk completion. *Circulation.* 2005;112(17): 2619–2626.

19. Carroccio A, Spielvogel D, Elozy SH, et al. Aortic arch and descending thoracic aortic aneurysms: experience with stent grafting for second -stage "elephant trunk" repair. *Vascular.* 2005;13(1):5–10.

20. Baldwin ZK, Chuter TAM, Hiramoto JS, Reilly LM, Schneider DB. Double-barrel technique for endovascular exclusion of an aortic arch aneurysm without sternotomy. *J Endovasc Ther* 2008;15(2):161–165.

21. Ohrlander T, Sonesson B, Ivancev K, et al. The chimney graft: a technique for preserving or rescuing aortic branch vessels in stent-graft sealing zones. *J Endovasc Ther* 2008;15(4): 427–432.

22. Oderich GS, Ricotta JJ. Modified fenestrated stent grafts: device design, modifications, implantation, and current applications. *Perspect Vasc Surg Endovasc Ther* 2009;21(3):157 -167.

23. Sonesson B, Resch T, Allers M, Malina M. Endovascular total aortic arch replacement by in situ stent graft fenestration technique. *J Vasc Surg* 2009;49(6):1589–1591.

23. Manning BJ, Ivancev K, Harris PL. In situ fenestration in the aortic arch. *J Vasc Surg* 2010; 52(2):491–494.

24. McWilliams RG, Murphy M, Hartley D, Lawrence-Brown MMD, Harris PL. In situ stent-graft fenestration to preserve the left subclavian artery. *J Endovasc Ther* 2004;11(2):170–174.

25. Murphy EH, Dimaio JM, Dean W, Jessen ME, Arko FR. Endovascular repair of acute traumatic thoracic aortic transection with laser-assisted in-situ fenestration of a stent-graft covering the left subclavian artery. *J Endovasc Ther* 2009;16(4):457–463.

26. Inoue K, Hosokawa H, Iwase T, et al. Aortic arch reconstruction by transluminally placed endovascular branched stent graft. *Circulation.* 1999;100(90002):II-316–321.

27. Saito N, Kimura T, Odashiro K, et al. Feasibility of the Inoue single-branched stent-graft implantation for thoracic aortic aneurysm or dissection involving the left subclavian artery: Short- to medium-term results in 17 patients. *J Vasc Surg* 2005;41(2):206–212.

28. Schneider DB, Curry TK, Reilly LM, et al. Branched endovascular repair of aortic arch aneurysm with a modular stent-graft system. *J Vasc Surg* 2003;38(4):855–855.

29. Ferreira M, Chuter T, Hartley D, et al. Hybrid repair of aortic arch aneurysms: A totally extrathoracic approach with branched endografts in two patients. *Vascular.* 2007;15(2):79 -83.

30. Chuter TAM, Buck DG, Schneider DB, Reilly LM, Messina LM. Development of a branched stent-graft for endovascular repair of aortic arch aneurysms. *J Endovasc Ther* 2003;10(5): 940–945.

31. Dorros G, Cohn JM. Adenosine-induced transient cardiac asystole enhances precise deployment of stent-grafts in the thoracic or abdominal aorta. *J Endovasc Surg* 1996;3(3):270–272.

32. Greenberg RK, Qureshi M. Fenestrated and branched devices in the pipeline. *J Vasc Surg* 2010;52(4 Suppl):15S-21S.

27

Thoracic Endovascular Aortic Repair (TEVAR): Complications and Failures

Ali Azizzadeh, MD, Kristofer Charlton-Ouw, MD, Samuel S. Leake, BS, Anthony L. Estrera, MD and H. J. Safi, MD

INTRODUCTION

Aortic aneurysms are the 13th leading cause of death in the United States. The prevalence of aortic aneurysms appears to be increasing secondary to heightened awareness, improvements in imaging, and an aging population.[1] The incidence of thoracic aortic aneurysms (TAA) is 5.9 new cases per 100,000 person-years.[2] The mean age at diagnosis ranges between 59 and 69 years, with a male-to-female ratio of 2:1 to 4:1.[3] Natural history studies suggest that after diagnosis, 74% of thoracic aneurysms rupture at a median interval of 2 years (range 1 month to 16 years).[2] Patients with thoracic aneurysms often have significant comorbidities including hypertension, coronary artery disease, chronic obstructive pulmonary disease, and congestive heart failure.[3] Descending thoracic aortic aneurysms are classified into three types (Figure 27–1): extent A (left subclavian artery to 6th rib), extent B (6th rib to diaphragm) and extent C (left subclavian artery to diaphragm).[4]

Since the 1950's, open surgical repair using a prosthetic graft has been the main treatment for patients with TAA. Open surgery involves thoracotomy, aortic cross-clamping, and major blood loss with potentially significant impacts on the heart, lung, kidneys, brain and the spinal cord. As a result, this approach is associated with significant morbidity and mortality with variable results in different centers.[5-8] Thoracic endovascular aortic repair (TEVAR), first developed in 1990's, has been adopted as a minimally invasive alternative for treatment of TAA.[9] The first thoracic device was approved in the United States by the Food and Drug Administration (FDA) in 2005.[10] Two additional devices were later approved.[11, 12] In all three pivotal trials, endovascular repair compared favorably to the traditional open repair for management of degenerative aneurysms. Published experience with TEVAR is rapidly accumulating. More

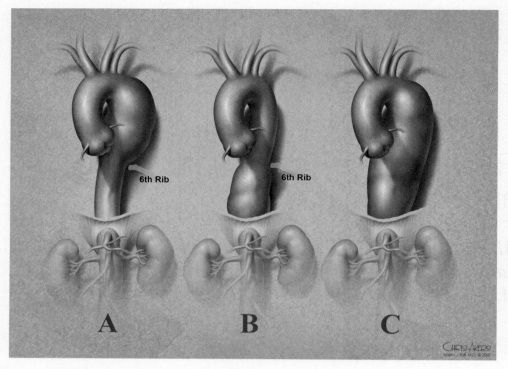

Figure 27–1. Classification of descending thoracic aortic aneurysms.

complex aneurysms extending to the aortic arch vessels are now commonly treated with endovascular repair (Figure 27–2). A recent systematic review and meta-analysis of comparative studies found that TEVAR, compared to open surgery, may reduce early death, paraplegia, renal insufficiency, transfusions, reoperation for bleeding, cardiac complications, pneumonia, and length of stay.[13] The aim of this chapter is to address the complications and failures after this procedure. These include mortality, stroke, spinal cord ischemia, retrograde dissection, device malfunction, access complications, endoleak, migration, infection, and aortobronchial fistula.

COMPLICATIONS

- **Mortality**
  According to a systematic review and meta-analysis which included 42 non-randomized studies (38 comparative, 4 registries) involving 5888 patients, the cumulative 30-day risk of mortality was 5.8% for TEVAR compared to 13.9% for open repair (P<.00001).[13] The cumulative all-cause mortality at 1, 2, and 3 years did not differ significantly between the two groups. Although TEVAR patients were significantly older, other baseline characteristics including coronary artery disease, diabetes, chronic obstructive pulmonary disease, hypertension and renal insufficiency were not significantly different between the two groups.

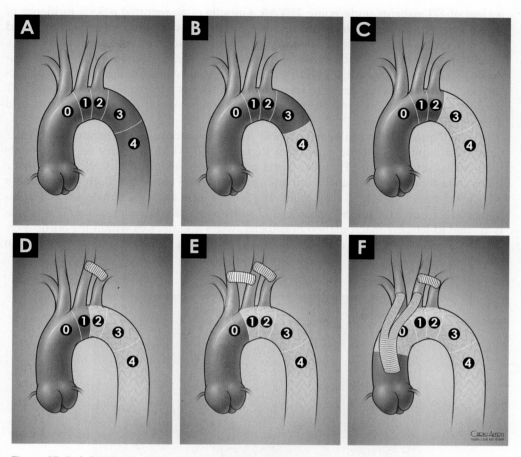

Figure 27–2. A Distribution of landing zones for TEVAR. Zone 0: repair involving the innominate artery. Zone 1: involving the left carotid artery. Zone 2: involving the left subclavian artery. Zone 3: involving the proximal third of the descending thoracic aorta. Zone 4: involving the distal two thirds of the descending thoraci aorta. **B&C** Placement of a device in zone 3 or 4 without any revascularization. **D** Coverage of the left subclavian artery with a left carotid subclavian bypass. **E** Coverage of the left carotid and subclavian arteries with a carotid-carotid and carotid subclavian bypass. **F** Complete arch coverage with ascending aorta to inominate and left carotid bypass as well as a left carotid subclavian bypass.

- **Stroke**

  Although TEVAR has a pattern of complications that are unique to endovascular procedures, perioperative stroke has a similar rate in both open and endovascular interventions (6.2% vs. 5%).[13] Stroke is among the most feared and devastating complications of endovascular and open repairs of the thoracic aorta. Perioperative stroke after TEVAR may be related to systemic factors (hypotension, hypertension, anticoagulation), intracranial causes (hemorrhage, edema, CSF drainage) or emboli (air, atheroma, thrombus).[14]

  Embolization may be related to the use and advancement of wires, catheters, and devices into a diseased atheromatous aortic arch, with dislodgement of atherosclerotic plaque to the brain. As a result, patients with a significant atherosclerotic burden and those with aneurysms close to the aortic arch are inherently at higher risk. In a 2007 review of 171 patients undergoing TEVAR, Gutsche el al. reported a 5.8% incidence of stroke.[15] Severe atheromatous aortic disease (>5 mm protrusion into aortic lumen), found in 7 of 8 perioperative stroke patients, was strongly associated with stroke (P=.0016). Combining a history of prior stroke with extent A coverage carried a 60% stroke incidence, while extent C resulted in a 15% incidence. After reviewing these data, 3 risk factors for perioperative stroke were identified: 1) a history of preoperative stroke; 2) CT grade IV atheroma (>5 mm) in the aortic arch or proximal descending aorta; and 3) extent A or C coverage.

In a 2007 prospective multicenter report from the European Collaborators on Stent/Graft Techniques for Aortic Aneurysm Repair (EUROSTAR) registry on 606 patients with endovascular repair of thoracic aorta pathologies (aneurysm, dissection, traumatic injury, anastomotic pseudoaneurysm and infectious/non specified), Buth et al. found a 3.1% incidence of stroke.[16] Using multivariate regression analysis, female sex and duration of procedure >160 min were associated with an increased risk for stroke. This is likely related to lengthy manipulation of catheter, wires and devices within the aortic arch. Figure 27–3 demonstrates a completion angiogram from a patient on our service with an

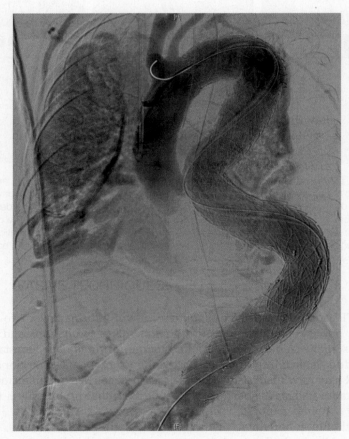

Figure 27–3. A completion angiogram from a patient with an extent C aneurysm who suffered a perioperative left hemispheric stroke. A total of 5 devices were placed through an extremely tortuous anatomy.

extent C aneurysm. A total of 5 devices were placed through an extremely tortuous anatomy. The patient suffered a perioperative left hemispheric stroke.

In a 2007 review of 153 patients, Khoynezhad et al. reported a stroke rate of 4.3%.[17] Using univariate analysis, they found that obesity (body mass index >30 kg/m^2), vascular thrombosis, embolization and significant blood loss carried a statistically significant risk for perioperative stroke.

Feezor et al. reported on the risk factors for perioperative stroke during TEVAR.[18] The study included 196 patients treated with TEVAR with an incidence of 4.6%. Seven (78%) of these patients had coverage of zones 0-2, while only 2 (22%) had coverage of zones 3-4; all patients with coverage of zones 0 or 1 had an elective arch revascularization performed. Five out of these nine patients (55.6%) had documented intraoperative hypotension (systolic BP < 80 mm Hg). Six patients (66.7%) had posterior circulation strokes, all of them with zones 0-2 coverage, and only one of them underwent a carotid-subclavian bypass. Since January 2006, all the patients considered for LSA coverage underwent preoperative CTA or MRA of the head and neck for evaluation of the posterior cerebral circulation. Those patients with a dominant left vertebral artery or incomplete circle of Willis underwent a prophylactic carotid-subclavian bypass. The patients who underwent TEVAR before the institution of this policy had a stroke rate of 6.4%, which decreased to 2.3% after a preoperative imaging protocol was instituted (P=.03). The authors concluded that stroke after TEVAR was multifactorial and appeared to be related to the coverage of the LSA and intraoperative hypotension. They recommended the elective revascularization of the LSA (carotid-subclavian bypass) in the setting of a dominant left vertebral artery or an incomplete circle of Willis.

- ## Spinal Chord Ischemia (SCI)

The incidence of paraplegia/paraparesis after TEVAR is 3.4%, compared to 8.2% for open repair (P<.0001).[13] The incidence of permanent paraplegia is also significantly different between the two modalities (1.4% vs. 4.9%, P=.001). SCI has been related to several risk factors, including aortic aneurysmal disease, extent of aortic repair or coverage,[19] previous abdominal aortic aneurysm repair,[20] compromised hypogastric artery inflow,[17] and left subclavian artery coverage.[16] Several diagnostic and therapeutic adjunctive methods have been used, including cerebrospinal fluid (CSF) drainage, to reduce the arterial-CSF gradient.[21] On our service, all patients undergoing elective TEVAR for a descending thoracic aortic aneurysm receive a CSF drainage catheter intraoperatively. Due to our large throacoabdominal experience, we have been able to carry out this protocol with a low (1.5%) complication rate.[22] The catheter is clamped and removed on postoperative day one if the patient remains neurologically intact. In patients who develop postoperative SCI, we drain the CSF to maintain a pressure <10 mm Hg, transfuse to a target hemoglobin of 12 gm/dL, and maintain a relatively high mean arterial pressure.

The EUROSTAR study reported a SCI incidence of 2.5%.[16] The use of 3 or more stent grafts (correlating with the length of coverage) was significant in patients experiencing SCI (paraplegia-paraparesis) with a 53% vs. 19% in the control group (P= .009). Coverage and occlusion of the T10 level intercostal arteries was also more frequent in patients with SCI than in those without neurological symptoms (40% vs. 18%). LSA coverage was also found to be an important risk factor for neurological complications. LSA was covered in 159 patients, of whom 40 had a revascularization procedure (transposition or bypass). The group without LSA revascularization experienced a 40% incidence of paraplegia-paraparesis vs. 19% in the revascularized group. The rate of combined neurologic complications (paraplegia or stroke) was 8.4% in the group without LSA revascularization compared to a 0% rate in the revascularized group. Multivariate regression analysis showed independent correlation of SCI with the number of stent grafts used (>3), coverage of the LSA, renal function impairment and simultaneous abdominal aortic repair. The authors recommended routine, prophylactic revascularization of the LSA in patients who required coverage of this vessel by the endograft at the proximal landing zone.

In a review of 153 patients, Khoynezhad et al. report a 4.3% incidence. The most significant risk factors in this study for developing SCI were: aortic aneurysm, the need for an iliac conduit, and an occluded or excluded hypogastric artery.[17]

- **Retrograde Dissection**

Retrograde type A aortic dissection (RAAD) is a rare and lethal complication of TEVAR procedures. It is defined as an intimal tear distal to the transverse arch with retrograde extension into the ascending aorta. (Figure 27–4) The risk for RAAD after TEVAR has been reported between 1.9% to as high as 6.8% in single-center series.[24-26] In these studies, RAAD has been related to several factors, including: 1) the TEVAR procedure itself (trauma caused by manipulation of wires/sheaths and stent graft balloon dilatation, large bore stent graft delivery system); 2) device properties (semi-rigidity and proximal bare spring, excessive radial force due to oversizing > 20%); 3) aortic wall friability (acute/chronic aortic dissection); and 4) Connective tissue diseases (Marfan syndrome, Ehler Danlos syndrome).

Eggebrecht et al. analyzed the 13-y experience from the European Registry on Endovascular Aortic Repair Complications, reporting an RAAD incidence of 1.33% (63/4,750 cases).[27] Of these, 48 patients (48/3,714 cases) had complete data sets for the analysis. Thirty-nine of the 48 patients (81%) underwent TEVAR for aortic dissection (acute 54%, chronic 27%). TEVAR was performed as an emergency in 16 (33%) patients and electively in 32 (67%). Four patients (8%) had Marfan syndrome. Forty patients (83%) had a proximal bare spring stent graft placed. RAAD occurred during the TEVAR procedure in 7 patients (15%), before the procedure during the index hospitalization in 10 (21%), and after discharge during follow-up in 31 (65%) patients. In 22 patients (46%), RAAD occurred within 30 days after the procedure and beyond 3 months in 15 patients (31%), with a median of 35 days (range 0 to 1050 days). Among the cohort, 58% of the patients experienced symptoms (chest pain or syncope), 19% had sudden death, and 25% were asymptomatic. Management consisted of emergency surgical repair in 25 patients (64%) and elective surgery in 5 patients (13%). Nine patients (23%) were treated medically with anti-impulse therapy. Overall mortality was 42% (20/48 patients). Causes included the stent graft (60%), manipulation of guide wires and sheaths (15%), and progression of underlying aortic disease (15%). The majority of the RAAD cases were reportedly associated with the use of proximal bare spring stent grafts, with direct evidence of device-related injury at surgery or autopsy in half of the patients.

Dong et al. reported a 2.5% (11 patients) incidence of RAAD in a series of 443 patients treated with TEVAR for type B dissection (acute 25%, chronic 75%).[28] The stent grafts were landed in zones 2 (2 patients) and 3 (9 patients). RAAD developed intraoperatively in 2 patients and postoperatively in the rest (2 hours to 36 months). Clinical manifestations included syncope, hypotension, dyspnea, hypoxemia, chest pain and sudden death. Three patients had Marfan syndrome. The site of new entry was identified at the tip of the proximal bare spring in 9 patients (81.1%) and within the area of anchorage in 1 patient by intraoperative angiogram, CT or open surgery. Three patients died perioperatively (27.3%). Authors concluded that RAAD is not a rare complication after endovascular repair of type B aortic dissection. Predisposing factors may include aortic wall fragility, disease progression, and stent graft-related causes.

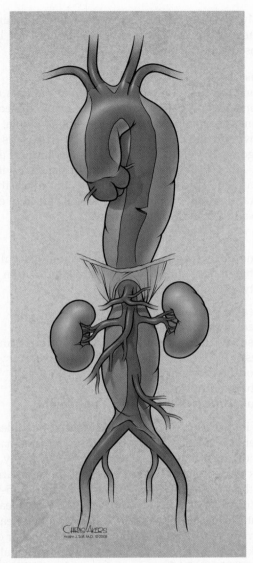

Figure 27–4. Retrograde dissection is defined as an intimal tear distal to the transverse arch with retrograde extension into the ascending aorta.

- **Device Malfunction**

  In relation to the abdominal aorta, the complexity of device delivery and deployment in the thoracic aorta is related to several factors including larger hemodynamic forces, more tortuous anatomy, and larger devices delivered over a relatively longer distance. In a comprehensive summary of failure modes of aortic endografts, Lee discusses their prevention and management.[29] Intraoperative factors include inability to advance the delivery system, unintended device movement and maldeployment.[30] Device infolding is likely related to oversizing and/or lack of apposition to the inner curvature of the aortic arch. This has been reported in the literature and can usually be salvaged with endovascular techniques. Additional endografts and bare stents can be placed to increase the radial force.[31, 32] Finally, all endografts are subject to material failure. These include metal fractures and fabric tears. This further highlights the need for long-term surveillance imaging of all endovascular aortic repairs.

- **Access Complications**

Vascular complications have been reported in 13% of patients undergoing TEVAR.[13] These complications include arterial thrombosis, occlusion, dissection, or rupture ("iliac on a stick"), hematoma, pseudoaneurysm, arteriovenous fistula, retroperitoneal bleeding, embolism, and wound infection. Some vascular disease is inherently present in many patients undergoing TEVAR. Attention to proper surgical and endovascular techniques is paramount. Liberal use of iliac conduits in patients with borderline anatomy cannot be overemphasized. This further underlines the necessity of performing these procedures in an operating room by a team that is well versed in open and endovascular bail-out techniques to address these complications.

- **Endoleak**

Endoleak remains one of the principal reasons for endovascular repair failure. It is defined as persistent blood flow outside the endograft and within the aneurysm sac, and it is classified in four types:[33]

I   a. Inadequate seal at proximal end of endograft
    b. Inadequate seal at distal end of endograft
II   Flow from vessel without attachment site connection (intercostals, LSA, bronchial arteries).
III a. Flow from module disconnection
     b. Flow from fabric disruption
IV   Flow from porous fabric (>30 d after graft placement)

There is paucity of information on the true incidence of endoleaks outside of the few clinical trials. The overall incidence of endoleaks from a meta-analysis of reported studies is 12.1%.[13] This, however, may be an overestimate, as many studies do not report endoleaks. The results of the three published US trials are summarized below:

Makaroun et al. in the WL Gore TAG pivotal trial, compared 5-year results of TEVAR with the TAG device (n=191) to surgical controls (n=94).[34] Endoleak occurred in 10.6% of patients at some point during the 5-year follow up. Most endoleaks were thought to be type I. Three patients required 5 endovascular reinterventions for endoleaks. These additional procedures took place from 45 to 1525 days after the original repairs.

Fairman el al. in the VALOR Trial reported the results of TEVAR using the Medtronic Vascular Talent Thoracic Stent Graft System (Medtronic Vascular, Santa Rosa, CA).[12] Among the 195 patients enrolled, the incidence of endoleak at 1 month follow- up was 25.9% (type 1: 4%; type II: 15.5%; type III: 1.7%; type IV: 0%). Fourteen procedures were performed to resolve the endoleak. At the 12-month follow-up, the incidence of endoleak was 12.2% (types I: 4.9%; type II 4.9%; type III and IV: 0%).

Matsumura et al. reported the results of TEVAR in the Zenith TX2 (William Cook, Europe) trial.[11] The outcomes of 160 TEVAR patients using the Zenith TX2 graft were compared to 70 patients treated with open surgery. The incidence of endoleak at predischarge, 30 days, 6 months, and 12 months were 13%, 4.8%, 2.6%, and 3.9%, respectively. Most of the endoleaks were type II. Most type I and III endoleaks were addressed in the first year with endovascular reintervention, and none required conversion. Overall, 4.4% of patents underwent secondary procedures through 12 months of follow-up.

Morales et al., in a retrospective review of 200 TEVAR patients for the etiology and outcomes of endoleaks at the Cleveland Clinic, found a 19.5% (39/200) incidence of endoleaks in follow-up (mean of 30 months).[35] These were classified as primary or secondary depending on whether they were noted or not in the first post-implantation CT. Fourteen patients developed a type I endoleak (11 primary and 3 secondary), 7 developed a type III (5 primary and 2 secondary); these were treated with a secondary endovascular intervention or conservatively. Sixteen patients developed a type II endoleak (13 primary and 3 secondary), thought to arise from the intercostal arteries, patent covered LSA, celiac and bronchial arteries. Glue embolization was performed in three patients with covered LSA endoleak, the rest were treated conservatively. The factors associated with endoleaks were presence of a carotid-LSA bypass (P=.0001), and longer aortic coverage by the stent graft (P=.005). Authors concluded that conservative treatment is adequate for type II endoleaks, while most type I and III endoleaks require a secondary intervention.

- **Migration**

Migration is defined as a >10 mm movement of the endograft relative to anatomical landmarks, or any migration leading to symptoms or requiring therapy.[33] Similar to the data on endoleak, there is a paucity of information outside clinical trials on device migration.

In the Gore TAG trial, migration occurred in one patient (incidence of 0.7%).[34] This patient underwent an open arch aneurysm repair for endoleak and migration at 5 months. The authors linked this to poor proximal neck anatomy. In the Medtronic VALOR trial, four stent graft migrations were reported in 12 months (incidence 2.1%).[12] Two migrations involved the proximal end of the graft moving distally, and two involved the distal end of the graft moving proximally. One of these patients reportedly required an additional intervention related to the migration. In the Cook TX2 trial, migration was reported in 2.8% of patients at 12 month follow-up. There were two cases of caudal migration of the proximal graft and one case of cranial migration of the distal graft. These cases were not associated with endoleak or increase in aneurysm diameter. None of the patients required a secondary intervention.[11]

- **Aortobronchial Fistula**

Development of an aortobronchial fistula is among the most serious and grave complications after TEVAR. In a retrospective review of 1113 TEVAR procedures performed over 10 years, the incidence of aorto-esophageal (AEF) or aortobronchial fistulae (ABF) was 1.7% (19 patients).[36] Among the indications for TEVAR, aortic pseudo-aneurysm was associated with the development of late AEF/ABF (P = 0.009). In addition, emergent and complicated procedures resulted in increased risk of AEF/ABF (P = 0.008 and P < 0.001, respectively). Eleven patients underwent surgical treatment, with a perioperative mortality of 64%. The remaining 8 patients who were treated conservatively died within 30 days. The overall survival at a mean follow-up time of 17.7 +/- 12.5 months was 16%.

- **Infection**

Graft infection is a very rare but serious complication of endovascular repair. The reported incidence ranges from 1-5%.[37-39] Etiological factors include perioperative contamination, hematogenous seeding, and local bacterial translocation.[37] One study reported a higher incidence in patients treated in an emergency setting.[38] The reported median time from the index procedure to the diagnosis of infection ranges from 115 to 244 days.[38,39] Commonly isolated organisms reported include *Staphylococcus* species, *Streptococcus* species, *Propionibacterium* species, *Enterobacter cloacae*, *Escherichia coli*, and *Pseudomonas aeruginosa*.[38,39] Treatment involves antimicrobial therapy, surgical explantation of the infected graft, and in situ homograft or antibiotic impregnated Dacron graft placement. At our institution, the new graft is also covered with an omental flap. Lifelong antibiotic therapy is often required. The reported mortality rate ranges from 25-60%.[38, 39]

CURRENT OPEN RESULTS

Although endovascular therapies are an attractive alternative to open repair for thoracic aortic pathologies, excellent results can still be achieved with open surgery at cardiovascular centers specializing in aortic work. Hybrid debranching as well as total endovascular repair of the transverse arch using branched or fenestrated technologies assumes that an anatomically feasible landing zone is present. For this reason most repairs of the ascending aorta are not amenable to endovascular repair and isolated arch aneurysms may be present in less than 10% of all repairs of the ascending and transverse aortic arch.[40] Excellent results with open repair of the ascending and aortic arch can be achievable with an incidence of stroke of 2.8% when the adjunct of retrograde cerebral perfusion is used and an early mortality of 3%.[41] Furthermore, excellent results can be achieved with open repair of descending thoracic and thoracoabdominal aortic aneurysm repair. Recent work has achieved an early mortality for DTAA and TAAA of less than 6% and a permanent paraplegia incidence of 2%.[42]

CONCLUSION

TEVAR is an excellent alternative to open surgery in properly selected patients with descending thoracic aortic aneurysms. The accumulated evidence shows that TEVAR can reduce mortality, paraplegia, and overall complications compared with open surgery. The long-term survival, durability and cost effectiveness of TEVAR remains to be determined. Appropriate recognition and management of TEVAR complications can improve long-term outcome of these patients.

REFERENCES

1. LaRoy LL, Cormier PJ, Matalon TA, Patel SK, Turner DA, Silver B. Imaging of abdominal aortic aneurysms. *AJR* 1989;152:785–792.
2. Bickerstaff LK, Pairolero PC, Hollier LH, et al. Thoracic aortic aneurysms: a population-based study. *Surgery* 1982;92:1103–1108.
3. Coady MA, Rizzo JA, Goldstein LJ, Elefteriades JA. Natural history, pathogenesis, and etiology of thoracic aortic aneurysms and dissections. *Cardiol Clin* 1999;17:615–635.
4. Estrera AL, Rubenstein FS, Miller CC, 3rd, Huynh TT, Letsou GV, Safi HJ. Descending thoracic aortic aneurysm: surgical approach and treatment using the adjuncts cerebrospinal fluid drainage and distal aortic perfusion. *Ann Thorac Surg* 2001;72:481–486.
5. Estrera AL, Miller CC, 3rd, Chen EP, et al. Descending thoracic aortic aneurysm repair: 12-year experience using distal aortic perfusion and cerebrospinal fluid drainage. *Ann Thorac Surg* 2005;80:1290–1296.

6. DeBakey ME, McCollum CH, Graham JM. Surgical treatment of aneurysms of the descending thoracic aorta: long-term results in 500 patients. *J Cardiovasc Surg* 1978;19:571–576.

7. Coselli JS, LeMaire SA, Conklin LD, Adams GJ. Left heart bypass during descending thoracic aortic aneurysm repair does not reduce the incidence of paraplegia. *Ann Thorac Surg* 2004;77:1298–1303.

8. Svensson LG, Crawford ES, Hess KR, Coselli JS, Safi HJ. Variables predictive of outcome in 832 patients undergoing repairs of the descending thoracic aorta. *Chest* 1993;104:1248–1253.

9. Dake MD, Miller DC, Semba CP, Mitchell RS, Walker PJ, Liddell RP. Transluminal placement of endovascular stent-grafts for the treatment of descending thoracic aortic aneurysms. *New Engl J Med* 1994;331:1729–1734.

10. Makaroun MS, Dillavou ED, Kee ST, et al. Endovascular treatment of thoracic aortic aneurysms: results of the phase II multicenter trial of the GORE TAG thoracic endoprosthesis. *J Vasc Surg* 2005;41:1–9

11. Matsumura JS, Cambria RP, Dake MD, Moore RD, Svensson LG, Snyder S. International controlled clinical trial of thoracic endovascular aneurysm repair with the Zenith TX2 endovascular graft: 1-year results. *J Vasc Surg* 2008;47:247–257.

12. Fairman RM, Criado F, Farber M, et al. Pivotal results of the Medtronic Vascular Talent Thoracic Stent Graft System: the VALOR trial. *J Vasc Surg* 2008;48:546–554.

13. Cheng D, Martin J, Shennib H, et al. Endovascular aortic repair versus open surgical repair for descending thoracic aortic disease a systematic review and meta-analysis of comparative studies. *J Am Coll Cardiol* 2010;55:986–1001.

14. Matsumura JS, Lee WA, Mitchell RS, et al. The Society for Vascular Surgery Practice Guidelines: management of the left subclavian artery with thoracic endovascular aortic repair. *J Vasc Surg* 2009;50:1155–1158.

15. Gutsche JT, Cheung AT, McGarvey ML, et al. Risk factors for perioperative stroke after thoracic endovascular aortic repair. *Ann Thorac Surg* 2007;84:1195–1200.

16. Buth J, Harris PL, Hobo R, et al. Neurologic complications associated with endovascular repair of thoracic aortic pathology: Incidence and risk factors. A study from the European Collaborators on Stent/Graft Techniques for Aortic Aneurysm Repair (EUROSTAR) registry. *J Vasc Surg* 2007;46:1103–1110.

17. Khoynezhad A, Donayre CE, Bui H, Kopchok GE, Walot I, White RA. Risk factors of neurologic deficit after thoracic aortic endografting. *Ann Thorac Surg* 2007;83:S882–889.

18. Feezor RJ, Martin TD, Hess PJ, et al. Risk factors for perioperative stroke during thoracic endovascular aortic repairs (TEVAR). *J Endovasc Ther* 2007;14:568–573.

19. Safi HJ, Miller CC, 3rd, Carr C, Iliopoulos DC, Dorsay DA, Baldwin JC. Importance of intercostal artery reattachment during thoracoabdominal aortic aneurysm repair. *J Vasc Surg* 1998;27:58–66.

20. Gravereaux EC, Faries PL, Burks JA, et al. Risk of spinal cord ischemia after endograft repair of thoracic aortic aneurysms. *J Vasc Surg* 2001;34:997–1003.

21. Safi HJ, Hess KR, Randel M, et al. Cerebrospinal fluid drainage and distal aortic perfusion: reducing neurologic complications in repair of thoracoabdominal aortic aneurysm types I and II. *J Vasc Surg* 1996;23:223–228.

22. Estrera AL, Sheinbaum R, Miller CC, et al. Cerebrospinal fluid drainage during thoracic aortic repair: safety and current management. *Ann Thorac Surg* 2009;88:9–15.

23. Cooper DG, Walsh SR, Sadat U, Noorani A, Hayes PD, Boyle JR. Neurological complications after left subclavian artery coverage during thoracic endovascular aortic repair: a systematic review and meta-analysis. *J Vasc Surg* 2009;49:1594–1601.

24. Eggebrecht H, Nienaber CA, Neuhauser M, et al. Endovascular stent-graft placement in aortic dissection: a meta-analysis. *Eur Heart J* 2006;27:489–498.

25. Fattori R, Lovato L, Buttazzi K, Di Bartolomeo R, Gavelli G. Extension of dissection in stent-graft treatment of type B aortic dissection: lessons learned from endovascular experience. *J Endovasc Ther* 2005;12:306–311.

26. Neuhauser B, Czermak BV, Fish J, et al. Type A dissection following endovascular thoracic aortic stent graft repair. *J Endovasc Ther* 2005;12:74–81.

27. Eggebrecht H, Thompson M, Rousseau H, et al. Retrograde ascending aortic dissection during or after thoracic aortic stent graft placement: insight from the European registry on endovascular aortic repair complications. *Circulation* 2009;120(11 Suppl):S276–281.

28. Dong ZH, Fu WG, Wang YQ, et al. Retrograde type A aortic dissection after endovascular stent graft placement for treatment of type B dissection. *Circulation* 2009;119:735–741.

29. Lee WA. Failure modes of thoracic endografts: Prevention and management. *J Vasc Surg* 2009;49:792–799.

30. Lee WA, Martin TD, Hess PJ, Beaver TM, Huber TS. Maldeployment of the TAG thoracic endograft. *J Vasc Surg* 2007;46:1032–1035.

31. Rodd CD, Desigan S, Hamady MS, Gibbs RG, Jenkins MP. Salvage options after stent collapse in the thoracic aorta. *J Vasc Surg* 2007;46:780–785.

32. Steinbauer MG, Stehr A, Pfister K, et al. Endovascular repair of proximal endograft collapse after treatment for thoracic aortic disease. *J Vasc Surg* 2006;43:609–612.

33. Chaikof EL, Blankensteijn JD, Harris PL, et al. Reporting standards for endovascular aortic aneurysm repair. *J Vasc Surg* 2002;35:1048–1060.

34. Makaroun MS, Dillavou ED, Wheatley GH, Cambria RP. Five-year results of endovascular treatment with the Gore TAG device compared with open repair of thoracic aortic aneurysms. *J Vasc Surg* 2008;47:912–918.

35. Morales JP, Greenberg RK, Lu Q, et al. Endoleaks following endovascular repair of thoracic aortic aneurysm: etiology and outcomes. *J Endovasc Ther* 2008;15:631–638.

36. Chiesa R, Melissano G, Marone EM, Marrocco-Trischitta MM, Kahlberg A. Aorto-oesophageal and aortobronchial fistulae following thoracic endovascular aortic repair: a national survey. *Eur J Vasc Endovasc Surg* 2010 Mar;39(3):273–9. Epub 2010 Jan 21.

37. Chiesa R, Tshomba Y, Kahlberg A, Marone EM, Civilini E, Coppi G, Psacharopulo D, Melissano G. Management of thoracic endograft infection. *J Cardiovasc Surg (Torino)* 2010 Feb;51(1):15–31.

38. Cernohorsky P, Reijnen MM, Tielliu IF, Sterkenburg SM, van den Dungen JJ, Zeebregts CJ. The relevance of aortic endograft prosthetic infection. *J Vasc Surg* 2011 Mar 10.

39. Heyer KS, Modi P, Morasch MD, Matsumura JS, Kibbe MR, Pearce WH, Resnick SA, Eskandari MK. Secondary infections of thoracic and abdominal aortic endografts. *J Vasc Interv Radiol* 2009 Feb;20(2):173–9. Epub 2008 Dec 20.

40. Milewski RK, Szeto WY, Pochettino A, Mosser GW, Moeller P, Bavaria JE. Have hybrid procedures replaced open aortic arch reconstruction in high-risk patients? A comparative study of elective open arch debranching with endovascular stent graft placement and conventional elective open total and distal aortic arch reconstruction. *J Thorac Cardiovasc Surg* 2010 Sep;140(3):590–7.

41. Safi HJ, Miller CC 3rd, Lee TY, Estrera AL. Repair of ascending and transverse aortic arch. *J Thorac Cardiovasc Surg* 2011 Jan 24. [Epub ahead of print].

42. Estrera AL, Sheinbaum R, Miller CC 3rd, Harrison R, Safi HJ. Neuromonitor-guided repair of thoracoabdominal aortic aneurysms. *J Thorac Cardiovasc Surg* 2010 Dec;140(6 Suppl): S131–5; discussion S142–S146.

28

TEVAR for Descending Thoracic Aortic Emergencies

Cheong J. Lee, MD, Mark L. Keldahl, MD and Mark K. Eskandari, MD

Initially developed to treat degenerative aneurysms of the descending thoracic aorta, the application of thoracic endovascular aortic repair (TEVAR) has rapidly expanded to the entire spectrum of thoracic aortic pathologies in both the elective and emergent settings. Particularly in the acute setting, TEVAR offers the potential for a durable repair while avoiding the morbidity of a thoracotomy, aortic cross-clamping and single-lung ventilation required for an open approach in a physiologically compromised patient. Although device considerations may differ depending on the pathology needing to be treated, TEVAR has gained wide acceptance by surgeons as the treatment of choice in potentially catastrophic situations of the descending thoracic aorta.[1-4] We review the stent graft devices and current data on its application in several thoracic aortic emergencies, including ruptured descending thoracic aortic aneurysms, traumatic aortic injuries, acute aortic dissections, and symptomatic penetrating aortic ulcers.

AVAILABLE DEVICES

Three commercial endografts are currently approved for use in the United States by the FDA: Gore TAG (W.L. Gore, Inc., Flagstaff, Arizona), TALENT (Medtronic, Santa Rosa, California), and Zenith TX 2 (William Cook, ApS, Bjaeverskov, Denmark). W.L. Gore developed the first commercially available thoracic aortic endoprosthesis to undergo a feasibility trial in the US in 1998, followed by a pivotal trial in 1999. Initial studies were halted in 2001 after the discovery of longitudinal wire fractures in the stent body, leading to voluntary withdrawal of the device from distribution. After structural modifications, the redesigned device was named the Gore TAG stent graft and underwent a confirmatory trial in late 2003. The multicenter phase II study showed that perioperative mortality was significantly lower (2.1% vs 11.7%; P = .007), as was spinal cord ischemia (SCI; 3% vs 14%; P = .003), when TEVAR was compared to open repair of descending thoracic aneurysms.[5] The overall and aneurysm-related mortality rates at 2 years for open surgery versus TEVAR were reported to be 25% and 3%, respectively. In a more recent comparative study using the same cohort of patients at 5-year follow-up, aneurysm-related mortality was again found to be lower for TAG patients (2.8% vs 11.7%), however, all-cause mortality was not significantly different (68% vs 67%) between the two groups.[6] The FDA approved commercial use of the Gore TAG endoprosthesis in March 2005 for the treatment of aneurysms of the descending thoracic aorta in patients who have appropriate anatomy including adequate ilio-femoral access, aortic inner diameter in the range of 23–37 mm, and 2 cm of non-aneurysmal aorta proximal and distal to the aneurysm.[7]

In 2005, the Vascular Talent Thoracic Stent Graft System for the Treatment of Thoracic Aortic Aneurysms (VALOR) trial, using the Medtronic Talent endoprosthesis, completed enrollment.[8] Patients were considered for inclusion in the phase II trial if they had a fusiform thoracic aneurysm >5 cm or >2 times the diameter of the non-aneurysmal aorta, as well as focal saccular aneurysms or penetrating atherosclerotic ulcers. The trial enrolled 195 patients for endovascular repair and their results were compared to 189 patients who underwent open repair at centers of excellence that were identified retrospectively. The operative mortality for TEVAR was 2.1%, paraplegia 1.5%, and stroke 3.6%. At 1 year, all-cause mortality was 16.1% and aneurysm-related mortality was 3.1% compared to 11% for open repair.[8] The results of the study led to FDA approval of the device in 2008 for the treatment of fusiform and saccular aneurysms as well as penetrating thoracic aortic ulcers in patients having appropriate anatomy, including ilio-femoral access vessel morphology that is compatible with vascular access techniques, non-aneurysmal aortic diameter in the range of 18–42 mm, and non-aneurysmal aortic proximal and distal neck lengths >20 mm.[7]

Matsumura et al reported a phase II study of TEVAR using the Zenith TX2 endovascular graft (n = 130) versus open surgery (n = 70) for patients with descending thoracic aortic aneurysms and large ulcers.[9] The 30-day mortality (1.9% vs 5.7%) was lower with TEVAR and major perioperative adverse events were less common (9.4% vs 33%; P < .01). Stroke, paraplegia, and paraparesis were lower in the TEVAR group (2.5% vs 8.6%; P = .07, 1.3% vs 5.7%; P = .07, and 4.4% vs 0%; P = .10, respectively). At 1-year follow-up there was a trend of improved overall mortality and aneurysm-related mortality with TEVAR, however, the results were not statistically significant: overall mortality (8.4% vs 14.5%, p = 0.12) and aneurysm-related mortality (5.8% vs 11.8%, p = 0.15). The authors concluded that TEVAR with the TX2 device is a safe and effective alternative to open surgical repair for the treatment of anatomically suitable descending aortic aneurysms and ulcers. This led to FDA approval of the device the same year for the treatment of patients with aneurysms or ulcers of the descending thoracic aorta having vascular morphology suitable for endovascular repair, including adequate ilio-femoral access compatible with the required introduction systems, non-aneurysmal aortic segments proximal and distal to the aneurysm or ulcer, length of at least 25 mm, and with a diameter measured outer wall to outer wall of not greater than 38 mm and no less than 24 mm.[7]

RUPTURED DESCENDING THORACIC AORTIC ANEURYSMS

Thoracic aortic aneurysm rupture is a rare, but catastrophic, event that has an estimated incidence of 5.0 per 100,000 people per year.[10] Ruptured descending thoracic aortic aneurysms (rDTAA) account for approximately 30% of all ruptured aneurysms of the thoracic aorta and overall mortality rates for these patients reach upwards of 90%.[10] Risk factors for rupture of thoracic aortic aneurysms are increasing age, female gender, chronic obstructive pulmonary disease (COPD), and, most importantly, increasing thoracic aortic diameter. Elective intervention is generally recommended in aneurysms greater than 6 cm, the point at which the annual risk of aneurysm related death, rupture, or dissection reaches 15%.[11]

Open surgical resection followed by an interposition graft has been the standard of care for decades for treatment of rDTAA. Despite improvements in surgical and critical care techniques, open surgical repair for thoracic aortic disease is still associated with significant morbidity and mortality. In the current literature, the perioperative mortality rates after open repair for descending thoracic aortic aneurysms is reported to be approximately 10%-20% for elective cases and 45% for ruptured cases.[12,13] Associated complications, including paraplegia, disabling stroke, and renal failure, are significant in the range of 30%-50%.[12,13] Implementation of TEVAR has demonstrated the anticipated reduction in perioperative mortality and morbidity in elective cases of thoracic aneurysms. Given its rare incidence, however, current literature is still limited to small series of rDTAA managed with TEVAR.

Jonker et al recently published a multi-institutional analysis comparing open surgery versus TEVAR for ruptured descending thoracic aneurysms.[2] A total of 161 patients with rDTAA were included from seven participating institutions, of which 92 were treated with TEVAR and 69 with open surgery. The 30-day mortality was 24.6% after open surgery compared with 17.4% after TEVAR (odds ratio [OR], 0.64; 95% confidence interval [CI], .30–1.39; $P = .260$).[2] The composite outcome of death, stroke, or permanent paraplegia occurred in 36.2% of the open repair group, compared with 21.7% of the TEVAR group (OR, 0.49; 95% CI, .24-.97; $P = .044$).[2] Although not statistically significant, the aneurysm-related survival of patients treated with open repair was 64.3% at 4 years, compared with 75.2% for patients treated with TEVAR ($P = .191$).[2] In 2010, Jonker and colleagues published a comprehensive meta-analysis collated from 24 studies involving 143 patients treated by TEVAR and 81 patients with open surgery.[13] The authors found a significantly lower 30-day mortality rate in the TEVAR group: 19% for patients treated with TEVAR for rDTAA compared to 33% for patients treated with open repair, which was significant (OR, 2.15, $P = .016$). The 30-day occurrence rates of myocardial infarction (11.1% vs 3.5%; OR, 3.70, $P < .05$), stroke (10.2% vs 4.1%; OR, 2.67; $P = .117$), and paraplegia (5.5% vs 3.1%; OR, 1.83; $P = .405$) were increased after open repair vs TEVAR, but this failed to reach statistical significance for stroke and paraplegia. Long-term follow-up, however, revealed 5 aneurysm-related deaths in the TEVAR group after 30 days, while no patients died of aneurysm-related causes in the open group after the same period. This comparison was limited in that 83% of patients in the open surgery group were lost during follow-up.

Despite low early operative morbidity and mortality, late complications such as endoleaks, graft migration, stent fractures, and aneurysm-related death, are much more common with TEVAR than those reported for the gold standard open procedure.[14] Nevertheless, data suggest endovascular repair of rDTAA is associated with a lower risk of a composite of death, stroke, and paraplegia, compared with traditional approaches.

TRAUMATIC AORTIC INJURY

Up to 15% of all deaths following motor vehicle collisions are due to injury to the thoracic aorta.[15] It has been estimated that over 80% of traumatic aortic injury (TAI) patients die at the scene and for those patients who arrive alive to the hospital the estimated mortality rate is 30%.[15] The proximal descending aorta, where the relatively mobile aortic arch can move against the fixed descending aorta (ligamentum arteriosum) is at greatest risk from the shearing forces of sudden deceleration. Since the early 1990s, the approach has been to delay definitive repair of TAI surgery for patients under tight blood pressure control using beta-blockers with or without vasodilators to maintain a systolic blood pressure of approximately 100 mmHg and a pulse rate of <100 beats per minute.[16] Even with adequate blood pressure control, however, the risk of free rupture remains as high as 5%–13%.[17,18] Open repair of TAI has been the standard of care with mortality rates ranging from 5% to 28% and paraplegia rates secondary to spinal cord ischemia ranging from 2.3% to 14%.[1,18] In 1997, Kato et al revolutionized the management of TAI with their published report of endoluminal stent grafting in a traumatic aortic aneurysm.[19] Implementation of TEVAR has the theoretical advantages of avoiding thoracotomy, aortic cross clamping, single lung ventilation, and the use of systemic heparinization in a patient with concomitant multi-organ trauma. Although no randomized data exist on the impact of TEVAR for TAI, collective observational data from institutions continue to amass in support of endoluminal approaches.

A recent meta-analysis of data from 17 studies published between 2003 and 2007 identified 369 patients who underwent open repair and 220 who underwent TEVAR for traumatic descending thoracic aortic rupture.[20] All studies were non-randomized retrospective cohort studies and there was limited data on baseline characteristics of the two groups. The injury severity score was reported to be significantly higher in patients who underwent TEVAR than open repair. Despite this, procedure-related and 30-day overall mortality rates were both significantly lower in the TEVAR group than in the open repair group. In addition, overall complication rates were significantly lower for patients who underwent endoluminal repair for TAI. Another large retrospective analysis conducted by Jonker et al using data from the New York Statewide Planning and Research Cooperative System was recently published.[21] In this database, 328 patients were found to have undergone open surgery (79.6%) or TEVAR (20.4%) for traumatic thoracic aortic injury between 2000 and 2007. Although there were more major injuries for patients in the TEVAR group, the authors reported a significantly lower mortality rate (6.0% vs 16.9%, p = 0.024) and fewer pulmonary complications (23.9% vs 37.9%) when compared to the open surgery group.

In comparison to the larger observational reports, the Northwestern experience also attests to the advantages of TEVAR in the management of TAI.[22] A retrospective 7-year review from January 2001 to December 2008 identified 24 patients with acute blunt thoracic aortic injury treated with TEVAR. TEVAR was successful in treating the aortic injury in all patients and there were no instances of procedure-related death, stroke, or paraplegia. Access to the aorta was obtained through a femoral/iliac cut-down (n=7) or an entirely percutaneous groin approach (n=17). Systemic heparin was not used in 84% of cases. One patient required secondary intervention for device collapse that was treated successfully with repeat endografting. There have been no delayed device failures or complications among the entire cohort at mid-term follow-up.

Earlier this year, the Society for Vascular Surgery pursued development of clinical practice guidelines for the management of traumatic thoracic aortic injuries with thoracic endovascular aortic repair.[23] In order to formulate these practice guidelines, the Society selected a panel of experts and conducted a systematic review and meta-analysis of the literature, which included 7,768 patients. The panel found that the mortality rate was significantly lower in patients who underwent endovascular repair, followed by open repair and nonoperative management (9%, 19%, and 46%, respectively, $P < .01$).[23] No significant difference in event rate across the three groups was noted for stroke. The risk of spinal cord ischemia (SCI) and end stage renal disease (ESRD) was higher in open repair compared with endovascular repair and nonoperative management (SCI: 9% open vs 3% endovascular and 3% nonoperative, $P < .01$; ESRD: 8% open vs 5% endovascular and 3% nonoperative, $P < .01$).[23] Compared with endovascular repair, open repair was associated with increased risk of graft infection and systemic infections, most commonly pneumonia. With a median follow-up of 2 years, there was a trend toward increased risk of a secondary procedure in endovascular compared with open repair ($P<.07$).[23] Given the limited quality of evidence in the literature, the consensus was formulated with a grading of level 2C (Table 28–1) for the application of TEVAR in traumatic aortic injuries. The overall view of the panel was that TEVAR is associated with improved outcomes compared with open repair; especially with regards to mortality and incidence of spinal cord ischemia.[23]

TEVAR in the setting of traumatic aortic injury has important limitations. Sizing the aorta for stent graft selection in the setting of hypovolemia, hemodynamic collapse, or early resuscitation may result in significant inaccuracy (>10%), leading to an increased risk of endograft collapse or migration.[24] The native aorta is known to increase in size with age. Patients with TAI tend to be younger and this natural growth may increase the potential risk for device migration and late endoleak. In addition, the need for continued imaging surveillance after TEVAR is problematic in younger patients with regards to radiation exposure and they are often lost to follow-up. The current lack of suitable devices that can accommodate the unique anatomy of these patients occasionally resulted in severe procedure-related complications. Specifically,

TABLE 28–1. GUIDELINES FOR TEVAR IN TRAUMATIC AORTIC INJURIES

Guideline	Consensus	Grade of recommendation 1—strong; 2—weak	Quality of evidence A—high; B—moderate; C—low or very low
Choice of treatment	We suggest that endovascular repair be performed preferentially over open surgical repair or nonoperative management.	2	C
Timing of repair	We suggest urgent (<24 hours) repair and, at the latest, prior to hospital discharge.	2	C
Management of minimal aortic injury	We suggest expectant management with serial imaging for type I injuries.	2	C
Type of repair in the young patient	We suggest endovascular repair regardless of age if anatomically suitable.	2	C
Management of left subclavian artery	We suggest selective revascularization of the left subclavian artery.	2	C
Systemic heparinization	We suggest routine heparinization but at a lower dose than in elective TEVAR.	2	C
Spinal drainage	We do not suggest routine spinal drainage.	2	C
Choice of anesthesia	We suggest general anesthesia.	2	C
Femoral access technique	We suggest open femoral exposure.	2	C

collapse of the stent graft due to the acute angle of the arch and limited size of the femoral arteries causing injuries at the access site has been described.[25] Although correctable with secondary interventions, initial endoleaks after TEVAR for TAI are reported to occur frequently (9–14%).[1,21]

Considering the inherent limitation for the treatment of thoracic aortic injury, the data demonstrate improved overall outcomes for TEVAR in the management of TAI. Further studies are required to establish long-term trends and outcomes to fuel the needed evolution of current device technologies and surveillance protocols.

ACUTE COMPLICATED TYPE B DISSECTION

Acute thoracic aortic dissection is an uncommon but potentially lethal disease with an incidence of 3 cases per 100,000 patients.[26] The risk factors for aortic dissection are multifactorial and include male gender, arterial hypertension, connective tissue disorders, steroid and cocaine use, bicuspid aortic valve, and deceleration trauma. Stanford class Type B dissections represent 40% of the cohort and can be further categorized into type B dissection without complications and type B dissection with complications of rupture, signs of impending rupture, and/or end-organ malperfusion from true lumen collapse following preferential pressurization of the aortic false lumen (Figure 28–1). In patients with complicated Type B dissection (cTBD), mortality is increased 3-fold over the uncomplicated cohort and constitutes a surgical emergency.[26] Emergency treatment options include open surgical thoracic aortic graft replacement, interventional or surgical flap fenestration and true lumen stenting, catheter reperfusion or extra-anatomic surgical

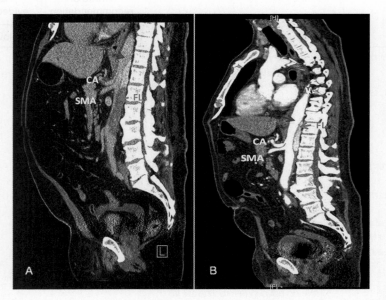

Figure 28-1. Acute Complicated Type B Aortic Dissection. **a.** Preferential pressurization of the false lumen leading to true lumen collapse and subsequent distal aortic occlusion. **b.** Following TEVAR of entry tear, re-expansion of the true lumen is seen with restoration of distal aortic perfusion.
CA = Celiac Artery; SMA = Superior Mesenteric Artery; TL = True Aortic Lumen; FL = False Aortic Lumen

bypass, and TEVAR. Salvage open surgical repair has been associated with high morbidity and mortality (24–34%) because these patients are frequently in extremis.[27] The primary objective of endografting for acute Type B dissections is to cover the primary entry tear with the intention of obliterating flow in the false lumen and directing flow back into the true lumen. In the acute setting, this abrogates end organ malperfusion and controls hemorrhage. In the mid- to long-term, it is anticipated that TEVAR promotes early aortic remodeling by accelerating false lumen thrombosis and preventing aneurysmal aortic degeneration.[28]

The use of TEVAR for type B dissection originates from an initial report by Dake and colleagues in 1999.[29] This study examined 19 patients who underwent TEVAR for type A (n = 4) or type B (n = 15) dissection. The authors reported a 100% technical success rate for stent placement, with complete thrombosis at the thoracic aortic false lumen being achieved in 80% of patients and partial thrombosis in the remaining 20%.[29] The 30-day mortality rate was 16%, with no deaths or incidence of aneurysm rupture during the subsequent follow-up period of 13 months.[29] A decade later, however, the majority of the subsequent data regarding TEVAR for cTBD is yet based on single-center outcomes. As with other centers of excellence, a 7-year review of Northwestern's experience with TEVAR for acute complicated Type B dissections demonstrated promising outcomes for its application in these circumstances. Twenty patients were identified and treated for cTBD. The average time from onset of symptoms to intervention was 5 days (0–17 days). Thirty-day death, stroke, and paraplegia rates were 0%, 10%, and 5% respectively. Success at sealing the rupture or reversing malperfusion was 100%. Three patients required early conversion and one patient required late conversion to open repair. Patient survival was 90% with a mean follow-up of 16 months (1–54 months).[30]

The largest collated data published is a meta-analysis of 29 studies performed by Parker et al in 2008, which included 942 patients over a 10-year period who underwent TEVAR for acute type B dissection with complications.[4] In that study, the in-hospital (30-day) mortality was 9% and other major complications (i.e., stroke, paraplegia, conversion to type A dissection, bowel infarction, major amputation) occurred in 8.1%.[4] During a mean follow-up duration of 20 months, re-intervention was required in 10.4% and aortic rupture was reported in 0.8%.[4] Mean overall survival was 88% at 20 months.

Recently, the Society for Vascular Surgery Outcomes Committee published their report on the results of TEVAR for acute cTBD. The study analyzed 1-year outcomes collected from five physician-sponsored investigational device exemption (IDE) clinical trials between 2000 and 2008. There were 99 cTBD patients, 85 who were acute (< 14 days from admission before malperfusion and/or rupture). Early adverse events included pulmonary (36.5%), vascular (28.2%), renal (25.9%), and neurologic (23.5%). Early major adverse events occurred in 37.6% of patients, including death (10.6%), stroke (9.4%), renal failure (9.4%), and paralysis (9.4%); late adverse events included vascular (15.8%), cardiac (10.5%), gastrointestinal (6.6%), and hemorrhage (5.3%). The point-estimate mortality rate was 10.8 (95% CI, 4.1–17.5) at 30 days and 29.4 (95% CI, 18.4–40.4) at 1 year.[31] Based on these findings, the committee concluded that emergency TEVAR for patients with cTBD (malperfusion or rupture) provided acceptable mortality and morbidity results out to 1 year.

Although data is far from definitive, TEVAR for acute complicated type B dissection is associated with acceptable and early outcome and midterm survival relative to conventional therapy.

PENETRATING AORTIC ULCERS AND INTRAMURAL HEMATOMA

Penetrating atherosclerotic ulcer (PAU) is defined by an ulceration of an aortic atherosclerotic plaque penetrating through the internal elastic lamina into the aortic media. Complications of PAU include development of (localized) intramural hematoma due to erosion of aortic vasa vasorum by the ulcer, pseudoaneurysm formation (Figure 28–2), progression to overt aortic dissection, or rupture in up to 40% of patients.[32] The natural history and pathophysiology of PAU, overall, is poorly understood.

There is debate as to whether intramural hematoma (IMH) is a distinct entity from PAU. IMH is commonly defined as bleeding into the outer layers of the aortic media, thought to be caused by the rupture of aortic vasa vasorum due to alterations from chronic arterial hypertension.[33] By definition, IMH lacks a detectable intimal tear or disruption, therefore, no communication with the true aortic lumen exists. This definition of IMH as being a "dissection without a tear" continues to be challenged as current high resolution imaging modalities allow better characterization of the aortic wall irregularities. As with PAU, the natural history and pathophysiology of IMH is not fully understood.

Penetrating ulcers and IMH both belong to the spectrum of aortic pathology deemed "acute aortic syndrome", which is inclusive of classical aortic dissection. Both PAU and IMH can progress to aortic dissection or rupture.[32] As with aortic dissections, the indication to consider TEVAR in patients with acute aortic syndrome has been reserved for those with involvement of the ascending aorta or in those who are symptomatic despite optimal medical treatment. Symptomatic patients presenting with acute aortic syndrome are generally believed to have a worse prognosis.

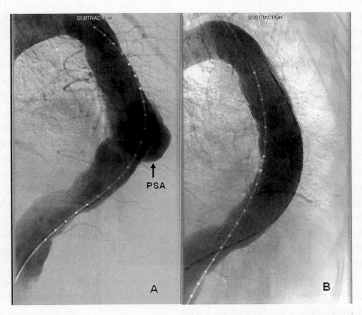

Figure 28-2. Penetrating Aortic Ulcer with Resultant Pseudoaneurysm. **a.** Patient with large symptomatic pseudoaneurysm of the descending thoracic aorta. **b.** Successful coverage of the pseudoaneurysm using TEVAR.
PSA = Pseudoaneurysm

In 2009, Eggebrecht et al reviewed the currently available literature and analyzed the data of 209 patients who underwent TEVAR for PAU and IMH.[3] All data were from institutional observational reports. The technical failure was reported to be 2%, with complete sealing of PAU and IMH achieved in 96% of patients. The overall in-hospital mortality was 7%, with an additional 2% aorta-related mortality rate during the mean follow-up period of 14.3 months. Although there is no agreed first-line treatment for incidental PAU, the authors of this study concluded that TEVAR should be indicated in symptomatic patients complicated by pseudoaneurysm formation or rupture. Similarly, progression of IMH towards overt dissection or rupture warrants treatment. A study by Patel et al, however, warns of technical challenges of sizing grafts and ballooning of landing zones when TEVAR is employed in the setting of IMH. Friable aortic wall in the setting of an IMH may lead to endograft erosion through the aortic wall when the graft is oversized beyond 10%.[34]

CONCLUSION

TEVAR is becoming the treatment of choice for acute surgical emergencies involving the descending thoracic aorta and has revolutionized the approach to the management of these difficult circumstances. Although device technology continues to rapidly evolve, the existing devices can be readily and successfully applied to the pathologies outlined above. Randomized studies may not be realistic given the acuity and the rarity of these clinical entities; regardless, emerging evidence continues to forecast encouraging results. The excitement has to be tempered by the critical lack of mature clinical data on the long-term outcomes of TEVAR and, as such, conclusive statements on the evolving modality remain to be elucidated.

REFERENCES

1. Demetriades D, Velmahos GC, Scalea TM, et al. Operative repair or endovascular stent graft in blunt traumatic thoracic aortic injuries: results of an American Association for the Surgery of Trauma Multicenter Study. *J Trauma* 2008;64:561–70; discussion 570–1.
2. Jonker FHW, Verhagen HJM, Lin PH, et al. Open surgery versus endovascular repair of ruptured thoracic aortic aneurysms. *J Vasc Surg* 2011;53:1210–6.
3. Eggebrecht H, Plicht B, Kahlert P, et al. Intramural hematoma and penetrating ulcers: indications to endovascular treatment. *Eur J Vasc Endovasc Surg* 2009;38:659–65.
4. Parker JD, Golledge J. Outcome of endovascular treatment of acute type B aortic dissection. *Ann Thorac Surg* 2008;86:1707–12.
5. Makaroun MS, Dillavou ED, Kee ST, et al. Endovascular treatment of thoracic aortic aneurysms: results of the phase II multicenter trial of the GORE TAG thoracic endoprosthesis. *J Vasc Surg* 2005;41:1–9.
6. Makaroun MS, Dillavou ED, Wheatley GH, et al. Five-year results of endovascular treatment with the Gore TAG device compared with open repair of thoracic aortic aneurysms. *J Vasc Surg* 2008;47:912–8.
7. Garcia-Toca M, Eskandari MK. Regulatory TEVAR clinical trials. *J Vasc Surg* 2010;52:22S–5S.
8. Fairman RM, Criado F, Farber M, et al. Pivotal results of the Medtronic Vascular Talent Thoracic Stent Graft System: the VALOR trial. *J Vasc Surg* 2008;48:546–54.

9. Matsumura JS, Cambria RP, Dake MD, et al. International controlled clinical trial of thoracic endovascular aneurysm repair with the Zenith TX2 endovascular graft: 1-year results. *J Vasc Surg* 2008;47:247–57; discussion 257.

10. Johansson G, Markstrom U, Swedenborg J. Ruptured thoracic aortic aneurysms: a study of incidence and mortality rates. *J Vasc Surg* 1995;21:985–8.

11. Elefteriades JA, Botta DM Jr. Indications for the treatment of thoracic aortic aneurysms. *Surg Clin North Am* 2009;89:845–67, ix.

12. Schermerhorn ML, Giles KA, Hamdan AD, et al. Population-based outcomes of open descending thoracic aortic aneurysm repair. *J Vasc Surg* 2008;48:821–7.

13. Jonker FH, Trimarchi S, Verhagen HJ, et al. Meta-analysis of open versus endovascular repair for ruptured descending thoracic aortic aneurysm. *J Vasc Surg* 2010;51:1026–32, 1032.e1–32.e2.

14. Geisbusch P, Hoffmann S, Kotelis D, et al. Reinterventions during midterm follow-up after endovascular treatment of thoracic aortic disease. *J Vasc Surg* 2011;53:1528–33.

15. Fabian TC, Richardson JD, Croce MA, et al. Prospective study of blunt aortic injury: Multicenter Trial of the American Association for the Surgery of Trauma. *J Trauma* 1997;42:374–80; discussion 380–3.

16. Fabian TC, Davis KA, Gavant ML, et al. Prospective study of blunt aortic injury: helical CT is diagnostic and antihypertensive therapy reduces rupture. *Ann Surg* 1998;227:666–76; discussion 676–7.

17. Holmes JH 4th, Bloch RD, Hall RA, et al. Natural history of traumatic rupture of the thoracic aorta managed nonoperatively: a longitudinal analysis. *Ann Thorac Surg* 2002;73:1149–54.

18. Neschis DG, Scalea TM, Flinn WR, et al. Blunt aortic injury. *N Engl J Med* 2008;359:1708–16.

19. Kato N, Dake MD, Miller DC, et al. Traumatic thoracic aortic aneurysm: treatment with endovascular stent-grafts. *Radiology* 1997;205:657–62.

20. Xenos ES, Abedi NN, Davenport DL, et al. Meta-analysis of endovascular vs open repair for traumatic descending thoracic aortic rupture. *J Vasc Surg* 2008;48:1343–51.

21. Jonker FH, Giacovelli JK, Muhs BE, et al. Trends and outcomes of endovascular and open treatment for traumatic thoracic aortic injury. *J Vasc Surg* 2010;51:565–71.

22. Garcia-Toca M, Naughton PA, Matsumura JS, et al. Endovascular repair of blunt traumatic thoracic aortic injuries: seven-year single-center experience. *Arch Surg* 2010;145:679–83.

23. Lee WA, Matsumura JS, Mitchell RS, et al. Endovascular repair of traumatic thoracic aortic injury: clinical practice guidelines of the Society for Vascular Surgery. *J Vasc Surg* 2011;53:187–92.

24. Jonker FH, Verhagen HJ, Mojibian H, et al. Aortic endograft sizing in trauma patients with hemodynamic instability. *J Vasc Surg* 2010;52:39–44.

25. Canaud L, Alric P, Desgranges P, et al. Factors favoring stent-graft collapse after thoracic endovascular aortic repair. *J Thorac Cardiov Surg* 2010;139:1153–7.

26. Hagan PG, Nienaber CA, Isselbacher EM, et al. The International Registry of Acute Aortic Dissection (IRAD): new insights into an old disease. *JAMA* 2000;283:897–903.

27. Bozinovski J, Coselli JS. Outcomes and survival in surgical treatment of descending thoracic aorta with acute dissection. *Ann Thorac Surg* 2008;85:965–70; discussion 970–1.

28. Conrad MF, Crawford RS, Kwolek CJ, et al. Aortic remodeling after endovascular repair of acute complicated type B aortic dissection. *J Vasc Surg* 2009;50:510–7.

29. Dake MD, Kato N, Mitchell RS, et al. Endovascular stent-graft placement for the treatment of acute aortic dissection. *N Engl J Med* 1999;340:1546–52.

30. Keldahl ML, Naughton P, Rodriguez H, et al. Single institutional review of endovascular treatment of complicated acute type B aortic dissection. Chicago Surgical Society, Chicago, IL, March 10, 2011.

31. White RA, Miller DC, Criado FJ, et al. Report on the results of thoracic endovascular aortic repair for acute, complicated, type B aortic dissection at 30 days and 1 year from a multidisciplinary subcommittee of the Society for Vascular Surgery Outcomes Committee. *J Vasc Surg* 2011;53:1082–90.

32. Tittle SL, Lynch RJ, Cole PE, et al. Midterm follow-up of penetrating ulcer and intramural hematoma of the aorta. *J Thorac Cardiov Surg* 2002;123:1051–9.
33. Svensson LG, Labib SB, Eisenhauer AC, et al. Intimal tear without hematoma: an important variant of aortic dissection that can elude current imaging techniques. *Circulation* 1999; 99:1331–6.
34. Patel HJ, Williams DM, Upchurch GR Jr, et al. The challenge of associated intramural hematoma with endovascular repair for penetrating ulcers of the descending thoracic aorta. *J Vasc Surg* 2010;51:829–35.

29

Endograft Repair of Blunt Aortic Injury

David G. Neschis, MD, Marshall E. Benjamin, MD and William R. Flinn, MD

Blunt aortic injury has been a leading cause of death in victims of a motor vehicle crash, second only to head trauma.[1] The often cited autopsy report by Greendyke, estimated that one of every six victims of fatal auto accidents sustained aortic rupture.[2] Parmley and colleagues noted rupture or laceration of the aorta was more common than previously appreciated, and it was estimated that about 85% of individuals with this injury died at the scene. Further, of the 15% of cases who made it to the hospital alive, the majority would die within 24 hours if repair was not performed.[3] Since those reports, increased awareness and significant improvements in diagnostic imaging has led to more timely diagnosis of blunt aortic injury which has allowed more successful treatment.

One of the most dramatic advances in the treatment of blunt aortic injury has been the use of endograft repair. Prior to 1997, when the first case of endovascular repair of traumatic aortic injury was described, the only treatment for this life-threatening condition was open surgical repair.[4] The modern experience with open repair of blunt aortic injury (coincidentally published the same year as publication of the first endograft) was summarized in a prospective study conducted by the American Association for the Surgery of Trauma (AAST) over a 2.5-year time period in 50 trauma centers in North America. In 274 cases of open repair of blunt aortic injury, the overall mortality of patients who arrived at the hospital alive was 31%, with a paraplegia rate of 8.7%.[5] This study led to improvements in the surgical management of these cases but also to the recognition that endovascular graft treatment of blunt aortic injury could represent a major breakthrough in treatment for these injuries.

Thereafter, the results of a second study (AAST2) was reported in 2008.[6] While no patients in the original report had endovascular repair, in AAST2, 65% of patients were selected for endograft repair and only 35% underwent open repair. Significant improvements were noted in outcomes for patients undergoing open repair; mortality dropped to 23.5% and the rate of paraplegia was 2.9%.[6] The results in endograft repair in these patients were notably even more encouraging, with a mortality of 7.2% and a paraplegia rate of 0.8%.[6] At that time however these more successful outcomes were offset by a 20% device complication rate, including a initial 14.4% incidence of endoleak. Additionally, one-third of these endoleak patients ultimately required open repair.[6] Nevertheless, this observed significant reduction in perioperative mortality and the incidence of paraplegia has been confirmed in other single-center experiences.[7,8] Meta-analyses of recent reports comparing open and endograft repair of blunt aortic injury have clearly demonstrated the benefits of endovascular repair noting significant improvements in procedure related mortality and rates of paraplegia.[9,10]

In our own comparison of open versus endovascular repair, endografting was associated with a significantly shorter length of stay, less intraoperative blood loss, and a lower incidence of postoperative tracheostomy compared with patients undergoing open repair.[11] In our experience of 43 consecutive cases of endograft repair, mortality was 11.6% and the paraplegia rate was 0%. However, similar to the findings in AAST2, there was a 14.3% endoleak rate, of which 50% of these endoleaks required open repair.[12] It has become clear that short-term results in anatomically appropriate patients are excellent; however, newer devices are required that will conform more effectively to the aortic anatomy of the young injured patient.

INITIAL EVALUATION

Prior to the development of modern CT angiography, all patients suspected of having a blunt aortic injury were evaluated with catheter-based angiography with the obvious disadvantages of being an invasive study requiring time to assemble a specialized team and then only visualizing the aortic lumen not the wall that has been injured. It is now well recognized that helical CT provides more accurate diagnosis of blunt aortic injury with an estimated sensitivity of 100% as compared with 92% for angiography.[13]

Modern CT equipment is almost universally available in any trauma setting and has become the study of choice for the evaluation of blunt aortic injury. Other modes of imaging include MRI and both transesophageal and intravascular ultrasonography. Intravascular ultrasound can be a very useful adjunctive study for accurate evaluation and sizing of the injured aorta that can be performed at the time of endovascular repair.[14] CT angiography can be very accurate in identifying an aortic injury suitable for endograft repair, but these scans are often performed early in the patient's admission when they are still in shock. Aortic measurements made off of an early CT scan may underestimate the aortic diameter and possibly lead to inaccurate endograft sizing.[15]

In the past when the diagnosis of traumatic aortic injury was made, immediate repair was recommended. More recent studies have documented the safety and usefulness of delaying aortic repair to allow treatment of other complex injuries.[16] In a large prospective study of patients with blunt aortic injury and a coexisting head injury, pulmonary injury, or cardiac insufficiency, initial treatment with beta blockers (with or without vasodilators) to maintain a stable systolic blood pressure (100-120mmHg) and pulse rate (<100), no patient had a fatal aortic rupture while awaiting repair.[13] While this approach may facilitate delayed repair in many patients it may be compromised in patient with concomitant brain injury. Patients with brain injury often require optimizing the cerebral perfusion pressure by elevation of the patient's systemic blood pressure. Early endograft repair in these cases can be more safely performed than open repair and resolve this treatment dilemma.

OPERATIVE APPROACH

Endovascular aortic repair is now a familiar procedure to most vascular surgeons, but several technical notes are worth mentioning. Ideally patients with traumatic aortic injuries requiring endograft repair are treated in an operative endovascular suite with fixed imaging equipment. Modern portable equipment can be used and may be particularly useful if the patient's head requires elevation due to brain trauma where a more flexible operative table may be required. Spinal drainage is not routinely employed due to the short area of aorta expected to be covered as these injuries do not typically affect the distal thoracic aorta.

Primary access is usually obtained via surgical exposure of the common femoral artery and a puncture for angiography on the contralateral side. Access site choice will be affected by other injuries, including pelvic and femoral fractures. Percutaneous access for the main device in the trauma setting has been reported.[17] An arch angiogram is performed initially to assess the overall anatomy and in particular to assess for the presence of vertebral artery dominance. Successful endograft repair of traumatic aortic injuries may require partial or complete coverage of the left subclavian artery and thereby compromise flow to a dominant left vertebral artery. If the left vertebral artery is significantly larger than the right and imaging of the aortic injury suggest that coverage of the left subclavian artery will be required, consideration should be given to preservation of left subclavian/vertebral flow, either via a pre-endograft carotid-subclavian bypass or plans made for a chimney-style stenting of the left subclavian artery at the time of endograft placement. It has been our experience that CT reconstructions often underestimate the degree of aortic angulation and repair complexity and, frequently, last minute adjustments in the endograft plan may have to be made at the time of angiography.

Overall, trauma victims are younger and the average age of patients with blunt aortic injury has been approximately 44 years.[12] The vascular anatomy of the aortic arch in these younger patients differs significantly from the elderly patient with thoracic aortic aneurysmal disease. Access vessels also tend to be smaller in younger patients and are more prone to spasm when manipulated, but this is offset by their relatively disease-free state. These arteries also tend to be fairly elastic and will usually allow passage of the endovascular device. It has been our experience and that of others that for patients with particularly small access vessels sheathless advancement of the Gore Excluder device can be safely performed.[12,18]

The young aorta is often sharply angulated at the aortic arch with an overall small diameter. A Lunderquist wire may often be too stiff and bend in some of the very acute angled arches. An Amplatz wire in these cases can maintain adequate stiffness with sufficient flexibility.[19] It is our practice to form a pigtail catheter in the distal thoracic aorta and pass this formed pigtail up past the area of injury to avoid the wire engaging the damaged area and causing further injury to the aorta.

Another controversy in the treatment of traumatic aortic injuries is the use of Heparin anticoagulation. In our early experience, we were reluctant to perform the endograft repair without Heparin for fear of creating limb thrombosis or stroke. This obviously delayed aortic repair in cases of significant head or intra-abdominal injury where heparin was initially contraindicated. The evolving experience with endograft repair of traumatic aortic ruptures has demonstrated that repair can be safely performed without the use of Heparin anticoagulation.[20] We now avoid the use of anticoagulation in selective cases, where anticoagulation would be hazardous due to

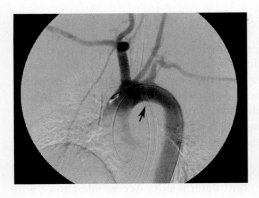

Figure 29–1. Classic "bird beak" appearance (arrow) when endograft extends into the horizontal portion of the aortic arch and does not fully co-opt to the lesser curve. This configuration allows flow between the aortic wall and the graft, which, when extreme, can result in endoleak or graft collapse.

associated traumatic injuries, and in which the aortic anatomy was uncomplicated. This approach has allowed timely repair in patients with an ongoing bleeding risk.[12]

The area of necessary aortic coverage to achieve successful repair will be determined by the length of uninjured aorta required to obtain a satisfactory seal, the location of the left subclavian artery with respect to the injury, and the overall acuity of the aortic arch angle. While it is desirable to maximize the proximal seal length, this may be compromised by the necessity to cover the left subclavian artery or by having the aortic graft extend into the horizontal portion of the aortic arch creating a "bird beak" effect (Figure 29–1).

Extension of the proximal portion of the graft into the horizontal portion of the aortic arch has been associated with graft collapse.[21] Although originally associated with over-sizing of the graft, collapse has been found to occur even with proper endograft sizing.[22] This collapse effect, although usually described as a relatively early complication, has also been described as late as 38 months after the initial repair.[23]

In our experience, the average native aortic diameter at the planned proximal ending zone was 22.7mm, with a range of 19 to 30mm.[12] This was obviously a problem early in our experience when the Gore TAG device was the only available device and the smallest thoracic device diameter was 26mm. This would have resulted in significant over-sizing in a number of patients. Prior to the availability of thoracic devices available in smaller diameters, we utilized proximal cuffs designed for use in abdominal aortic aneurysms. Our experience and the experience of others were that these proximal aortic abdominal cuffs were very helpful with respect to their relatively small introducer diameter and their ability to conform to the aortic angulation.[12,18] An obvious disadvantage of extension cuffs is their short length. Stacking of several overlapping cuffs is often required which has the theoretical potential for separation between cuffs. We have not experienced this particular complication however.

It has been our preference to accept a shorter than standard (2cm) landing zone rather than perform routine coverage of the left subclavian artery. This has generally been more due our attempt to avoid the bird-beaking effect in the transverse portion of the aortic arch (described above), rather than a specific concern about coverage of the left subclavian artery. In our experience, 21% of cases required partial or complete subclavian artery coverage and there have been no sequelae in those patients.[12] We will selectively perform left subclavian revascularization preferentially prior to repair of the aortic injury in patients with a narrow or absent right vertebral artery or in patients with a left internal mammary artery bypass to the coronary circulation in which left subclavian artery coverage might be required. We accept a short landing zone in cases of traumatic aortic repair, as it is expected that the site of injury should heal over time and would unlikely dilate as in the case of aneurysmal repair. There has been documented healing of the site of injury in an autopsy endograft explant three months after injury.[24] We have achieved successful repair with a coverage length as short as 5mm without short or mid-term failure.[12]

In young trauma patients arterial pulsations are hyperdynamic and can become a particular problem when device placement requires millimeters of precision. A variety of techniques have been described to reduce the arterial pressures within the aorta at the time of deployment, including the use of Adenosine to induce hypotension or the use of rapid ventricular pacing.[25,26] We have found the use of Adenosine to create a temporary asystole to be helpful and safe in this situation and have used Adenosine to augment placement in 50% of patients. Doses as high as 18mg to 24mg are often required to achieve the desired effect.[12]

Follow-up CT angiography is generally performed within a week of endograft placement or before the patient's discharge. Patients are instructed to return for a follow-up visit within two weeks following discharge for evaluation of groin wounds and pulses and to establish a point of contact for future visits. Follow-up CT angiography and PA and lateral chest radiographs are obtained at six months and then yearly thereafter. However, due to the young age of these patients, the risk of radiation exposure over time can be significant. It has been estimated that a single CT scan obtained in a 20-year-old patient carries a 0.06% lifetime risk of an associated malignancy.[27] We, therefore, have increased the intervals between visits to more than one year in selected cases with repairs that appear to be stable.

PATTERNS OF GRAFT FAILURE

As noted earlier, the significantly lower mortality and paraplegia rates for endograft repair of traumatic aortic injury seen both in our own experience as well as that of the prospective AAST2 trial, were offset by an approximately 20% device complication rate.[6] The endoleak rate was 14.4%, half of which required open exploration for resolution.[6] Our experience has been similar with respect to endoleaks and their subsequent requirement for endograft explant. Some common pitfalls were described earlier, however, even when devices are properly sized and care is taken to minimize the bird beak effect, device failure and endoleaks do occur. In evaluating patterns of graft failure in our own experience, we identified that the distance from the left subclavian artery to the area of injury and the acuity of the aortic arch angle were both significantly associated with device failure (Figure 29–2). The mean distance from the origin of the left subclavian artery to the site of injury was 2.2cm in repairs without graft failure and 1.2cm in repairs that experienced graft failure, such as endoleak or device collapse ($p = 0.04$).[12] Additionally, the aortic angulation was 92.8 degrees in the device failure group versus 111 degrees in the success group ($p = 0.03$). In further evaluating patterns of graft failure, we identified that the morphological features of the injured aorta can be grouped into four categories (Figure 29–3). In our series, 50% of cases were of the type 1 variety, 7.5% were type 2, 32.5% were type 3, and 10% were type 4. There were no device failures in types 1, 2 and 3 aortas. However, all endograft repairs performed in type 4 lesions required major interventions. Based on our experience, we would recommend the use of caution when attempting endograft repair in a tightly angulated aorta in which the most extreme bend in the aorta is in the planned landing zone and that landing zone is less than 2cm in length.[12]

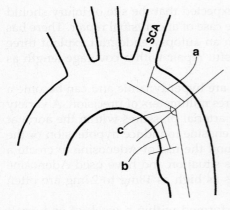

Figure 29-2. Anatomic relationships of aorta in setting of blunt injury. A, distance from the left subclavian artery to the sharpest bend in the descending thoracic aorta. B, distance form the bend to the site of injury. C, angle made at sharpest bend in the descending thoracic aorta. From Neschis DG, Moainie S, Flinn WR, Scalea TM, Bartlett ST, Griffith BP. Endograft repair of traumatic aortic injury-a technique in evolution: a single institution's experience. Annals of surgery 2009;250(3):377–82.

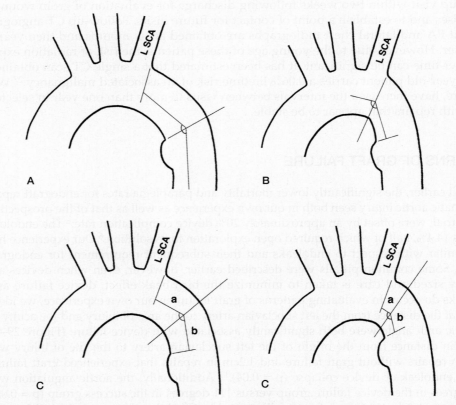

Figure 29-3. a. Type 1 aortic injury – There is a variable distance form the left Subclavian artery (LSCA) to the bend. The site of injury is at the bend. **b.** Type 2 aortic injury – The bend is at the level of the L SCA. There is a variable distance from the bend to the site of injury **c.** Type 3 aortic injury - There is a variable distance between the L SCA and the bend (a) and between the bend and the site of injury (b). a+b is 2 cm or greater. **d.** Type 4 aortic injury – this situation exists when a+b <2cm, and is especially troublesome when the angulation at the bend is <90⁰.
From: Neschis DG, Moainie S, Flinn WR, Scalea TM, Bartlett ST, Griffith BP.
Endograft repair of traumatic aortic injury-a technique in evolution: a single institution's experience. Annals of surgery 2009;250(3):377–82.

MINIMAL AORTIC INJURY

As imaging modalities have improved, ever more subtle aortic injuries are being identified. A classification scheme for severity of aortic injury is demonstrated in Figure 29–4. Using this classification scheme, a minimal aortic injury would be that of a small intimal defect without evidence of intramural hematoma or pseudoaneurysm. This classification system, however, does not differentiate between large pseudoaneurysm versus punctate pseudoaneurysm one or two millimeters in diameter.

Using a definition of minimal aortic injury as an intimal tear of less than one centimeter with no or minimal periaortic hematoma, it is estimated that this type of injury can be present in approximately 10% of patients with blunt aortic injury.[28] Based on evidence that most of these type 1 injuries heal spontaneously, practice guidelines of the Society for Vascular Surgery for traumatic thoracic aortic injury recommend expectant management with serial imaging for this type of lesion.[29] Serial imaging is required as, in one study of minimal aortic injury, 50% of such injuries that were followed up had developed pseudoaneurysms by eight weeks after injury.[28]

Cases of pseudoaneurysm of just a few millimeters in diameter may pose more of a treatment decision dilemma. Technically these would be type 3 severity lesions and endovascular repair recommended. It is our practice to weigh in the overall status of the patient and, in particular, the anatomic complexity that would go along with repair. In situations where patients would be good candidates from an anatomic standpoint and the chances of success high, we typically will perform endograft repair. In cases where the anatomy is more unfavorable and carries a higher risk for technical failure, observation and serial imaging are recommended.

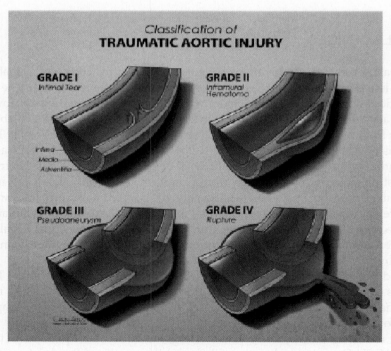

Figure 29-4. Classification system for traumatic aortic injury. From: Azizzadeh A, et al. J Vasc Surg 2009;49: 1403–8

MID-TERM RESULTS

The relatively recent more widespread adoption of endovascular repair for blunt aortic injury makes long-term performance data at this point unavailable. This may also be in part due to the well recognized difficulties with long term follow up of trauma patients. However, some reports of mid-term results are available. McPhee et al. reported no evidence of endoleak or stent graft migration following endograft repair of aortic injury in five patients after a mean follow-up of 16.6 months.[30] Canaud et al. reported a series of 27 patients with a remarkable 100% follow-up rate. After a median follow-up of 40 months, they observed no case of endograft migration or perigraft leak.[31] In our experience there have been no case of endograft failure in the mid and long term in 35 patients.[12] Our longest follow-up patient is now six years status post repair with stacked Gore aortic cuffs and is doing well without evidence of leak or migration.

Understandably, one of the concerns raised about endograft repair for traumatic aortic injury is the unknown changes that may occur in the aorta over time. Concerns have been raised regarding potential dilatation of the aorta with aging, which theoretically could lead to graft migration. The study of Siegenthaler et al. followed aortic growth in the aorta of piglets having undergone endograft stent placement in the proximal descending thoracic aorta. They observed that while the aorta proximal and distal to the stented segment grew in diameter, the segment that underwent stenting did not. There was also evidence of intimal hyperplasia and focal fibrosis in the inner media adjacent to the stent.[32] These findings suggest that thoracic endovascular stent grafting may inhibit aortic dilatation, and that endograft migration may not be a significant concern, even in the long term.

AVAILABLE DEVICES

Over the past several years, alterations have been made in the currently available devices to address issues related to graft size and conformability in the aortic arch. The first available thoracic endograft in the United States was the Gore TAG graft, first approved for use in thoracic aortic aneurysms and available in 2004. Currently this graft is available in diameter ranges from 26mm to 45mm and sheath sizes ranges from 20 to 24 French. The advantages of this device include the potential to allow sheathless delivery if necessary from an access standpoint and the relative simplicity of deployment. Disadvantages include that the smallest diameter is 26mm, which would result in significant over-sizing in a significant percentage of trauma patients. Additionally, the covered flares proximal and distal to the graft create encroachment of fabric several millimeters proximal to the initial seal zone. This can become a particular issue if the graft needed to be deployed just distal to the origin of the left common carotid artery. Additionally, this graft may be more prone to device collapse; however, this has not been borne out in any specific study.

To address these issues, a more conformable version of the Gore TAG graft (C-TAG) is currently in trials. This newer graft addresses some of the issues mentioned above by having a wider range of diameters available. The graft is also designed to be more conformable to the aortic arch, and the flares proximally and distally have been essentially removed. At the time of this writing, the initial set of patients in the trauma arm of the C-TAG study has been enrolled, and the results of this study will be forthcoming.

The Zenith TX2 thoracic endograft developed by Cook, Incorporated, is also available. Currently available sizes range from 28mm to 42mm in diameter, with introducer sheaths ranging from an outer diameter of 22 to 24 French. The current version of this graft includes the Pro-Form design, which allows the proximal-most stent to remain constrained until the remainder of the graft is deployed. This allows the proximal stent to conform to the angle of the aortic arch and is deployed last. The authors have found in selected patients that this Pro-Form design has allowed very accurate placement and excellent apposition to the aortic wall. Disadvantages include a minimal diameter of 28mm, which would create over-sizing in a significant portion of trauma patients. Additionally, the length of the individual stent components may limit where this device can be placed in tortuous anatomy.

The Talent thoracic stent graft comes in a range of diameters from 22mm to 46mm. This represents the widest range of currently available thoracic aortic graft diameters. The current version of the graft includes the Captivia delivery system, which allows the proximal springs to be constrained until the remainder of the graft is delivered. This allows the proximal portion of the graft to conform to the angulated aorta. At the time of this writing, there are registries involving trauma patients treated with the Talent thoracic graft, the results of which should be forthcoming.

There is little question that endograft repair has been the most dramatic recent advancement in the treatment of traumatic aortic injury with strikingly lower rates of patient death or permanent disability due to spinal; cord ischemia.[33] At present however, it appears that these significant improvements in early outcomes may be accompanied by an increased rate of device failure. Our experience with analysis of aortic arch configuration suggests that the incidence of device failure can be reduced with more rigorous case selection and beyond that, innovations in device engineering will provide more graft size variability and grafts that can more easily conform to the sharply angulated small aorta. The long-term durability and natural history of thoracic endograft devices remain unknown at present. We recommend continued regular follow-up, although this can be difficult in a young population of patients. As noted in the SVS clinical practice guidelines, the optimal follow-up strategy remains in evolution, considering the concerns of accumulated radiation, iodinated contrast exposure, and late endograft collapse. For now, follow-up most likely should be individualized to the particular patient considering their age, aortic anatomy, and perceived stability of the endograft.[29]

REFERENCES

1. Smith RS, Chang FC. Traumatic rupture of the aorta: still a lethal injury. *Am J Surg* 1986; 152(6):660–3.
2. Greendyke RM. Traumatic rupture of aorta; special reference to automobile accidents. *JAMA* 1966;195(7):527–30.
3. Parmley LF, Mattingly TW, Manion WC, Jahnke EJ, Jr. Nonpenetrating traumatic injury of the aorta. *Circulation* 1958;17(6):1086–101.
4. Semba CP, Kato N, Kee ST, et al. Acute rupture of the descending thoracic aorta: repair with use of endovascular stent-grafts. J *Vasc Interv Radiol* 1997;8(3):337–42.
5. Fabian TC, Richardson JD, Croce MA, et al. Prospective study of blunt aortic injury: Multi-center Trial of the American Association for the Surgery of Trauma. *J Trauma* 1997;42(3): 374–80; discussion 80–3.

6. Demetriades D, Velmahos GC, Scalea TM, et al. Operative repair or endovascular stent graft in blunt traumatic thoracic aortic injuries: results of an American Association for the Surgery of Trauma Multicenter Study. *J Trauma* 2008;64(3):561–70; discussion 70–1.

7. Ott MC, Stewart TC, Lawlor DK, Gray DK, Forbes TL. Management of blunt thoracic aortic injuries: endovascular stents versus open repair. *J Trauma* 2004;56(3):565–70.

8. Midgley PI, Mackenzie KS, Corriveau MM, et al. Blunt thoracic aortic injury: a single institution comparison of open and endovascular management. J *Vasc* Surge 2007;46(4):662–8.

9. Tang GL, Tehrani HY, Usman A, et al. Reduced mortality, paraplegia, and stroke with stent graft repair of blunt aortic transections: a modern meta-analysis. J *Vasc Surg* 2008; 47(3):671–5.

10. Xenos ES, Abedi NN, Davenport DL, et al. Meta-analysis of endovascular vs open repair for traumatic descending thoracic aortic rupture. J *Vasc* Surge 2008;48(5):1343–51.

11. Moainie SL, Neschis DG, Gammie JS, et al. Endovascular stenting for traumatic aortic injury: an emerging new standard of care. *Ann Thorac Surg* 2008;85(5):1625–9; discussion 9–30.

12. Neschis DG, Moainie S, Flinn WR, Scalea TM, Bartlett ST, Griffith BP. Endograft repair of traumatic aortic injury-a technique in evolution: a single institution's experience. *Ann Surg* 2009;250(3):377–82.

13. Fabian TC, Davis KA, Gavant ML, et al. Prospective study of blunt aortic injury: helical CT is diagnostic and antihypertensive therapy reduces rupture. *Ann Surg* 1998;227(5):666–76; discussion 76–7.

14. Azizzadeh A, Valdes J, Miller CC, 3rd, et al. The utility of intravascular ultrasound compared to angiography in the diagnosis of blunt traumatic aortic injury. J *Vasc Surg* 2011; 53(3):608–14.

15. van Prehn J, van Herwaarden JA, Muhs BE, Arnofsky A, Moll FL, Verhagen HJ. Difficulties with endograft sizing in a patient with traumatic rupture of the thoracic aorta: the possible influence of hypovolemic shock. J *Vasc Surg* 2008;47(6):1333–6.

16. Pate JW, Fabian TC, Walker W. Traumatic rupture of the aortic isthmus: an emergency? World journal of surgery 1995;19(1):119–25; discussion 25–6.

17. Tehrani HY, Peterson BG, Katariya K, et al. Endovascular repair of thoracic aortic tears. *Ann Thorac Surg* 2006;82(3):873–7; discussion 7–8.

18. Rosenthal D, Wellons ED, Burkett AB, Kochupura PV, Hancock SM. Endovascular repair of traumatic thoracic aortic disruptions with "stacked" abdominal endograft extension cuffs. J *Vasc Surg* 2008;48(4):841–4.

19. Neschis DG, Moaine S, Gutta R, et al. Twenty consecutive cases of endograft repair of traumatic aortic disruption: lessons learned. *J Vasc Surg* 2007;45(3):487–92.

20. Hoornweg LL, Dinkelman MK, Goslings JC, et al. Endovascular management of traumatic ruptures of the thoracic aorta: a retrospective multicenter analysis of 28 cases in The Netherlands. *J Vasc Surg* 2006;43(6):1096–102; discussion 102.

21. Idu MM, Reekers JA, Balm R, Ponsen KJ, de Mol BA, Legemate DA. Collapse of a stent-graft following treatment of a traumatic thoracic aortic rupture. *J Endovasc Ther* 2005;12(4): 503–7.

22. Steinbauer MG, Stehr A, Pfister K, et al. Endovascular repair of proximal endograft collapse after treatment for thoracic aortic disease. *J Vasc Surg* 2006;43(3):609–12.

23. Shukla AJ, Jeyabalan G, Cho JS. Late collapse of a thoracic endoprosthesis. *J Vasc Surg* 2011;53(3):798–801.

24. Mattison R, Hamilton IN, Jr., Ciraulo DL, Richart CM. Stent-graft repair of acute traumatic thoracic aortic transection with intentional occlusion of the left subclavian artery: case report. *J Trauma* 2001;51(2):326–8.

25. Dorros G, Cohn JM. Adenosine-induced transient cardiac asystole enhances precise deployment of stent-grafts in the thoracic or abdominal aorta. *J Endovasc Surg* 1996;3(3):270–2.

26. Pornratanarangsi S, Webster MW, Alison P, Nand P. Rapid ventricular pacing to lower blood pressure during endograft deployment in the thoracic aorta. *Ann Thorac Surg* 2006; 81(5):e21–3.

27. Brenner DJ, Hall EJ. Computed tomography—an increasing source of radiation exposure. The New England journal of medicine 2007;357(22):2277–84.

28. Malhotra AK, Fabian TC, Croce MA, Weiman DS, Gavant ML, Pate JW. Minimal aortic injury: a lesion associated with advancing diagnostic techniques. *J Trauma* 2001;51(6):1042–8.

29. Lee WA, Matsumura JS, Mitchell RS, et al. Endovascular repair of traumatic thoracic aortic injury: clinical practice guidelines of the Society for Vascular Surgery. *J Vasc Surg* 2011; 53(1):187–92.

30. McPhee JT, Asham EH, Rohrer MJ, et al. The midterm results of stent graft treatment of thoracic aortic injuries. *J Surg Res* 2007;138(2):181–8.

31. Canaud L, Alric P, Branchereau P, Marty-Ane C, Berthet JP. Lessons learned from midterm follow-up of endovascular repair for traumatic rupture of the aortic isthmus. *J Vasc Surg* 2008;47(4):733–8.

32. Siegenthaler MP, Celik R, Haberstroh J, et al. Thoracic endovascular stent grafting inhibits aortic growth: an experimental study. *Eur J Cardiothorac Surg* 2008;34(1):17–24.

33. Neschis DG, Scalea TM, Flinn WR, Griffith BP. Blunt aortic injury. *New Engl J Med* 2008; 359(16):1708–16.

30

Outcomes of Planned Celiac Artery Coverage During TEVAR

Manish Mehta, MD, MPH

INTRODUCTION

It has been over a decade since the introduction of thoracic endovascular aneurysm repair (TEVAR), and today there is ample evidence suggesting early and midterm advantages of this endovascular procedure over the traditional open thoracic aortic reconstruction in anatomical suitable patients.[1–3] Anatomically suitability during TEVAR implies that patients with descending thoracic aortic aneurysms (TAA) have adequate proximal and distal thoracic stent graft landing zones which according to "instructions for use" of thoracic stent grafts would include a 2 cm aneurysm free normal thoracic aorta distal to the left common carotid artery, and similarly a 2 cm aneurysm free normal thoracic aorta proximal to the celiac artery. Although extensions of the proximal thoracic stent graft landing zones that include coverage of the left subclavian artery with or without extra-anatomic left carotid-subclavian bypass, or even the left carotid artery coverage with extra-anatomic right to left carotid-carotid and left carotid-subclavian bypass have been considered relatively safe, other extra-anatomic visceral reconstructions that include celiac/superior mesenteric bypass or 'debranching' to extend the distal landing zones have been associated with significant morbidity and mortality.[4]

The importance of collateralization through the visceral arterial tree has been well understood, and it is rare for symptoms of visceral/intestinal ischemia to develop with stenosis or even occlusion of one of the mesenteric arteries.[5] There are several important collateral pathways between the celiac and the superior mesenteric artery that supply blood flow to the abdominal viscera, and when either of these 2 arteries is narrowed or occluded the collateral pathways across the pancreaticoduodenal arteries become vital. With critical stenosis or occlusion of the celiac artery, blood flow to the liver, spleen, stomach, and duodenum proceeds from the superior mesenteric artery (SMA) to the pancreaticoduodenal collaterals to the hepatic artery. Furthermore, the incidence of a replaced right hepatic artery that originates from the SMA is 15–20%, which helps provide collateral blood flow between the two visceral arteries.[6] When dealing with TAA, in the 'real world" clinical scenarios, patients sometimes present with extensive aneurysmal involvement that extends up to the distal thoracic aorta, precluding an adequate distal stent graft landing zone, and coverage of the celiac artery to facilitate adequate stent graft fixation and seal is necessary. Visceral artery revascularizations during TEVAR are complex procedures and their associated morbidity and mortality. In light of the complexity of visceral revascularization in TAA patients, and the fact that the celiac and the SMA have a rich collateral network has set the stage for us to evaluate the feasibility and efficacy of celiac artery coverage without revascularization during TEVAR. We report our experience of planned celiac artery coverage during endovascular repair of complex TAA.

THE VASCULAR INSTITUTE FOR HEALTH & DISEASE, ALBANY MEDICAL CENTER EXPERIENCE

Methods

Since 2004, 228 patients underwent TEVAR for treatment of lesions in the thoracic aorta. Early in our experience, TEVAR was preformed for patients with distal stent graft landing zone of at least 2 cm, in accordance with the "indications for use" of the FDA approved and commercially available thoracic stent grafts. As our experience evolved and we were faced with patients with complex TAA that extended up to the celiac artery, we were forced to evaluate the outcomes of celiac artery coverage during TEVAR in treating these high risk patients.

Patients with inadequate distal stent graft landing zones above the celiac artery underwent a detailed evaluation of the gastroduodenal collateral circulation between the SMA and the celiac artery by CTA. When CTA was non-demonstrable for well developed gastroduodenal collaterals or failed to indicate an aberrant replaced right hepatic artery originating from the SMA, pre-operative and/or intra-operative selective arteriogram was performed to further delineate the existence of these collaterals. The arteriogram was obtained in the anterior-posterior as well as lateral projections, and when selective catheterization failed to indicate gastroduodenal-pancreaticoduodenal collaterals, temporary celiac artery occlusion with a 5–6mm balloon was obtained prior to superior mesenteric arteriogram.

TEVAR procedures were performed using general or spinal anesthesia using TAG thoracic stent graft (WL Gore & Associates, Flagstaff, AZ), or Talent thoracic stent graft (Medtronic Ave., Santa Rosa, CA). Cerebral spinal fluid (CSF) drainage was used selectively, and in general reserved for patients with prior abdominal aortic reconstructions via open surgical or endovascular means, or in patients that required extensive coverage of the thoracic aorta during TEVAR. The sequence of placement of the thoracic stent grafts, be it proximal to distal or vice versa, was up to the discretion of the vascular surgeon. Patients with celiac artery stent graft coverage that presented with critical SMA stenosis or when further lengthening of the distal thoracic stent graft landing zone was needed to obtain and adequate seal and the SMA was partly covered with the stent graft, access into the SMA was obtained via a 6 Fr. Guide sheath or a 4–5 mm balloon catheter prior to stent graft deployment and subsequently a balloon expandable stent was routinely deployed in the proximal SMA to maintain patency.

At the completion of TEVAR, patient assessment included an arteriogram to identify distal stent graft seal, with careful evaluation for the presence of distal type Ib endoleak, or type II endoleak via retrograde flow into the TAA from the celiac artery. During the postoperative period clinical parameters suggesting presence of visceral ischemia or malperfusion were evaluated, including the development of lactic acidosis, leukocytosis, fever, and abdominal pain. Postoperative follow-up included routine clinical evaluation at 1 month and every 6 months thereafter, and initial CTA at 1 month, 6 month, 12 month, and yearly thereafter. During follow-up, any endoleaks noted at the distal thoracic aortic stent graft attachment site were treated by coil embolization procedures. Via a transfemoral approach, a guide catheter was traversed across the distal stent graft attachment site in between the stent graft and thoracic aortic wall. The catheter was advanced into the distal thoracic aortic aneurysm and coils were placed in proximity to the celiac artery, or the site of the endoleak channel. All data was prospectively collected in a vascular registry and Institutional Review Board approval was obtained for evaluation of all patient outcomes data.

Results

Patients considered high risk for open surgical thoracoabdominal aortic reconstructions were considered for TEVAR with coverage of celiac artery to achieve a seal at the distal stent graft landing zone. Over a 5 year period, 31 (14%) of 228 patients with TEVAR required celiac artery stent graft coverage, and 12 (39%) of these 31 patients required additional partial coverage of the SMA. All 12 patients with complete celiac artery coverage and partial SMA coverage underwent balloon expandable stent placement in the SMA.

The demographics and operative findings are listed in Table 30–1; majority of patient were females (65%), the mean age was 74 years (range 55–87 years), the mean TAA size was 6.5 cm, and the mean estimated blood loss was 379 cc. During the postoperative period, on postoperative day 1 complications of visceral ischemia developed in 2 patients (6%); one patient developed shock liver and required emergent right renal to hepatic artery revascularization, and died. A second patient developed acalculus cholecystitis and underwent a successful open surgical cholecystectomy. One other patient developed ischemic colitis affecting the sigmoid colon; at the time of sigmoid resection, the stomach, small bowel, and the proximal colon were not ischemic. Two (6%) patients developed paraplegia; one had a prior infrarenal abdominal aortic aneurysm repair 3 years prior to the TEVAR. The 30-day operative mortality was 6%; one patient died with complications of visceral ischemia, and the second patient suffered complications of myocardial infarction (Table 30–2).

TABLE 30–1. PATIENT DEMOGRAPHICS

TEVAR with celiac artery coverage	31
Male/Female	11 (35%), 20 (65%)
Mean age	74.2 years
Mean TAA size	6.5 cm
Coronary artery disease	18 (58%)
Hypertension	28 (90%)
Chronic obstructive pulmonary disease	12 (39%)
Pre-existing renal failure (dialysis)	4 (12%)
Mean estimated blood loss	379 cc

TABLE 30-2. COMPLICATIONS IN TEVAR PATIENTS WITH CELIAC COVERAGE

TEVAR with celiac artery coverage	31	Outcome
Visceral ischemia	2 (6%)	
– Shock liver	1 (3%)	Death
– Acalculus cholecystitis	1 (3%)	Cholecystectomy
Paraplegia	2 (6%)	1 Death
30-day mortality	2 (6%)	
Type 1b endoleak @ distal attachment site	2 (6%)	Coil embolization
Type II endoleak: Celiac artery retrograde flow	3 (10%)	Coil embolization

During the postoperative follow-up, endoleaks were noted on CTA evaluations in 9 (29%) patients, 4 (13%) patients had type II endoleaks from intercostal arteries, 3 (10%) patients had a type II endoleak vial retrograde flow from the celiac artery, and w(6%0 patient had a type Ib endoleak from distal stent graft attachment site. All 5 (16%) patient with endoleaks from retrograde flow via the celiac artery or from the distal stent graft attachment site were treated successfully by coil embolization. The embolization procedure was performed via a transfemoral approach, and an angled/directional catheter was directed between the stent graft and the aortic wall and used to access the aneurysm sac. The catheter was placed in proximity of the celiac artery and/or the endoleak channel and coils were selectively placed. At a mean follow-up of 15 months, 2 (6%) patients with stent graft migration from distal attachment site required additional stent graft extensions. Over a mean follow-up of 15 months, there have been no other complications of mesenteric ischemia, spinal cord ischemia, SMA in-stent stenosis, or conversion to open surgical repair.

Discussion

TEVAR has evolved to become a viable option for treatment for aortic lesions that affect the descending thoracic aorta. When thoracic aneurysms are extensive and expand beyond the limitations of currently available thoracic endoprosthesis, surgeons and interventionalists are often forced to make improvements that are technically and technologically driven to facilitate repair of these complex and extensive aneurysms that if untreated or treated by surgical reconstruction are associated with a significant morbidity and mortality.[7,8] In evaluating our single center experience of 31 TEVAR patients with intentional celiac artery coverage, the findings suggest that the incidence of complication of visceral ischemia in these patients is 6%, and the incidence of death with associated visceral ischemia is 3%. In considering the alternative of treating these patients with surgical visceral artery debranching, the morbidity and mortality of intentional celiac artery coverage during TEVAR in patients that on CTA and/or arteriography have demonstrated the presence of visceral collateral pathways between the celiac and the SMA would seem acceptable.

Although our experience of intentional celiac artery coverage to facilitate distal stent graft seal zone during TEVAR is the largest to-date, several other centers have published data with comparable results.[9–11] Their findings also suggest the feasibility and short term efficacy of celiac artery stent graft coverage to facilitate TEVAR with a caveat that selective celiac and SMA arteriography alone might not readily predict the complications of visceral ischemia.

When planning TEVAR for complex thoracic aortic aneurysms that have limited distal supraceliac stent graft landing zone, several recommendations can be made based on the currently available data, these include:

1. A thorough evaluation of the celiac and SMA collaterals via CTA and/or arteriography should be considered essential prior to planning TEVAR and celiac artery coverage. Studies evaluating CTA and standard arteriography have indicated that accuracy of CTA for depicting visceral arterial anatomy and identifying branches of the gastroduodenal and pancreaticoduodenal arteries that are the collateral communications between the celiac and the SMA is >90%.[12] When CTA fails to demonstrate well developed visceral collaterals between the celiac and the SMA, selective arteriogram is necessary and often requires temporary occlusion of the celiac artery with a 5 to 6mm balloon catheter prior to selective superior mesenteric arteriography to assess the visceral collaterals.

2. Placement of cerebral spinal fluid (CSF) drainage catheters should be considered in these patients since these procedures require significant coverage of the thoracic aorta, and the distal extent of the stent grafts usually extends to the T12-L1 level which could potentially also cover the artery of Adamkiewicz.[13,14] Although the etiology for developing complications of spinal cord ischemia (SCI) during TEVAR are multifactorial and not necessarily just related to coverage of the artery of Adamkiewicz, significant coverage of the thoracic aorta during TEVAR does increase the risk for developing SCI and should be evaluated during these procedures.

3. Co-existing occlusive disease in the SMA should be evaluated via angiography prior to stent graft deployment. Instance when celiac artery coverage with stent graft is needed and the presence of severe SMA occlusive disease is identified, even when asymptomatic, placement of a balloon expandable stent in the SMA should be considered. Theoretically this could help prevent mesenteric/visceral ischemia that might otherwise develop in patients as their abdominal organs rely on the SMA with critical stenosis as the sole blood supply. In our experience, 39% of the patients with celiac artery coverage had either co-existing severe SMA occlusive disease or partial stent graft coverage of the SMA, and underwent balloon expandable stent placement to maintain patency of the SMA. We have no comparative data to evaluate what might the outcomes have been if the SMA did not undergo stent placement, however since none of these patients have developed symptoms of visceral ischemia, we have continued to employ this strategy when managing these complex TAAs.

4. Preoperative evaluation of patient for the presence of symptoms of chronic mesenteric ischemia, as subtle as they might be, should be thoroughly evaluated prior to embarking on these procedures. Furthermore, during the postoperative period, signs and symptoms of mesenteric ischemia should be carefully evaluated by subjective clinical examinations, as well as objective data such as assessment of leukocytosis, lactic acidosis, elevation of amylase/lipase, and liver function tests. Finally, patients that develop signs and/or symptoms of visceral ischemia should undergo prompt visceral revascularization.

5. Finally, CTA alone might be inadequate in differentiating between a type Ib endoleak (inadequate distal stent graft seal) and a type II endoleak (persistent retrograde celiac artery flow into the TAA), and selective transfemoral angiography if often needed to differentiate between the endoleak types. In such instance,

when postoperative CTA suggests an endoleak in proximity to the distal stent graft attachment site, selective SMA catheterization and arteriogram with anterior-posterior and lateral imaging can be used to identify type II endoleak via retrograde flow from the celiac artery. For treatment of these endoleaks, an embolization procedure can be performed via a transfemoral approach. An angled/ directional catheter is directed between the stent graft and the aortic wall and used to access the aneurysm sac. The catheter is placed in proximity to the celiac artery and/or the endoleak channel and appropriately sized coils are selectively deployed. If a persistent type II endoleak from celiac artery is suspected prior to TEVAR, selective coil embolization of the celiac artery can be performed prior to or during TEVAR.

In conclusion, TEVAR has become an acceptable means for managing patients with TAA and is generally considered to be associated with less morbidity and mortality when compared to open surgical repair of complex thoracic aortic aneurysms. Our initial experience of 31 patients with celiac artery coverage during TEVAR suggests an acceptably low incidence of visceral ischemic complication in select patients with demonstrable pancreaticoduodenal and gastroduodenal arterial collaterals between the celiac and SMA. We believe preoperative CTA and selective visceral angiography area complementary in identifying visceral collateral circulation and should be thoroughly evaluated until we fully recognize the strengths and limitations of these procedures in predicting visceral ischemia. Patients with planned celiac artery stent graft coverage that have preexisting severe SMA stenosis should be considered for SMA stent placement at the time of TEVAR to optimize visceral collateral circulation. Finally, although these results are promising, currently available data only suggests that celiac artery coverage to facilitate lengthening the distal stent graft seal zone is feasible with limited morbidity and mortality in select patients, and its ling term efficacy remains to be evaluated.

REFERENCES

1. Dake MD, Miller DC, Semba CP, Mitchell RS, et al. Transluminal placement of endovascular stent-grafts for the treatment of descending thoracic aortic aneurysms. *N Engl J Med* 1994; 331:1729–34.
2. Leurs LJ, Bell R, Degrieck Y, et al. Endovascular treatment of thoracic aortic disease: Combined experience from the EUROSTAR and United Kingdom Thoracic Endograft registries. *J Vasc Surg* 2004;40:670–9; discussion 679–80.
3. Makaroun MS, Dillavou ED, Wheatly GH, et al. Five-year results of endovascular treatment with Gore TAG device compared with open repair of thoracic aortic aneurysms. *J Vasc Surg* 2008 May; 47(5):912–18.
4. Murphy ED, Beck AW, Clagget GP et al. combined aortic debranching and thoracic endovascular aneurysm repair (TEVAR) effective but at a cost. *Arch Surg* 2009 Mar;144(3): 22–7.
5. Valentine RJ, Martin JD, Myers SI, et al. Asymptomatic celiac and superior mesenteric artery stenosis are more prevalent among patients with unsuspected renal stenosis. *J Vasc Surg* 14:195, 1991.
6. Olofsson PA, Connelly DP, Stoney RJ: Surgery of the celiac and mesenteric arteries. In Maimovici H (ed): *Vascular Surgery: Principles and Techniques.* Norwalk, Conn, Appleton Lange, 1989, p750.
7. Bakaeen FG, Chu D, Huh J, et al. Contemporary outcomes of open thoracic aortic surgery in a veteran population: do risk models exaggerate mortality. *Am J Surg* 2009 Dec;198(6): 889–94.

8. Patel R, Cairad MF, Paruchuri V, et al. Thoracoabdominal aneurysm repair: hybrid versus open repair. *J Vasc Surg* 2009 Jul;50(1)15–22.
9. Leon LR, Mills JL, Jordan W, et al. The risks of celiac artery coverage during endoluminal repair of thoracic and thoracoabdominal aortic aneurysms. *Vasc Endovascular Surg* 2009 Feb-Mar;43(1):51–60.
10. Belenky A, Haddan M, Idov I, et al. Celiac trunk embolization as a means of elongating descending thoracic aortic aneurysm neck prior to endovascular aortic repair. *Cardiovasc Intervent Radiol* (2009) 32:923–27.
11. Vaddineni SK, Taylor SM, Patterson MA et al. Outcomes after celiac artery coverage during endovascular thoracic aortic aneurysm repair: Preliminary results. *J Vasc Surg* 2007;45: 467–71.
12. Savastano S, Teso S, Corra S, et al. Multislice CT angiography of the celiac and superior mesenteric arteries: Comparison with arteriographic findings. *Radiol Med.* 2002 may-Jun: 103(5–6):456–63.
13. Lazorthes G: Arterial vascularization of the spinal cord. *J Neurosurg* 1971;35;253–262.
14. Freezor RJ, Martin TD, Hess PJJr, et al. Intent of aortic coverage and incidence of spinal cord ischemia after thoracic endovascular aneurysm repair. *Ann Thorac Surg* 2008 Dec;86(6): 1809–14.

Complex Venous Problems

31

Iliofemoral Venous Stenting

Sean P. Lyden, MD

INTRODUCTION

Chronic venous insufficiency describes a condition that affects the venous system of the lower extremities caused by venous hypertension producing limb pain, swelling, edema, skin changes, and ulcerations. Risk factors found to be associated with CVI include age, sex, a family history of varicose veins, obesity, pregnancy, phlebitis, and previous leg injury.[1,2] Venous outflow obstruction appears to play a more significant role in the pathogenesis of CVI and its clinical expression than previously appreciated.[3] Venous outflow obstruction can lead to venous valvular insufficiency, ambulatory venous hypertension and chronic venous insufficiency. Some common etiologies of iliofemoral venous outflow obstruction include deep venous thrombosis (DVT), May-Thurner syndrome, extrinsic compression from abdominal and pelvic tumors and radiation induced injury. Regardless of the etiology, therapy of iliofemoral deep venous stenoses and occlusions can be beneficial to the patient when successful.

Iliofemoral thrombosis is a common cause of venous outflow obstruction. Thrombolysis for this problem has been practiced by interventionalists for well over two decades and been shown to restore valvular function eliminating venous reflux when successful.[5] This therapy improves outcomes and reduces the long term incidence of chronic venous insufficiency.[4] This fact has been reinforced by the recent acknowledgement of catheter directed thrombolytic treatment of acute (<14 days) iliofemoral deep venous thrombosis as beneficial to reduce acute symptoms and post thrombotic morbidity by the 2008 Chest guidelines (Class 2B recommendation).[5] This change in the Chest guidelines has raised awareness of the usefulness of catheter directed thrombolysis and eventual iliofemoral venous stenting among primary care physicians.

The thrombotic disorders center on disturbances of Virchow's Triad, which includes endothelial injury, hypercoagulability and circulatory stasis. In patients with acute iliofemoral DVT and an associated risk factor, there should be no need to evaluate for a hypercoagulable state. In the absence of an identifiable risk factor for DVT or anatomic etiology, blood work to evaluate for a coagulation defect is important in determining the length of time needed to treat with anticoagulation after successful clot removal.

325

TREATMENT TECHNIQUE FOR PATIENTS WITH ACUTE ILIOFEMORAL DVT

For iliofemoral venous occlusions due to fresh (<1 month old) thrombus, the use of thrombolysis can allow dissolution of thrombus and allow successful endovascular treatment. In treating patients, the first thing to decide is the site of access. Preoperative duplex imaging is imperative to identify the level and extent of acute thrombosis. Access below the level of thrombosis will lead to improved outcomes. Typically this will mean combined tibial and popliteal access from a prone position in most patients who present with severe clot burden of the entire iliac and femoral system. The use of tibial access at the ankle will improve resolution of the popliteal clot and will improve flow through the femoral veins decreasing acute rethrombosis risk and hopefully increasing long term patency. When inferior vena cava clot is present, bilateral simultaneous access to the iliofemoral and cava segment should be used to establish good flow into the cava from both sides. After dissolution of clot, endovascular treatment with stenting of residual disease should be performed.

For the patients without femoral thrombus burden a supine femoral approach can be used. In the occasional patient where the clot cannot be crossed from an infrainguinal approach, a jugular or arm approach may be successful. The difficulty in approaching the disease from above is that once the femoral level is reached, remaining competent valves if present can make crossing more difficult.

Pharmacological thrombolysis is traditionally infused through catheters and infusion wires which have multiple side holes to diffuse the agent over a large area. Single level, dual level (or more) infusions are performed with the goal of bathing the entire clot in plasminogen activator. Concomitant low dose heparin (500 units per hour) is typically infused through the access sheath to prevent thrombosis around the sheath. Larger doses of heparin were previously used in order to obtain systemic anticoagulation, but this has been suggested to increase the risk of hemorrhage.

MECHANISM OF ACTION OF PLASMINOGEN ACTIVATORS

All pharmacologic thrombolytic agents (streptokinase, urokinase, tPA, and rPA) work through plasmin mediated fibrin dependent mechanisms. They are all forms of plasminogen activators and none of the agents directly degrade fibrin. All of the agents convert plasminogen to plasmin, which subsequently degrades fibrin. All of the drugs have varying degrees of fibrin specificity (or the ability to distinguish between circulating and bound plasminogen). Higher fibrin specificity was hoped to lower systemic bleeding complications, however, large trials have shown no difference in bleeding rates.

LIMITATIONS OF PLASMINOGEN ACTIVATORS

Many limitations exist for use of urokinase, tPA, and rPA for thrombolysis. The current thrombolytic agents have needed a mean duration of >24 hours to achieve flow in both the STILE and TOPAS trial for arterial lesions.[6,7] Typically longer infusion times are needed to treat venous clot than arterial clot, which most likely is due to the lower flow rates seen in the venous circulation. Clots rich with plasminogen activator inhibitor 1 (PAI-1) or platelet-rich clots may be resistant to thrombolysis. Finally, even with localized delivery of drug, systemic circulation of the drug occurs which can create a systemic "lytic state" from the resulting hypofibrinogenemia. Low fibrinogen levels have been associated with an increased risk of hemorrhage. In fact, 5 to 16% of patients treated with pharmacologic thrombolysis experience major hemorrhage and a 1–2% incidence of intracranial hemorrhage. Besides intracranial bleeding, retroperitoneal, gastrointestinal, and catheter entry site bleeding can occur. This has been the Achilles heel of currently available agents. The need to overcome this problem has spurred the development of mechanical thrombectomy devices.

MECHANICAL THROMBECTOMY

In order to expand treatment and to address concerns regarding the time needed for dissolution of thrombus by pharmacologic means, and to diminish the amount of pharmacologic agent used mechanical thrombectomy devices have been developed and marketed over the past decade. The vast majority of mechanical thrombectomy devices now work by active aspiration based on the Venturi effect.[8] The Angiojet device (Medrad Minneapolis, MN) has been arguably the most successful and commonly used device in current practice. Saline jets injected within the device tip create a Venturi effect that removes thrombus. Use of the AngioJet device close to the heart uncommonly results in bradyarrhythmias of uncertain etiology.[9] Large particulate debris and well organized emboli are still problematic for most devices, and embolization can occur with all mechanical thrombectomy devices.[10,11]

The Trellis device (Bacchus Vascular, Santa Clara, CA) is unique in that it attempts to limit the delivery of thrombolytic agent to a controlled area coupled with mechanical fragmentation. The device contains a proximal and distal occlusion balloon to localize delivery of pharmacologic agents. A dispersion wire is driven by a motor unit which fragments the clot. After the clot is dissolved, the proximal balloon is deflated to allow aspiration.

ULTRASOUND ENHANCED THROMBOLYSIS

One of the newest ideas being marketed is the use of sound waves to speed thrombolysis. Low frequency ultrasound has been shown to mechanically fragment clots and to augment enzymatic fibrinolysis.[12–14] Several devices have been developed to try to increase the efficacy of clot dissolution using these principles. The EKOS Ekosonic Mach 4e (Ekos, Bothel, WA) device delivers sound waves to the clot in the hopes of accelerating the speed and completeness of thrombolysis. The system generates ultrasound waves in the treatment zone of the catheter through the piezoelectric conversion of radiofrequency energy. The ultrasound emanates radially from the treatment zone to improve the dispersion of infused physician-specified fluids. To date no randomized trial has been completed to support its use or efficacy. Once the acute clot burden is eliminated by either pharmacologic or mechanical means treatment of the underlying etiology of the occlusion can occur.

CHRONIC TOTAL OCCLUSIONS

In the absence of acute thrombosis, chronic total occlusions (CTO) are treated by crossing followed by direct stenting. Ipsilateral and contralateral femoral and popliteal, internal jugular and brachial venous access routes can all be used successfully to cross iliofemoral and caval occlusions. The most commonly used technique to cross a CTO is spinning a hydrophilic guide wire with catheter or balloon support. Use of braided catheters and dedicated crossing catheters (e.g. Quick-Cross Spectranetics, Colorado Springs, CO) has diminished the need for using angioplasty balloons for support. Due to the lack of calcification, subintimal re-entry tends to be easier for venous disease than arterial occlusions.

ILIOFEMORAL STENTING

Identification of the etiology and site of the occlusion may be done in many instances by venography. (Figure 31–1 A and B) However it can be difficult from direct venographic imaging. The presence of residual collateral vessels is a hallmark of residual obstruction and should prompt more studies to identify the location and allow treatment. Imaging in other orientations such as steep right anterior and left anterior oblique angles may show the area of residual stenosis. When the area has not been identified further investigation with other modalities is mandatory. Simple pull back pressure measurements may identify the level of residual disease. The drop in pressure across the area of disease will typically be much smaller than that found for arterial disease due to the low pressure in the venous system.[15]

INTRAVASCULAR ULTRASOUND

Intravascular ultrasonography (IVUS) is probably the best modality to identify residual disease and ensure correction of the problem. In patients with May-Thurner syndrome, the crossing artery can be clearly identified as well as the normal venous diameter proximal to

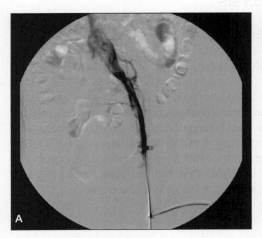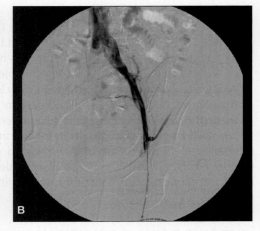

Figure 31–1. a/b. Venogram of patient with chronic left iliofemoral DVT from May-Thurner Syndrome found on CT venogram. The area of the origin of the occlusion is difficult to ascertain and was confirmed by intravascular ultrasound. Dilated collateral vessels draining the left iliac system are noted.

the problem. In the area of occlusion in May-Thurner, chronic webs may also be seen. Intravascular ultrasound can be used to size the reference vessel to ensure a correctly sized stent is chosen. This technique will also allow completion imaging to make sure that the entire area of concern has been treated. Neglen documented the importance of IVUS in chronic iliac venous occlusive disease of the pelvis when he compared assessment with IVUS against transfemoral venography in 304 consecutive limbs. He noted that with IVUS, fine intraluminal and mural details were detected (e.g., trabeculation, frozen valves, mural thickness, and outside compression) that were not seen with venography. The median stenosis (with diameter reduction) on venographic results was 50% vs. IVUS where it was 80%. The actual stenotic area was more severe when measured directly with IVUS. No preoperative or intraoperative pressure test adequately measured the hemodynamic significance of the stenosis. When collaterals were present he noted a more severe stenosis was observed.[16]

Self-expanding stents remain the mainstay of treatment for iliofemoral venous occlusions. Due to the thin wall of veins and increased elastic recoil, angioplasty alone is seldom sufficient treatment. Self-expanding nitinol stents have accuracy in placement, flexibility, and crush resistance; all of which are important characteristics for stents in the venous system. Stents are typically oversized 1mm larger than the reference vessel they are intended to treat. Nitinol stents do not come larger than 14mm in the United States, thus for larger diameter vessels usage of the Wallstent (Boston Scientific, Natick, MA) and Gianturco Z stent (Cook, Bloomington, IN) have predominated.[17] I use tend to use Wallstents for larger diameter vena cava and iliac vein lesions. Self-expanding stents may be post dilated after placement. Imaging with either venography should show expansion of the stent with loss of collateral filling. If distal collaterals still fill, further interrogation should be done to identify and treat the unidentified residual stenosis (Figure 31–2 and 31–3) Durable results can be expected with adequate treatment of the occlusive process. (Figure 31–4)

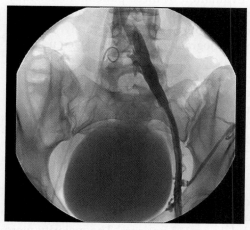

Figure 31–2. Improved common iliac vein after self-expanding stent. Note the persistent dilated distal collaterals originating still off the femoral vein suggesting residual stenosis.

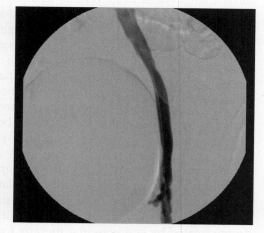

Figure 31–3. Resolution of collateral filling after stenting into the left external iliac vein

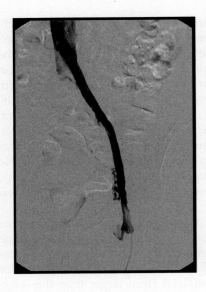

Figure 31–4. Continued patency of the iliofemoral stent of same patient with May-Thurner syndrome at 13 month venographic follow up.

TREATMENT OUTCOMES

May-Thurner

May-Thurner syndrome is used to describe anatomic compression of the left iliac vein.[18] The left common iliac vein is usually located posterior to the right iliac artery and can be compressed between the artery and the fifth lumbar vertebrae. Compression from the left common iliac and internal iliac artery can also occur as the etiology.[19,20] Compression of the right iliac vein from the left common iliac artery has also been documented.[21] Symptoms from this compression can include left lower extremity edema, pain, varicosities, venous stasis changes, and deep venous thrombosis. Evaluation of these patients historically included a venous duplex scan to rule out deep venous thrombosis and an abdominal computed tomography (CT) scan to rule out pelvic mass followed by venography. Contrast enhanced CT venography and magnetic resonance venography have both proven useful as a sole diagnostic test for this condition.[22,23]

One study, noted outcomes for ten patients treated with urokinase thrombolysis and Wallstents for May-Thurner syndrome. Patients received thrombolysis for an average of 52 hours, clearly longer than for most arterial problems. One patient with a concomitant hypercoagulable state rethrombosed at one month and was retreated with thrombolysis and one patient had an asymptomatic reocclusion found at 36 month follow up.[24] Another retrospective study of 39 patients with May-Thurner found all patients presented with leg pain or edema. Over half (20) presented with chronic symptoms and were treated with angioplasty and stent alone. The overall patency rate at 1 year was 79% with 85% of patients symptoms completely or partially improved.[25]

A review of six studies containing at least five patients with May-Thurner syndrome treated by endovascular therapy found data on 113 patients. The majority were females (72%) presenting with DVT (77%), most of which was acute in onset (73%). Therapy consisted of catheter-directed thrombolysis and subsequent stent placement in the majority of patients, resulting in a mean technical success of 95% and a mean 1-year patency of 96%.[26]

Iliofemoral Thrombolysis and Stenting

Semba and colleagues reported on thrombolytic therapy followed by angioplasty and stenting of 21 patients with iliofemoral DVT almost twenty years ago with a technical and clinical success rate of 85%.[27] Another early study reported outcomes of stents for 59 stenoses and occlusions of the vena cava and iliofemoral veins from 1996 for pelvic malignancy, trauma, surgery, or pregnancy; and idiopathic stenoses. Patients underwent anticoagulation therapy for 3-6 months after stent placement. Overall primary and secondary 1-year patency rates were 50% and 81%, respectively. Primary and secondary 4-year patency rates were and 50% and 75%, respectively. Notably, one-year secondary patency rates were statistically significantly lower (P = .05) for patients with malignant disease.[28]

Follow up was also documented in a study by Bjarnason, who treated 87 limbs with a technical success rate of 86% for iliac veins and 63% for femoral veins. The primary and secondary patency rates at 1 year were 63% and 78%, respectively, for the iliac veins, and 40% and 51%, respectively, for the femoral veins. They importantly noted the technical success rates were lower in patients who had had symptoms for more than 4 weeks compared to those who had a more recent onset of symptoms.[29]

Mewissen reported a registry of patients with symptomatic lower limb DVT. Iliofemoral DVT was present in 71% and femoral-popliteal DVT in 25%. They used urokinase infusions (mean, 7.8 million i.u.) for a mean of 53.4 hours. This study again reinforces the finding of the longer infusion times than for arterial lesions. After thrombolysis, about half of the iliac lesions were treated with stents. Complete lysis was achieved in 31% infusions; 50%-99% lysis in 52% and <50% lysis in 17%. Complete lysis occurred in 34% of cases of acute thrombosis whereas only 19% of cases of chronic DVT (P < .01). At 1 year, the primary patency rate was 60%. Major bleeding complications occurred in 11% most often at the puncture site, with 1% developing pulmonary emboli.[30] With very low risk of pulmonary embolism, most authors have continued to not use prophylactic inferior vena cava filters either permanent or temporary when treating patients with iliofemoral thrombosis.

With the removal of urokinase from the US market, most investigators began to gain experience with tPA for thrombolysis. Verhaeghe and colleagues noted 24 consecutive patients with acute iliofemoral DVT underwent infusion of alteplase at 3 mg/hour.[31] As time has continued we have found that significantly lower dosages will achieve the same effect. I currently use 0.5mg to 1.5mg per hour for catheter directed thrombolysis. The tPA dosage chosen depends on the overall clot burden and the number and level of infusions used.

Neglen and coauthors reported 139 consecutive lower extremities stented for chronic iliac venous obstruction (61 limbs with primary disease and 78 with post-thrombotic disease). They found postoperative (8%) and late occlusions (3%) occurred only in post-thrombotic limbs. Primary, primary-assisted and secondary cumulative patency rates of the stented area at 2 years were 52%, 88% and 90%, respectively, in the primary disease group as compared to 60%, 100% and 100% in the post-thrombotic group. The importantly noted the importance of IVUS in both diagnosis and treatment since phlebography was unreliable. Stenting after balloon dilation was emphasized for all venoplasties as well as placement of stents well into the IVC when treating iliocaval junction stenosis.[32] Neglen also has emphasized the absence of collateral vessels does not exclude the existence of significant obstruction, and their presence may indicate an obstruction not visualized.[33]

In an attempt to stress the success of thrombolysis and stenting over anticoagulation therapy for iliofemoral DVT, Aburahma documented results for 51 patients treated during a 10-year period. 33 patients were treated with anticoagulation while 18 patients were treated with thrombolysis and stenting. Initial lysis was achieved in 89% those with residual stenoses were treated with stenting with a success rate of 90%. Two patients in treated with anticoagulation had a symptomatic pulmonary embolism vs. none treated with thrombolysis. At 30 days, venous patency and symptom resolution were achieved in 1 of 33 patients (3%) treated with anticoagulation versus 15 of 18 (83%) treated with intervention. Kaplan-Meier analysis showed primary iliofemoral venous patency rates at 1, 3, and 5 years of 24%, 18%, and 18% and 83%, 69%, and 69% for groups the anticoagulation and interventional therapy groups respectively.[34]

In the early part of this decade, we began to see the use of percutaneous mechanical thrombectomy (PMT) with iliofemoral disease. A study in 2002 used catheter-directed thrombolysis with adjunctive PMT to treat 28 symptomatic limbs with lower extremity deep vein thrombosis. Mean per-limb infusion time was 16.8 hours +/− 12.8, much shorter than many prior studies. Similarly, mean per-limb total doses of thrombolytic agents were lower than those reported in published studies of DVT thrombolysis. They noted minimal thrombus removal when using PMT alone.[35] Several reports also show similar results with uncommonly used devices such as the Helix and Arrow-Trerotola devices.[36,37]

A study compared catheter directed thrombolysis (CDT) versus rheolytic mechanical thrombectomy using the AngioJet catheter with infusion of thrombolytic agent over an 8 year period. CDT or PMT was performed in 46 (47%) and 52 (53%) procedures, respectively. In the CDT group, complete or partial thrombus removal was accomplished in 32 (70%) and 14 (30%) cases, respectively. In the PMT cohort, complete or partial thrombus removal was accomplished in 39 (75%) and 13 (25%) cases, respectively. Significant reductions in the intensive care unit and hospital lengths of stay was noted in the PMT group (0.6 and 4.6 days) when compared to the CDT group (2.4 and 8.4 days). The primary patency rates at 1 year of CDT and PMT groups were not significantly different at 64% and 68%, respectively. Hospital cost analysis showed significant cost reduction in the PMT group compared to the CDT group (P < .01).[38]

Dietzek reported on a company sponsored registry using the Trellis(R) Peripheral Infusion System. Demographic, thrombus characterization, and procedural data were collected during the treatment of 2203 extremity DVTs in 2024 patients via case-report forms submitted by the treating physicians. Thrombi were iliofemoral in 25.1%; iliofemoral to popliteal in 19.3%; inferior vena cava only or IVC and infrainguinal lower extremity in 18.7%; femoral to popliteal in 12.2%; isolated femoral in 6%, iliac in 6% or popliteal 0.6%.; and upper extremity (12.1%). Thrombus chronicity was reported as acute in 34.5%, acute-on-chronic in 41.5%, subacute in 10.4%, subacute-on-chronic in 9.8%, and chronic in 3.8%. The thrombolytic agent chosen by the physician most often was tissue plasminogen activator; (95.8%) at an average total dose per patient of 14.9 +/−8.3 mg. Combined Grade III and II venous patency following treatment across all thrombus chronicities was 95.5% and was achieved in a single setting in 83.3% of patients with an average PMT run time of only 22.3 +/−9.4 minutes. Sixteen percent of patients' limbs required additional catheter-directed thrombolysis (CDT); 75% required angioplasty and/or stent. No major bleeding complications, symptomatic pulmonary embolism (PE), or other significant adverse events occurred during the procedures.[39] Although the data is self-reported from a company registry, the study clearly shows diminished need for pharmacological thrombolytic agent and treatment time as compared to catheter directed therapy and once again shows little to no risk of pulmonary embolism. Similarly Martinez Trabal found significantly more thrombus was removed with the Trellis device in less than half the time and with 39% less plasminogen activator than with catheter directed thrombolysis. However, the reduction in treatment time did not translate into lower length of stay in the intensive care unit or hospital.[40]

The use of the Trellis and Possis device for treatment of iliofemoral DVT in patients with traditional contraindications for catheter directed thrombolysis was reported by Rao. Of 43 patients 15 (35%) had a high risk for bleeding. Eighty-one percent presented with lower extremity DVT despite anticoagulation. Sixty-three percent were treated in one session, but 16 patients required a lytic infusion after suboptimal PMT. Iliac stenting was required in 35% of limbs treated. Successful lysis (>50%) was achieved in 95% of patients and symptom resolution in 93%. Importantly there were no major systemic bleeding complications, only two access site hematomas and worsening of pre-existing rectus sheath hematoma requiring transfusion in another two. Freedom from DVT recurrence and reintervention was 95% at 9 months by life-table analysis.[41]

Titus reported 36 patients from the Cleveland Clinic undergoing iliofemoral venous angioplasty and stenting over a 4-year period until 2008. Thrombolysis was performed in 52.8% of patients. The majority of patients who had a recognized underlying etiology were diagnosed with May-Thurner syndrome (42%) but an etiology was not determined in 25%. Patency rates at 6, 12, and 24 months were 88%, 78.3%, and 78.3%, respectively. Secondary patency rates for the same time frames were 100%, 95%, and 95%. Better outcomes were seen in stenting for May-Thurner syndrome and idiopathic causes, whereas external compression and thrombophilia seemed to portend less favorable outcomes (P < .001).[42]

CONCLUSIONS

Iliofemoral stenoses and occlusions are an important etiology of chronic venous insufficiency that should be treated. In the setting of acute thrombosis, catheter directed thrombolysis and percutaneous mechanical thrombectomy are useful in removing the acute clot allowing treatment of underlying disease. In comparison to arterial thrombosis, thrombolytic doses are higher and treatment times are longer with CDT when treating venous diseases. Use of PMT reduces the dose and treatment time with pharmacological agents but does not necessary decrease length of stay. In certain select instances PMT can facilitate treatment of acute iliofemoral thrombosis in patients with traditional contraindications for CDT. May-Thurner is a common anatomic problem leading left sided iliofemoral venous pathology. Self-expanding stents are the mainstay of treatment after removal of acute clot and liberal use of intravascular ultrasonography will optimize outcomes. Venographic identification of residual collateral vessels should prompt further investigation for untreated underlying disease.

REFERENCES

1. Scott TE, LaMorte WW, Gorin DR, et al. Risk factors for chronic venous insufficiency: a dual case-control study. *J Vasc Surg* Nov 1995;22(5):622–628.
2. Jawien A. The influence of environmental factors in chronic venous insufficiency. *Angiology* Jul-Aug 2003;54 Suppl 1:S19–31.

3. Neglen P, Thrasher TL, Raju S. Venous outflow obstruction: An underestimated contributor to chronic venous disease. *J Vasc Surg* Nov 2003;38(5):879–885.

4. Comerota AJ, Gravett MH. Iliofemoral venous thrombosis. *J Vasc Surg* Nov 2007;46(5): 1065–1076.

5. Kearon C, Kahn SR, Agnelli G, et al. Antithrombotic therapy for venous thromboembolic disease: American College of Chest Physicians Evidence-Based Clinical Practice Guidelines (8th Edition). *Chest* Jun 2008;133(6 Suppl):454S-545S.

6. Ouriel K, Veith FJ, Sasahara AA. Thrombolysis or peripheral arterial surgery: phase I results. TOPAS Investigators [see comments]. *J Vasc Surg* 1996;23(1):64–73; discussion 74–65.

7. Results of a prospective randomized trial evaluating surgery versus thrombolysis for ischemia of the lower extremity. The STILE trial. *Ann Surg* Sep 1994;220(3):251–266; discussion 266–258.

8. Kasirajan K, Gray B, Ouriel K. Percutaneous AngioJet thrombectomy in the management of extensive deep venous thrombosis. *J Vasc Interv Radiol* Feb 2001;12(2):179–185.

9. Jeyabalan G, Saba S, Baril DT, et al. Bradyarrhythmias during rheolytic pharmacomechanical thrombectomy for deep vein thrombosis. *J Endovasc Ther* Jun 2010;17(3):416–422.

10. Arko FR, Davis CM, 3rd, Murphy EH, et al. Aggressive percutaneous mechanical thrombectomy of deep venous thrombosis: early clinical results. *Arch Surg* Jun 2007;142(6):513–518; discussion 518–519.

11. Stahr P, Rupprecht HJ, Voigtlander T, et al. A new thrombectomy catheter device (AngioJet) for the disruption of thrombi: An in vitro study. *Catheter Cardiovasc Interv* Jul 1999;47(3): 381–389.

12. Francis CW, Suchkova VN. Ultrasound and thrombolysis. *Vasc Med* 2001;6(3):181–187.

13. Francis CW, Blinc A, Lee S, et al. Ultrasound accelerates transport of recombinant tissue plasminogen activator into clots. *Ultrasound Med Biol* 1995;21(3):419–424.

14. Suchkova V, Carstensen EL, Francis CW. Ultrasound enhancement of fibrinolysis at frequencies of 27 to 100 kHz. *Ultrasound Med Biol* Mar 2002;28(3):377–382.

15. Neglen P, Raju S. Proximal lower extremity chronic venous outflow obstruction: recognition and treatment. *Semin Vasc Surg* Mar 2002;15(1):57–64.

16. Neglen P, Raju S. Intravascular ultrasound scan evaluation of the obstructed vein. *J Vasc Surg* Apr 2002;35(4):694–700.

17. Michel C, Laffy PY, Leblanc G, et al. [Treatment of Cockett syndrome by percutaneous insertion of a vascular endoprosthesis (Gianturco)]. *J Radiol* May 1994;75(5):327–330.

18. May R, Thurner J. The cause of the predominantly sinistral occurrence of thrombosis of the pelvic veins. *Angiology* Oct 1957;8(5):419–427.

19. Steinberg JB, Jacocks MA. May-Thurner syndrome: a previously unreported variant. *Ann Vasc Surg* Nov 1993;7(6):577–581.

20. Uchino A, Maeoka N, Ohno M, et al. [A variation of May-Thurner syndrome: a case report]. *Rinsho Hoshasen* Sep 1989;34(9):1043–1045.

21. Abboud G, Midulla M, Lions C, et al. "Right-sided" May-Thurner syndrome. *Cardiovasc Intervent Radiol.* Oct 2010;33(5):1056–1059.

22. Oguzkurt L, Tercan F, Pourbagher MA, et al. Computed tomography findings in 10 cases of iliac vein compression (May-Thurner) syndrome. *Eur J Radiol* Sep 2005;55(3):421–425.

23. Wolpert LM, Rahmani O, Stein B, et al. Magnetic resonance venography in the diagnosis and management of May-Thurner syndrome. *Vasc Endovascular Surg* Jan-Feb 2002;36(1): 51–57.

24. Patel NH, Stookey KR, Ketcham DB, et al. Endovascular management of acute extensive iliofemoral deep venous thrombosis caused by May-Thurner syndrome. *J Vasc Interv Radiol* Nov-Dec 2000;11(10):1297–1302.

25. O'Sullivan GJ, Semba CP, Bittner CA, et al. Endovascular management of iliac vein compression (May-Thurner) syndrome. *J Vasc Interv Radiol* Jul-Aug 2000;11(7):823–836.

26. Moudgill N, Hager E, Gonsalves C, et al. May-Thurner syndrome: case report and review of the literature involving modern endovascular therapy. *Vascular* Nov-Dec 2009;17(6): 330–335.

27. Semba CP, Dake MD. Iliofemoral deep venous thrombosis: aggressive therapy with catheter-directed thrombolysis. *Radiology* May 1994;191(2):487–494.
28. Nazarian GK, Bjarnason H, Dietz CA, Jr., et al. Iliofemoral venous stenoses: effectiveness of treatment with metallic endovascular stents. *Radiology* Jul 1996;200(1):193–199.
29. Bjarnason H, Kruse JR, Asinger DA, et al. Iliofemoral deep venous thrombosis: safety and efficacy outcome during 5 years of catheter-directed thrombolytic therapy. *J Vasc Interv Radiol* May-Jun 1997;8(3):405–418.
30. Mewissen MW, Seabrook GR, Meissner MH, et al. Catheter-directed thrombolysis for lower extremity deep venous thrombosis: report of a national multicenter registry. *Radiology* Apr 1999;211(1):39–49.
31. Verhaeghe R, Stockx L, Lacroix H, et al. Catheter-directed lysis of iliofemoral vein thrombosis with use of rt-PA. *Eur Radiol* 1997;7(7):996–1001.
32. Neglen P, Berry MA, Raju S. Endovascular surgery in the treatment of chronic primary and post-thrombotic iliac vein obstruction. *Eur J Vasc Endovasc Surg* Dec 2000;20(6):560–571.
33. Neglen P, Raju S. Balloon dilation and stenting of chronic iliac vein obstruction: technical aspects and early clinical outcome. *J Endovasc Ther* Apr 2000;7(2):79–91.
34. AbuRahma AF, Perkins SE, Wulu JT, et al. Iliofemoral deep vein thrombosis: conventional therapy versus lysis and percutaneous transluminal angioplasty and stenting. *Ann Surg* Jun 2001;233(6):752–760.
35. Vedantham S, Vesely TM, Parti N, et al. Lower extremity venous thrombolysis with adjunctive mechanical thrombectomy. *J Vasc Interv Radiol* Oct 2002;13(10):1001–1008.
36. Vedantham S, Vesely TM, Sicard GA, et al. Pharmacomechanical thrombolysis and early stent placement for iliofemoral deep vein thrombosis. *J Vasc Interv Radiol* Jun 2004;15(6):565–574.
37. Lee KH, Han H, Lee KJ, et al. Mechanical thrombectomy of acute iliofemoral deep vein thrombosis with use of an Arrow-Trerotola percutaneous thrombectomy device. *J Vasc Interv Radiol* Mar 2006;17(3):487–495.
38. Lin PH, Zhou W, Dardik A, et al. Catheter-direct thrombolysis versus pharmacomechanical thrombectomy for treatment of symptomatic lower extremity deep venous thrombosis. *Am J Surg* Dec 2006;192(6):782–788.
39. Dietzek AM. Isolated pharmacomechanical thrombolysis of deep venous thrombosis utilizing a peripheral infusion system: Manuf. *Int Angiol* Aug 2010;29(4):308–316.
40. Martinez Trabal JL, Comerota AJ, LaPorte FB, et al. The quantitative benefit of isolated, segmental, pharmacomechanical thrombolysis (ISPMT) for iliofemoral venous thrombosis. *J Vasc Surg* Dec 2008;48(6):1532–1537.
41. Rao AS, Konig G, Leers SA, et al. Pharmacomechanical thrombectomy for iliofemoral deep vein thrombosis: an alternative in patients with contraindications to thrombolysis. *J Vasc Surg* Nov 2009;50(5):1092–1098.
42. Titus JM, Moise MA, Bena J, et al. Iliofemoral stenting for venous occlusive disease. *J Vasc Surg* Mar 2011;53(3):706–712.

32

Endovascular Treatment of Inferior Vena Caval Occlusions

Praveen R. Anchala, MD and Scott A. Resnick, MD

Central venous occlusion is an increasingly prevalent and often profoundly symptomatic medical entity.[1] This increase in prevalence appears to be associated with the more frequent use of chronic central venous access devices, as does the overall increase in clinically relevant large vessel venous occlusions.[1] While malignancy and long term dialysis catheter placement are likely the most common etiologies of central venous occlusion, there are numerous other causes.[1] Even though extensive venous collateral networks are able to at least partially decompress many of these lesions, occlusion of the caval veins are difficult to bypass and can often be particularly symptomatic.

Obstructive lesions of the inferior vena cava (IVC) can be associated with chronic symptoms, but some total occlusions can be completely silent.[2] These lesions that remain silent for long periods of time can present acutely with distal thrombosis,[2] making it necessary to look for signs and symptoms of caval occlusion in any case of distal thrombosis. Symptoms of obstruction in the lower extremities can be extremely variable in type and intensity, and can be difficult to predict. As the prevalence of IVC occlusion continues to increase, diagnosing and treating these lesions can have a profound impact on chronic venous disease management.

VENA CAVAL SYNDROMES

While we will primarily focus on the IVC in this chapter, it is important to compare and contrast superior vena cava (SVC) and inferior vena cava occlusions as each have their own set of characteristic signs and symptoms. SVC syndrome, the more common of the two caval occlusions, can present with face, neck, and upper extremity swelling. SVC syndrome can also lead to dyspnea as the fixed caval lesion leads to diminished venous return and decreased preload.[1] In contrast, IVC disease is often much more subtle in nature with a more chronic disease course. The classing finding of IVC occlusion is lower extremity edema, but signs and symptoms can vary greatly depending on the location of the lesion. Scrotal swelling is a common feature of IVC disease due to the potential for fluid to accumulate within the scrotum, and IVC obstruction should be explored in these cases if it cannot be readily explained. In addition, ascites, anasarca, and hepatic and renal dysfunction can occur with more proximal IVC lesions.

PATHOPHYSIOLOGY OF VENA CAVAL OCCLUSION

Diseases that cause vena caval obstruction can be divided into three main groups: (1) extrinsic compression, (2) chronic catheterization, and (3) other etiologies. The majority of SVC cases are caused by extrinsic compression or chronic venous catheterization.[1] Malignant compression of the superior vena cava is especially common, likely due to its thin wall and low intravascular pressure, as well as the numerous structures immediately adjacent to its course.[1] This pathogenesis is well known with the superior vena cava since its course through the relatively rigid mediastinal structures makes compression more likely. On the other hand, chronic catheterization for dialysis, TPN, or chemotherapy can result in thrombosis via Virchow's triad.[3] The concurrent formation of a fibrin sheath, intimal injury, and hemodynamic stasis associated with chronic catheterization provides a nidus for thrombus.

Uncomplicated catheterization alone rarely results in large vessel obstruction unless a significant underlying lesion was already present. In the short term, central venous devices can cause intimal injury due to focal areas of endothelial denudation.[4] This can be further compounded with the long term use of devices as vein wall thickening, increased smooth muscle cells, and focal catheter attachments to the vein wall with thrombus and collagen occur.[4] The etiology of these changes is not completely understood, but it is likely primarily related to repetitive mechanical irritation and injury to the endothelium.

While the IVC is also subject to external malignant compression, catheter related obstruction is much less common than in the SVC. This is primarily related to the fact that chronic lower extremity catheterization is relatively infrequent. While femoral, transhepatic, or direct caval access catheters are occasionally placed, their use is avoided if possible. In addition, lower extremity catheters have been shown to have increased risk of line infections, so their clinical use is of last resort. Nonetheless, these procedures continue to be performed, especially in patients who have lost upper extremity access, making the patient's history particularly important in achieving the diagnosis.

Central venous devices of the upper extremities observed under fluoroscopy demonstrate continuous motion due to the movement of mediastinal structures created by cardiac wall motion and respiratory variations. These indwelling devices are often large in caliber and stiff leading to intimal thickening as the inner wall of the vessel is continuously injured by the mobile catheter or wire. While this continuous motion should primarily be thought of as affecting devices in the SVC due to their location, this can also be a method of pathogenesis in IVC devices, especially if they extend above the diaphragm (Figure 32–1).

While there is overlap between the causative factors of SVC and IVC occlusions, the prevalence of these etiologies can vary greatly. While SVC disease is frequently

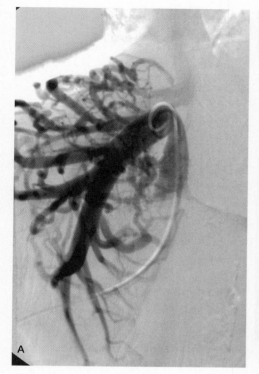 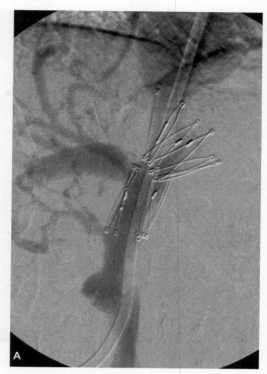

Figure 32–1. a. IVCgram via pigtail catheter placed via tract of existing translumbar catheter shows intrahepatic IVC occlusion with extensive intrahepatic venous collaterals reconstituting patent suprahepatic IVC **b.** IVCgram following intrahepatic IVC Z-configuration stenting and thru placement of new tunneled translumbar dialysis catheter extending above diaphragm into right atrium shows improved but still stenotic IVC lumen.

malignant in origin, occlusion of the IVC is more often benign in etiology. The most common of these benign etiologies is thrombosis of an existing caval filter, occurring in 2–10% of treated patients.[5] (Figure 32–2) Other specific benign causes that affect predominantly the IVC include, but are not limited to, liver transplant anastamotic lesions and Budd-Chiari syndrome. Additionally, there are a number of specific abdominal malignancies that invade, rather than compress, the IVC. This is usually attributed to renal cell carcinoma invading the cava via malignant spread from the renal vein; hepatoma and adrenal cortical carcinoma are also known to spread in this manner.

While we have explored a number of etiologies that can cause caval occlusion, these entities do not usually occlude the cava directly. Rather, they narrow the vessel and the subsequent slow-flow state within the cava leads to the formation of a superimposed thrombus. This thrombus worsens the obstructive qualities of the initial lesion by further reducing the effective luminal diameter, creating a larger segment of flow irregularities, and by recruiting the formation of additional thrombus. This frequent presence of superimposed thrombus, along with the large caliber of the caval veins, makes the treatment of caval occlusions difficult. This thrombus also has the potential to detach from its origin, leading to pulmonary emboli, and leading to one of the more dire complications of intervention.

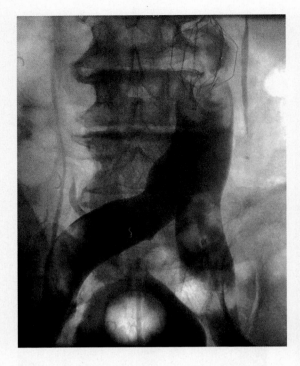

Figure 32–2. Iliocavagram showing completely thrombosed Trapeze IVC filter and bilateral iliac vein thrombus.

EMBRYONIC DEVELOPMENT OF THE IVC

The adult IVC develops from an array of paired longitudinal embryonic veins and the interconnections between them.[6] The embryonic structure is particularly complex near the liver and diaphragm as offshoots from the hepatic and infrarenal IVC have to anastomose. This area has been described to be prone to developmental abnormalities such as webs and strictures.[3] Parts of this formative system disappear while others have remnants such as the azygous and thoracolumbar veins. All remnants interconnect with each other to create an extensive collateral network. In cases of IVC obstruction, the thoracolumbar vein receives drainage directly from the common iliac vein through an opening that has been described as more prominent in cases of IVC obstruction.[3] Thus, the natural collateral network can bypass the occluded segment of IVC to some extent. This is in contrast to the almost always symptomatic case of occluded common iliac veins.[7] Logically, cases of combined common iliac and IVC occlusion are likely to exhibit poor collateral compensation.[3] This natural network of collaterals around the embryonic formation of the IVC may explain the variance in symptoms seen with IVC occlusions (Figure 32–3).

NATURAL HISTORY

A retrospective study by Raju et al on 120 obstructive lesions of the IVC revealed that IVC occlusion is more common among women.[3] In addition, limb symptoms were only bilateral in 33% of the cases, while unilateral symptoms were found in the remaining 67% of patients.[3] Four of these 120 patients developed acute distal thrombosis below a chronically

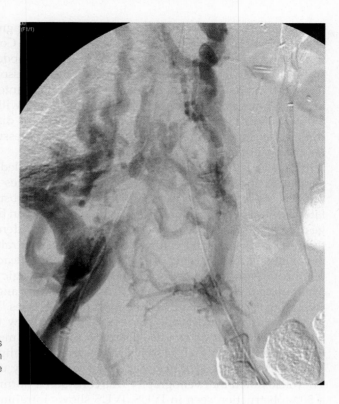

Figure 32–3. Iliocavagram demonstrates complete IVC occlusion (wire from each iliac passing through cava) with extensive right and left iliac vein origin collaterals.

occluded IVC, and all of these patients had unilateral leg complaints.[3] The occlusive segment of the IVC can vary greatly based on the etiology, but general pathology shows that a majority of lesions are infrarenal (82%), followed by suprarenal below the diaphragm (14%) and further extension into the thoracic IVC (4%).[3] Additionally, disease is rarely found limited to the IVC proper and usually includes distal extension into the common iliac vein or beyond.[3]

Clinical features of patients with IVC occlusion typically fall into three groups: (1) asymptomatic or cosmetically symptomatic, (2) acutely symptomatic, and (3) chronically symptomatic. Asymptomatic patients can have transient symptoms with little functional impairment, and can experience limb, scrotal, or abdominal varices. Transient leg pain and swelling can be common complaints in this subset of patients. Acutely symptomatic patients usually present with the distal thrombosis, and will have acute unilateral leg pain and swelling that is persistent. Chronically symptomatic patients can have indolent leg swelling and pain, ulceration, impaired hepatic or renal function, or changes in skin pigmentation secondary to hemosiderin deposition.

DIAGNOSIS OF IVC OCCLUSION

Testing for inferior vena cava obstruction is often omitted in the evaluation of venous patients, but can provide valuable information in some cases. Ultrasound evaluation is notoriously unreliable in detecting obstruction and thrombosis of the vena cava. Evaluation of the vena cava using computed tomography and magnetic resonance imaging has been well described in the literature with excellent results.[8] Computed tomography is currently the method of choice when considering non-invasive modalities.[8]

Unlike the arterial system, pressure gradients associated with venous stenosis are often in the range of 2-3 mm Hg and are difficult to interpret.[9] In addition, obstructions in the venous system can be difficult to evaluate with the patient at rest or supine. Small pressure gradients could indicate significant disease, and a normal evaluation does not exclude the presence of disease. Instead, pressure gradients are used primarily for end point determination.

This lack of accurate hemodynamic testing has led to the diagnosis and treatment of obstruction to be based on morphologic changes in venography. Often, venous outflow obstruction can be identified by definitive obstruction and the presence of collaterals. However, in some instances, the findings can be very subtle, and are only suggestive of disease. These findings can include widening of the iliac or caval veins, thinning of the injected contrast column, partial intraluminal filling defects, or filling of collaterals. The subtlety of findings can at times lead to the misdiagnosis or nondetection of significant venous stenosis. Morphologic assessment is improved with multi-oblique venography, and the use of multiple angled evaluations should be considered the standard in all but the most obvious cases.[10]

Intravascular ultrasonography (IVUS) is a new technique in the evaluation of venous stenosis. It allows the detection of venous morphology and a more accurate estimation of the degree of stenosis. Neglen et al compared the use of IVUS to venography in these cases.[10] They found that venography underestimates stenosis by 30%. They also noted that venography was considered normal in one-fourth of cases despite a 50% obstruction seen in IVUS. IVUS shows intraluminal details that can be missed with contrast studies. IVUS appears to be the best available method for diagnosing significant caval obstruction, but it is a more invasive diagnostic method.

RISK FACTORS FOR COAGULOPATHY

A risk factor for venous thromboembolism, either hereditary or acquired, can now be identified in 80% of patients.[11] In addition, some patients are found to have multiple risks. Inherited thrombophilia is a genetic tendency to venous thromboembolism that usually presents in young patients and is recurrent. It is estimated that an inherited thrombophilic condition can now be identified in over 50% of patients with juvenile or idiopathic thrombosis.[11] The most frequent hereditary causes of coagulopathy are factor V Leiden mutations and prothrombin gene mutations, accounting for 50–60% of cases.[11] Factor V Leiden, an autosomal dominant trait, is estimated to be prevalent in 4–6% of the general population[12] while prothrombin mutations are found in 1.7–3% of European descendants.[13] The remaining cases are primarily composed of defects in protein S, protein C, and antithrombin.

In a study of 2,132 venous thromboembolism patients by Mateo et al, 12.9% had an anticoagulant protein deficiency. These protein deficiencies consisted of protein S deficiency (7.27%), protein C deficiency (3.19%), and antithrombin defects (0.5%). Additionally, antiphospholipid antibodies account for 4.1% of inherited coagulopathies.[14] The causes of acquired thrombophilia are too numerous for discussion, but include, among others, malignancy, obesity, pregnancy, surgery, trauma, oral contraceptives, chronic liver disease, and smoking. While there is no specific evaluation of these risk factors in the occurrence of IVC occlusions, it is likely that given the systemic nature of thrombophilia the rate of thrombosis in the IVC is similar.

TREATMENT

While a variety of surgical techniques have been attempted in cases of IVC occlusion, bypass has been the most used surgical approach.[15] Surgical procedures are invasive and have had disappointing results, with patency rates ranging from 54–88% after a mean follow-up period of 19.5 months.[15] Endovascular techniques such as balloon angioplasty and stenting have gained favor over these more invasive surgical procedures since their first reported use in 1995.[16] Furthermore, reliance on endovascular techniques is critical given the large caliber of the vessels in question, limited surgical access to caval segments, and the palliative nature of many caval procedures. This also limits the ability for a surgical conversion if endovascular procedures are unsuccessful or if complications arise. We will explore the current state of endovascular management in the treatment of inferior vena cava occlusion.

Technical Challenges

The presence of an overlying thrombus on the primary lesion makes endovascular treatment of caval occlusions challenging. While traversal of the occluded segment is critical for success, superimposed vessel thrombus can lengthen the necessary crossing distance while also masking the fixed underlying lesion. Finally, given the thin walled nature of the cava, care must be taken during endovascular procedures since creating an extravascular communication is a realistic possibility.

In most cases a hydrophilic guidewire and hydrophilic catheter is the lesion crossing combination of choice. However, more aggressive crossing techniques are sometimes required, especially when complete occlusion is present. Alternatives such as hydrophilic guidewire back ends and even sharp recanalization with steerable needles can be utilized in these instances. These aggressive options should be used with great care and only after careful consideration of the potential management pitfalls. When in doubt, cross-sectional imaging of the area in question should be obtained prior to aggressive traversal techniques to ensure that no vital intervening structures are present.

Thrombectomy and/or Thrombolysis

Once guidewire traversal has been achieved, if superimposed thrombus is present, initial attention should be directed towards its removal. Vessel manipulation prior to clot removal can result in fatal pulmonary embolization. Thrombectomy or thrombolysis should ideally take place with limited clot manipulation, as can be achieved with lytic agents in a flow-directed manner. While this is readily performed via upper extremity venous access in the case of SVC obstruction, the frequent association with iliac or iliofemoral occlusion in IVC obstruction usually necessitates more caudal lower extremity access. Atraumatic percutaneous entry into the popliteal, lesser saphenous, or tibioperoneal veins can be achieved with ultrasound guidance. The large vessel diameter of the vena cava makes thrombolysis or thrombectomy far less effective than in smaller caliber lumens. It is difficult to administer thrombolytic agents from the intralumenal catheter all the way to the vessel wall in these large caliber vessels. Utilizing vigorous manual pulse spray and power pulse spray are beneficial in achieving deeper lytic penetration into the thrombus and to the caval wall, but experience suggests that complete resolution of clot burden is infrequent. Remaining clot is often found adherent to the vessel wall.

Similarly, suction thrombectomy or mechanical thrombectomy devices are usually able to clear a variable diameter channel through a thrombosed caval lumen but rarely are able to create a diameter wide enough to expose the vessel wall. While these debulking procedures can be helpful, they are rarely definitive and significant mural thrombus remains in most cases. Given the low pressure and slow-flow within the caval systems, the possibility of rethrombosis is quite high unless a smooth flow channel is created (Figure 32–4).

Percutaenous Transluminal Angioplasty

Percutaneous transluminal angioplasty (PTA) provides a nonsurgical method of returning blood flow through the inferior vena cava. The necessity for a clear flow channel with no

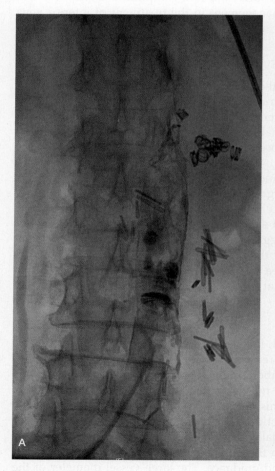
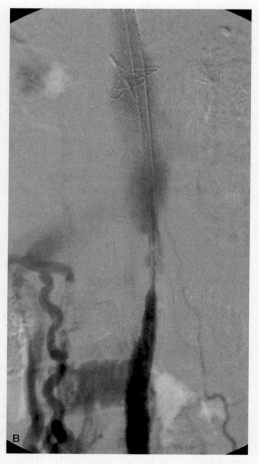

Figure 32–4. a. IVCgram demonstrates complete caval thrombosis. Although there is no underlying lesion visualized the thrombosed segment appears to taper at the cephalad terminus. **b.** IVCgram following extensive thrombolysis and mechanical thrombectomy shows resolution of overlying thrombus and demonstrates causative caval stenotic lesion.

residual pressure gradient often requires the use of mechanical displacement as an adjunctive technique. This technique is utilized throughout the treated segment, not just at the level of the underlying lesion. By using an expandable balloon, PTA allows the operator to create mechanical displacement of the clot burden. This should allow recanalization of the inferior vena cava as the lesion in question is traversed. Angioplasty without stenting initially showed promising results but long term patency rates have been disappointing and so angioplasty alone is only performed in select cases.[17]

Stents

One way of improving the efficacy of angioplasty in the treatment of IVC occlusion while diminishing the rate of restenosis is through insertion of a stent in association with balloon dilation of the inferior vena cava. Stents provide a radial force that maintains vascular patency by offsetting the recoil forces of the vasculature and providing a clear flow channel.[18] Stent technology and design advancements have been associated with improved patency rates and decreased need for reintervention.[19]

The threshold for endovenous stent placement should be low, and often numerous large diameter stents are needed to achieve the desired result. It is crucial to completely resolve any hemodynamically significant pressure gradient across the treated area. However, there are few reports of using pressure measurements to evaluate hemodynamic significance of venous stenosis.[20] Instead, one should strive to resolve any collateral venous flow, which could be an indicator of resolving pressure gradients.

Results for the use of PTA with stenting have been encouraging. Rates of initial technical success in recanalization of the IVC have been between 85 and 100% of cases.[21,22] Published rates of patency have been similarly encouraging. In their study of 44 patients, Hartung et al reported the rates of primary, assisted primary, and secondary patency rates to be 73.2%, 87.6%, and 89.9%, respectively at 36 and 60 months.[21] Additionally, they reported survival rates to be 100% at 12 months and 97.3% at 60 months.[21] Te Riele et al found the primary patency rate to be 78% and the 9 month occlusion free survival rate to be 56% in their study of nine patients.[22] The rate of perioperative stent migration has ranged from 0–5% in most studies.[21,22] The risk of death or major pulmonary embolism due to the endovascular procedure is rare, with the majority of studies not encountering these dire complications.[21,22]

While the technical challenges in creating a smooth flow lumen are well known, a number of specific issues arise when endovascular stenting of caval occlusions are attempted. The large diameter of the vena cava requires careful stent selection. While the relatively soft and conformable nitinol stents, which possess significant radial force, have ideal characteristics for venous use, they have a limited selection of sizes. The largest manufactured diameter of 14 mm precludes it from use in the majority of inferior vena caval lesions; however, many caval lesions also involve the iliac venous confluences. Nitinol stents are ideally suited for these areas and can be used in the "kissing" stent configuration and continued into the vena cava in a "double barrel" stent configuration (Figure 32–5). This configuration sacrifices some luminal caliber, but the conformability of nitinol is so well suited to the venous system that its use outweighs this downside (Figure 32–6). Additionally, this configuration is advantageous when "through stenting" of a thrombosed caval filter is desired (Figure 32–7).

Alternatively, confluence lesions can be treated with "kissing" configuration stents that extend into a large caliber single stent in the cava itself, similar to an aortic stent graft configuration (Figure 32–8). The options for stent placement within the large

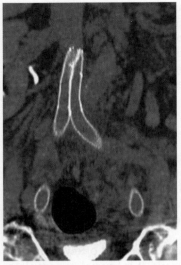

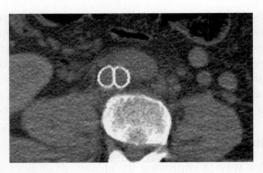

Figure 32–6. Noncontrast CT axial image following reconstruction shows kissing double-barrel configuration caval stents. Note the double "D", rather than double "O" configuration of the conformable nitinol stents results in limited lumen caliber loss.

Figure 32–5. Noncontrast CT coronal reformatted image following iliocaval reconstruction shows kissing iliac venous confluence stent configuration continued into the IVC as a stented double-barrel caval lumen.

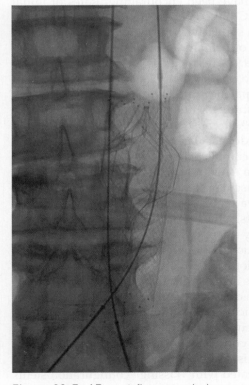

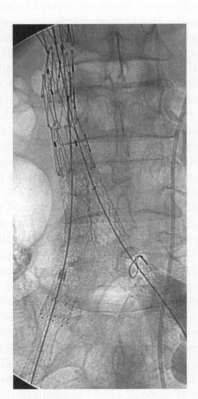

Figure 32–8. AP spot fluoroscopic image demonstrates iliocaval reconstruction with kissing iliac venous confluence nitinol stent configuration into Z-configuration caval stents.

Figure 32–7. AP spot fluoroscopic image demonstrates Trapeze filter in place with kissing-configuration nitinol stents passing through, and conforming to, filter strut interspaces.

lumen cava are limited. The Z-configuration stent is well suited to the large caliber caval lumen, and the significant radial force makes it an excellent candidate for displacement of extrinsic tumor compression or an intraluminal nidus such as a thrombosed caval filter. Gaines et al used Z stents in 20 patients with 90% initial success, and 65% of these patients maintained primary patency while 75% maintained secondary longer term patency.[23]

Care must be taken to not oversize the stent excessively as kinking or tenting of the relatively thin walled and unsupported cava can occur, and may necessitate placement of one or more overlapping stents to create a smooth taper between the oversized stent and true caval diameter. A number of large diameter balloon-expandable stents are available, and the rigid nature of the stent cage makes sizing critical. Since IVC diameters vary significantly with a large number of variables, such as hydration and valsalva, stent stability is not guaranteed unless the cage is pressed against the underlying lesion or other supporting structure. Extreme care must be used with balloon-expandable stents to ensure the stent is placed at the site of a fixed lesion. These stents should be used with great caution when the primary goal is residual thrombosis displacement rather than fixed lesional dilation as migration of a balloon expandable stent supported only or mostly by thrombus is a distinct possibility. In these instances, alternative stent platforms should be considered.

Although the sharp tines at the end of a woven Wallstent (Boston Scientific, Natick, Massachusetts) are concerning for vessel wall injury and subsequent restenosis, and the radial force of larger stents are limited, the large range of diameters and the woven nature make them ideal for residual thrombus displacement. While self expanding nitinol-based stents also displace residual thrombus effectively, their manufactured size range and laser cut rather than woven design limits their use in some instances. Kumar et al describe their selection of Wallstents in the majority of cases to be due to the size availability of stents and the ability to use the stent across branchpoints since the stent has a woven open-celled structure.[24] Wallstents show primary patency results of 71% and secondary patency rates of 82% at 24 months.[3,25]

Stent grafts are another option that offers certain theoretical advantages, such as broad size ranges and thrombus displacement, but there are few reports of its use in the venous system outside of arterialized dialysis circuits and TIPS procedures. Further studies of their use in cases of inferior vena cava obstruction are needed before their use in this instance can be evaluated.

Once stent choice and treatment options have been decided and therapy is undertaken, care should be used to monitor for caval-specific hemodynamic issues. Relief of caval occlusion, especially in the IVC, can lead to immediate and massive volume redistribution from the trunk and lower extremities to the right heart with subsequent heart strain and eventual cor pulmonale. Monitoring blood pressure, heart rate, and EKG can provide valuable information about the occurrence of this condition. Operators should consider placement of a central venous pressure monitoring catheter following relief of any high IVC occlusion as the de-compensation associated with such massive volume redistribution can be quite rapid.

One common concern about stenting of the inferior vena cava arises when addressing lesions traversing the renal veins. Traditionally, great care has been taken to prevent coverage of the renal vein ostia for fear of inducing renal dysfunction. In these cases, many operators utilize Wallstents as previously mentioned, although the wider interstices of Z-configuration stents make their use more logical. However, there has been some evidence that stent implantation across the renal vein ostia does not cause renal impairment.[26] Still, this should be something taken into consideration when implanting a stent.

It is important to remember that many caval reconstruction procedures are palliative in nature. The goals of the procedure can vary widely depending on the specific patient's case and treatment plan. The procedural outcome will differ between palliation of an obstructing malignant process and relief of a benign caval occlusion. When treating malignant disease, stent coverage of otherwise significant venous structures may be acceptable. Specifically, stent placement across the renal veins can usually be performed without significant sequelae in palliative cases since collateral drainage is present and long term prognosis is not of as much consequence. Clearly, the palliative nature of the procedure dictates the outcome goals. With malignant obstruction, return to native baseline diameter is often not possible (Figure 32–9). Stents with larger radial force can be used preferentially in these cases in an attempt to primarily relieve symptoms in the purpose of palliation. Use of Wallstents in these patients has been reported with good results. Zamora et al showed complete revascularization and disappearance of collateral circulation in the 5 cases of malignant obstruction they treated with Wallstents.[27] Four of these five patients showed clinical improvement with amelioration of their congestive symptoms, while one did not. All of these patients eventually died from their malignant disease.[27]

The use of Z-configuration stents in inferior vena caval obstruction is not well described in the literature, but is used by many operators, especially in cases of malignant obstruction. Z-configuration stents provide excellent radial force and can be

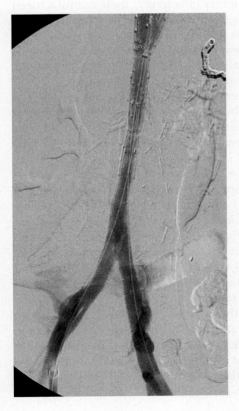

Figure 32-9. IVCgram following iliocaval reconstruction with stent placement for extrinsic compression and occlusion by metastatic germ cell tumor. Note lack of return to baseline IVC diameter (compare with caliber of iliac veins) in this palliative procedure.

placed across ostia without concern due to the wide spaced interstices. The anchoring hooks and barbs surrounding the stent provide a secure placement; however, these large interstices also make it more likely for extrusion of clot out of the stent and the delivery system of the Z-configuration stent is quite large. In comparison, the Wallstent has a much smaller delivery system for a similar stent diameter. Its woven nature provides excellent clot displacement but also provides less radial force. Also due to its woven composition, incomplete expansion of the Wallstent creates differences in lengths and a focal stricture across one segment of the stent drastically alters the luminal diameter across the entire stent. While Wallstents are well studied in the literature with good results, the use of Z-configuration stents should be further explored.

Dilation of the offending malignant obstructive tumor frequently causes significant patient discomfort. While these procedures can be done with deeper sedation or even general anesthesia, this is not recommended as the discomfort should be a signal to the operator that impending vessel rupture is possible if more aggressive dilation is performed. Thus, discomfort should never be ignored. Should a caval tear occur, neither surgical nor endovascular options for treatment are reliably effective. It is this limit on final vessel diameter that lies behind the decision to create single, rather than dual, channel drainage in some cases of malignant obstruction.

While endovascular techniques have been used for palliation in patients with underlying malignancy causing IVC obstruction, venous occlusion due to benign causes poses a difference challenge since long term patency must be maintained. In the vast majority of benign caval occlusion, the goal is reconstruction and recreating not only the original venous relationships but also the original venous lumen diameter whenever possible. In many instances the treated vessel will be immediately recatheterized with another chronic central venous device at the end of the procedure. This is often the case in chronic hemodialysis patients where maintenance of a patent central venous system is equivalent to maintenance of a lifeline. Unfortunately, this ultimately leads to the same restenotic process that occluded the vessel in the first place. The need for repeated treatments is the expectation in this patient population.

Antiplatelet and Anticoagulation Therapy

Minimizing restenosis is a primary endpoint in the treatment of benign lesions, and every attempt at long term durability and viability should be made. Initiation of adequate antiplatelet therapy with aspirin and clopidogrel should be considered prior to attempting relief of caval obstruction. Additionally, continued antiplatelet therapy as well as anticoagulation with warfarin should be considered once reconstruction is achieved. Anticoagulation in silent lesions is particularly controversial, and there is some thought that anticoagulation is particularly important in this patient population since distal thrombosis can occur.[3]

MANAGEMENT OF BUDD-CHIARI SYNDROME CAUSED BY IVC OCCLUSION

Budd-Chiari syndrome is characterized by hepatic venous outflow obstruction from the level of the hepatic veins proximal to the junction of the IVC and the right atrium.[28] Subsequent hepatic congestion can lead to significant stenosis of the intrahepatic caval segment. Decompression of this hepatic congestion, often through TIPS creation, rather than therapy directed towards the caval stenosis, is the treatment of choice. However, when treatment of the associated caval stenosis is deemed indicated, angioplasty with stenting in these patients has shown excellent results with primary patency of 70–100%.[29] However, PTA in these patients has been of particular concern due to the large amount of thrombus that can be present in these cases, and the higher risk of clinically significant pulmonary embolism. In fact, mortality secondary to pulmonary embolism has been reported as high as 11%.[30] Li et al pre-treated 16 Budd-Chiari patients with warfarin and found that after 1 year spontaneous fibrinolysis of IVC thrombus occurred in the majority of these patients. Those who did not have spontaneous resolution with warfarin, 2 of the 16 patients, underwent subsequent PTA with excellent results. No patients evaluated were noted to have a pulmonary embolism during this time period.[31] It appears that anticoagulation prior to PTA is an effective treatment of IVC obstruction in this subset of patients. More widespread studies are needed before this can be extrapolated to other benign conditions of IVC occlusion.

MANAGEMENT OF IVC OCCLUSION IN LIVER TRANSPLANTATION

IVC obstruction following liver transplantation is a complication that occurs in 1–2% of liver transplantations. Early occlusion usually occurs in the first several months following transplantation and is secondary to technical factors at or adjacent to the anastomotic segment causing stenosis, torsion, or compression of the IVC.[32] Late occlusion occurs from intimal hyperplasia or fibrosis at the anastomosis.[32] Early or late occlusion can present with ascites, lower extremity edema, transaminitis, and abdominal pain. If not treated, IVC occlusion above the hepatic venous inflow can result in passive hepatic congestion and can lead to liver graft failure.

Treatment options of IVC obstruction secondary to liver transplants include surgical revision of the anastomotic site, retransplantation, and endovascular angioplasty with or without stent placement.[33] Due to the high rate of morbidity and mortality associated with invasive surgical revisions, endovascular management of the occlusion is preferred in many cases.[33] The endovascular approach does carry specific concerns for the risk of anastomotic disruption or dehiscence during balloon expansion, especially in the early postoperative period.[34]

Endovascular management of these cases has continued to gain favor over surgical options in recent years, and now usually consists of angioplasty with primary stent placement.[33] Lee et al evaluated 14 patients with IVC occlusion after liver transplantation. The median interval between transplantation and stent placement was 32 days. Stent placement was successful in all patients, with continued patency seen on computed tomography 65.3 months after IVC stent placement.[35] IVC stent placement appears to be a safe and effective treatment in the management of IVC occlusion secondary to liver transplantation, with excellent long term patency rates.

POST PROCEDURE FOLLOW-UP

A regular regimen of noninvasive vascular imaging should be undertaken to assess for restenosis and allow for early reintervention prior to recurrent complete occlusion. While redilation or restenting of an in-stent stenosis is a routine procedure, recanalization of a reoccluded stent lumen can be far more difficult. It is important to warn patients about signs of recurrent stenosis should they arise, as this may lead to higher rates of compliance with follow-up visits. Although the initial procedures are often technically challenging and often provide only temporary clinical relief, endovascular treatment of caval occlusions is a highly rewarding endeavor that can result in dramatic symptom improvement for patients with few other options. With close clinical and imaging follow-up and early intervention for recurrent disease, endovascular therapy can often provide durable long-term symptomatic relief.

REFERENCES

1. Rice TW, Rodriguez RM, Light RW. The superior vena cava syndrome: clinical characteristics and evolving etiology. *Medicine* 2006. 85(1):37–42.
2. Siegfried MS, Rochester D, Bernstein JR, Miller JW. Diagnosis of inferior vena cava anomalies by computerized tomography. *Comput Radiol* 1983;7:119–123
3. Raju S, Hollis K, Neglen P. Obstructive lesions of the inferior vena cava: clinical features and endovenous treatment. *J Vasc Surg* 2006; 44(4):820–7.
4. Forauer AR, Theoharis C. Histologic changes in the human vein wall adjacent to indwelling central venous catheters. *J Vasc Interv Radiol* 2003;14(9 Pt 1):1163.
5. Grassi CJ, Swan TL, Cardella JF, et al. Quality improvement guidelines for percutaneous permanent inferior vena cava filter placement for the prevention of pulmonary embolism. *J Vasc Interv Radiol* 2001;12:137–141.
6. McClure CFW, Butler EG. The development of vena cava inferior in man. *Am J Anat* 1925; 35:331–383.
7. Raju S, Fredericks R. Venous obstruction: an analysis of one hundred thirty-seven cases with hemodynamic, venographic, and clinical correlations. *J Vasc Surg* 1991;14:305–313.
8. Kandpal H, Sharma R, Gamangatti S, Srivastava DN, Vashisht S. Imaging the inferior vena cava: a road less traveled. *Radiographics* 2008 May-Jun;28(3):669–89.
9. Gillespie DL. Iliocaval stenting. In: Kibbe MR, Pearce WH, Yao JST, editors. *Modern Trends in Vascular Surgery: Venous Disorders.* Connecticut: People's Medical Publishing House; 2010. pp. 273–280.
10. Neglen P, Thrasher TL, Raju S. Venous outflow obstruction: An underestimated contributor to chronic venous disease. *J Vasc Surg* 2003;38(5):879–885.
11. Anderson FA, Spencer FA. Risk Factors for Venous Thromboembolism. *Circulation* 2003; 107(23 Suppl 1):I9–16
12. Koster T, Rosendaal FR, de Ronde H, et al. Venous thrombosis due to poor anticoagulant response to activated protein C: Leiden Thrombophilia Study. *Lancet* 1993;342:1503–1506.
13. Poort SR, Rosendaal FR, Reitsma, et al. A common genetic variation in the 3 -untranslated region of the prothrombin gene is associated with elevated plasma prothrombin levels and an increase in venous thrombosis. *Blood* 1996;88:3698–3703.
14. Mateo J, Oliver A, Borrell M, Sala N, Fontcuberta J. Laboratory evaluation and clinical characteristics of 2,132 consecutive unselected patients with venous thromboembolism--results of the Spanish Multicentric Study on Thrombophilia (EMET-Study). *Thromb Haemost* 1997; 77(3):444.
15. Alimi YS, DiMauro P, Fabre D, Juhan C. Iliac vein reconstructions to treat acute and chronic venoocclusive disease. *J Vasc Surg* 1997;25:673–81.
16. Juhan C, Hartung O, Alimi Y, et al. Treatment of nonmalignant obstructive iliocaval lesions by stent placement: mid-term results. *Ann Vasc Surg* 2001;15:227–32.
17. Sato M, Yamada R, Tsuji, et al. Percutaneous transluminal angioplasty in segmental obstruction of the hepatic inferior vena cava: long-term results. *Cardiovasc Inter Rad* 1990;13:189–92.
18. Hendricks DE, Hagspiel KD. Cryoplasty for the Treatment of In-Stent Renal Artery Stenosis? *Tex Heart Inst J* 2008;35:489–491.

19. Neglen P, Raju S. Balloon dilation and stenting of chronic iliac vein obstruction: technical aspects and early clinical outcome. *J Endovasc Ther* 2000;7:79–91.
20. Funaki et al. Using pullback pressure measurements to identify venous stenoses persisting after successful angioplasty in failing hemodialysis grafts. *AJR Am J Roentgenol* 2002;178(5): 1161–65.
21. Hartung O, Otero A, Boufi M, et al. Mid-term results of endovascular treatment for symptomatic chronic nonmalignant iliocaval venous occlusive disease. *J Vasc Surg* 2005 Dec;42(6): 1138–44.
22. Te Riele WW, Overtoom TT, van der Berg JC, et al. Endovascular recanalization of chronic long-segment occlusions of the inferior vena cava: midterm results. *J Endovasc Ther* 2006; 13(2):249–53.
23. Gaines PA, Belli AM, Anderson PB, et al. Superior vena caval obstruction managed by the Gianturco Z stent. *Clin Radiol* 1994;49:202–6.
24. Kumar NG, Dugan MM, Illig KA, et al. Lower extremity arteriovenous fistula with central venous stenosis iliocaval stenting to treat venous outflow obstruction. *J Vasc Surg* 2011; 53(2):487–8.
25. Oderich GS, Treiman GS, Schneider P, et al. Stent placement for treatment of central and peripheral venous obstruction: a long term multi-institutional experience. *J Vasc Surg* 2000; 32:760–9.
26. O'Sullivan GJ, Lohan DA, Cronin CG, et al. Stent implantation across the ostia of the renal veins does not necessarily cause renal impairment when treating inferior vena cava occlusion. *J Vasc Interv Radiol* 2007;18(7):905–8.
27. Zamora CA, Sugimoto K, Mori T, et al. Use of the wallstent for symptomatic relief of malignant inferior vena cava obstructions. *Radiat Med* 2005;23(5):380–5.
28. Janssen HL, Garcia-Pagan JC, Elias E, et al. Budd-Chiari syndrome: a review by an expert panel. *J Hepatol* 2003;38(3):364–71.
29. Venbrux AC, Mitchell SE, Savander SJ, et al. Long-term results with the use of metallic stents in the inferior vena cava for treatment of Budd-Chiari syndrome. *J Vasc Interv Radiol* 1994;5: 411–6.
30. Baijal SS, Roy S, Phadke RV, et al. Management of idiopathic Budd-Chiari syndrome with primary stent placement: early results. *J Vasc Interv Radiol* 1996;7(4):545–53.
31. Li T, Zhang WW, Bai W, et al. Warfarin anticoagulation before angioplasty relieves thrombus burden in Budd-Chiari syndrome caused by inferior vena cava anastomotic obstruction. *J Vasc Surg* 2010;52(5):1242–5.
32. Berger H, Hilbertz T, Zuhlke K, Forst H, Pratschke E. Balloon dilatation and stent placement of suprahepatic caval anastomotic stenosis following liver transplantation. *Cardiovasc Inter Rad* 1993;16(6):384–387.
33. Tasse J, Borge M, Pierce K, Brems J. Safe and effective treatment of early suprahepatic inferior vena caval outflow compromise following orthotopic liver transplantation using percutaneous transluminal angioplasty and stent placement. *Angiology* 2011;62(1):46–8.
34. Saeb-Parsy K, Jah A, Butler A, et al. Use of a donor aortic interposition allograft to treat stenosis of the suprahepatic inferior vena cava after liver transplantation. *Liver Transpl* 2009; 15(6):662–665.
35. Lee JM, Ko GY, Kyu-Bo G, et al. Long-term efficacy of stent placement for treating inferior vena cava stenosis following liver transplantation. *Liver Transpl* 2010;16(4):513–9.

33

The Importance of Iliofemoral Thrombosis on Chronic Venous Disease

Emily A. Wood, MD, Rafael D. Malgor, MD, RPVI, Nicos Labropoulos PHD, DIC, RVT and Antonios P. Gasparis MD, RVT

INTRODUCTION

Deep vein thrombosis (DVT) is an important cause of disability and mortality in Western societies.[1] Risk factors for developing acute DVT include recent surgery, immobilization, pregnancy, malignancy, trauma, and obesity.[2] The incidence of post-thrombotic syndrome (PTS) and venous ulcers continues to rise, generating an estimated annual cost of 200 million dollars.[3]

Understanding the pathophysiology of DVT is essential for prompt diagnosis and appropriate treatment. Recently, several authors have demonstrated the impact of location and amount of thrombus, or thrombus load, on post-thrombotic sequelae.[4-6] Patients with proximal DVT, mainly those with iliac vein thrombosis, have an increased risk of pulmonary embolism (PE), recurrence of venous thromboembolism (VTE), and PTS.[5-9]

In this chapter, we expand upon the clinical presentation that is specific to iliac vein thrombosis discussing its implications with regard to outcomes and available treatment options.

NATURAL HISTORY

Chronic venous disease (CVD) is caused by venous hypertension as a result of reflux, obstruction, or a combination of reflux and obstruction. Secondary venous disease resulting from a venous thrombosis with endothelial and valve damage with or without reflux or unresolved obstruction is a well-established etiology.[10-11] Predictive factors of severity in patients sustaining DVT include extensive thrombosis at first episode, ipsilateral recurrent

DVT, and sub-therapeutic levels of anticoagulation.[12] The prevalence of primary venous disease accounts for over 70% of all CVD. Attention should also be paid to secondary CVD, as it progresses much more rapidly than primary.[13]

Calf DVT and iliac vein thrombosis are described as different stages along the same continuum.[14] In about 15-20% of symptomatic untreated calf DVT, thrombus may extend into the proximal veins. Therefore, the understanding of continuity and propagation of thrombus from calf veins must prompt close surveillance or more prompt treatment in selected patients. In addition to that knowledge, distal thrombi rarely cause symptomatic PE, while iliofemoral vein thromboses cause PE that can be diagnosed clinically in about half of the patients. Patients who have symptomatic PE have a DVT in about 70% of the cases, with two-thirds of these being proximal.[15] Iliofemoral thrombosis is more common on the left side with a left: right ratio of 2:1 to 3:1. This is because compression of the iliac veins is more common on the left side.[16]

DVT recanalization rate differs according to location of thrombosis. The recanalization rate between proximal and distal DVT was assessed in 51 patients over a 5-year period by Asbeutah *et al*. Twenty-six limbs with proximal involvement had slower thrombus resolution rate at 1 week and at 6 months compared to 28 limbs with isolated distal DVT (34% and 85% versus 67% and 100%). However, similar recanalization rates at 5 years (96% versus 100%) were reported.[17] Limbs with proximal DVT had worse clinical outcome with 56% developing skin damage (CEAP 4-6) at 60 months, while only 11% of the limbs with distal DVT were found to have skin damage.[17] Reflux was present in 96% of patients with proximal DVT and in only 36% of those with distal DVT.[17]

Recurrence is a very important factor in the natural history of DVT that must be considered while planning treatment. Unprovoked DVT is the strongest risk factor for recurrence.[4, 18] Other series also showed that a *combination* of proximal and distal thrombus increases the risk of recurrent DVT.[5] In a prospective, multicenter study enrolling 387 patients, risk for recurrence was also higher in patients with proximal DVT compared to those with distal DVT (univariate HR, 2.4 [CI, 1.1 to 5.6]; $P < 0.036$).[6]

IMPACT AND SIGNIFICANCE

Proximal thrombi have an important impact on social and economic aspects of our society.[19] They result in more severe and long-lasting patient morbidities than those with popliteal or below knee DVT.[9] The incidence of recurrence is higher in proximal DVT than in distal DVT. Recanalization in post-thrombotic veins results in chronic luminal changes such as valve dysfunction, stenosis and webs in about two-thirds of the patients, who may then go on to develop a combination of partial obstruction and reflux.[7, 10] The thrombus load is much greater in proximal veins. van Ramshorst *et al* in a prospective longitudinal study showed an exponential thrombus regression rate in the femoropopliteal segments and an even greater rate in distal segments.[20]

The amount of residual disease and the degree of recanalization depend upon the vein segment involved with a higher recanalization rate in calf veins due to the calf muscle pump. The impact of thrombus location and a higher incidence of PE associated with iliofemoral DVT compared to other locations was shown by Douketis *et al* in a study of 1,149 patients with symptomatic proximal DVT.[21] At 3 months, the rate of iliofemoral venous thromboembolic events, including PE, was 5.1% in patients with popliteal DVT, 5.3% in patients with femoral DVT, and 11.8% in patients with iliofemoral DVT.[21] More importantly, iliofemoral DVT resulted in a two-fold increased risk of recurrent VTE (OR 2.4, $p= 0.06$).[21] Examples of iliofemoral thrombosis are shown in Figure 33–1.

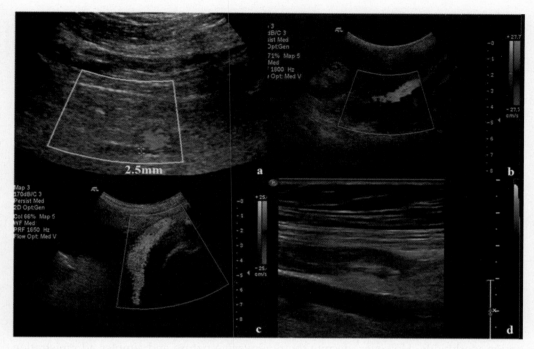

Figure 33–1. Examples of iliofemoral vein obstruction. **A** Acute iliac vein thrombosis in a patient that underwent spine surgery and presented with left lower extremity pain and swelling. The left common iliac vein is compressed by the right common iliac artery. At the site of compression the vein lumen measured 2.5mm. **B** Acute iliofemoral thrombosis in a patient who presented with significant thigh swelling. The iliac vein is seen below the artery. It is dilated and has echolucent material, indicating acute thrombosis. **C** Chronic iliofemoral obstruction on a patient who had skin discoloration (CEAP C4) and venous claudication. He had a documented episode of DVT 5 years earlier extending from the common iliac to the calf veins. **D** Acute on chronic thrombosis of the femoral vein on a patient who had a documented iliofemoral thrombosis extending into the popliteal vein. The vein is dilated and has echolucent (fresh thrombus) and echogenic (chronic thrombus) material.

To determine the chronological changes of venous physiology following proximal DVT, one study followed 20 patients with acute iliofemoral vein thrombosis for over 5 years who received conventional anticoagulation. The results of the study revealed that even after 5 years, 70% of the patients had obstructive lesions of the iliac veins with only minor changes occurring during that time. Furthermore, they concluded that although venous outflow continuously improves with conventional anticoagulation following iliofemoral thrombosis, valvular competence and muscle pump function are consistently pathological. This creates severe venous hypertension with a risk of PTS sequelae.[22] PTS occurs in as many as 30% to 60% of patients presenting with proximal DVT.[4]

Outcomes of patients with DVT also depend to a great degree on both location and single versus multiple thrombosed segments. The likelihood of recanalization and, in turn, the likelihood of avoiding the development of PTS sequelae decreases as the location of the thrombosed segment moves proximally.[7] Some studies found that nearly 95% of popliteal or calf DVT and >50% of femoral DVT recanalize spontaneously and completely.[23] In contrast, less than 20% of iliac vein thromboses recanalize, rendering the vein completely patent with no luminal obstructions.[24]

Development of PTS is more frequently seen in patients sustaining iliofemoral DVT than those who have either popliteal or calf DVT.[6-7, 25] Labropoulos *et al* analyzed 120 limbs with a first episode of DVT and found a higher incidence of PTS in patients with thrombosis in multiple segments. Venous claudication was present only when iliac veins were involved (7/37 iliofemoral DVT vs. 0/40 femoropopliteal DVT, p=0.004).[7] No patient with isolated common femoral, iliac or IVC thrombosis developed venous claudication. Another prospective study of 1,412 patients with an initial DVT episode revealed a 1.3-fold higher risk of developing PTS when a patient sustains an iliofemoral DVT compared to a popliteal vein DVT (RR 1.3, 95% CI 1.1– 1.6).[25] A multicenter Canadian study enrolling 387 patients showed that patients with more severe PTS (as measured by the Villalta score) were found to have a common femoral or iliac vein DVT rather than a calf DVT (2.23 increase in score for iliofemoral versus distal DVT; P< 0.001).[6]

TREATMENT AND OUTCOMES

The ultimate goal of treating iliofemoral vein thrombosis is to prevent venous reflux and/or obstruction, recurrent thrombosis and the development of PTS. Current available treatment options are anticoagulation, venous thrombectomy, and systemic or catheter-directed thrombolysis (CDT). Anticoagulation is the most commonly used treatment option worldwide. However, despite the noninvasive nature and simpler administration protocols, the efficacy of unfractionated heparin or LMWH for iliac thrombosis is modest due to its slow acting-mechanism, particularly when a large thrombus burden is present.

The first operative procedure employed to attempt thrombus removal was open venous thrombectomy. The procedure is associated with incomplete thrombus removal and significant local wound complications. Currently, it is reserved for patients who are not candidates for endovenous thrombolysis and risk impending venous gangrene, with the specific aim of limb salvage. A multicenter trial enrolling 51 patients randomized for anticoagulation and thrombectomy showed higher iliac vein patency (76% vs 35%; P<.03) and preservation of valve function (52% vs 26%; P<.05) in patients treated with venous thrombectomy with temporary arteriovenous fistula.[26] Hybrid open-endovascular technique using balloon angioplasty and stenting following open venous thrombectomy has also been described with good results.[27]

CDT has been shown to be more efficient in removing thrombus than systemic intravenous thrombolysis. The local delivery of thrombolytics allows a higher concentration of medication within the thrombus which decreases the risk of bleeding. Pharmacomechanical thrombolysis (PhMT) has been added to CDT to further decrease infusion time and bleeding complications and improve results by fragmenting the thrombus and thus increasing surface contact with the thrombolytics. In comparing PhMT to CDT in 93 patients, Lin *et al* found similar treatment success, with a mean thrombolytic infusion time in the CDT group of 18 ± 8 hours compared to 76 ± 34 minutes with PhMT. There was a decreased blood transfusion requirement in the PhMT group compared to the CDT patients (0.2 packed red blood cell units vs. 1.2 units, p< 0.05) and a decreased ICU stay (0.6 days vs. 2.4 days, p<0.04).[28]

In the current treatment scenario of iliac vein thrombosis, endovenous thrombectomy and thrombolysis has gained popularity due to its minimally invasive approach, higher local concentration of thrombolytic medication and consequently faster thrombus load dissolution. Patients with extensive acute iliofemoral DVT, less than 14 days from onset of symptoms or acute findings on DUS, life expectancy >1 year with good functional status, and low risk of bleeding are potential candidates.[29-30]

Two trials looked at venous patency and reflux following thrombolysis. Elsharawy *et al* in a randomized trial of 35 patients comparing CDT with anticoagulation to anticoagulation alone demonstrated that CDT offered better short-term outcome.[31] Patients were followed with duplex and at 6 months those treated with CDT had a better patency rate (72% vs. 12%, p< 0.001). Venous reflux was higher in patients treated with anticoagulation than with CDT (41% vs. 11%, p= 0.04). Schweizer *et al* randomized 250 patients to thrombolysis or anticoagulation, comparting local versus systemic therapy in both study arms. They found that systemic thrombolysis had higher rates of recanalization and lower rates of reflux and PTS at 12 months of follow-up than anticoagulation alone.[32]

The resolution of the thrombus load in patients sustaining iliac or iliofemoral vein DVT who underwent CDT compared to those who were only anticoagulated with heparin was demonstrated by the randomized control trial CaVenT (**Ca**theter-directed **Ve**nous **T**hrombolysis). In this study of 118 patients, the iliofemoral patency was higher (64% vs 36%; $P<0.004$) and the functional venous obstruction rate lower (20% vs 49%; $P<0.004$) in the CDT group compared to patients on anticoagulation.[33]

Improvement in venous function may help prevent development of PTS and thus improve quality of life. Comerota *et al* compared 68 patients treated for proximal DVT with CDT (identified through a registry from multiple institutions) to 30 patients treated with anticoagulation (identified through medical chart review). Patients who underwent thrombolysis reported better overall physical functioning, fewer stigmata, less health distress and fewer post-thrombotic symptoms when compared to the anticoagulation group. Quality-of-life results were directly related to the initial success of thrombolysis.[34] In a review of patients with iliofemoral acute DVT undergoing PhMT, Gasparis *et al* had comparable findings with 13 of 14 patients (93%) having minimal or no disability (venous disability score, VDS < 1)) as well as low venous clinical severity score (VCSS). None of the patients had advanced clinical signs of venous insufficiency (C4-C6), with only two patients (14%) having persistent swelling (C3) during follow-up.[35]

Chronic venous outflow obstruction following iliofemoral DVT plays a significant role in the development of PTS and venous claudication. When looking at patients with advanced CVD (C5-6), Marston *et al* reported that 37% of imaging studies[36] demonstrated ilio-caval venous outflow obstruction of at least 50%, and 23% had obstruction of >80%. This has significant impact in the management of patients with advanced CVD. Recognizing that these patients may have an underlying obstruction in the proximal segment should lead to further investigation.

Treatment with endovenous techniques to relieve the underlying obstruction can result in significant clinical improvement with relief of venous claudication, improvement in leg pain and swelling, and healing of venous ulcers if recent. Delis *et al* evaluated 23 limbs in 16 patients who underwent iliac vein stenting and compared results to those of the control group (contralateral limbs).[37] At 8.4 months (IQR, 2-11.8 months), venous outflow and calf muscle pump function had both improved (P < 0.001). The CEAP status had also improved (P < 0.05) from a median class C3 [range, C3-C6; IQR, C3-C5 (distribution, C6; 6; C4: 4; C3: 13)] before intervention to C2 [range, C2-C6; IQR, C2-C4.5 (distribution, C6: 1; C5: 5; C4: 4; C2: 13)] after intervention. Incapacitating venous claudication noted in 62.5% (10 of 16, 95% CI, 35.8%–89.1%) of patients (15 of 23 limbs; 65.2%, 95% CI, 44.2%–86.3%) before stenting was eliminated in all after stenting (P < 0.001).[37]

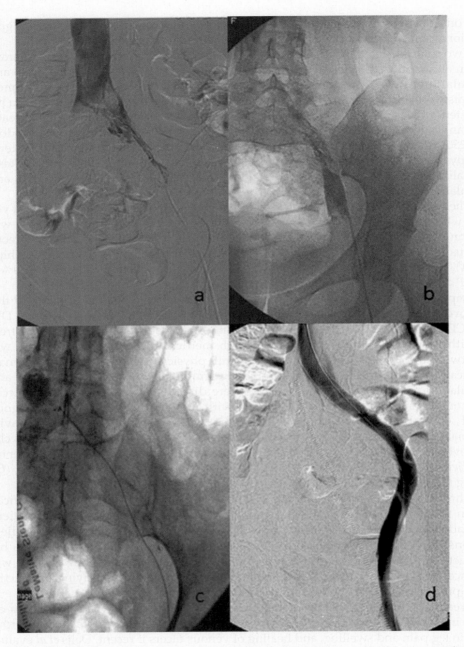

Figure 33–2. Venographic images of a 55 year-old female patient who presented with left lower extremity edema and pain. **A,B** Extensive iliofemoral DVT is depicted in the diagnostic venogram. **C** Pharmaco-mechanical thrombectomy with a 30-cm Trellis® catheter parked proximal to the thrombus with the proximal balloon inflated to isolate the segment to be thrombectomized. **D** Completion venogram following deployment of 16x60mm Wallstent showing no stenosis or residual thrombus.

CONCLUSION

Iliac vein thrombosis carries a significant negative socioeconomic impact, generating a substantial financial burden on the healthcare system. It also entails a higher likelihood of developing PTS and pulmonary emboli.

While direct evidence of the influence of proximal thrombosis on chronic venous disease is not available, its significant contribution can be inferred at this time. Two ongoing prospective clinical trials will help elucidate its impact. The Dutch CaVA trial (**Ca**theter **V**ersus **A**nticoagulation Alone for Acute Primary Iliofemoral DVT) aims to show improvement in health-related quality of life (HRQOL)—in particular, a reduction in the incidence of PTS—by using early thrombolysis instead of conventional anticoagulation medical therapy for treatment of acute iliofemoral DVT (http://clinical trials.gov/ct2/show/NCT00970619). Similarly, the ATTRACT trial (**A**cute Venous **T**hrombosis: **T**hrombus **R**emoval with **A**djunctive **C**atheter-Directed **T**hrombolysis) is designed to determine if the initial use of CDT in symptomatic patients with acute proximal DVT reduces the incidence of PTS, within a 2-year follow-up period.[38]

Understanding the limitations of anticoagulation in patients with iliac vein thrombosis who have a large thrombus load, as well as prompt identification of situations in which endovascular thrombectomy and thrombolysis are indicated, may reduce the incidence of PTS in the future.

REFERENCES

1. Prandoni P, Kahn SR. Post-thrombotic syndrome: prevalence, prognostication and need for progress. *Br J Haematol* 2009;145(3):286–295.
2. Heit JA, Silverstein MD, Mohr DN, Petterson TM, O'Fallon WM, Melton LJ, 3rd. Risk factors for deep vein thrombosis and pulmonary embolism: a population-based case-control study. *Arch Intern Med* 2000;160(6):809–815.
3. Heit JA, Rooke TW, Silverstein MD, Mohr DN, Lohse CM, Petterson TM, O'Fallon WM, Melton LJ, 3rd. Trends in the incidence of venous stasis syndrome and venous ulcer: a 25-year population-based study. *J Vasc Surg* 2001;33(5):1022–1027.
4. Prandoni P, Noventa F, Ghirarduzzi A, Pengo V, Bernardi E, Pesavento R, Iotti M, Tormene D, Simioni P, Pagnan A. The risk of recurrent venous thromboembolism after discontinuing anticoagulation in patients with acute proximal deep vein thrombosis or pulmonary embolism. A prospective cohort study in 1,626 patients. *Haematologica* 2007;92(2):199–205.
5. Labropoulos N, Jen J, Jen H, Gasparis AP, Tassiopoulos AK. Recurrent deep vein thrombosis: long-term incidence and natural history. *Ann Surg* 2010;251(4):749–753.
6. Kahn SR, Shrier I, Julian JA, Ducruet T, Arsenault L, Miron MJ, Roussin A, Desmarais S, Joyal F, Kassis J, Solymoss S, Desjardins L, Lamping DL, Johri M, Ginsberg JS. Determinants and time course of the postthrombotic syndrome after acute deep venous thrombosis. *Ann Intern Med* 2008;149(10):698–707.
7. Labropoulos N, Waggoner T, Sammis W, Samali S, Pappas PJ. The effect of venous thrombus location and extent on the development of post-thrombotic signs and symptoms. *J Vasc Surg* 2008;48(2):407–412.
8. Yamaki T, Nozaki M. Patterns of venous insufficiency after an acute deep vein thrombosis. *J Am Coll Surg* 2005;201(2):231–238.
9. Stain M, Schonauer V, Minar E, Bialonczyk C, Hirschl M, Weltermann A, Kyrle PA, Eichinger S. The post-thrombotic syndrome: risk factors and impact on the course of thrombotic disease. *J Thromb Haemost* 2005;3(12):2671–2676.

10. Meissner MH, Eklof B, Smith PC, Dalsing MC, DePalma RG, Gloviczki P, Moneta G, Neglen P, T OD, Partsch H, Raju S. Secondary chronic venous disorders. *J Vasc Surg* 2007;46 Suppl S: 68S-83S.

11. Raffetto JD, Khalil RA. Mechanisms of varicose vein formation: valve dysfunction and wall dilation. *Phlebology* 2008;23(2):85–98.

12. Ziegler S, Schillinger M, Maca TH, Minar E. Post-thrombotic syndrome after primary event of deep venous thrombosis 10 to 20 years ago. *Thromb Res* 2001;101(2):23–33.

13. Labropoulos N, Gasparis AP, Pefanis D, Leon LR, Jr., Tassiopoulos AK. Secondary chronic venous disease progresses faster than primary. *J Vasc Surg* 2009;49(3):704–710.

14. Kearon C. Natural history of venous thromboembolism. *Circulation* 2003;107(23 Suppl 1): I22–30.

15. Kearon C, Ginsberg JS, Hirsh J. The role of venous ultrasonography in the diagnosis of suspected deep venous thrombosis and pulmonary embolism. *Ann Intern Med* 1998;129(12): 1044–1049.

16. Mewissen MW, Seabrook GR, Meissner MH, Cynamon J, Labropoulos N, Haughton SH. Catheter-directed thrombolysis for lower extremity deep venous thrombosis: report of a national multicenter registry. *Radiology* 1999;211(1):39–49.

17. Asbeutah AM, Riha AZ, Cameron JD, McGrath BP. Five-year outcome study of deep vein thrombosis in the lower limbs. *J Vasc Surg* 2004;40(6):1184–1189.

18. Palareti G, Cosmi B. Predicting the risk of recurrence of venous thromboembolism. *Curr Opin Hematol* 2004;11(3):192–197.

19. Kahn SR, Shbaklo H, Lamping DL, Holcroft CA, Shrier I, Miron MJ, Roussin A, Desmarais S, Joyal F, Kassis J, Solymoss S, Desjardins L, Johri M, Ginsberg JS. Determinants of health-related quality of life during the 2 years following deep vein thrombosis. *J Thromb Haemost* 2008;6(7):1105–1112.

20. van Ramshorst B, van Bemmelen PS, Hoeneveld H, Faber JA, Eikelboom BC. Thrombus regression in deep venous thrombosis. Quantification of spontaneous thrombolysis with duplex scanning. *Circulation* 1992;86(2):414–419.

21. Douketis JD, Crowther MA, Foster GA, Ginsberg JS. Does the location of thrombosis determine the risk of disease recurrence in patients with proximal deep vein thrombosis? *Am J Med* 2001;110(7):515–519.

22. Akesson H, Brudin L, Dahlstrom JA, Eklof B, Ohlin P, Plate G. Venous function assessed during a 5 year period after acute ilio-femoral venous thrombosis treated with anticoagulation. *Eur J Vasc Surg* 1990;4(1):43–48.

23. Thomas ML, McAllister V. The radiological progression of deep venous thrombus. *Radiology* 1971;99(1):37–40.

24. Mavor GE, Galloway JM. Iliofemoral venous thrombosis. Pathological considerations and surgical management. *Br J Surg* 1969;56(1):45–59.

25. Tick LW, Kramer MH, Rosendaal FR, Faber WR, Doggen CJ. Risk factors for post-thrombotic syndrome in patients with a first deep venous thrombosis. *J Thromb Haemost* 2008;6(12):2075–2081.

26. Plate G, Einarsson E, Ohlin P, Jensen R, Qvarfordt P, Eklof B. Thrombectomy with temporary arteriovenous fistula: the treatment of choice in acute iliofemoral venous thrombosis. *J Vasc Surg* 1984;1(6):867–876.

27. Hartung O, Benmiloud F, Barthelemy P, Dubuc M, Boufi M, Alimi YS. Late results of surgical venous thrombectomy with iliocaval stenting. *J Vasc Surg* 2008;47(2):381–387.

28. Lin PH, Zhou W, Dardik A, Mussa F, Kougias P, Hedayati N, Naoum JJ, El Sayed H, Peden EK, Huynh TT. Catheter-direct thrombolysis versus pharmacomechanical thrombectomy for treatment of symptomatic lower extremity deep venous thrombosis. *Am J Surg* 2006;192(6):782–788.

29. Kearon C, Kahn SR, Agnelli G, Goldhaber S, Raskob GE, Comerota AJ. Antithrombotic therapy for venous thromboembolic disease: American College of Chest Physicians Evidence-Based Clinical Practice Guidelines (8th Edition). *Chest* 2008;133(6 Suppl):454S-545S.

30. Klein SJ, Gasparis AP, Virvilis D, Ferretti JA, Labropoulos N. Prospective determination of candidates for thrombolysis in patients with acute proximal deep vein thrombosis. *J Vasc Surg;* 51(4):908–912.

31. Elsharawy M, Elzayat E. Early results of thrombolysis vs anticoagulation in iliofemoral venous thrombosis. A randomised clinical trial. *Eur J Vasc Endovasc Surg* 2002;24(3): 209–214.

32. Schweizer J, Kirch W, Koch R, Elix H, Hellner G, Forkmann L, Graf A. Short- and long-term results after thrombolytic treatment of deep venous thrombosis. *J Am Coll Cardiol* 2000;36(4): 1336–1343.

33. Enden T, Klow NE, Sandvik L, Slagsvold CE, Ghanima W, Hafsahl G, Holme PA, Holmen LO, Njaastad AM, Sandbaek G, Sandset PM. Catheter-directed thrombolysis vs. anticoagulant therapy alone in deep vein thrombosis: results of an open randomized, controlled trial reporting on short-term patency. *J Thromb Haemost* 2009;7(8):1268–1275.

34. Comerota AJ, Throm RC, Mathias SD, Haughton S, Mewissen M. Catheter-directed thrombolysis for iliofemoral deep venous thrombosis improves health-related quality of life. *J Vasc Surg* 2000;32(1):130–137.

35. Gasparis AP, Labropoulos N, Tassiopoulos AK, Phillips B, Pagan J, Cheng L, Ricotta J. Midterm follow-up after pharmacomechanical thrombolysis for lower extremity deep venous thrombosis. *Vasc Endovasc Surg* 2009;43(1):61–68.

36. Marston W. Summary of evidence of effectiveness of primary chronic venous disease treatment. *J Vasc Surg* 2010;52(5 Suppl):54S-58S.

37. Delis KT, Bjarnason H, Wennberg PW, Rooke TW, Gloviczki P. Successful iliac vein and inferior vena cava stenting ameliorates venous claudication and improves venous outflow, calf muscle pump function, and clinical status in post-thrombotic syndrome. *Ann Surg* 2007;245(1):130–139.

38. Comerota AJ. The ATTRACT trial: rationale for early intervention for iliofemoral DVT. *Perspect Vasc Surg Endovasc Ther* 2009;21(4):221–224; quiz 224–225.

34

Endovascular Treatment of Pulmonary Embolism

Marlene Mathews, MD and David L. Gillespie, MD

INTRODUCTION

Acute major pulmonary embolism (PE) has a high mortality rate despite recent advances in diagnosis and treatment. Although the lethality of PE is comparable to that of acute myocardial infarction, its mortality has changed relatively little in thirty years.[1] Patients who present with hemodynamic shock can have a mortality rate of up to 58%, and the majority of deaths from acute massive PE occur within 1 hour of presentation.[2]

The spectrum of pulmonary embolism ranges widely, from asymptomatic patients with microemboli in small peripheral pulmonary arterioles, to hemodynamically unstable patients with large saddle emboli obstructing the proximal pulmonary trunk. The primary difficulty with recommending the optimal treatment strategy for PE lies with correctly identifying the patient population that will derive the most benefit from intervention.[3] Outcomes vary widely depending on patient characteristics. Clinical evidence for catheter-directed interventions (CDI) suffers from a lack of randomized and controlled trials, consisting mostly of retrospective reviews, single-institution experiences and case reports. However, many of the studies that cite no difference in outcome between CDI and systemic thrombolysis are low in patient numbers and do not adequately compare a combination of catheter-directed fibrinolysis and fragmentation with systemic treatment.[2]

Here we will review the pathophysiology and definitions of PE, discuss current clinical guidelines and outline the most recent clinical data regarding endovascular treatment.

PATHOPHYSIOLOGY AND CLASSIFICATION

The majority of pulmonary emboli originate from thrombus in the deep veins of the lower extremity and pelvis. Thrombus can embolize through the inferior vena cava (IVC) and right heart, compromising gas exchange and hemodynamic function.[4] The clinical impact of the embolism depends on the severity of the obstruction, the patient's anatomy, the patient's baseline cardiopulmonary status and a variety of compensatory neurohumoral responses.

Most patients who die from acute massive PE suffer from severe pulmonary vascular resistance and right ventricular (RV) afterload as a result of their hypoxemia and compensatory pulmonary vasoconstriction.[5] Indeed, RV failure and increased pressure can impair LV preload and increase myocardial oxygen demand whilst concomitantly limiting its flow. Ventilation-perfusion mismatch, increases in total dead space and right-to-left shunting result in gas exchange abnormalities. These abnormalities are typically an increased alveolar-arterial oxygen gradient and arterial hypoxemia in the setting of hyperventilation and respiratory alkalosis.[6]

Interpreting the guidelines and outcomes data for PE requires a recognition that treatment recommendations depend highly on patient characteristics and clinical presentation. To tailor medical and interventional therapies for PE to the appropriate patients, definitions for subgroups of PE are required. However, these definitions have not been clearly delineated in the literature and this exacerbates the controversy regarding the clinical data.

The 2008 publication by the American College of Chest Physicians, *Evidence-Based Clinical Practice Guidelines Regarding Treatment of PE*, as well as a separate consensus guideline by the *2008 European Society of Cardiology Task Force Regarding PE management*, share many of the same recommendations regarding categorizing patients with massive vs. submassive PE. In March 2011, the American Heart Association assembled a group of physicians to compose a scientific statement on the management of massive and submassive PE. Not unlike the ACCP or European Society, the AHA defines acute *massive* PE as a condition "with sustained hypotension (systolic blood pressure <90 mm Hg for at least 15 minutes or requiring inotropic support, not due to a cause other than PE, such as arrhythmia, hypovolemia, sepsis, or left ventricular [LV] dysfunction), pulselessness, or persistent profound bradycardia (heart rate <40 bpm with signs or symptoms of shock)." Early risk stratification is essential to properly identifying patients with massive PE, who very often have echocardiographic evidence of right heart failure/hypokinesis and CT angiography demonstrating PA dilation in addition to sustained hypotention. *Submassive* PE, on the other hand, is defined as acute PE without systemic hypotension (systolic blood pressure >90mmHg) but with either RV dysfunction (on echo, by increased BNP or EKG changes) or myocardial necrosis (TpnI >0.4ng/mL or TpnT >0.1ng/mL).[3]

Risk stratification of patients with symptomatic PE has been shown to be helpful in deciding which patients are at the highest risk and may therefore benefit from a more aggressive approach. In the ICOPER Registry (International Cooperative Pulmonary Embolism Registry), Goldhaber et al[7] reported on 2454 consecutive eligible patients with acute PE registered from 52 hospitals in seven countries in Europe and North America. The primary outcome measure was all-cause mortality at 3 months. The prognostic effect of baseline factors on survival was assessed with multivariate analyses. This study revealed that patients with RV hypokinesis had a much higher mortality rate (20.9%) than counterparts with normal RV size and function (14.8%)

Similarly, Schoepf et al[8] found Right ventricular enlargement on chest computed tomography to be a predictor of early death in acute pulmonary embolism. *In* 431 consecutive patients with CT diagnosis of PE they found 64% of PE patients had RV enlargement. These patients had higher 30-day mortality than patients with normal

RV size. This subset of PE patients experienced a higher rate of adverse outcomes when compared with patients who had normal RV size

Therefore, based on these definitions, it is preferable to refer to *massive* PE as a PE characterized by dramatic sudden onset of hypotension, tachycardia and respiratory distress. Risk stratification is possible through the use of echocardiography, CT angiography and close hemodynamic monitoring. Submassive PE, on the other hand, can be recognized as PE-related right ventricular (RV) dysfunction and troponin elevation despite normal arterial pressure. Discussions surrounding resuscitation, medical therapy and advanced interventions for PE are specific to these classifications.

OVERVIEW OF TREATMENT STRATEGIES

For patients with hemodynamic instability caused by massive PE, systemic thrombolysis is considered to be the standard of care.[5,9,10] However, contraindications to systemic thrombolysis and the limiting effect of time (at least 2 hours) render this treatment modality implausible in some situations. Clinical evidence for utilizing catheter-directed thrombolysis in patients with massive PE remains scarce.[2,11] A variety of endovascular interventions, including catheter-based thrombolysis and fragmentation, percutaneous pulmonary embolectomy, and IVC filter placement have been reported in the literature for patients with acute PE. The reported mortality rates based on these endovascular techniques vary from 0% to 25%.[1] Because of the variety of endovascular treatment strategies and the lack of a controlled trial, the most efficacious treatment strategy remains unclear. However, a growing body of institutional-specific evidence and retrospective studies is demonstrating safe and beneficial use of catheter-directed interventions (CDIs) for patients with massive PE and hemodynamic compromise. In patients with submassive PE, however, systemic anticoagulation and a case-by-case selection of systemic thrombolysis remains the mainstay of treatment.

SYSTEMIC ANTICOAGULATION AND THROMBOLYSIS

To understand current advances in the treatment of acute massive PE and the need for larger prospective trials comparing endovascular intervention with systemic medical therapy, an appreciation of the clinical evidence in favor of and against these therapeutic modalities is necessary.

For more than 30 years, systemic heparin has been the foundation of treatment for venous thromboembolism (VTE), including both deep vein thrombosis (DVT) and PE.[1] It is still the primary and preferred treatment for patients with submassive PE and those stratified into a low-risk category without significant hemodynamic instability, Heparin prevents thrombus propagation and activates endogenous fibrinolysis to facilitate thrombus dissolution over a time period of weeks to months. Its pharmacokinetics, however, make its titration to therapeutic levels quite a difficult task. Several studies have since shown low-molecular-weight heparin to be as effective or superior to intravenous administration of unfractionated heparin.[12]

The use of thrombolytic agents in acute PE was first reported more than 3 decades ago. In contrast to heparin, thrombolytic agents actively promote hydrolysis of fibrin molecules. All fibrinolytic drugs approved by the FDA are enzymes that convert the patient's native circulating plasminogen into plasmin. Plasmin is a serine protease that cleaves fibrin at several sites, liberating fibrin-split products, including the D-dimer fragment, resulting in rapid thrombus dissolution and more rapid improvement in pulmonary flow with oxygenation as well as RV function. The rationale for fibrinolysis in acute PE is to rapidly reverse hemodynamic compromise and gas exchange dysfunction. In 2010, the FDA label for alteplase (Activase, Genentech, San Francisco, CA) explicitly stated that the agent is indicated for "... massive pulmonary emboli, defined as obstruction of blood flow to a lobe or multiple segments of the lung, or for unstable hemodynamics, i.e., failure to maintain blood pressure without supportive measures."

Despite its widespread use, the benefit of systemic thrombolytic therapy has not been established in prospective randomized trials. The controversy regarding systemic thrombolysis for PE can be attributed to the heterogeneity of studies and their treatment populations. Thirteen placebo-controlled randomized trials of fibrinolysis for acute PE have been published, but only a subset evaluated *massive* PE specifically.[3,13] These trials included 480 patients randomized to fibrinolysis and 464 randomized to placebo; 6 of the 13 trials study alteplase, representing only 56% of all patients. To complicate matters, these 6 studies used variable infusion regimens. Four studies have used intravenous streptokinase, in total only enrolling 94 patients.

A recent meta-analysis of the literature by Wan et al[14] corroborates the lack of a clear role for systemic thrombolysis in the treatment of pulmonary embolus. This study of 11 different trials failed to show any benefit of systemic thrombolysis vs heparin. This study however had a mix of high and low risk patients. A subgroup analysis of pts with major (hemodynamically unstable) pulmonary embolism in the 5 trials however was associated with a significant reduction in pulmonary embolism or death compared to heparin alone (9.4% versus 19.0%; OR 0.45, 95% CI 0.22 to 0.92, number needed to treat 10) but no benefit in the 6 trials that excluded these patients

The decision to administer a fibrinolytic agent in addition to heparin anticoagulation, therefore, requires judicious and educated decision-making on an individual basis to assess benefits versus risks. Potential benefits include more rapid resolution of symptoms (e.g., dyspnea, chest pain, and psychological distress), improvement of respiratory and cardiovascular function without need for mechanical ventilation or vasopressor support, and increased probability of survival. However, major hemorrhage from systemic tissue plasminogen activator (tPA) is approximately 20%, with a 3-5% rate of intracerebral hemorrhage.[15] The current potpourri of clinical data provides limited guidance in establishing contraindications to the use of fibrinolytic agents in PE. Contraindications must therefore be extrapolated from author experience and from guidelines for ST-segment elevation myocardial infarction.

For patients with massive PE who have major contraindications for thrombolysis, such as recent operation, trauma or stroke, urgent pulmonary embolectomy has been described as a viable option.[16-19] This procedure includes a median sternotomy incision, cardiopulmonary bypass, control of the main pulmonary artery and surgical removal of thrombus in the pulmonary artery. The results of embolectomy will be optimized if patients are referred before the onset of cardiogenic shock. Due to a paucity of centers willing to perform successful pulmonary embolectomy for patients with acute massive PE and contraindications to thrombolysis, the data for this operation is fraught by low numbers. However, recent studies, such as those by Vohra et al[18], Fukuda et al[16] and Kawahito et al[17] stress that pulmonary embolectomy is an acceptable treatment modality in a carefully selected patient population with highly specialized and skilled surgeons. It is imperative to avoid blind instrumentation of the fragile pulmonary arteries. Extraction is limited to directly visible thromboembolus, which can be accomplished through the level of the segmental pulmonary arteries. The decision to proceed with surgical embolectomy requires interdisciplinary teamwork, discussion that involves the surgeon and interventionalist, and an assessment of the local expertise. Most of these studies have found that although short-term complication rates are relatively high, once patients recover from the initial insult they have good long-term survival and functional outcomes.

An understudied treatment for quickly decompensating PE-related RV failure or cardiogenic shock is endovascular intervention with either catheter-directed thrombolysis or percutaneous mechanical thrombectomy. Employing treatment paradigms established within the iliofemoral deep vein thrombosis literature, endovascular interventions are seemingly ideal in that they target clot burden directly without incurring the risks of hemorrhage identified with systemic thrombolysis. However, case reports, single-center experiences, retrospective reviews and meta analyses comprise the bulk of the clinical data highlighting these techniques. The field requires larger prospective trials. Despite this limitation however, endovascular interventions should be strongly considered in selected patient populations for *acute massive PE.*

OVERVIEW OF ENDOVASCULAR INTERVENTIONS

Percutaneous techniques to relieve complete and partial occlusions in the pulmonary trunk are potentially life-saving in correctly selected patients with acute massive PE. A variety of endovascular treatment strategies have been reported in the literature for PE,[2,20–22] and although many of the reports are low in patient number, their beneficial outcomes are difficult to ignore. The quandary, however, is that these catheter-directed interventions (CDIs) hinge on careful patient selection and are largely operator-dependent. Large centers with specialists are frequently the only places able to offer these interventions. The implementation of a multi-center prospective trial to demonstrate the efficacy of endovascular treatment of massive PE over systemic thrombolysis has not yet been done. What we can gain from the literature, however, is confidence in the outcomes of massive PE treated with CDI by skilled interventionalists and surgeons. CDI is hugely beneficial in patients with hemodynamic compromise and contraindications to systemic thrombolysis, and when thrombolysis has failed to improve hemodynamics. Combination therapy that includes both catheter-based clot fragmentation and local thrombolysis is an emerging strategy. There are four general categories of percutaneous intervention for removing pulmonary emboli and decreasing thrombus burden: (1) catheter infusion of intrapulmonary thrombolysis, (2) aspiration thrombectomy, (3) thrombus fragmentation, and (4) rheolytic thrombectomy (a combination). The goals of catheter-based therapy are to reduce RV strain and pulmonary vascular resistance, in turn increasing systemic perfusion, limiting the alveolar-arterial oxygen gradient and reversing RV failure.

Catheter-Directed Thrombolysis

Catheter-directed thrombolysis with intrapulmonary thrombolytic infusion in patients with acute massive PE has been reported in several studies with overall success.[1] CDT involves selective infusion catheter placement in the pulmonary artery, followed by continuous infusion of thrombolytic drugs over a period of time. The treatment objective is to accelerate thrombus dissolution and achieve rapid reperfusion of the pulmonary arteries.

However, findings from the ICOPER suggested that patients with massive PE treated with in situ thrombolysis might not experience any survival advantage or reduction in major cardiovascular events. A partial explanation for this data is that in situ thrombolysis still carries significant hemorrhage risk without allowing thrombolytics to adequately access the clot. Schmitz-Rode et al[23] demonstrated with in vitro and in vivo flow studies that an obstructing pulmonary embolus causes a proximal vortex that prevents a drug infused upstream from reaching the downstream embolus; instead there is rapid washout of thrombolytics into the pulmonary vasculature. In an ideal scenario, this catheter-directed intervention results in hemodynamic improvement with restoration of RV hypokinesis, normalization of RV size, and reduction of abnormally high pulmonary arterial pressures, but in reality this may not be the case. Instead, newer catheter-directed therapies, designed to increase the surface area of contact between the clot and the thrombolytics, are becoming increasingly favorable.

Aspiration Thrombectomy

Aspiration thrombectomy uses sustained suction applied to the catheter tip to secure and remove the thrombus.[3,24] The Greenfield suction embolectomy catheter (Meditech/Boston Scientific, Natick, MA) was the first FDA-approved device. The device is 10F in caliber and contains a steerable catheter with a 5-mm or 7-mm plastic suction cup at the tip. The device removes the centrally located fresh embolus by manual suction with a large syringe and requires the retrieval of the device and the thrombus as a unit through an open femoral or jugular venotomy. Because of its introduction in the 1970s, clinical reports have shown that more than 100 patients with massive PE have been successfully treated using this device. Clinical success using this device in extracting pulmonary thrombus was as high as 83% of patients with massive PE, with the majority of them experiencing immediate hemodynamic improvement. The 30-day mortality rate ranged from 5% to 30%.[24]

In addition to the Greenfield, the Aspirex PE thrombectomy device (Aspirex; Straub Medical, Wangs, Switzerland) was specifically designed and developed for percutaneous interventional treatment of massive PE in pulmonary arteries with calibers of 6–14 mm. The central part of the catheter system is a high-speed rotational coil within the catheter body that creates negative pressure through an L-shaped aspiration port at the catheter tip, macerates aspirated thrombus, and removes macerated thrombus. Aspirated blood cools and lubricates the catheter system. A recent clinical study that included 13 patients with acute massive PE revealed successful thrombus aspiration in the pulmonary arteries without cardiovascular deaths or recurrent PE during a mean follow-up period of 12 months. This device is ideally suited for patients with massive PE with contraindications for thrombolysis.

The most significant drawback of aspiration embolectomy is technical: pieces of the clot that are older, more hardened, or unable to be broken up by physical perturbation are not amenable to removal.

Thrombus Fragmentation

Thrombus fragmentation has been performed with balloon angioplasty, a pigtail rotational catheter or a more advanced fragmentation device, the Amplatze catheter (ev3 Endovascular, Plymouth, MN), which uses an impeller to homogenize the thrombus, have been widely described.[11,25] The rotatable pigtail catheter (Cook, Bloomington, IN) is a common technique used in this approach and can be used synergistically with adjunctive techniques. It is a modified 5F pigtail catheter with a radiopaque tip, with 10 side holes for contrast material injection. An oval side hole in the outer aspect of the pigtail loop allows direct passage of a 0.035-inch guidewire through the hole to act as a central axis around which the catheter rotates. The catheter rotates bimanually to break apart large fresh clots. One disadvantage of the pigtail catheter is that the tip of the catheter disrupts the clot in multiple smaller fragments, which can embolize distally in the pulmonary circulation. Ideal thrombectomy catheters for use in the pulmonary circulation must be readily maneuverable, effective in removal of thromboemboli, and safe by virtue of minimizing distal embolization, mechanical hemolysis, or damage to cardiac structures and pulmonary arteries.

The advantages of the rotating pigtail, however, are many. First it is widely availability and has low cost relative to mechanically-driven thrombectomy devices. As previously alluded to, thrombus fragmentation also effectively increases the available thrombus surface area for effective thrombolysis. Several in vivo hemodynamic studies have shown that, once a large pulmonary thrombus is fragmented into multiple smaller thrombi, the redistribution of larger central clots into the peripheral pulmonary bed may immediately increase total pulmonary blood flow and relieve RV afterload, which can improve oxygenation and hemodynamic oxygen perfusion. In a study that examined 20 patients with massive PE on whom this endovascular technique was used, catheter intervention with the pigtail rotational catheter showed a 33% recanalization rate by thrombus fragmentation without thrombolytic therapy.[26] Although numerous clinical studies using the pigtail catheter fragmentation technique have shown significant hemodynamic improvement in patients with massive PE, these studies have not demonstrated survival benefits using this treatment approach.

By far one of the most common endovascular approaches for iliofemoral DVT is rheolytic therapy, a modality that combines mechanical fragmentation with thrombolysis. The adjunctive infusion of thrombolytic therapy significantly improves thrombus dissolution and relieves clot burden. Several studies have examined this technique in massive pulmonary embolism.

Rheolytic Therapy

Rheolytic thrombectomy catheters include the AngioJet Xpeedior thrombectomy device (Possis/Medrad; Minneapolis, MN), Hydrolyser (Cordis, Miami, FL), and Oasis (Meditech/ Boston Scientific, Natick, MA) catheters, which use a high-velocity saline jet to fragment adjacent thrombus by creating a Venturi effect and removing the debris into an evacuation lumen.[3]

The AngioJet catheter is a 6F over-the-wire catheter that permits simultaneous infusion of the thrombolytic agent, along with a Venturi effect to remove debris. This technique is termed "pharmacomechanical thrombectomy" and dissolves the clot by both thrombolysis and mechanical thrombectomy. The pharmacomechanical thrombectomy technique using this device is widely adapted in DVT interventions, particularly iliofemoral. Short-acting, newer-generation fibrinolytic drugs, such as alteplase (10 to 20 mg), reteplase (2.5 to 5 U), or tenecteplase (5 to 10 mg), may be used for the pharmacomechanical thrombectomy approach. One of the greatest limitations to AngioJet in the pulmonary vasculature, however, is that the catheter is not designed to treat vessels greater than 12 mm in diameter. Procedural-related complications and deaths have been reported using this device in PE interventions.[27] In one study, the rheolytic AngioJet device was associated with a high rate of complications, including 5 procedure-related deaths.

One of the most plausible explanations for the adverse outcomes using AngioJet is that efficacious removal of a large clot burden in the pulmonary artery results in a neurohormal release that may cause refractory hypotension leading to impaired consciousness, syncope, seizures, or cardiac arrest. Overall, the excellent thrombus aspiration capacity of AngioJet seems to be counterbalanced by deleterious systemic side effects. Because of these reported complications, the FDA has issued a block-box warning on the device label. Based on safety concerns, the AngioJet device should not be used as the initial mechanical treatment in patients with acute massive PE.[1,27]

Ultrasound-Accelerated Thrombolytic Therapy

Although very little data has been published on this technique for thrombolysis in general, much less for acute PE, ultrasound-accelerated catheter-directed thrombolysis is a novel treatment strategy that is emerging to relieve clot burden.[28] Using the EkoSonic Endovascular System (EKOS, Seattle, WA), a 5.2-F multilumen side-port infusion catheter, with infusion lengths of 6 to 50 cm depending on the length of the thrombotic occlusion, is used to infuse thrombolytics and emit ultrasound energy to accelerate the thrombolytic cascade. Once the EkosSonic catheter is positioned in the pulmonary artery over a 0.035-inch guidewire, the guidewire is exchanged for a matching ultrasound core wire containing a series of ultrasound transducer elements (2.2 MHz, 0.45 W), which are distributed approximately 1.0 cm apart along its leading tip to evenly deliver ultrasound energy radially along the coaxial infusion zone. A control unit provides continuous monitored variables, including temperature and ultrasound energy power output in the treatment zone, by means of thermocouples incorporated in the catheter and automatically adjusts power to optimize lysis of the intravascular thrombosis. The acoustic streaming energy dissociates the fibrin and increases the fibrin porosity without causing distal embolization, which also facilitates the penetration of thrombolytic agents into the thrombus for receptor binding. Despite the novelty of this technique, only two case reports demonstrate successful outcomes using EKOS and further investigation is warranted.

IVC Filter Placement

Since the approval of retrievable IVC filters by the FDA in the past decade, IVC filter placement has been widely expanded under the auspices of filter retrievability. However, retrieval rates are often less than 50% and the incidence of fatal PE has not declined with any significance.[29] For patients with hemorrhagic conditions or contraindications to anticoagulation, placement of a retrievable IVC filter may be appropriate. However, defining a "contraindication to anticoagulation" requires prudence that takes into account that hemorrhage risk following major trauma declines after 4 days. The two primary indications for IVC filter are major hemorrhage that precludes anticoagulation and recurrent PE despite anticoagulation. Multiple randomized controlled trials have convincingly demonstrated the efficacy of IVC filters in the reduction of PE recurrence, however, using the IVC filter as the primary means of PE prevention is not recommended[3]. Complications of IVC filter placement are uncommon but still happen with relative significance, because the outcomes can be filter. These complications include filter migration, IVC perforation, and IVC thrombosis.

COMPARISON OF ENDOVASCULAR TECHNIQUES

In a systematic review of available cohort data comprising a total of 348 patients, clinical success with percutaneous therapy alone for patients with acute massive PE was 81% (aspiration thrombectomy 81%; fragmentation 82%; rheolytic thrombectomy 75%) and 95% when combined with local infusion of thrombolytic agents (aspiration thrombectomy 100%; fragmentation 90%; rheolytic thrombectomy 91%).[30] In a retrospective report of 51 patients with massive or submassive PE (28% with shock, 16% with hypotension, and 57% with echocardiographic evidence of RV dysfunction) treated with AngioJet rheolytic thrombectomy, technical success was achieved in 92%, 8% experienced major bleeding, and in-hospital mortality was 16%.[27,31] Patients with submassive PE treated with rheolytic thrombectomy had similar improvement, with decreased obstruction, improved perfusion, and improved Miller indices. Lin et al,[32] Krichavsky et al[33,34] and Gao et al[31] have all recently demonstrated efficacy of catheter-directed fragmentation combined with thrombolysis and aspiration, but the numbers are low. In summary, the preferred endovascular approach to pulmonary embolism still necessitates more clinical evidence, but at the time our institution recommends mechanical fragmentation using a rotational pigtail catheter in a carefully selected group of patients with *massive* PE.

CONCLUSIONS

Mortality from pulmonary embolism in the United States remains high despite advances in its treatment. Current data regarding catheter-directed interventions (CDI) for the treatment of acute massive PE are limited by the ambiguous definitions of massive PE vs. submassive PE, the small sample size and the heterogeneity of treatment regimes implemented.

Based on recommendations by the American Heart Association and ACCP, it is preferable to refer to *massive* PE as characterized by dramatic sudden onset of hypotension, tachycardia and respiratory distress. *Submassive* PE, on the other hand, can be recognized as PE-related right ventricular (RV) dysfunction and troponin elevation despite normal arterial pressure.

Taking into account these different classifications, the burden of data is in favor of CDI for acute massive PE, although large prospective trials are necessary to confirm this. Despite this, systemic anticoagulation and thrombolysis remain the mainstay of treatment for acute massive PE, even in the setting of imminent hemodynamic and cardiovascular collapse. More emphasis should be placed on investigating the clinical efficacy of CDI not only in acute massive PE but also submassive PE. CDI enables a high concentration of thrombolytic agents to be infused directly into the thrombus, resulting in shorter infusion times and reduced doses of the thrombolytic drug needed for thrombus resolution, which theoretically decreases the risk of hemorrhagic complications compared with systemic thrombolysis.

At large centers with experienced operators, catheter-based interventions should be considered for patients who present with RV failure and hemodynamic instability. Patients with massive PE who have contraindications to fibrinolytic therapy who present to centers unable to offer catheter or surgical embolectomy should be considered for urgent transfer to a center with these services available so that they can be evaluated for this therapy. There should be a plan in place for expedition of such transfers.

Institutions with expertise in advanced intervention for PE should be identified in advance so that criteria and procedures for transfer can be agreed on explicitly. To ensure transfer is safe, only appropriately trained and equipped ambulance crews should be used to transfer these critically ill unstable patients.

A variety of endovascular interventions, including catheter-based thrombolysis and fragmentation, percutaneous pulmonary embolectomy, and IVC filter placement have been reported in the literature for patients with acute PE and should be considered as first-line treatment strategies at institutions equipped with the appropriate skill and expertise.

REFERENCES

1. Lin PH, Chen H, Bechara CF, Kougias P. Endovascular interventions for acute pulmonary embolism. *Perspect Vasc Surg Endovasc Ther* 2010;22:171–82.
2. Kuo WT, Gould MK, Louie JD, Rosenberg JK, Sze DY, Hofmann LV. Catheter-directed therapy for the treatment of massive pulmonary embolism: systematic review and meta-analysis of modern techniques. *J Vasc Interv Radiol* 2009;20:1431–40.
3. Jaff MR, McMurtry MS, Archer SL, et al. Management of Massive and Submassive Pulmonary Embolism, Iliofemoral Deep Vein Thrombosis, and Chronic Thromboembolic Pulmonary Hypertension: A Scientific Statement From the American Heart Association. *Circulation* 2011;123:1788–830.
4. Piazza G, Goldhaber SZ. Fibrinolysis for acute pulmonary embolism. *Vasc Med* 2010;15:419–28.
5. Agnelli G, Becattini C. Acute pulmonary embolism. *N Engl J Med* 2010;363:266–74.
6. Liu P, Meneveau N, Schiele F, Bassan JP. Predictors of long-term clinical outcome of patients with acute massive pulmonary embolism after thrombolytic therapy. *Chin Med J* (Engl) 2003;116:503–9.
7. Goldhaber SZ, Visani L, De Rosa M. Acute pulmonary embolism: clinical outcomes in the International Cooperative Pulmonary Embolism Registry (ICOPER). *Lancet* 1999;353:1386–9.
8. Schoepf UJ, Kucher N, Kipfmueller F, Quiroz R, Costello P, Goldhaber SZ. Right ventricular enlargement on chest computed tomography: a predictor of early death in acute pulmonary embolism. *Circulation* 2004;110:3276–80.
9. Meneveau N. Therapy for acute high-risk pulmonary embolism: thrombolytic therapy and embolectomy. *Curr Opin Cardiol* 2010;25:560–7.
10. Zamanian RT, Gould MK. Effectiveness and cost effectiveness of thrombolysis in patients with acute pulmonary embolism. *Curr Opin Pulm Med* 2008;14:422–6.
11. Kuo WT, van den Bosch MA, Hofmann LV, Louie JD, Kothary N, Sze DY. Catheter-directed embolectomy, fragmentation, and thrombolysis for the treatment of massive pulmonary embolism after failure of systemic thrombolysis. *Chest* 2008;134:250–4.
12. Simonneau G, Sors H, Charbonnier B, et al. A comparison of low-molecular-weight heparin with unfractionated heparin for acute pulmonary embolism. The THESEE Study Group. Tinzaparine ou Heparine Standard: Evaluations dans l'Embolie Pulmonaire. *N Engl J Med* 1997;337:663–9.
13. Goldhaber SZ, Haire WD, Feldstein ML, et al. Alteplase versus heparin in acute pulmonary embolism: randomised trial assessing right-ventricular function and pulmonary perfusion. *Lancet* 1993;341:507–11.
14. Wan S, Quinlan DJ, Agnelli G, Eikelboom JW. Thrombolysis compared with heparin for the initial treatment of pulmonary embolism: a meta-analysis of the randomized controlled trials. *Circulation* 2004;110:744–9.
15. Meyer G, Gisselbrecht M, Diehl JL, Journois D, Sors H. Incidence and predictors of major hemorrhagic complications from thrombolytic therapy in patients with massive pulmonary embolism. *Am J Med* 1998;105:472–7.

16. Fukuda I, Taniguchi S, Fukui K, Minakawa M, Daitoku K, Suzuki Y. Improved outcome of surgical pulmonary embolectomy by aggressive intervention for critically ill patients. *Ann Thorac Surg* 2011;91:728–32.

17. Kawahito K, Adachi H. Balloon catheter pulmonary embolectomy under direct visual control using a choledochoscope. *Ann Thorac Surg* 2011;91:621–3.

18. Vohra HA, Whistance RN, Mattam K, et al. Early and late clinical outcomes of pulmonary embolectomy for acute massive pulmonary embolism. *Ann Thorac Surg* 2010;90:1747–52.

19. Digonnet A, Moya-Plana A, Aubert S, et al. Acute pulmonary embolism: a current surgical approach. *Interact Cardiovasc Thorac Surg* 2007;6:27–9.

20. Banovac F, Buckley DC, Kuo WT, et al. Reporting standards for endovascular treatment of pulmonary embolism. *J Vasc Interv Radiol* 2010;21:44–53.

21. Goldhaber SZ. Percutaneous mechanical thrombectomy for acute pulmonary embolism: a double-edged sword. *Chest* 2007;132:363–5.

22. Angel de Gregorio M, Laborda A, de Blas I, Medrano J, Mainar A, Oribe M. Endovascular treatment of a haemodynamically unstable massive pulmonary embolism using fibrinolysis and fragmentation. Experience with 111 patients in a single centre. Why don't we follow ACCP recommendations? *Arch Bronconeumol* 2011;47:17–24.

23. Schmitz-Rode T, Kilbinger M, Gunther RW. Simulated flow pattern in massive pulmonary embolism: significance for selective intrapulmonary thrombolysis. *Cardiovasc Inter Rad* 1998;21:199–204.

24. Greenfield LJ. Catheter pulmonary embolectomy. *Chest* 1991;100:593–4.

25. Goldhaber SZ. Percutaneous mechanical thrombectomy for massive pulmonary embolism: improve safety and efficacy by sharing information. *Catheter Cardio Inte* 2007;70:807–8.

26. Schmitz-Rode T, Janssens U, Schild HH, Basche S, Hanrath P, Gunther RW. Fragmentation of massive pulmonary embolism using a pigtail rotation catheter. *Chest* 1998;114:1427–36.

27. Bonvini RF, Righini M, Roffi M. Angiojet rheolytic thrombectomy in massive pulmonary embolism: locally efficacious but systemically deleterious? *J Vasc Interv Radiol* 2010;21: 1774–6; author reply 6–7.

28. Stambo GW, Montague B. Bilateral EKOS catheter thrombolysis of acute bilateral pulmonary embolism in a hemodynamically unstable patient. *Am J Emerg Med* 2010;28:983 e5–7.

29. Smoot RL, Koch CA, Heller SF, et al. Inferior vena cava filters in trauma patients: efficacy, morbidity, and retrievability. *J Trauma* 2010;68:899–903.

30. Skaf E, Beemath A, Siddiqui T, Janjua M, Patel NR, Stein PD. Catheter-tip embolectomy in the management of acute massive pulmonary embolism. *Am J Cardiol* 2007;99:415–20.

31. Chechi T, Vecchio S, Spaziani G, et al. Rheolytic thrombectomy in patients with massive and submassive acute pulmonary embolism. *Catheter Cardio Inte* 2009;73:506–13.

32. Lin PH, Annambhotla S, Bechara CF, et al. Comparison of percutaneous ultrasound-accelerated thrombolysis versus catheter-directed thrombolysis in patients with acute massive pulmonary embolism. *Vascular* 2009;17 Suppl 3:S137–47.

33. Krichavsky MZ, Rybicki FJ, Resnic FS. Catheter directed lysis and thrombectomy of submassive pulmonary embolism. *Catheter Cardio Inte* 2011;77:144–7.

34. Gao H, Huang GY, Ma LL, Wang LX. Combined catheter thrombus fragmentation and fibrinolysis for acute pulmonary embolism. *Intern Med J* 2011.

35

Quality of Life and Activities of Daily Living with Venous Disease

Thom W. Rooke, MD and Cindy L. Felty, MSN, CNP, CWS

Three key questions must be confronted when evaluating a patient with venous disease: (1) Does the patient need treatment; (2) If yes, what type of treatment (conservative[a] or aggressive[b]) should the patient receive; and (3) If the patient is treated (either conservatively or aggressively) will the recommended therapy be covered by a third-party payer? The first two questions are *medical* in nature and tend to be answered by health practitioners. The third is a *social* question and is often left to the discretion of third party payers. Not surprisingly, the factors that affect decision-making for the first two questions are not necessarily the same as those that affect decision-making for the third.

Before treatment decisions can be made, the health practitioner and/or third-party payers must obtain key pieces of information about the impact of the patient's venous disease on his/her well-being. There are several ways this information is obtained:

Objective Measures

These include *vascular laboratory testing* (duplex scanning and/or physiological testing) and the *physical examination*. The CEAP (for Clinical, Etiologic, Anatomic, and Pathophysiologic assessments) classification system provides a well-validated, widely accepted basis for objectively grading the clinical severity of venous disease.[1] Using CEAP, venous disease can be divided into objective categories (0–6, Figure 35–1) that correspond to signs ranging from "no venous disease" to "active venous ulcer."

Subjective Measures

The subjective assessment of venous disease is more difficult than the objective assessment and depends heavily on the use of various questionnaires (Figure 35–2). These question-

---

[a]Conservative – graduated elastic compression with wraps or stockings, periodic limb elevation, analgesics, non-elastic compression, etc.

[b]Aggressive – vein stripping, catheter ablation, revascularization of occluded veins, sclerotherapy, etc.

0 – No disease
1 – Telangiectases, small veins
2 – Varicose Veins
3 – Edema
4 – Stasis changes
5 – Healed ulcer
6 – Active ulcer

Figure 35–1. Clinical Categories of the CEAP Classification System

Generic
- 36-Item Short Form Health Survey (SF-36)
- Nottingham Health Profile (NHP)

Venous-specific
- Chronic Venous Insufficiency Questionnaire (CIVIQ)
- Venous Insufficiency Epidemiological and Economic Study (VEINES)
- Aberdeen Varicose Vein Questionnaire (AVVQ)
- Charing Cross Venous Ulceration Questionnaire (CXVUQ)

Physician-generated tools
- Venous Severity Scoring (VSS) System
  - Venous Disability Score (VDS)
  - Venous Segmental Disease Score (VSDS)
  - Venous Clinical Severity Score (VCSS)

Figure 35-2. Tools for the Assessment of Chronic Venous Disease

naires provide a means of assessing the impact of venous disease on the patient's quality of life, activities of daily living, and other aspects of overall well-being.

Based on assessments that combine objective and subjective measures, there is little disagreement regarding the need to treat patients with clinically severe venous disease (C4–6).[2–4] As a group, these patients burden the economy (the cost of treating venous ulcers alone exceeds $ 2.5 billion, with more than 2 million work days missed annually because of disease)[5], and those afflicted experience pain, impaired function, loss of mobility, emotional distress, and social isolation that results in a decreased quality of life. Because there is general agreement regarding the seriousness of C4–6 venous disease, most practitioners and payers agree with conservative and, where possible, aggressive therapies for these patients.

The situation with regard to milder forms of venous disease is far less harmonious. *Should relatively "benign" disease categories (C1–3) also be treated aggressively? If so, should third party payers be expected to cover the cost of these therapies?*

The answers become especially problematic when we consider the relatively high prevalence of mild-moderate venous disease. Whereas active or healed venous ulcers occur in approximately one percent of the population[6] varicose veins are much more common and affect up to a quarter of the population (more in selected demographic groups). The situation is even worse for spider veins, which affect up to 80% of people

18–64 years old[7]. The number of patients with milder forms of venous disease is staggering, and the potential cost of treating everyone is prohibitive.

To further complicate the decision-making process, the value of treatment is less certain for patients with mild-moderate venous disease than for patients with severe disease. *What are the short- and long-term benefits of treating patients with moderate edema? Or those who complain of pain? Or those with concerns that may be "significant" to the patient but are considered "cosmetic" by others?* In general, the uncertainty regarding the need for, or efficacy of, treatment has steered third party payers toward coverage for severe venous problems and away from coverage when patients have "only" mild-moderate venous disease. A quick tour of the internet demonstrates several recurring themes with regard to the coverage policies of most large insurance carriers[8]. Treatment is usually reimbursed when there are *intractable ulcers* caused by venous stasis, significant *hemorrhage* from veins, recurrent *superficial phlebitis,* and occasionally *severe pain and swelling* (such that it interferes with daily living and requires chronic analgesia). In most cases it is also a requirement that these situations persist despite a trial (typically three months) of conservative management using analgesia and prescription compression hose.

While it is admirable that most third party payers accept the need to treat patients with severe venous disease, they are much more reluctant to cover the costs of treatment for mild-moderate disease. In this setting reimbursement decisions often hinge on whether the practitioners can convince the payers that the disease is severe enough to adversely impact the patient's quality of life and activities of daily living. But how does one objectively assess signs and symptoms like "swelling", "cosmetic impairment", and "pain" when patients with these problems are not typically hospitalized, do not miss work because of them, and may not have demonstrable hemodynamic abnormalities. Swelling and cosmetic impairment are "objective" problems, but their impact is wide-open to interpretation. Pain, on the other hand, is purely subjective – so how does one "measure" pain objectively?

As mentioned earlier, one approach for "quantifying" *subjective* endpoints involves the use of questionnaires. A report by Launois, et al[9] describes the CIVIQ-20 questionnaire as a tool for assessing the clinical consequences of venous disease in terms of specific dimensions (such as physical burden, psychological burden, pain, etc). Their results demonstrate that the impact of venous disease in patients with C1 or C2 disease (spider and/or varicose veins) is minimal, but that patients with C3 disease (edema) have impairments in most dimensions that are of comparable severity to those seen in patients with C4 (stasis) disease.

This raises a number of questions regarding patients with venous disease who are troubled by *edema, pain,* or *cosmetic* concerns. For example:

Is *edema* associated with C3 disease a reasonable indication for aggressive therapy? As noted above, mild-moderate edema is often considered a mere nuisance since it doesn't cause hospitalization or work absences. But the flaws in this argument are not hard to find. Case in point – the detrimental effects of edema on job performance depend on not only the severity of edema, but also on the type of job one performs (a mattress tester can work despite huge amounts of edema, but a fashion model specializing in skinny jeans might wind up standing in the unemployment line as the result of otherwise trivial edema). Unfortunately, for most jobs it is difficult if not impossible to determine the extent to which edema interferes with a patient's performance.

The use of costly, invasive therapies for the indication of *pain* is a highly controversial issue for those being asked to reimburse for venous treatments. Pain is a major health problem in the United States (where problems such as headache, low back pain, etc. are leading causes of morbidity and lost work days), and if a practitioner is not going to be proactive about treating pain it might be best for them to find a new profession. It is generally accepted that pain severe enough to discourage walking and exercise can contribute to poor cardiovascular conditioning, obesity, and potentially diabetes; this means that patients with mild-moderate venous disease may be at higher risk for these morbidities.[c] Unfortunately, pain is a purely subjective symptom; patients may tell you that they are experiencing pain from their veins, but it is virtually impossible to assess this with much objectively. Third party payers tend to assume that all patients "exaggerate" when it comes to pain. For this reason, pain – perhaps the biggest, most prevalent, and most important consequence of varicose veins and other types of chronic venous disease – is frequently the most difficult indication to get covered by payers.

The *cosmetic* impact of venous disease is even harder to quantify, especially if problems that seem purely cosmetic at presentation can progress over time to significant venous disease (C4–6). For example, it is often asserted[10], that "treatment could reduce the risk of ulcers if performed early in the course of chronic venous disease" – a direct argument in favor of offering treatment for venous disease while it is still at the relatively asymptomatic cosmetic stage.

The issue of cosmesis warrants an even closer look. Is *cosmesis* alone ever a reasonable indication for reimbursing the cost of treating venous disease? At first glance, the answer seems to be "never," and not surprisingly insurance generally does not provide coverage for problems that are purely cosmetic. Exceptions may be made in extreme situations – payers often cover for cosmetic treatment involving burns, mastectomy, birth defects, and other conditions in which the cosmetic problems are truly "severe." But doesn't venous disease encompass a similar spectrum with regard to severity? Large congenital venous malformations, Klippel-Trenaunay-Weber Syndrome, and many other conditions can be disfiguring, and treatment of these lesions is frequently (and appropriately) covered by payers. But at what point can a venous abnormality be legitimately called "disfiguring?" It is conceivable that even small cosmetic impairments could interfere with our previously mentioned fashion model's livelihood. To the extent that cosmetic imperfections may legitimately exert an adverse effect on quality of life, or the ability to perform one's job (as in the case of the fashion model), or on other activities of daily living, it's appropriate to ask "when should the cost of treating these lesions – including those deemed 'mild' by others – be covered by payers?"

Both data and common sense suggest that mild-moderate venous disease (C1–3) has the potential to reduce quality of life and interfere with activities of daily living, so logic dictates that symptomatic veins should be treated when possible. But exactly *how* should they be treated? Does it make sense to treat these veins aggressively with stripping/ablation/sclerotherapy/stenting or other invasive modalities? Or should conservative care (compression stockings) be used? Third party payers almost invariably suggest that the cheapest (i.e., stockings) be offered.[d] But is "cheapest" appropriate in this setting? In order to assess the choice of therapy (aggressive versus conservative) for mild-moderate venous disease, four variables ought to be assessed: *effectiveness*, *availability*, *cost*, and patient *acceptability*.

---

[c]Isn't this a serious handicap for which aggressive therapy should be offered?

[d]Of course, the cost of stockings is conveniently *not* covered by third-party payers in most cases.

The *effectiveness* of venous therapy depends on the modality used. Few would attempt to argue that surgical stripping, catheter ablation, or sclerotherapy are ineffective; they clearly destroy unwanted veins and eliminate problems such as varicose veins. In contrast, elastic compression improves the hemodynamics in many types of venous disease but doesn't treat the underlying problem ("stockings never cured anybody.")[e]

Availability of therapy, once a major concern, is clearly no longer an issue. Vein clinics have proliferated like lawyers and coffee houses, and in many parts of the country it is impossible to find a street corner that does not have two or three vein clinics on it. The quality of care provided by some of these establishments remains, not surprisingly, an issue.

Cost is an obvious concern. Invasive therapies are relatively expensive and "conservative" therapies are relatively cheap (although it should be pointed out that stockings are not really "cheap" – they're just "cheaper" than aggressive therapies). Unfortunately, in today's medical environment big decisions may hinge on small differences in cost.

Perhaps the most controversial questions revolve around the issue of patient *acceptability* with regard to various venous treatment options. Fairly or not, invasive therapies (especially vein stripping) have a bad reputation, having been besmirched by patient's mothers (and grandmothers and great-grandmothers) as being among the most "terrible" tortures ever devised by medicine. Fortunately, modern techniques such as ambulatory phlebectomy, catheter ablation, and sclerotherapy have rendered aggressive procedures minimally invasive and universally well-tolerated. In contrast, the most commonly recommended form of "conservative" therapy (i.e., compression stockings), once considered relatively "benign," is now among the most *hated* therapies in America today. Patients inevitably complain that stockings are hot, tight, and uncomfortable. Those with advanced age, arthritis, or other physical limitations cannot don or doff them without difficulty. And men will not wear them above the knee, largely due to social conventions. Did I mention they look ugly?

Lurie and Kistner recently reported at the American Venous Forum on their findings with regard to patient's preference for conservative versus surgical management in the treatment of primary chronic venous disease[11]. In this study of 150 patients with mild-moderate (C2–4) venous disease, patient's symptoms and quality of life were assessed using the SQOR-V tool. All patients were treated initially with stockings; three-fourths reported improved symptoms and one-fourth did not improve. All patients were then given the choice of proceeding with a surgical procedure to address their venous problem. Amazingly, 80 percent of all patients chose to discontinue their stockings (many despite the fact that their stockings had produced an improvement in their symptoms) and proceed with surgery. A patient's chances of improving with surgery were 21 times greater if they had improvement with the use of stocking as compared to those who did not improve with stocking use.

The implications of this study are not subtle. Conventional wisdom (in this case, the wisdom advocated by most third party payers) suggests that essentially all patients

---

[e]There is considerably more controversy regarding the effectiveness of other types of therapies (such as the various oral agents available for treating vein disease) or the effectiveness of "prevention" in general as a means of modifying the progression of venous disease, but these issues are beyond the scope of this chapter.

with venous disease/varicose veins should be treated first with elastic compression, and if they improve the compression should be continued indefinitely. Only those patients that don't improve (or can't tolerate compression) are generally approved for invasive therapies. However, the findings of Lurie and Kistner suggest that it might be more logical to treat patients initially with stockings, and then surgically treat those who improve (stockings therefore become a type of *diagnostic* test – if a patient improves with stocking use, it's very likely that they will improve with surgery). But if this is true, does it make any sense to recommend a trial of "conservative" care with graduated elastic compression stockings? Why not take patients with mild-moderate venous disease (C1–3) and proceed *directly* to definitive treatments, resorting to stocking use only if this approach fails to provide adequate relief of symptoms?

CONCLUSIONS

1. In most patients, severe venous disease (C4–6) reduces quality of life and interferes with activities of daily living.
2. In many patients, mild-moderate venous disease (C1–3) likewise reduces quality of life and impairs activities of daily living, but the impact is variable; some patients are essentially asymptomatic and stable, while others are debilitated and/or miserable.
3. Patients with venous disease (especially varicose veins) tolerate/accept surgery (aggressive, invasive therapy) better than stockings (conservative therapy).

In view of this, perhaps we need to rethink our treatment algorithms. It may make sense to treat all forms of venous disease (mild, moderate, and severe) as aggressively as possible using whatever invasive means are appropriate (stripping, catheter ablation, sclerotherapy, etc.). Only when aggressive (invasive) measures fail should consideration turn to conservative measures (like elastic stockings). This strategy is likely to be met with 1) greater patient acceptance, 2) improved quality of life/activity of daily living, and, unfortunately, 3) resistance from third-party payers.

REFERENCES

1. Eklöf B, Rutherford RB, Bergan JJ, et al. Revision of the CEAP classification for chronic venous disorders: Consensus statement. *J Vasc Surg* 2004; 40:1248–52.
2. Phillips T, Stanton B, and Lew R. A study of the impact of leg ulcers on quality of life: Financial, social, and psychologic implications. *Journal of the American Academy of Dermatology* 1994; 31(1):49–53.
3. van Korlaar I, Vossen C, Rosendaal F, et al. Quality of life in venous disease. *Thromb Haemost* 2003 Jul; 90(1):27–35.
4. Kaplan RM, Criqui MH, Denenberg JO, et al. Quality of life in patients with chronic venous disease: San Diego population study. *J Vasc Surg* 2003; 37:1047–53.
5. Sen CK, Gordillo GM, Roy S, et al. Human skin wounds: A major and snowballing threat to public health and the economy. *Wound Repair Regen* 2009; Nov-Dec; 17(6):763–771.
6. Angle N, Bergan JJ. Chronic venous ulcer. *BMJ* 1997 314(7086):1019.
7. Evans CJ, Fowkes CV, Ruckley AJL. Prevalence of varicose veins and chronic venous insufficiency in men and women in the general population: Edinburgh vein study. *J Epidemiology Community Health* 1999; 53:149–153.

8. Aetna Clinical Policy Bulletin: Varicose Veins. http://www.aetna.com/cpb/medical/data/ 1_99/0050.html. Accessed 3/29/2011.
9. Launois R, Mansilha A, Jantet G. International psychometric validation of the chronic venous disease quality of life questionnaire (CIVIQ-20). *Eur J Vasc Endovasc Surg* (2010)40, 783–789.
10. Bergan JJ, Schmid-Schönbein GW, Coleridge Smith PD, et al. Chronic venous disease. *N Engl J Med* 2006; 355:488–498.
11. Lurie F, Kistner RL. Trends in Patient Reported Outcomes of Conservative and Surgical Treatment of Primary Chronic Venous Disease Contradict Current Practices. Abstract presented at AVF, 2011.

Hemodialysis

36

Minimally Invasive Basilic Vein Arteriovenous Fistula Transposition for Hemodialysis Vascular Access

William C. Jennings, MD, FACS,
Kip W. Dorsey, MD and Jason D. Alder, MD

INTRODUCTION

Establishing an arteriovenous fistula (AVF) for vascular access is the consensus recommendation for hemodialysis patients.[1,2] Individuals with autogenous vascular access have lower mortality and morbidity rates in addition to fewer interventions than patients with other methods of dialysis access. Medicare cost for dialysis per patient per year is also lower with AVFs as opposed to AV grafts or catheter-based dialysis.

The original radiocephalic AVF remains the first choice for dialysis vascular access in appropriate patients since first reported in 1966 by Cimino, Appell, and colleagues. However, some authors have reported over 40% of these access operations failed or failed to mature. We find few patients in our referral practice to be good candidates for radiocephalic AVFs and feel careful patient selection to be the key element for success.[3] Antebrachial fistulas, based on brachial artery or proximal radial artery inflow, are generally viewed as the second preferred options among vascular access surgeons; but even these procedures are not feasible in many patients due to chronic illness with the loss of common superficial venous outflow options. Individuals are frequently referred for vascular access with complex medical histories associated with many past intravenous catheters and venipunctures, leaving the cephalic and medial antebrachial veins unsuitable for incorporation into a successful vascular access. The basilic vein is frequently spared in these patients and is generally considered as the third recommended option for autogenous access when transposed to a safe and reliable position for cannulation.[1,2]

The first basilic vein transposition for vascular access was reported by Dagher, et al. in 1976.[4] This operation is most often performed with a lengthy longitudinal incision in the medial aspect of the arm (openAVF-T) (Figure 36–1).[5] The forearm basilic

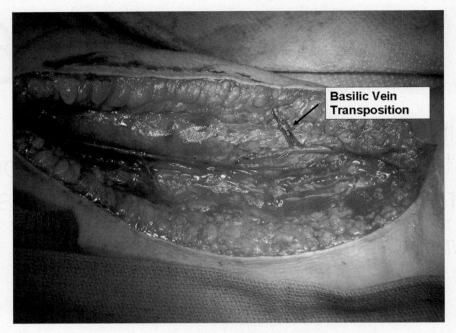

Figure 36–1. A standard incision for an open basilic vein arteriovenous fistula transposition is shown in this photo. Many surgeons feel the risk of wound complications is substantial.

vein is less commonly of adequate size and is therefore used infrequently for transposition but also offers a successful access conduit in appropriately selected patients. As expected, the incidence of wound complications associated with these standard openAVF-T procedures is considerably higher than with simple AVFs.[6,7] A simple and less invasive technique for basilic vein harvest prior to tunneled AVF transposition incorporates segmental bridged incisions for basilic vein mobilization. This may avoid or moderate some of the wound complications reported in standard openAVF-T operations (Figure 36–2).[8,9]

MINIMALLY-INVASIVE TECHNIQUES

Surgical care has moved steadily toward minimally invasive operations and procedures during the past decades and vascular surgery is no exception. Interventional or minimally invasive procedures such as intraluminal balloon angioplasties, stents, and endograft placements have become standard common practice. Peritoneal dialysis patients have also benefited by minimally invasive laparoscopic catheter placement with improved outcomes and more precise surgical procedures. Endoscopic saphenous vein harvest was first reported by Jordan, et al. in 1997.[10] This was rapidly followed by other centers describing fewer wound complications and less discomfort for patients with endoscopic vein harvest as opposed to open procedures.[11] Gazoni and others extended this concept to vein harvest for lower extremity arterial bypass operations; finding fewer wound complications, shortened hospital stays, and equivalent outcomes when compared to standard open procedures.[12]

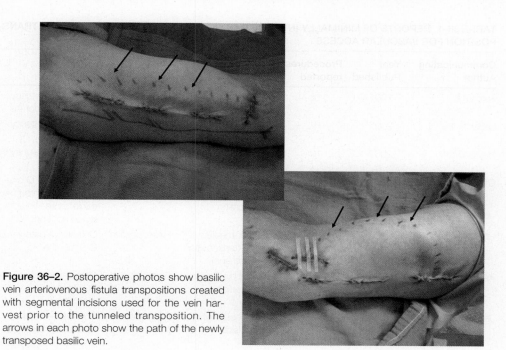

Figure 36–2. Postoperative photos show basilic vein arteriovenous fistula transpositions created with segmental incisions used for the vein harvest prior to the tunneled transposition. The arrows in each photo show the path of the newly transposed basilic vein.

Other minimally invasive techniques for vein retrieval have been reported, including the use of a laryngoscope.[13] Endoscopic harvest of vein or artery conduits for cardiac or peripheral vascular bypass has become common with endoscopic saphenous vein harvest for cardiac bypass procedures used in up to 80–95% of the cases in some reports.[14,15] Coronary artery bypass grafting using the radial artery with endoscopic harvest has been reported by several authors finding equivalent or improved results when compared to open harvest procedures. An initial criticism of endoscopic vein harvest was that more time was required for the procedure; however, improvement in technology and experience have allowed most practitioners to experience acceptable harvest times similar to open procedures, and in some cases, faster retrieval of the venous conduit.[11]

Endoscopic AVF basilic vein transposition (endoAVF-T) was first reported by Martinez, et al. in 2001.[16] This was followed by other reports of endoAVF-Ts utilizing various devices and minimally invasive techniques for endoscopic vein harvest.[16,17,18,19,20,21] Other authors have reported alternative minimally invasive techniques for harvesting the basilic vein for transposition, including a vein inversion technique using balloon catheters.[22] Reports of minimally invasive basilic vein transposition series are shown in Table 36–1. Our surgical vascular access group reviewed our experience with endoAVF-Ts and compared those outcomes with those of our immediate preceding traditional open AVF-T operations.[20] We found no difference in primary, assisted, or cumulative patency rates between the endoAVF-T patients and open AVF-T patients. In addition, our study found initial access utilization was sooner for both primary and staged endoAVF-Ts (p < 0.01). Figure 36–3 shows patency rates for endoAVF-T procedures from this report.

Several devices using varying techniques have been available for endoscopic vein harvest, including Terumo VirtuoSaph™° ® (Terumo Cardiovascular Systems Corporation, Ann Arbor, Michigan, USA), Sorin ClearGuide® (SorinGroup, Milan, Italy),

TABLE 36–1. REPORTS OF MINIMALLY INVASIVE BASILIC VEIN ARTERIOVENOUS FISTULA TRANS-POSITION FOR VASCULAR ACCESS

Communicating Author	Year Published	Procedures reported	Technique Used	Study Type	Outcomes
Tordoir[18]	2001	12	Endoscopic Basilic Transposition	Retrospective	Cumulative patency 100% @ 12 months
LeSar[16]	2001	9	Endoscopic Basilic Transposition	Retrospective	Cumulative patency 89% @ 19 months
Hayakawa[17]	2002	10	Endoscopic Basilic Transposition	Retrospective	Cumulative patency 60% @ 12 months
Oto[19]	2003	5	Endoscopic saphenous vein Translocation	Retrospective	All successful @ one month. One thrombecto-my required, Total fol-lowup not specified.
Hill[22]	2005	32	Catheter-mediated basilica transposition (vein inversion)	Retrospective	Cumulative patency 72% @ 9 months
Keuter[21]	2005	6	Endoscopic Basilic Transposition	Retrospective	Cumulative patency 90% @ 12 months and 24 months
Jenninas[20]	2010	98	Endoscopic Basilic Transposition	Retrospective	Cumulative patency 96.0% and 88.9% @ 12 and 24 months, respec-tively

Maquet VasoView® (Maquet GmbH & Co., Rastatt, Germany), and others. The Terumo device has been utilized extensively in our medical center for saphenous vein harvesting and has been our preferred device for vascular access basilic vein transposition procedures in addition to the less common saphenous vein harvest for a translocation autogenous fistula. These devices were developed and approved for saphenous vein

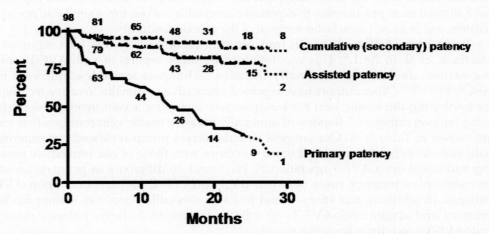

Figure 36–3. Endoscopic AVF Transposition: Kaplan-Meier patency curve. Dotted lines are used to indicate when patient numbers fell below 10% and the curve becomes imprecise. From: Paul EM, Sideman MJ, Rhoden DH, Jennings WC. Endoscopic basilic vein transposition for hemodialysis access. *J Vasc Surg.* 2010;51(6): 1451–56. © Elsevier Inc.

harvest, and their use for other venous conduit procedures should be considered as an "off label" application.

In our experience, not all vascular access patients are well suited for endoAVF-Ts. Brachial vein harvest and short basilic segments where the basilic vein enters the brachial venous system in the distal arm are examples of vascular access procedures where we use an open technique with segmental bridged incisions.[23] Transposition of basilic veins with multiple large side branches veins or double channel veins may be best accomplished with segmental harvesting incisions located at key sites identified with preoperative US. When a cephalic or median antebrachial vein AVF in obese individuals is too deep for reliable cannulation, we prefer a lipectomy technique rather than transposition or elevation.[24] However, when a basilic vein transposition is necessary in obese patients; endoAVF-T may offer significant benefit.

Ultrasound (US) is a key element of our vascular access practice. Venous mapping and arterial evaluation with US are well established recommendations prior to AVF construction.[1,2] We feel the combination of physical and US examinations conducted by the surgeon offers the most information in selecting the preferred vascular access procedure and avoiding operations likely to fail. Although not the topic of this chapter, US is also an important part of postoperative access evaluation for our vascular access patients. Decisions on maturation, cannulation timing, detection of dysfunction when present, and more are enhanced with US examination and access flow measurements.

TECHNICAL CONSIDERATIONS FOR ENDOSCOPIC BASILIC VEIN TRANSPOSITION

The necessary equipment includes a forward viewing endoscope and digital camera with a standard endoscopic cart including monitor, insufflator, and light source. We position the cart just above the patients shoulder so the entire team is able to visualize the screen. Figure 36–4 shows screen positioning and the operating surgeon. The patient's arm is elevated on 2–3 folded towels to allow maneuvering of the harvesting tools. A 5.5 mm forward viewing proprietary endoscope is necessary with the Terumo device. The vein harvesting device pack contains two main components, the dissector and the harvester; in addition to an insertion cannula for the working channel, insufflation tubing, and cautery connecting equipment.

EndoAVF-Ts may be constructed with local anesthetic and sedation along with the addition of a regional block administered by the surgeon through the axillary incision at the start of the procedure. This small incision in the axilla allows identification of the basilic vein, along with the medial antebrachial, intercostal brachial, and other regional cutaneous nerves targeted for the block. Dissection is minimized during this step, leaving the investing fascia intact until the endoscopic mobilization and side branch division is completed to insure adequate insufflation of the working channel. This regional anesthetic technique also works well with openAVF-Ts or may be provided by the anesthesiologist using a more proximal block, in appropriate patients, usually accomplished with US guidance.

A brief US evaluation in the operating room before an endoAVF-T confirms the operative plan, marks the basilic vein path, identifies the location and size of branching veins, and allows for precise planning of incisions (Figure 36–5). Harvesting basilic

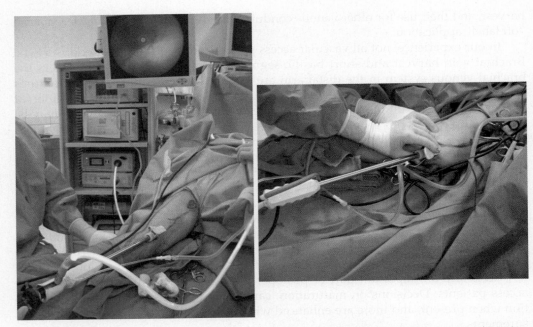

Figure 36–4. Photos show equipment and patient positioning for endoscopic basilic vein harvest prior to tunneled transposition.

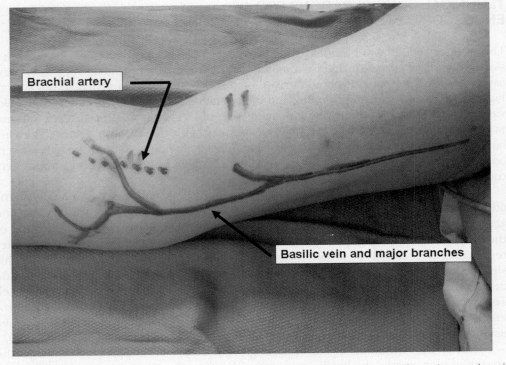

Figure 36–5. A brief preoperative ultrasound evaluation by the surgeon confirms the vascular anatomy and surgical plan in addition to selecting the incision sites.

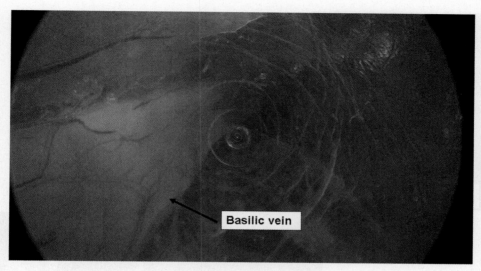

Figure 36–6. Endoscopic image of initial basilic vein dissection, separating the surrounding areolar soft tissue from the vein.

veins endoscopically was markedly improved with the development of specific systems and devices for saphenous vein harvest. We utilized varying techniques and equipment, however, our most experience has been with the Terumo endoscopic device and we currently use it for endoscopic vein harvest of the basilic vein. We rarely use the saphenous vein for vascular access but when needed, in appropriate patients, we harvest it endoscopically.

The basilic vein is exposed through a small incision in the distal arm and side branches are ligated 2–3 mm from the vein wall. The anterior vein wall is exposed proximally in the adventitial plane for a few centimeters to allow placement of the working insertion cannula to facilitate easy introduction and exchange of the vein harvesting tools. The distal vein is not divided at this time. The initial endoscopic tool (the dissecting rod) is inserted through the cannula and used to separate the surrounding areolar soft tissue from the vein (Figure 36–6). Use of the relatively atraumatic dissection device and avoidance of direct pressure on the vein minimizes vessel manipulation during mobilization. CO_2 is delivered at the tip of the device allowing low pressure insufflation of the working tunnel. Tunnel insufflation pressures below 10 mm Hg (and often less) support adequate visualization using the non-occlusive insertion cannula. The CO_2 insufflation is placed on standby when not in use. The anterior surface of the vein is mobilized initially and the dissecting instrument is then passed along both sides and behind the vein. The dissector is advanced in a parallel plane to the vein, not applying pressure on the vein wall with the dissecting tip and avoiding an angulated approach. As the dissection is continued proximally, the trunk and branches of the median antebrachial nerve are visualized and gently separated from the vein atraumatically, as in an open procedure. The endoscope light may be visualized through the skin as the device is advanced, monitoring the progress of the dissection.

After the soft tissue surrounding the vein has been separated with the dissecting rod, the endoscope is exchanged into the vein harvesting tool. With low pressure insufflation of the established working tunnel, the harvesting device is introduced through

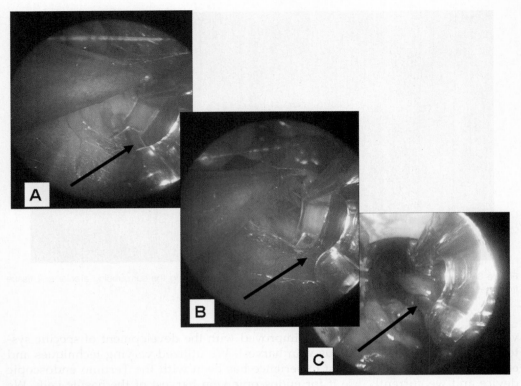

Figure 36–7. The arrows show the vein keeper segment of the harvester rod. **A** The harvester rod is advanced into the axilla with the vein keeper closed. **B** The vein keeper is opened and positioned to accept the basilic vein. **C** The captured vein may now be maneuvered to expose side branches for division.

the cannula and advanced along the vein to the proximal (axillary) site of dissection. Once advanced into the axilla, the vein keeper device is opened, the vein positioned within an atraumatic holder, and the containment pin is closed to secure the vein (Figure 36–7). As the harvester is withdrawn, side branches are isolated and divided with a bipolar maneuverable cautery that allows simultaneous cutting and coagulation. Side branches are displayed and divided well away from the basilic vein to avoid thermal injury to the vein wall (Figure 36–8). Gentle retraction and rotation of the harvesting device exposes the branches several millimeters from the basilic vein.

After the basilic vein has been mobilized and all branches divided, the introducing cannula is removed and additional vein length may be harvested distally through the same incision. A branching site at the most distal portion of the vein that is of adequate size and condition for transposition is selected for the division point, when possible. This distal harvest site was identified by ultrasound prior to the procedure and considered in positioning and orientation of the distal incision. Selecting a distal branch point for division, when feasible, allows creation of create a broad venous flare or "branch patch" for the AVF anastomosis. The vein is irrigated with heparinized solution after distal mobilization and transaction.

The basilic vein is then identified within the axillary incision and withdrawn proximally. Prior to tunneling, all branch sites are reevaluated by gentle, low-pressure distention and irrigation of the vein and each individual side branch is secured by ligature

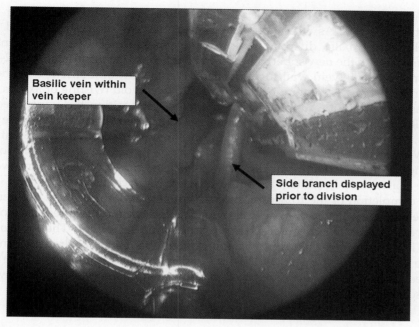

Figure 36–8. Side branches are displayed and divided well away from the basilic vein to avoid thermal injury to the vein wall.

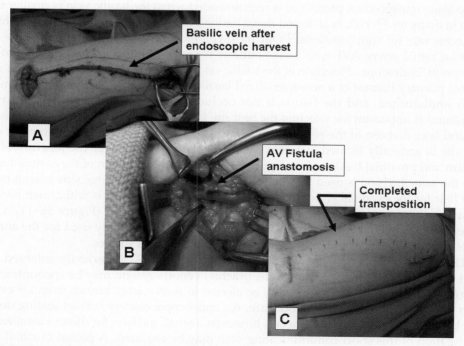

Figure 36–9. The surgical photos show: **A** The basilic vein after endoscopic harvest prior to the tunneled transposition. **B** An end-to-side anastomosis establishes the AVF flow. **C** The dashed line marks the path of the tunneled transposition.

or clip. Figure 36–9 shows the basilic vein after endoscopic harvest and prior to the tunneled transposition. As with all transpositions, the vein must be mobilized proximally, well into the axilla, dividing the investing fascia and side branches to ensure a smooth transition to the new superficial position. Branches are securely ligated 2–3 mm away from the basilic vein wall to avoid the development of a stricture as the vein matures and enlarges. The anterior surface is marked to avoid twisting or axial rotation during passage through a tunneler. The surgeon must position the transposed vein such that it is located both anteriorly and superficially to ensure safe and reliable use of the access, 4–6 millimeters deep within the subcutaneous tissue but not adherent to the dermis. We prefer to use the radial artery for vascular access inflow, when possible, minimizing the risk of steal syndrome.[32] If a brachial artery AVF is necessary, we limit size of the anastomosis in relation to the diameter of the brachial artery.

After completion of the transposition and prior to wound closures, the vein harvest tunnel site is evaluated to ensure adequate hemostasis. Gentle pressure along the vein-harvested pathway expresses any irrigation fluid or blood. The incisions are closed in layers of absorbable suture. Compression dressings and drains are not utilized. The patient's arm is evaluated for both adequate AVF flow through the newly transposed vein, and to ensure that distal arterial perfusion is maintained without signs of ischemia.

STAGED TRANSPOSITIONS

A two stage transposition procedure is recommended when the basilic vein is smaller than 4 mm in diameter.[5,20] Hill, et al. found that a basilic vein diameter ≥ 4 mm predicted a higher success rate for transpositions.[22] Our most common first stage inflow procedure is a proximal radial artery AVF with access outflow through the median cubital vein into the basilic vein. Endoscopic dissection of the basilic vein after a previous first stage AVF is similar to a primary harvest of a non-arterialized basilic vein. The first stage AVF anastomosis is left undisturbed, and the fistula is not occluded during endoscopic mobilization. Ultrasound is important for selecting the best site for initiating the endoscopic vein dissection and later division of the vein for tunneling. The small incision for the endoscopic cannula site is generally located just proximal to the cubital fossa over the juncture of the forearm and proximal basilic veins (Figure 36–10). After mobilization of the mature basilic vein, the same incision is used for vein division incorporating the large side branch into a wide flair for the eventual end-to-end anastomosis. The basilic vein is withdrawn into the axillary incision and tunneled into the new transposed position (Figure 36–11). CV-8 Gortex (W.L. Gore and Associates, Flagstaff, Ariz) suture is routinely used for the anastomosis with a posterior running suture and anterior interrupted sutures.

During the endoscopic harvest for a staged endoAVF-T, a markedly enlarged and short communicating vein branch to the brachial venous system may be encountered in the mid arm. The surgeon will usually be alerted to such a large branch from US evaluation just prior to the surgical procedure. An endoscopic cautery/vessel sealing device may be used for these larger branches, however, a small incision for direct visualization and ligation of this short communicating vein may be required. A paired brachial vein will be present, so ligation and division of the connecting brachial vein site is appropriate, if necessary, to avoid narrowing the basilic vein during harvest.

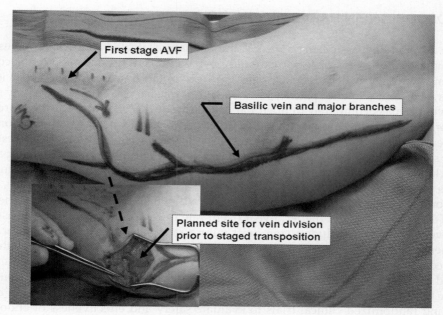

Figure 36–10. Preoperative ultrasound maps the basilic vein for this second stage transposition. The confluence of the forearm basilic vein and the median cubital vein (inflow from the first stage AVF) is selected as the incision site for endoscopic harvest and vein division prior to transposition tunneling. Figure K. shows the completed procedure.

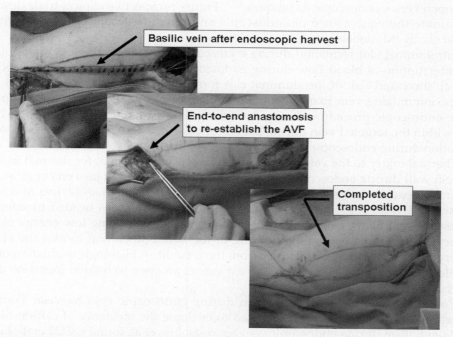

Figure 36–11. The surgical photos show a second stage endoscopic basilic vein transposition. **A** The basilic vein after endoscopic harvest prior to the tunneled transposition. **B** An end-to-end anastomosis re-establishes AVF flow. **C** The new tunneled path of the staged transposition.

ENDOSCOPIC VEIN HARVEST CONTROVERSIES

Lower extremity bypass patency: Several authors have evaluated endoscopic versus open saphenous vein harvest for lower extremity bypass procedures and reported successful outcomes with equivalent patency rates.[12] However, a recent retrospective review by Walker, et al. found inferior patency rates for endoscopic harvest in lower extremity saphenous vein bypass compared to open harvest techniques.[26] Contrary to their previous reports, the authors found no difference in length of stay or wound complication rates between the two groups. Individual surgeon preference accounted for the harvest technique selected. They continue to use endoscopic vein harvest in non-diabetic patients with claudication and employ open techniques or segmental (skip) incisions in other bypass patients.

Coronary artery bypass grafting: Lopes, et al. in a secondary analysis of the PRE-VENT IV trial reported a higher 3-year event rate in the primary outcome measures.[27] The events analyzed included vein graft failure rates, deaths, myocardial infarctions, and need for revascularization. The original report was not randomized and the harvest techniques, surgical experience, and devices used were not specified. They concluded that endoscopic vein harvesting was independently associated with vein graft failure in the original study and was associated with adverse clinical outcomes, recommending randomized clinical trials to evaluate safety and effectiveness of endoscopic vein harvesting. Barnard and Keenan responded in 2011, suggesting that the statistical analysis was misleading and that endoscopic vein harvest technique is comparable with open harvesting techniques in both short and long-term outcomes.[28] Other reports by Dacey, et al. and a meta analysis by Athanasiou, found no difference in patency with open verses endoscopic techniques.[15,29] Future prospective clinical trials designed to evaluate the equivalence of endoscopic and open vessel harvesting techniques should clarify this debate.

Intraluminal clot formation during endoscopic vein harvest: Vessel manipulation and interruption of blood flow during endoscopic vein harvest may to be associated with an increased risk of intraluminal clot formation. As in open vein harvest techniques, minimizing vein manipulation and vein wall trauma should be incorporated in the endoscopic procedure. Using a working trocar that avoids obstructing blood flow within the targeted vein during harvest should also help minimize the risk of clot formation during endoscopic vein harvesting.[30]

Thermal injury to the vein wall during harvest: The potential for thermal injury to the vein wall during endoscopic harvest has been evaluated. Rojas-Pena et al. studied thermal spread in endoscopic vein harvesting of pigs using two devices and found that when dividing side branches, a margin of only 1 mm was needed to safeguard against thermal injury extending to the main vessel.[31] Delivering low energy electrocautery at the tunnel wall allows sealing of the vein branch and locates the electrocautery transection point safely away from the conduit. A histologic evaluation of vein samples obtained with endoscopic harvest versus an open technique found no difference between the vessels studied.

Potential carbon dioxide embolism during endoscopic vein harvest: Transesophageal echocardiography has been used to evaluate the incidence of carbon dioxide (CO_2) embolism during endoscopic vein harvests. Lin, et al. found a CO_2 embolus rate of 17.1% using a closed harvesting system with insufflation pressure of 15mmHg.[32] Using lower insufflation pressure (< 12mmHg), they later reported detection of CO_2

embolism decreased to 10.6%, of which only the first 3 out of 143 occurrences showed any clinical symptoms.[33] Kim, et al. and other authors found no hemodynamic effects during endoscopic vein harvest using CO2 insufflation with a pressure limit of 12 mmHg.[49,50] Chavanon, et al. demonstrated the importance of CO2 insufflation for endoscopic harvest, reporting increased vein trauma and wound hematomas when CO2 insufflation was not used in harvesting.[35] Avoiding a closed endoscopic system and using low pressure insufflation seems prudent for endoscopic vein harvest.

Cost and endoscopic skills: Equipment costs for endoscopic vein harvest for transposition AVFs are important but may be outweighed by potential savings in several areas including operative wound closure times, a decrease in wound complications avoiding some hospitalizations, earlier removal of dialysis catheters, and patient comfort. A learning curve for endoscopic vein harvest is variable and most likely related to previous endoscopic experience. In centers with an established cardiac or peripheral vascular program substantial institutional experience and training opportunities may be in place.

REFERENCES

1. National Kidney Foundation (NKF-K/DOQI)®. Clinical practice recommendation 8: vascular access in pediatric patients. *Am J Kidney Dis.* 2006 Jul;48 Suppl 1:S274–6.
2. Fistula First: National Vascular Access Improvement Initiative [homepage on the Internet]. http://www.fistulafirst.org/
3. Jennings WC, Kindred MG, Broughan TA. Creating radiocephalic arteriovenous fistulas: technical and functional success. *J Am Coll Surg* 2009 Mar;208(3):419–25. Epub 2009 Jan 21.
4. Dagher F, Gelber R, Ramos E, Sadler J. The use of basilic vein and brachial artery as an A-V fistula for long term hemodialysis. *J Surg Res* 1976 Apr;20(4):373–6.
5. Arroyo MR, Sideman MJ, Spergel L, Jennings WC. Primary and staged transposition arteriovenous fistulas. *J Vasc Surg* 2008 Jun;47(6):1279–83.
6. Harper SJF, Goncalves I, Donughman T, Nicholson ML. Arteriovenous fistula formation using transposed basilic vein: extensive single centre experience. *Eur J Vasc Endovasc Surg* 2008;36:237–241.
7. Oliver, MJ., McCann, R.L., Indridason, O.S., Butterfly, D.W., & Schwab, SJ. Comparison of transposed brachiobasilic fistulas to upper arm grafts and brachiocephalic fistulas. *Kidney Int* 2001;60:1532–1539.
8. Kakkos SK, Haddad GK, Weaver MR, Haddad RK, Scully MM. Basilic vein transposition: what is the optimal technique? *Eur J Vasc Endovasc Surg* 2010 May;39(5):612–9. Epub 2010 Feb 20.
9. Carolyn Glass, John Porter, Michael Singh, David Gillespie, Kate Young, Karl Illig. A large-scale study of the upper arm basilic transposition for hemodialysis. *Ann Vasc Surg* 2010 Jan;24(1):85–91. Epub 2009 Jul 23.
10. Jordan WD Jr, Voellinger DC, Schroeder PT, McDowell HA. Video-assisted saphenous vein harvest: the evolution of a new technique. *J Vasc Surg* 1997 Sep;26(3):405–12; discussion 413–4.
11. Wang S, Tang H, Wilkinson V, Lukat T, Gelfand ET, Koshal A, Modry DL, Mullen JC, Hao C, Finegan BA. Saphenous vein harvest with SaphLITE® system versus conventional technique: a prospective, randomized study. *Ann Thorac Surg* 2005 Jun;79(6):2018–23.
12. Gazoni LM, Carty R, Skinner J, Cherry KJ, Harthun NL, Kron IL, Tribble CG, Kern JA. Endoscopic versus open saphenous vein harvest for femoral to below the knee arterial bypass using saphenous vein graft. *J Vasc Surg* 2006 Aug;44(2):282–7; discussion 287–8.

13. Basbug HS, Tasatargil A, Aksoy NH, Golbasi I, Turkay C, Mete A, Sadan G, Bayezid O. Minimally invasive saphenous vein harvesting using a laryngoscope: procedural, functional, and morphologic evaluation. *Heart Surg Forum* 2005;8(6):E425–430.

14. Aranki SF, ShopnickB. Demise of open vein harvesting. *Circulation* 2011; 123:127–128.

15. Dacey LJ, Braxton JH Jr, Kramer RS, Schmoker JD, Charlesworth DC, Helm RE, Frumiento C, Sardella GL, Clough RA, Jones SR, Malenka DJ, Olmstead EM, Ross CS, O'Connor GT, Likosky DS. Long-term outcomes of endoscopic vein harvesting after coronary artery bypass grafting. *Circulation* 2011 Jan 18;123(2):147–53. Epub 2011 Jan 3.

16. Martinez BD, LeSar CJ, Fogarty TJ, Zarins CK, Hermann G. Transposition of the basilic vein for arteriovenous fistula: an endoscopic approach. *J Am Coll Surg* 2001 Feb;192(2):233–6.

17. Hayakawa K, Tsuha M, Aoyagi T, Miyaji K, Hata M, Tanaka S, Tanaka A, Shiota J. New method to create a vascular arteriovenous fistula in the arm with an endoscopic technique. *J Vasc Surg* 2002 Sep;36(3):635–8.

18. Tordoir JH, Dammers R, de Brauw M. Video-assisted basilic vein transposition for haemodialysis vascular access: preliminary experience with a new technique. *Nephrol Dial Transpl* 2001 Feb;16(2):391–4.

19. Oto, T. Endoscopic saphenous vein harvesting for hemodialysis vascular access creation in the forearm: A new approach for arteriovenous bridge graft. *J Vasc Access* 2003 Jul-Sep;4(3): 98–101.

20. Paul EM, Sideman MJ, Rhoden DH, Jennings WC. Endoscopic basilic vein transposition for hemodialysis access. *J Vasc Surg* 2010;51(6):1451–56. Epub 2010 Mar 20.

21. Keuter XH, van der Sande FM, Kessels AG, de Haan MW, Hoeks AP, Tordoir JH. Excellent performance of one-stage brachial-basilic arteriovenous fistula. *Nephrol Dial Transpl* 2005;20:2168–2171.

22. Hill BB, Chan AK, Faruqi RM, Arko FR, Zarins CK, Fogarty TJ. Keyhole technique for autologous brachiobasilic transposition arteriovenous fistula. *J Vasc Surg* 2005 Nov;42(5):945–50.

23. Jennings WC, Sideman MJ, Taubman KE, Broughan TA. Brachial vein transposition arteriovenous fistulas for hemodialysis access. *J Vasc Surg* 2009 May; 49(5) (suppl):S5–S6.

24. Barnard KJ, Taubman KE, Jennings WC. Accessible autogenous vascular access for hemodialysis in obese individuals using lipectomy. *Am J Surg* 2010 Dec;200(6):798–802; discussion 802.

25. Jennings WC. Creating arteriovenous fistulas in 132 consecutive patients: exploiting the proximal radial artery arteriovenous fistula: reliable, safe and simple forearm and upper arm hemodialysis access. *Arch Surg* 2006 Jan;141(1):27–32; discussion 32.

26. Walker J, Katzen J, Nabozny M, Young K, Glass C, Singh MJ, Illig KA. Long-term results of endoscopic versus open saphenous vein harvest for lower extremity bypass. *Ann Vas Surg* 2011;25:101–107.

27. Lopes RD, Hafley GE, Allen KB, Ferguson TB, Peterson ED, Harrington RA, Mehta RH, Gibson CM, Mack MJ, Kouchoukos NT, Califf RM, Alexander JH. Endoscopic versus open vein-graft harvesting in coronary-artery bypass surgery. *New Engl J Med* 361(3): 235–44.

28. Barnard JB, Keenan DJM. Endoscopic saphenous vein harvesting for coronary artery bypass grafts: NICE guidance. *Heart* 2011; 97: 327–329.

29. Athanasiou T, Aziz O, Al-Ruzzeh S, Philippidis P, Jones C, Purkayastha S, Casula R, Glenville B. Are wound healing disturbances and length of hospital stay reduced with minimally invasive vein harvest? A meta-analysis. *Eur J Cardiothorac Surg* 2004;26:1015–1026.

30. Brown EN, Kon ZN, Tran R, Burris NS, Gu J, Laird P, Brazio PS, Kallam S, Schwartz K, Bechtel L, Joshi A, Zhang S, Poston RS. Strategies to reduce intraluminal clot formation in endoscopically harvested saphenous veins. *J Thorac Cardiov Surg* 2007;134:1259–1265.

31. Rojas-Pena A, Koch KL, Heitner HD, Hall CM, Bergin IL, Cook KE. Quantification of thermal spread and burst pressure after endoscopic vessel harvesting: A comparison of 2 commercially available devices, *J Thorac Cardiov Surg* 2010;09:1–6.

32. Lin T-Y, Chiu K-M, Wang M-J, Chu S-H. Carbon dioxide embolism during endoscopic saphenous vein harvesting in coronary artery bypass surgery. *J Thorac Cardiov Surg* 2003; 126:2011–15.

33. Chiu K-M, Chen C-L, Chu S-H, Lin T-Y. Endoscopic harvest of saphenous vein: a lesson learned from 1,348 cases. *Surgical Endoscopy* 2008;22:183–7.
34. Kim SH, Kim DK, Yoon TG, Lim JA, Woo NS, Kim TY. Haemodynamic effects during endoscopic vein harvest of the saphenous vein for off-pump coronary artery bypass grafting surgery. *Eur J Anaesthesiol* 2009;26(11):969–73.
35. Chavanon O, Ducharme B, Carrier M, Cartier R, Hasbert Y, Pagas P, Pellerin M, Pelletier LC, Perrault LP. Endoscopic saphenectomy for coronary artery bypass surgery: comparison of two techniques with and without carbon dioxide insufflation. *Can J Cardiol* 2000;16(6): 757–61

37

Novel Technique to Salvage Aneurysmal AVF

Timothy G. Canty, Jr., MD and Karen Woo, MD

INTRODUCTION

Over the last decade, K-DOQI guidelines have increasingly emphasized the importance of autogenous arteriovenous fistula (AVF) for dialysis access. While it is clear that ateriovenous fistula have lower rates of infection and thrombosis when compared to dialysis grafts, nearly one third of all ateriovenous fistula develop complications. A poorly defined complication of AVF is aneurysm formation. The incidence of aneurysm formation in autogenous arteriovenous fistula (AVF) ranges from 5% to as high as 30%, the majority of which occur in the upper arm.[1] The sequelae of aneurysm formation in AVF include skin breakdown, bleeding, rupture, thrombosis, poor flow resulting in inadequate dialysis, and infection.

K-DOQI guidelines recommend that intervention be performed on aneurysmal AVF and that aneurysmal AVF segments should not be cannulated.[2] Treatment strategies for AVF aneurysms include ligation, placement of prosthetic interposition, or more recently, use of percutaneous stent grafts. The aneurysms described in most reports using these techniques are focal or are pseudoaneurysms. There is, however, a subset of dialysis patients with diffuse, massive, and tortuous aneurysmal dilatation of their AVF who present a unique challenge. In an effort to maintain an all-autogenous access, we developed a procedure to treat diffusely aneurysmal AVF in which the luminal diameter is reduced, excess length is resected, and the newly reconstructed AVF is re-tunneled for continued use. In this chapter we examine the incidence of true aneurysms in AVF, the natural history and complications associated with aneurysmal AVF, put forth our treatment protocol and surgical technique as well as evaluate other published methods to treat aneurysmal AVF.

INCIDENCE

The true incidence of aneurysmal degeneration of AVF is difficult to determine. These aneurysms have a variable presentation ranging from unsightly appearance to acute bleeding and infection and thus do not always come to the attention of providers. Furthermore, the definition of an aneurysmal AVF is not well established. Pasklinsky defined an aneurysmal AVF as a dilatation more than three times the native vessel diameter with the reference segment not including the areas immediately before or after the aneurysms.[3] Their group, in an effort to discern aneurysms from local dilations, suggested a minimum diameter of at least 2 cm. This definition would be applicable to most of the patients treated in our series but not all. Several cephalic upper arm fistula we operated on had diffuse aneurysmal dilation from the arterial anastomosis through the entire cephalic arch, not allowing for any type of reference vessel diameter. The incidence reported in the literature ranges 5-7% up to 30%.[1,3] Most reports include focal dilations as well as pseudoaneuryms which appear to be much more common than true aneurysms of the venous wall.

ETIOLOGY

There are several theories as to why AVF become aneurysmal. Repeated punctures at access sites may progressively weaken the venous wall in a kind of "Swiss cheese" type effect resulting in gradual dilation of the outflow vein.[3] This causal mechanism would be a reasonable explanation for focal aneurysmal dilation of segments that are "over used" for a significant period of time. In contrast to this scenario, the series of aneurysms that we treated were all diffusely enlarged, affecting almost the entire length of the fistula from the anastomosis to its central outflow. Clearly, the etiology of this diffuse aneurysmal dilatation is not related to a focal problem with repeated cannulation.

Central or outflow vein stenosis can contribute to aneurysmal dilation by increasing the pressure in the fistula. In our series, less than 20% of the patients with aneurysmal AVF had central stenoses detected on pre-operative fistulagram. This incidence is consistent with a report by Pasklinsky of 23 aneurysmal AVF in which 17% of the patients were found to have a central outflow stenosis.[3] While it seems plausible that venous hypertension caused by central or outflow stenosis could contribute to aneurysmal dilation of AVF, it is apparent that the two are not mutually exclusive. Not all, or even a majority, of patients with aneurysmal AVF have a central stenosis, and the vast majority of dialysis patients found to have central stenosis do not have aneurysms of their AVF.

Interestingly, there were multiple patients in our series whose AVF developed diffuse aneurysmal dilation prior to the AVF even being punctured for dialysis. One such patient stated her new fistula grew rapidly and became aneurysmal within four to six months. These patients were all renal transplant patients with failing or failed transplants. In fact, 47% of the patients in our series had a history of renal transplantation. Pasklinsky also noted that 14 of 23 patients (61%) requiring management of aneurysmal AVF had received a kidney transplant.[3] We speculate that there may be an association between immunosuppression and fistula aneurysm formation. An association has been previously described in relation to immunosuppression and abdominal aortic aneurysm (AAA) enlargement. A series examining 1500 heart, liver and kidney transplant patients demonstrated that while the incidence of AAA in the transplant patients was no different from the normal population, the rate of growth and rupture was significantly higher.[4] Ammori reviewed the literature and found a mean aneurysm growth rate of 1.10 cm per year in aortic aneurysms that were diagnosed after cardiac transplantation.[5] In addition, a link between prednisone and aneurysm formation as well as rupture has been demonstrated in an animal model.[6]

There are also reports linking aneurysm formation in vein grafts occurring in patients with other known aneurysms suggesting some type of a systemic dilatory process or predisposition. This has been seen in vein grafts dilating after use for repair of popliteal aneurysms as well as leg grafts dilating in patients with known AAA.[7,8] While a vein graft and an AVF both have systemic pressure and high flow the local hemodynamics are different between the two groups.[3] In our series of 19 patients with diffuse aneurysmal dilation of their AVF, none of the patients had any other type of aneurysm known or in their history.

NATURAL HISTORY/COMPLICATIONS

Aneurysmal dilation of an AVF occurs over several years in most cases. The mean time a fistula was in use prior to intervention for aneurysm in our series was 48 months and 47 months in the series described by Pasklinsky.[3] The exact nature of how these occur and grow is largely unknown for several reasons. The dialysis units appreciate a large fistula as it is generally easy to stick. With a "if it ain't broke, don't fix it" mentality in most dialysis centers, it is difficult determine if there is a size at which problems can start to occur or at what size revision/reduction is indicated.

Well documented complications of aneurysmal AVF include skin breakdown, inflammation, pain, infection, thrombosis, poor flow, steal syndrome, venous hypertension, and high output congestive heart failure. Cannulation issues are also a common problem with aneurysmal AVF. The aneurysmal segments typically are lined with mural thrombus which can become significant, making access to the flow channel with standard dialysis needles difficult. In our series two patients were referred for "thrombosed" fistulas due to dark clot found in the needles. However, on further examination, the flow in the aneurysmal AVF was patent but the segments being punctured had thrombus over a centimeter thick.

There have been no reported cases of spontaneous rupture of an aneurysmal AVF. Histologic examination of the wall of an aneurysmal AVF demonstrates significant collagen infiltration and wall thickening making spontaneous rupture unlikely.[3] In contrast, there have been reports of rupture of an aneurysmal AVF after direct cannulation of the aneurysmal segment.[9] The National Kidney Foundation Disease Outcomes Quality Initiative guidelines recommend that direct cannulation of aneurysmal segments in AVF be avoided.[2]

Another potential serious complication of aneurysmal AVF is infection. The repeated puncture of aneurysmal fistula with sub-sterile technique in areas of poor quality, compromised skin can lead to superficial skin infections. In addition, the thrombus can become seeded with bacteria, leading to infections of the thrombus and the aneurysmal wall itself. This can lead to acute bleeding as well as intravascular infection. Three patients in our series had evidence of focal infection around the aneurysmal portion of their AVF. These patients were started immediately on antibiotics and their work up and surgical treatment was expedited to within 24-48 hours. In these patients, the infected portion of the aneurysmal AVF was resected, the area was copiously irrigated with antibiotic solution, and the reduction/revision surgery was carried out.

TREATMENT OPTIONS

One of the first descriptions of aneurysms of AVF was published in 1978 which included a series of five aneurysms which had formed in areas of repeated needle puncture.[10] The only management that was performed for these aneurysms was avoidance of these areas for future puncture. Subsequently, a variety of approaches have been described to treat AVF aneurysms with the majority involving resection of the aneurysmal portion of the AVF and performing an interposition repair with graft or other material. These approaches will all be discussed, in addition to a novel approach using only autogenous tissue which was developed by the authors.

The most straightforward approach to treating aneurysmal AVF is by simply ligating the fistula with or without resection of the aneurysmal portion.[3,11–13] This method eliminates the problem, however mandates that a new dialysis access be created. Given that the number of patients requiring a renal transplant continues to increase faster than the number of available donors and the median wait time to receive a renal transplant is four years, preserving sites for access has become paramount.[14]

One technique to preserve the fistula is to resect the aneurysmal portion and perform re-anastomosis.[9,11,15] This approach requires that there is adequate length in the fistula that can be mobilized to obtain a tension-free anastomosis. This technique works well for smaller, localized aneurysms.

For more extensive aneurysms, one of the most common techniques for repair is resection of the aneurysmal portion and replacement with an interposition graft. Polytetrafluoroethylene (PTFE) is regularly used as the interposition graft.[3,11,16] This approach preserves the access site but essentially converts the access into an arteriovenous graft with the associated risks of infection and decreased patency. Another option for interposition graft, is the saphenous vein.[3] In a series of seven patients where the aneurysmal AVF was replaced with great saphenous vein, six were still patent at a mean follow-up of 18 months with one thrombosis.[3] Although the authors do not provide a direct comparison of patency between saphenous vein and prosthetic graft, they do state that they preferentially use saphenous vein over prosthetic graft when saphenous vein is available.

Several techniques of aneurysmorrhaphy have been described with some involving implantation of an external graft. A case report of one patient involved a technique of longitudinally incising the aneurysm, oversewing the wall with prolene suture over a Hegar dilator, followed by wrapping of the segment in braided metal mesh.[15] This patient was successfully using the fistula and had no complications 15 months postoperatively with no evidence of aneurysm recurrence. Another series of four patients described a similar technique of oversewing the wall of the aneurysm and then wrapping the segment with a polyethylene terephthalate prosthesis to reduce the incidence of intimal hyperplasia.[17] One patient required removal of the external prosthesis during the post-operative period for infection. All four patients in the series were successfully using their fistulas for dialysis within four to six weeks of surgery. No long term follow up was provided on this group of patients. A third technique of aneurysmorrhaphy involves plication of the aneurysm.[18] In this technique, a clamp is placed longitudinally over the aneurysmal area and the excess wall is plicated using 4.0 prolene suture without resecting the excess. A series of 15 patients who underwent this procedure did not experience any thrombosis or graft failure in the post-operative period, but long-term follow up is not provided.[18]

An alternative technique for aneurysmorrhaphy has been performed using surgical staplers.[19,20] The stapler is used longitudinally to reduce the aneurysm, the excess wall is resected and the staple line is then oversewn with prolene suture. In a series of 12 patients treated in this fashion, during the mean follow up of 29 months, two patients developed recurrent aneurysms.[20] The AVF in the remaining ten patients remained patent without recurrence of aneurysm formation. A separate series of five patients managed with the stapler method had patent functional fistulas during the follow up of eight months to one year.[19]

More recently, with the increasing popularity of endovascular interventions, covered stents have been used to repair aneurysmal AVF. This technique is more commonly used in the treatment of arteriovenous graft pseudoaneurysms.[20–23] There is a report of two patients with AVF being treated in this fashion.[24] These two patients had their aneurysms excluded with a Wallgraft endoprosthesis (Boston Scientific Inc., Watertown, MA). One of the AVF failed at 3 months after the procedure. The other patient's AVF remained patent at six months with no flow outside the Wallgraft on ultrasound. The authors of this paper advised against puncturing the Wallgraft. This technique would be feasible in patients with localized aneurysms who have adequate landing zones for the stent graft as well as adequate length of remaining access to use for dialysis access puncture. While this technique does preserve future access sites, it again essentially converts an autogenous fistula into a prosthetic graft.

OUR TECHNIQUE

We have described a reduction/revision procedure for repair of aneurysmal AVF that involves using only autogenous tissue.[25] Our procedure is applicable to localized aneurysms, but as stated above was developed initially to address diffusely aneurysmal AVF. We have a standardized pre-operative work up for aneurysmal AVF. Initial consultation involves a detailed history and physical exam. We pay particular attention to the quality of the overlying skin noting any lesions, scabs or evidence of infection and erosion. The overall size of the arm was examined looking for any signs of central venous stenosis. Hand perfusion and neurologic function was examined to rule out any steal syndrome. The date the fistula was created and the date it was first used were determined as well as when the fistula first began to enlarge. The dialysis units were queried about the flow in the aneurysmal AVF during dialysis as well the effectiveness of the dialysis. Additional information about site of cannulation, difficulty with puncture, and prolonged bleeding after needle removal was also obtained.

All patients who present with aneurysmal fistula undergo a complete duplex exam in our vascular lab for characterization of the fistula and evaluation for stenoses. The fistula treated in our series all had very diffuse, not focal, aneurysms with significant tortuosity. In reconstruction and revision of aneurysmal AVF our technique involves resection of a significant length of fistula to achieve a new fistula that lies in a straight path. Pre operative duplex allows us to look at the entire aneurysmal fistula and determine the most diseased segments and thus plan which segments to target for resection.

After the intial duplex exam we recommend a preoperative fistulagram. While this again helps fully characterize the aneurysmal fistula, the primary purpose of this study is determine if there is a central venous or outflow vein stenosis or occlusion.

We feel this is important because if a patient has a central venous occlusion, we do not proceed with the revision and reduction procedure. Following our experience with this series of patients, we have changed our practice and opted not to perform the reduction/revision on patients with central venous or outflow vein stenoses or occlusions. The poor long term viability of an AVF with central occlusion and a high likelihood of aneurysm recurrence and arm edema are lessons that we learned from our initial experience. Symptomatic or problematic fistula aneurysms in patients with central venous occlusion are now treated with ligation and resection, and construction of a new dialysis access on the contralateral arm.

In our initial experience, patients with aneurysmal AVF and central venous or outflow vein stenosis were treated with angioplasty and then operated on. In our series, nearly 20% of the patients had central stenosis. These patients were treated with angioplasty utilizing a combination of a cutting balloon followed by a high pressure balloon. Those patients treated pre operatively for a central or outflow stenosis were studied between 3-6 weeks post operatively to reassess to stenosis and re-treat if necessary. In one patient with a massive aneurysmal cephalic AVF, a high grade 4 cm cephalic arch stenosis was identified. The reduction/revision surgery was completed and the new fistula was transected at the level of the cephalic arch and rotated into a small axillary incision where a new veno-veno anastomosis was created to allow for outflow via the axillary vein. The overall poor long term results in treating the cephalic arch stenosis in this manner with angioplasty and even stenting caused us to change the way we now approach these patients.

SURGICAL TECHNIQUE

Due to the length of the procedure and the extensive dissection, we routinely use general anesthesia for patient comfort during the reduction/revision procedure. We place a tunneled hemodialysis catheter at the time of the operation for use until the operative site has healed.

The first step of the procedure is to make a skin incision along the length of the aneurysmal fistula. The aneurysmal fistula is then circumferentially dissected out from the arterial anastomosis to a point where the fistula becomes normal in diameter. (Figure 37–1) A full dose of heparin is then given intravenously. Proximal and distal control of the fistula is obtained using vascular clamps. The aneurysmal fistula is then opened longitudinally along its entire length. (Figure 37–2) The excess length secondary to the tortuosity of the aneurysmal fistula is resected. (Figure 37–3) A back wall anastomosis is constructed using a 6-0 prolene suture in a running fashion. (Figure 37–4) In order to construct a fistula that is 8-10 mm in diameter, a 20 French red rubber catheter is inserted into either end of the fistula. Using the catheter as a guide, the excess wall of the fistula is resected. The fistula is then reconstructed over the catheter again using 6-0 prolene suture. (Figure 37–5) An effort is made to create the suture line on the lateral or medial aspect of the reconstructed fistula in order to avoid repeated puncture of the suture line when the fistula is used for dialysis. A new tunnel is created for the fistula. (Figure 37–6) The excess skin over the fistula is resected. (Figure 37–7) Any areas of skin breakdown or thinning of the skin are included in the excision. Finally, the skin is closed in two layers using absorbable sutures and a subcuticular skin closure. (Figure 37–8)

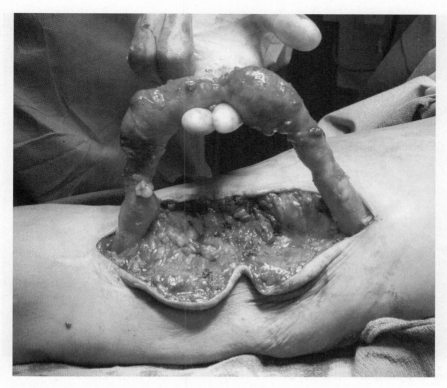

Figure 37–1. Circumferential dissection of aneurysmal fistula

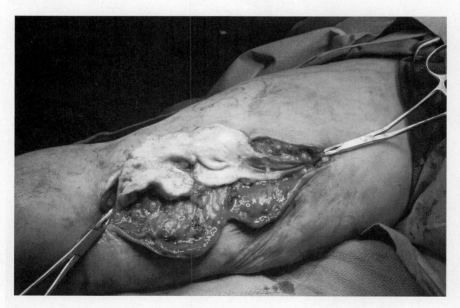

Figure 37–2. Longitudinal venotomy along length of fistula

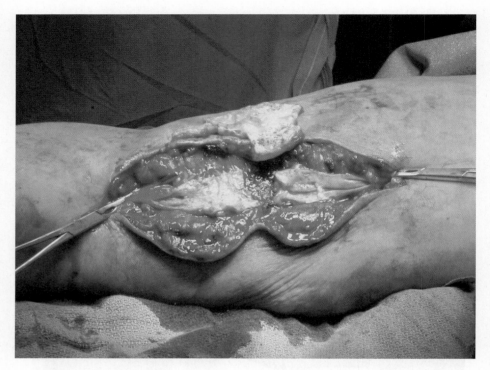

Figure 37–3. Resection of excess length

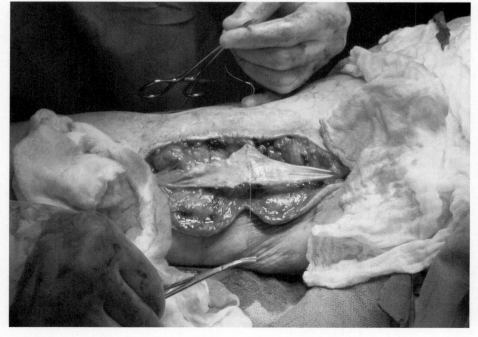

Figure 37–4. Back wall anastomosis

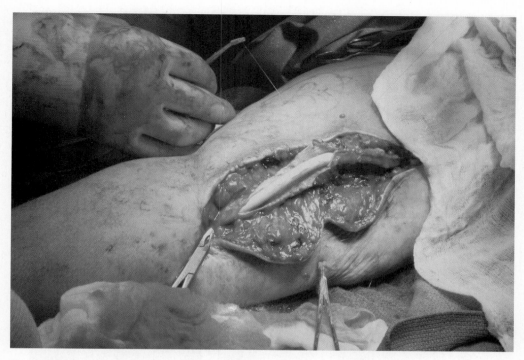

Figure 37–5. Reconstruction of fistula over red robinson catheter

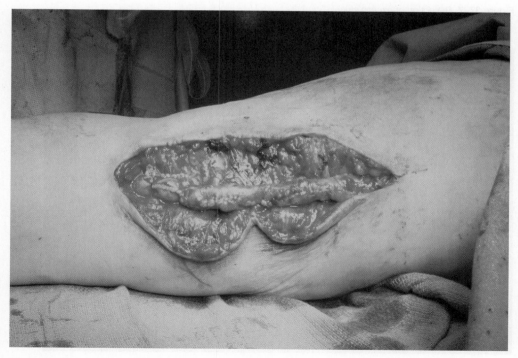

Figure 37–6. Reconstructed fistula

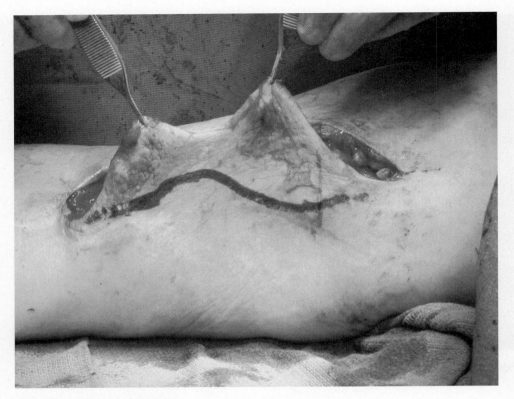

Figure 37–7. Resection of excess skin

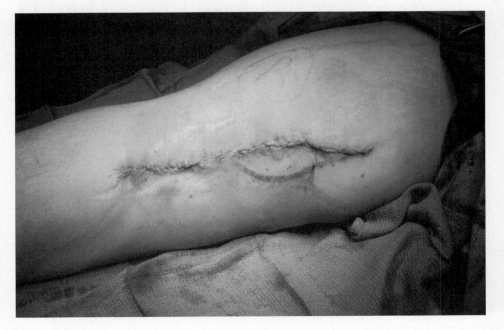

Figure 37–8. Skin closure

Patients are followed post-operatively by the vascular surgeon until the wound is healed. Once the wound is adequately healed, hemodialysis through the fistula is resumed. The tunneled catheter is removed when successful hemodialysis through the fistula is achieved.

In a series of 19 patients treated in this fashion over a 4 year period, the mean operative time was 188 minutes and the mean estimated blood loss was 268cc. The median follow up was 23 months. The median primary patency was 14 months with an interquartile range (IQR) of 24. The median secondary patency was 16.5 months, IQR 26. The mean post-operative length of stay was 1.1 and the mean time to removal of tunneled hemodialysis catheter was ten weeks.

During the follow-up period, three patients required percutaneous angioplasty of an outflow stenosis to maintain patency. One patient who had an infection pre-operatively developed an infection in the 30-day post-operative period and required removal of the fistula. There was one thrombosis at 15 months and one at 16 months. One late infection occurred at 27 months that required fistula ligation and there were two late deaths that were not related to the fistula. Three patients were lost to follow-up. Of the eleven patients still being followed at the end of the follow-up period, all had functional fistulas with no evidence of recurrence.

CONCLUSION

Aneurysms of arteriovenous fistulas are a relatively uncommon but potentially serious complication for end-stage renal disease patients who rely on hemodialysis. The indications for treatment include skin breakdown, difficulty with puncture, high output congestive heart failure and quality of life. A variety of approaches have been described for the surgical treatment of aneurysmal AVF, most of which are applicable to focal aneurysms and involve use of a type of interposition graft. Our novel approach of surgical resection of excess length, reduction of luminal diameter, and reconstruction is a viable option for the treatment of complicated diffusely aneurysmal AVF. Mid-term results of this novel procedure demonstrate acceptable patency and complication rates. This technique offers the ability to maintain the benefits of an all-autogenous dialysis access while conserving future dialysis sites.

REFERENCES

1. Salahi H, Fazelzadeh A, Mehdizadeh A, et al. Complications of arteriovenous fistula in dialysis patients. *Transplant Proc* 2006;38:1261–4.
2. KDOQI Clinical Practice Guidelines and Clinical Practice Recommendations for 2006 Updates: Hemodialysis adequacy, peritoneal dialysis adequacy and vascular access. *Am J Kidney Dis* 2006;48:S1–S322 (suppl 1).
3. Pasklinsky G, Meisner R, Labrropoulos N, et al. Management of true aneurysms of hemodialysis access fistulas. *J Vasc Surgery* 53:1291–1297.
4. Englesbe MJ, Wu AH, Clowes AW, et al. The prevalence and natural history of aortic aneurysms in heart and abdominal organ transplant patients. *J Vasc Surg* 2003;37:27–31.
5. Ammori BJ, Madan M, Bodenham AR, et al. A review of the management of abdominal aortic aneurysms in patients following cardiac transplantation. *Eur J Vasc Endovasc Surg* 1997;14:185–90.

6. Reilly JM, Savage EB, Brophy CM, et al. Hydrocortisone rapidly induces aortic rupture in a genetically susceptible mouse. *Arch Surg* 1990;125:707–9.
7. Peer Rm, Upson JF. Aneurysmal dilation in saphenous vein bypass grafts. *J Cardiovasc Surg* 1990;31:668–71.
8. Nishibe T, Muto A, Kaneko K, et al. True aneurysms in a saphenous vein graft placed for repair of a popliteal aneurysm: etiologic considerations. *Ann Vasc Surg* 2004:18:747–9.
9. Yang TH, Lee CH, Tsai CS, et al. Successful surgical treatment of a rupture to an arteriovenous fistula aneurysm. *Cardiovasc J Afr* 2009;20:196–7.
10. Mennes PA, Gilula LA, Anderson CB, et al. Complications associated with arteriovenous fistulas in patients undergoing chronic hemodialysis. *Arch Intern Med* 1978;138:1117–21.
11. Patel KR, Chan FA, Batista RJ, et al. True venous aneurysms and arterial steal secondary to arteriovenous fistulae for dialysis. *J Cardiovasc Surg* 1992;33:185–8.
12. Karabay O, Yetkin U, Silistreli E, et al. Surgical management of giant aneurysms complicating arteriovenous fistulae. *J Int Med Res* 2004;32:214–7.
13. Lam W, Betal D, Morsy M, et al. Enormous brachio-cephalic arteriovenous fistula aneurysm after renal transplantatation: case report and review of the literature. *Nephrol Dial Transplant* 2009;24:3542–4.
14. 2007 Annual Report of the U.S. Organ Procurement and Transplantation Network and the Scientific Registry of Transplant Recipients: Transplant Data 1994–2003. Department of Health and Human Services, Health Resources and Services Administration, Healthcare Systems Bureau, Division of Transplantation, Rockville, MD; United Network for Organ Sharing, Richmond, VA; Arbor Research Collaborative for Health, Ann Arbor, MI.
15. Georgiadis GS, Lazarides MK, Panagoutsos SA, et al. Surgical revision of complicated false and true vascular access related aneurysms. *J Vasc Surg* 2008;47:1284–91.
16. Grauhan O, Zurbrugg HR, Hetzer R. Management of aneurysmal arteriovenous fistula by a perivascular mesh. *Eur J Vasc Endovasc Surg* 2001;21:274–5.
17. Balaz P, Rokosny S, Dlein D, et al. Aneurysmorrhaphy is an easy technique for arteriovenous fistula salvage. *J Vasc Access* 2008;9:81–4.
18. Lo HY. Arteriovenous fistula aneurysm-plicate, not ligate. *Ann Acad Med* Singapore 2007;36:851–3.
19. Hakim NS, Romagnoli J, Contis JC, et al. Refashioning of an aneurysmatic arterio-venous fistula by using the multifire GIA 60 surgical stapler. *Int Surg* 1997;82:376–7.
20. Pierce GE, Thomas JG, Fenton JR. Novel repair of venous aneurysms secondary to arteriovenous dialysis fistulae. *Vasc Endovasc Surg* 2007;41:55–60.
21. Vesely TM. Use of stent grafts to repair hemodialysis graft-related pseudoaneurysms. *J Vasc Interv Radiol* 2005;16:1301–7.
22. Barshes NR, Annambhotla S, Bechara C, et al. Endovascular repair of hemodialysis graft-related pseudoaneurysm: an alternative treatment strategy in salvaging failing dialysis access. *Vasc Endovasc Surg* 2008;42:228–34.
23. Hausegger KA, Tiessenhausen K, Klimpfinger M, et al. Aneurysms of hemodialysis access grafts: treatment with covered stents: a report of three cases. *Cardiovasc Inte Rad* 1998;21:334–7.
24. Najibi S, Bush RL, Terramani TT, et al. Covered stent exclusion of dialysis access pseudoaneurysms. *J Surg Res* 2002;106:15–9.
25. Woo K, Cook PR, Garg J, et al. Mid-term results of a novel technique to salvage autogenous dialysis access in aneurysmal arteriovenous fistulas. *J Vasc Surg* 2010;51:921–925.

38

Management of Central Vein Obstruction

Shankar M. Sundaram, MD and Brian G. Peterson, MD

OVERVIEW

Obstruction of the central venous circulation and the superior vena cava (SVC) is an increasingly more common and widespread clinical problem worldwide. The SVC and the brachiocephalic veins bilaterally serve as the primary venous drainage system for the head, neck and upper extremities. The SVC is a low pressure thin walled structure in the middle mediastinum that is susceptible to external compression from the other more rigid structures in the area including the trachea, aorta, peritracheal and peribronchial lymph nodes, and the pulmonary artery. Prior to draining into the right atrium, the azygos vein joins the SVC, and it serves, along with the hemiazygos vein, intercostal veins, internal thoracic veins, and superior/inferior epigastric veins as important collateral pathways for the drainage of the head and neck and upper extremity. The clinical effects of venous congestion of the head and neck and upper extremities affects more than 15,000 individuals in the United States per year. In its most rare and severe form, facial and upper extremity edema, dilated chest wall venous collaterals, and dyspnea has been characterized as the SVC syndrome. Historically, malignant etiologies were the main cause of central vein obstruction (CVO), but non-malignant causes such as chronic indwelling intravenous catheter use and permanent pacemaker leads have surged in recent times. Treatment of CVO has traditionally been surgical, which enjoys great palliative and curative effects for both malignant and non-malignant etiologies. Endovascular therapies, however, have recently revolutionized the treatment of CVO, and now have been shown to be the first line treatment in many of these patients.

In this chapter, the etiology, pathophysiology, clinical signs, and diagnostic workup of CVO will be discussed, along with the detailed description and analysis of surgical and endovascular treatments for CVO.

ETIOLOGY

The first description of CVO was in 1757 by the Scottish anatomist William Hunter, which was due to a large thoracic aortic aneurysm.[1] Case reports throughout the next two centuries focused on this etiology, as well as infectious causes such as tuberculous and syphilitic lesions. With widespread tobacco use, thoracic malignancies were accountable for over 80% of the cases of CVO and subsequent SVC syndrome by the mid-twentieth century.[2] The advent of chronic indwelling catheters dramatically increased the number of non-malignant causes of CVO, especially among patients with end stage renal disease (ESRD), who develop intimal hyperplasia as well as venous thrombosis.

Pulmonary malignancies account for over 60% of the cases of CVO and SVC syndrome. These include both primary mediastinal and bronchogenic carcinomas. Bronchogenic carcinomas account for 77% of thoracic malignancy cases and 46% of all SVC syndrome cases. Cancers are almost equally divided between small cell and non-small cell lung malignancies. Lymphoma accounted for 8% of the total and germ cell tumors accounted for 3%. Although germ cell tumors are relatively rare, SVC syndrome developed in the highest percentage of these. Metastatic prostate cancer, thymic cancer, and adenocarcinoma of unknown primary are more rare malignant causes of CVO.[3]

Benign etiologies account for 40% of the cases of CVO. Of these, approximately 70% are from chronic indwelling central catheters.[6] The obstruction is internal and composed of thrombus, fibrosis or a combination of the two. The risk of CVO with the use of these catheters is cumulative, with increased number and duration of catheters having a higher risk. In addition, the particular access site for central venous catheter placement is important in terms of increasing risk. Catheters placed by subclavian access have a 42% incidence of CVO compared to internal jugular access, and left-sided accesses have increased rates of CVO as compared to right sided accesses.[4] Overall, 1–3% of patients with CVO proceed to SVC syndrome.[3]

Cardiac rhythm management devices (CRMD) encompass permanent pacemakers (PPM) and implantable cardiodefibrillators (ICD). These devices are usually placed percutaneously into the subclavian vein or via surgical cutdown into the cephalic vein. Either single or dual leads are placed into the central circulation, with the tips of the leads into the right atrium and/or ventricle. CVO secondary to CRMD has been documented for more than three decades. Early studies with first generation CRMD devices with bulky leads and larger introducing sheaths lead to a total occlusion rate of 32% and severe stenosis with collateral formation in 47%.[5] More recent studies have placed the rate of CVO in the range of 6–21%, and usually occur more than one month after implantation.[6] In addition, maturation of ipsilateral dialysis access sites are often hampered by the presence of CRMD, and the presence of both a CRMD and an indwelling venous catheter in an ipsilateral extremity doubles the rate of CVO and its sequelae of SVC syndrome.[7]

Mediastinal fibrosis was once the most common benign cause of CVO. The pathophysiology is either idiopathic or due to chronic Histoplasmosis infection. These bulky lesions expand from the lymph nodes in the middle mediastinum and paratracheal areas to occlude the SVC. Because of the slow nature of this growth, presentation is rarely emergent. Medical therapy, including corticosteroids are the mainstay of treatment, with interventional or surgical techniques applied to SVC syndrome or recurrent cases. Stent malpositioning and vessel injury are common with intervention on these lesions, as the firm nature of the compressing mass leads to migration, and a tendency to overinflate procedural balloons.[8]

PATHOPHYSIOLOGY

The mechanism of CVO is dependent on the underlying etiology that initiated the process. Extrinsic compression of the SVC and central veins has a different sequence of events than intrinsic endothelial changes from indwelling catheters, though both processes lead to the common result of CVO.

Extrinsic compression of the central veins leads to severe narrowing of the flow lumen. Given that the central veins have low pressure and flow, intravascular thrombus formation occurs quite readily, with the formation of cytokines and other inflammatory products that promote a fibrotic state.[9] If the extrinsic process invades the central veins, tumor emboli producing distal obstruction or occlusion can occur separate from the thrombotic reaction to the intravascular foreign body.

The presence of central venous catheters (CVC) causes a localized trauma to the venous endothelium that leads to a complex cascade of inflammatory events that combine with non-laminar flow and turbulence from the presence of the CVC itself within the lumen. Turbulence has been shown to cause platelet deposition and venous wall thickening.[10] Endothelial denudation occurs with the CVC placement, and platelet microthrombi develop in 24 hours, followed by the presence of smooth muscle cells in 7–8 days. With the continued presence of the CVC in the lumen of the vessel, over the next 2 weeks the microthrombi consolidate into organized thrombi. Over the long term (greater than 90 days), the continued inflammatory state results in vessel wall thickening, formation of a fibrin bridge and lumen narrowing.[10]

CLINICAL FINDINGS

CVO has various modes of presentation, depending on the primary etiology, the duration of the particular disease, and location of the stenosis or occlusion. For ESRD patients, they can present as asymptomatic and CVO's are only found on diagnostic central venography in conjunction with evaluation prior to access placement. CVO's can also present during access evaluation for poor maturation, bleeding, and flows on dialysis. Clinical signs of venous congestion secondary to subclavian vein pathology include edema and venous hypertension of the corresponding extremity or breast. If the brachiocephalic veins are involved, there is edema of the ipsilateral neck and face, and possibly of the ipsilateral extremity.[21] Both of these locations are many fold worse if there is a patent and functioning arteriovenous access on the side of the CVO. Besides the most common finding of ipsilateral edema, the next most common finding is extensive chest wall collateral vein formation.

The spectrum of clinical findings extends to perhaps the most dreaded clinical finding in CVO's, which is the SVC syndrome. It is characterized by bilateral innominate vein and SVC stenosis, which produces bilateral upper extremity and neck swelling, extensive collateral vein formation, dyspnea, orthopnea and shortness of breath leading to airway compromise. Other late findings include dysphagia and cognitive dysfunction, hemoptysis and hoarseness. Malignant patients will also present with weight loss and lethargy. Lymphoma patients will also have night sweats and fever. (Figure 38–1, Figure 38–2)

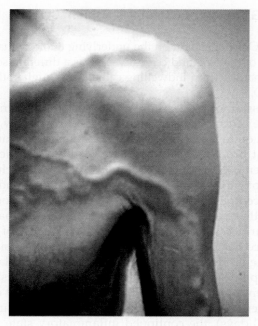

Figure 38–1. Chest wall collaterals due to CVO

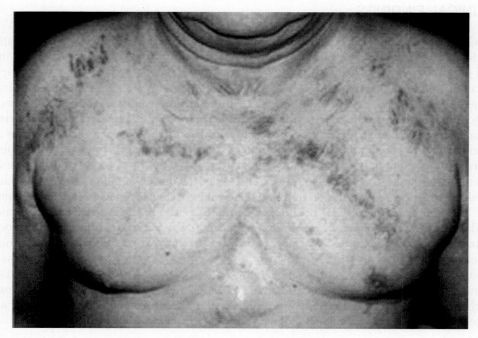

Figure 38–2. Bilateral chest wall collaterals
(Images from Wieser S, Kohler, M:QJM (2010) 103(9): 707)

DIAGNOSTIC EVALUATION

A detailed history and physical exam will almost always suggest the diagnosis of CVO, as well as allowing one to focus on the diagnostic treatment modalities. Obtaining in the patient's history the type, number and location of previous access sites in the extremity involved should be elucidated, as well as any previous PPM or cardiac devices. Weight loss, dyspnea, hemoptysis, night fever, sweats are other questions that should be solicited.

a) Plain x-rays

Helpful only for malignant and non-catheter causes of CVO, as mediastinal shift due to mass effect or an actual lung mass can be seen. In the absence of gross abnormalities such as these, the yield for plain chest x-rays is low.

b) Ultrasonography

Can be utilized to evaluate the extra-thoracic vessels such as the internal jugular, subclavian, and cephalic veins, as the brachiocephalic veins and SVC cannot be seen. An ultrasonic examination that is normal would reveal normal respiratory variation in the size of the central veins and polyphasic atrial waves.[11] (Figure 38–3a, 3b)

In the absence of polyphasic atrial waves, there is a high likelihood of CVO. Analysis of duplex waveforms reveal that when Doppler flow found atrial waveforms that were not polyphasic, central conduit occlusive disease was detected with a sensitivity of 79.6%. Monophasic atrial waveforms were associated with a 25% failure rate of catheterization due to central vein occlusive disease, whereas polyphasic atrial waveforms were correlated with a 100% success rate for catheter placement.[11]

c) CT and MRI

CT is most useful in the diagnostic workup of CVO due to extrinsic compression of the SVC and innominate veins due to tumor or fibrosis. It provides detailed three dimensional images of the structures surrounding the central vessels such as the trachea, bronchus and lymph nodes. In addition, with the addition of intravenous contrast, the flows in the venous vessels as well as collateral vessels can be visualized.

MR venography also can provide detailed images of the central venous circulation and surrounding structures. The advantages it has over CT is that it provides several several planes of view and has been shown to be 100% sensitive and specific in accurately diagnosing abnormalities of the central veins.[12] The drawback with MR is the contraindication of patients with pacemakers and other metallic implants, as well as cost, compliance, and the effect of gadolinium on the risk of developing nephrogenic systemic fibrosis. (Figure 38–4, Figure 38–5)

d) Contrast Venography

It is considered the gold standard for central vein anatomy and for the diagnosis of CVO, and provides a roadmap prior to either surgical or endovascular interventions, and delineates the venous collaterals as well. A commonly utilized venographic classification system has been developed by Doty and Stanford for assessing the degree of central vein obstruction. (Figure 38–6), (Figure 38–7A-D)

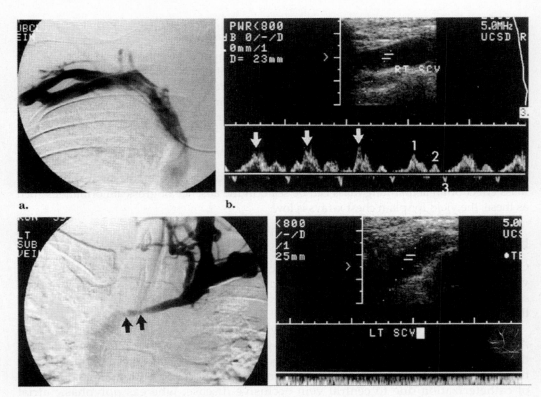

Figure 38–3. (above): Duplex ultrasonography reveals polyphasic atrial waves that correspond to normal venous outflow in the central veins by venography. **(below):** Duplex ultrasonography reveals continuous antegrade flow at all times with absence of transmitted atrial waveforms, consistent with the venogram showing obstruction of the left brachiocephalic veins.

Images from: S.C. Rose, T.B. Kinney and W.P. Bundens et al., Importance of Doppler analysis of transmitted atrial waveforms prior to placement of central venous catheters, J Vasc Interv Radiol 9 (1998), pp. 927–934

SURGICAL TREATMENT

Surgical therapy for CVO is reserved for specific situations non-amenable to endovascular intervention.

- Patients with extensive Type III or IV Stanford/Doty classification of SVC syndrome.
- Patients who have failed endovascular therapy.
- Patients with extensive intrathoracic malignancies with life expectancies greater than 1 year and who are good candidates.

Surgical therapy can be subdivided into extra-anatomic bypass and direct inline reconstruction. Extra-anatomic bypass is best reserved for isolated occlusions to the internal jugular and subclavian bypasses. For isolated proximal subclavian vein occlusions, the options are either ipsilateral internal jugular vein turndown, where the superior portion of jugular is ligated and brought down to the mid-subclavian level, or subclavian vein to jugular vein transposition. For complete brachiocephalic

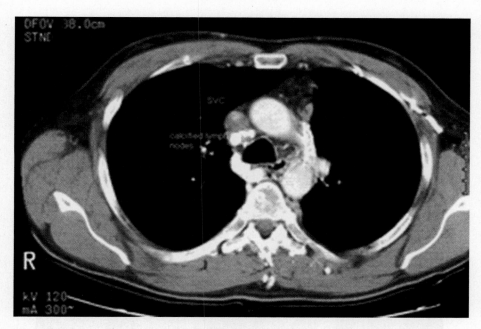

Figure 38–4. Large calcified lymph node in the middle mediastinum causing obstruction of the SVC.

and subclavian and SVC occlusions, extra-anatomic bypass from the ipsilateral axillary to femoral vein using GSV has been described.

There are many options for conduits in inline direct surgical bypass of the SVC and brachiocephalic veins. Limitations for autologous conduit include poor size mismatch for saphenous and other peripheral veins, as well as compression from small mediastinal width as well as tumor. Expanded polytetrafluoroethylene (ePTFE) is also a good choice in patients with contraindication or unavailability of autologous vein. Finally, use of cryopreserved or fresh homografts and other alternative conduits have been described.

- **Greater saphenous vein (GSV)**: Used mostly for extra-anatomic reconstruction when Type III/IV SVC syndrome exists in a patient who is not a candidate for endovascular AND open sterntomy techniques. It is thus harvested, reversed and placed from the ipsilateral internal jugular vein to the common femoral vein and tunnelled subcutaneously.[13] If central veins are of small caliber, GSV may be used in inline reconstructions.
- **Femoral vein**: Large size conduit for use and thus minimizes size mismatch between it and the central veins, but harvest of this vessel is tedious and is contraindicated in patients with deep vein thrombosis, underlying chronic venous insufficiency, or previous open lower extremity operations.[14]
- **ePTFE**: An excellent conduit for larger diameter reconstructions such as the brachiocephalic veins or SVC, as the flow through the vein is greater than 1 liter/minute. However, it is not as efficacious for small diameter vessels such as the external or internal jugular vein as slower flow and size mismatch could lead to early thrombosis. Following implantation, will need aspirin therapy daily.

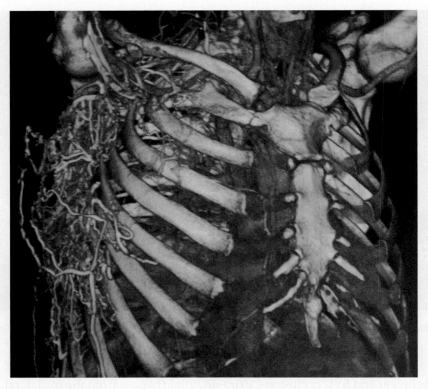

Figure 38–5. CT three dimensional reconstruction reveals the extensive chest wall collaterals with SVC and Brachiocephalic vein occlusion.

- **Spiral saphenous vein conduit**: The conduit of choice for central venous reconstructions as it is autologous tissue, has good size match to all vessels and has proven patency and efficacy over a greater than 30 year time period. It was first described by Chiu in 1974 in an animal model, and popularized soon after by Doty.[15,16] The operative detail of harvesting and creating the conduit and implantation will be discussed in detail.

The spiral saphenous vein graft (SSVG) is constructed by harvesting the GSV in the usual manner. A median sternotomy is performed and the distance between the confluence of the jugular vein and subclavian vein to the right atrial appendage is measured. Next, the diameter of the jugular vein is noted and this length will be the diameter of the SSVG. The length of SVG needed to perform the bypass is calculated by the following formula:[17]

$$\text{SVG length needed} = \frac{\text{Innominate vein diameter (mm) x length to right atrium (cm)}}{\text{Saphenous vein diameter (mm)}}$$

The harvested SVG is then incised longitudinally along its entire length, the valves excised and a chest tube that is the same diameter as the innominate vein is chosen as the stent to wrap the incised SVG over itself in a spiral configuration. The cut edges are sutured together with 7–0 polyprophylene sutures. (Figure 38–8)

Once the SSVG is constructed, weight based heparin bolus is given, vascular clamps are placed at the jugular-subclavian confluence, and the innominate vein is

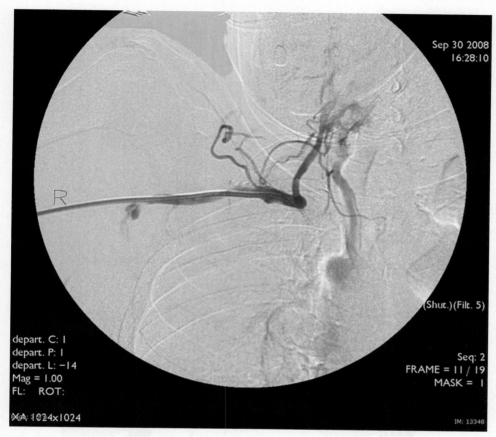

Figure 38–6. Diagnostic Venogram revealing CVO

divided. Any thrombus or intimal irregularities are removed, and proximal anastomosis is performed with 7–0 polyprophylene suture. Next, a side-biting clamp is placed on the right atrial appendage, and the tip of the appendage and any trabeculae are removed. The other end of the SSVG is then anastomosed to the right atrial appendage with 5–0 polyprophylene suture. (Figure 38–9)

Results of open surgical treatment of CVO are overall excellent. Outcomes are based on etiology of the CVO, length, and type of conduit utilized. Doty et al reported 10 year patency rates of 88%, while Gloviczki et al reported 86% secondary patency at 5 years with SSVG.[17,18] PTFE also has enjoyed good success with excellent secondary patency at 2 years at about 70%.[19] Better results occur when the PTFE is sutured to the larger innominate vein or SVC as opposed to the internal jugular or subclavian veins. In addition, addition of a brachial arteriovenous fistula to augment flow thru the graft improves outcomes as well. Bilateral reconstructions involving both innominate veins to the SVC in separate or spliced bypasses are no longer recommended, as unilateral revascularization is adequate for head, neck, and upper extremity decompression.[20] To date no studies have compared directly the results between malignant and benign etiologies. Postoperative surveillance consists of a contrast CT study 3–6 months after the procedure, and only due to recurrent symptoms thereafter.

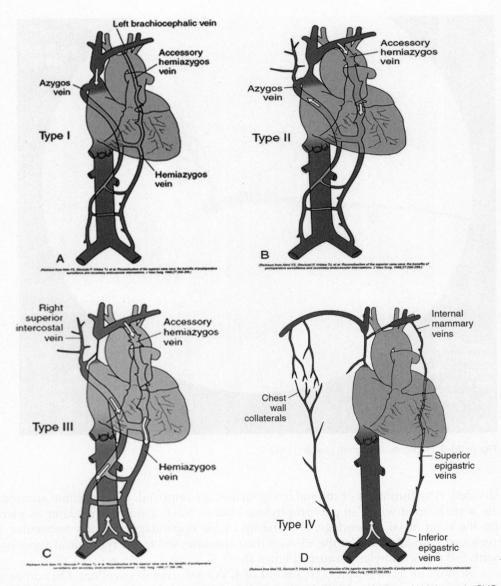

Figure 38–7. Venographic classification of superior vena cava (SVC) syndrome: **A**, Type I: high-grade SVC stenosis but still normal direction of blood flow through the SVC and azygos vein. There is increased collateral circulation through the hemiazygos and accessory hemiazygos veins in type I. **B**, Type II: greater than 90% stenosis or occlusion of the SVC but a patent azygos vein with normal direction of blood flow. **C**, Type III: occlusion of the SVC with retrograde flow in both the azygos and hemiazygos veins. **D**, Type IV: extensive occlusion of the SVC and innominate and azygos veins with chest wall and epigastric venous collaterals.

(Redrawn from Alimi YS, Gloviczki P, Vrtiska TJ, et al. Reconstruction of the superior vena cava: the benefits of postoperative surveillance and secondary endovascular interventions. J Vasc Surg. 1998;27:298–299.)

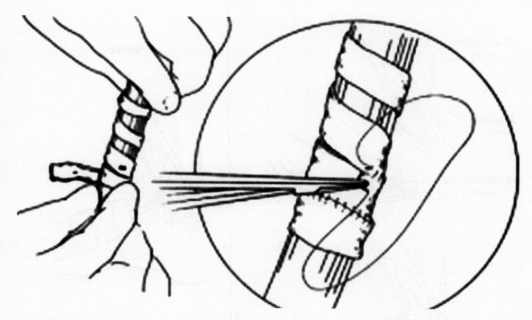

Figure 38–8. Adapted from Doty JR, Doty DB: Spiral saphenous vein bypass graft for superior vena cava obstruction. In Yang SC, Cameron DE, editors: Current Therapy in Thoracic and Cardiovascular Surgery, Philadelphia, Mosby, p. 184–186.

ENDOVASCULAR REPAIR

While open surgical reconstruction has excellent long term patency and has shown to be remarkably durable for most patients, it does have significant peri-procedural risks and short term morbidity, and not all patients can be considered candidates for these procedures. Endovascular repair (EVR) has over the past two decades become the first line treatment for all etiologies of CVOs, as recommended by the NKF-K/DOQI guidelines. The perceived advantages of endovascular interventions include less morbidity, shorter procedural time and shorter recovery times. Simultaneously with the advancement of EVR has been the enormous rise in the number of patients with CVO secondary to chronic indwelling venous catheters, mostly for dialysis access. While its immediate efficacy in treating CVO is well established, the long term effects and durability remain unknown.

Percutaneous transluminal angioplasty (PTA) for CVO was first performed in 1984 by Glanz.[21] Bare metal stents (BMS) were first placed by Gunther in 1989 for refractory SVC stenosis.[22] Covered stents were first described in 1996 by Sapoval for recurrent disease in an ESRD patient.[23] More recent additions to the armentarium include pharmacomechanical therapy and the HeRO catheter (Hemospere, Inc., Eden Prairie, MN).

Access

Obtaining access is a key first step in any endovascular procedure, and the treatment of CVO is no different. However, unlike many arterial procedures, dual access is frequently needed. This mainly involves an upper extremity and femoral venous access, and is very useful in facilitating antegrade and retrograde venograms, but also to cross the lesions. (Figure 38–10)

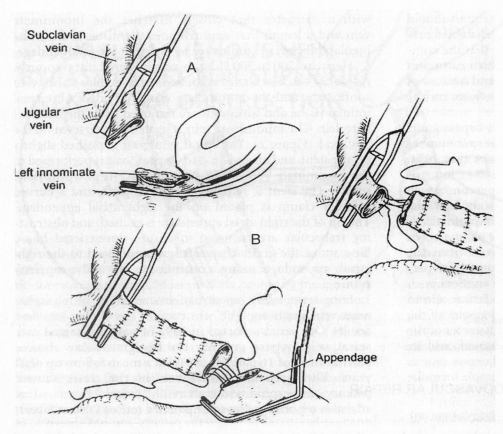

Figure 38–9. Adapted from Doty JR, Doty DB: Spiral saphenous vein bypass graft for superior vena cava obstruction. In Yang SC, Cameron DE, editors: Current Therapy in Thoracic and Cardiovascular Surgery, Philadelphia, Mosby, p. 184–186.

Once these accesses are obtained, the procedural sheath should be long (at least 45–55 cm) and be at least 8 French, so as to have full axial support close to the lesion, and have a conduit for both PTA and stenting. To further increase support, a guide catheter (RDC, JR, LIMA) can be placed through the procedural sheath prior to an attempt to cross the lesion. All patients should be systemically anticoagulated at this point and close monitoring of the activated clotting time (ACT) should be performed.

Crossing tools

The simplest tool to cross the lesion is a hydrophilic wire, either alone or with a catheter. The catheter can be either an angled hydrophilic catheter or straight crossing catheter. The technical success of crossing the lesion should be over 80% with the simple methods. If the lesion cannot be crossed with the wire/catheter combination, more advanced crossing tools are now required. There are many crossing tools in the market, mostly used in lower extremity arterial disease. They include:[24]

- Frontrunner XP CTO (Cordis Corp., Miami Lakes, Florida), with an actuating distal tip that creates a channel through occlusions via blunt microdissection.

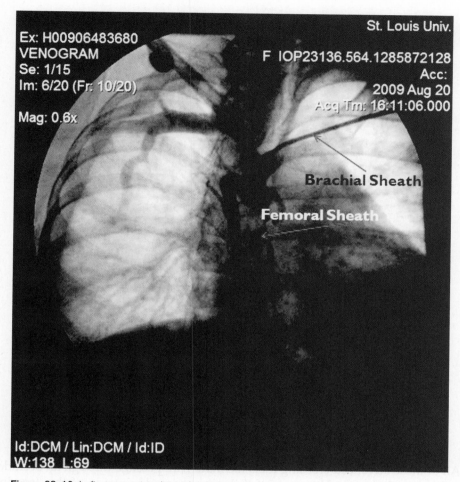

Figure 38–10. Left upper extremity and right femoral sheaths are shown into the central circulation and the corresponding venogram.

- PowerWire radiofrequency (RF) guidewire (Baylis Medical Company, Montreal, Quebec, Canada), which works through RF energy delivered through a nitinol core wire with PTFE coating.
- Crosser Catheter (FlowCardia, Inc., Sunnyvale, California), a rapid-exchange catheter delivering high-frequency vibration for recanalization.
- Avinger Wildcat 7 Fr Guidewire Support Catheter (Avinger, Inc., Redwood City, California), acts like a corkscrew, wedging through the blockage. By turning the catheter, the drill spins through the artery, enabling a guidewire to pass through the occluded area.
- Spectranetics Excimer Laser (Spectranetics, Inc., Colorado Springs, CO). Catheter provides kinetic and heat energy to break through the front "cap" of occlusions.
- Re-entry devices such as the Outback catheter (Cordis, Inc., Miami Lakes, FL), which utilizes a sharp needle that can be directed towards the front cap of the occlusion to allow wire passage or re-enter the true lumen beyond the lesion. (Figure 38–11)

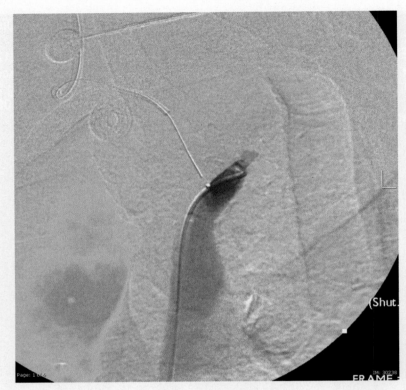

Figure 38–11. Laser catheter creating channel from right brachiocephalic vein into SVC. Venogram from sheath in right femoral vein provides roadmap to guide laser catheter.

All of these advanced crossing tools facilitate wire passage through an occluded or severely stenotic lesion. However, if the wire proceeds outside of the "roadmap" established by the antegrade or retrograde venograms, or the patient has chest and interscapular pain, one must immediately stop as there is a risk of perforation. Repeat venograms are done periodically to check progress as well as assuring that the true lumen has been re-entered after the lesion. Do not proceed without confirming true lumen re-entry.

Balloon Angioplasty and Stenting

Once the lesion has been successfully crossed, the hydrophilic wire is exchanged for a stiff wire such as the Amplatz (Boston Scientific, Natick, MA) or Lunderquist (Cook, Bloomington, IN) or a stiff Glidewire (Terumo, Inc., Somerset, NJ). The lesion is now ready to be intervened by PTA by a non-compliant balloon. The choice of sizes to be utilized depends on the location of the CVO. Subclavian and IJ lesions can be treated by a 8–10 mm rigid balloon, but innominate vein or SVC lesions require a 10–14 mm balloon. (Figure 38–12A, 12B)

Following PTA, venography should be performed to assess the efficacy and success of the procedure. The SVC and innominate veins should have more recoil from the balloon than the peripheral veins, as they are more elastic in nature. The indication for stent placement include suboptimal angioplasty (>30% narrowing with persis-

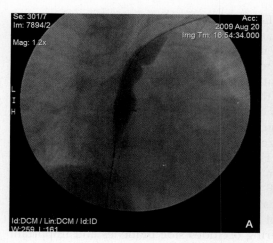
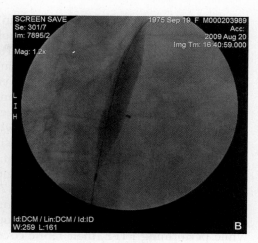

Figure 38–12. A PTA balloon with "waste" indicating the area of stenosis **B** Fully inflated balloon.

tent fillings of the venous collaterals), dissection, and recurrent stenosis requiring more than two interventions within 2 months.[25] As therapy for CVO has evolved, PTA has become more of an adjunctive procedure done prior to stenting in benign and malignant etiologies for SVC syndrome.[26] The long term benefit of this treatment paradigm has never been proven, however, in the dialysis access and CRMD populations. The main effect of stenting over PTA is increased immediate technical success and a bailout option after complications of PTA such as dissection, pseudoaneurysm, or perforation.

With regards to choice of stent, the two major choices are either a self-expanding stent that is post-dilated to coapt the vessel, or a balloon-expandable stent. Both of these choices have specific benefits as well as disadvantages. In addition, there are uncovered and covered stent grafts in each of the above two families of stents. In terms of stents that have had the most clinical experience, the four most commonly used stents for CVOs and SVC syndrome are the Gianturco Z-stent (Cook), Palmaz stent (Cordis), SMART stent (Cordis), and the Wallstent (Boston Scientific).

The Gianturco Z-stent is a stainless steel, balloon expandable device that was one of the first stents used in CVOs. It was originally created for use in malignant airway use. It comes in very large diameters,15–35 mm, and are 5 cm in length. It does require large 14–16 French procedural sheaths. This was first generation technology that had good radial strength in the middle segment of the stent, but had issues of stent fracture and metal fatigue.[27]

The Palmaz stent is a stainless steel, balloon expandable stent that comes in diameters of 8–12 mm, 3 cm in length, and requires a 10F sheath for placement. It has good radial strength, but like the Z stent it has problems with stent compressibility and their rigid stainless steel foundation does not lend itself to flexibility in tortuous areas, like the curve of the brachiocephalic veins.

The SMART stent is a self-expanding, nickel-titanium alloy (Nitinol) that is characterized by the property of thermal memory. When deployed, it reverts to its normal configuration and size when exposed to the temperature of the body. It comes in sizes up to 14 mm in diameter and 6 cm in length. It is useful in tortuous areas, but like any self-expandable stent, deployment has to be performed carefully, as it can foreshorten and jump forward.

The Wallstent is composed of the thin Elgiloy stainless steel wire mesh, and thus is a superalloy of Cobalt, Chromium, Nitinol, and stainless steel. It is self-expanding, and comes in diameters ranging from 10–16 mm and lengths of 2–9 cm. The primary advantage of the Wallstent is flexibility in tortuous areas and the ability to reconstrain and redeploy the device or remove it entirely. The disadvantages are poor radial strength and foreshortening, more so than the SMART stent.

Covered stents used in the central venous circulation include the BARD (Murray Hill, NJ) self-expanding Fluency stent, which is a PTFE covered device that requires a 8–9F procedural sheath and comes in sizes up to 10mm in diameter and 80mm in length. The iCAST stent (Atrium Medical, Hudson, NH) is a PTFE stent that is balloon expandable and comes in sizes up to 10mm in diameter and 38mm in length. It has the advantage of using a relatively small 7F procedural sheath. Stent grafts used for aneurysmal disease in the central venous circulation are an emerging technology. While covered grafts are useful as bailout devices for perforation and extravasation while performing PTFE, their fabric covering occludes side branches and important collaterals which could make the signs and symptoms of CVO worse with stent occlusion or thrombosis. However, their use could be more applicable in the subset of patients with malignant SVC syndrome, as they could potentially prevent tumor ingrowth. (Figure 38–13)

Role of Thrombolytics and Pharmomechanical Thrombectomy

Thrombolytic therapy for SVO has been well described, and can be used as stand alone therapy for acute occlusions or as adjunctive therapy with thrombolysis done first, followed

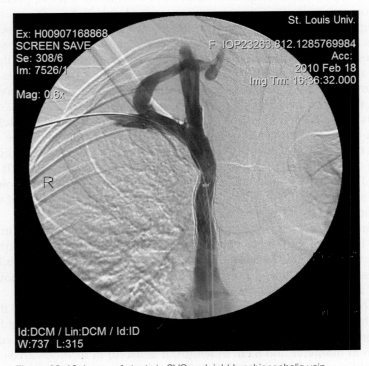

Figure 38–13. Image of stents in SVC and right brachiocephalic vein

by definitive PTA +/– stenting.[28] Catheter directed thrombolysis was first described with intravenous streptokinase and urokinase, and more recently with recombinant tissue plasminogen activator (rt-PA). In addition, more recently, thrombolysis has been combined with mechanical thrombectomy with various commercially available devices to create a pharmacomechanical thrombectomy that promotes clot lysis with clot maceration and removal and greatly shortens treatment times and amount of lytic agent required.[28]

The different devices include Angiojet (Medrad, Inc., Warrendale, PA) which utilizes a 6F rheolytic catheter that uses negative vacuum effect (Venturi) behind a series of saline jets. The unique aspect of Angiojet is that the direction of the jets can be reversed and a thrombolytic agent can be sprayed onto the thrombus. The Trellis system (Bacchus Vascular, Santa Clara, CA) utilizes two occluding balloons to isolate the thrombus and then disrupts the thrombus with a spinning wire while infusing thrombolytic agent. The area of thrombus is then suctioned and after suction is complete the balloons are deflated.

To best effect therapeutic benefit, acute lesions <5 days old and lesions due to benign etiologies are addressed, as malignant etiologies are usually more chronic and resistant to thrombolysis. Therapeutic yield is enhanced by crossing the lesion(s) in question and placing the catheter for thrombolysis within the lesion itself. (Figure 38–14A, 14B)

Catheter directed thrombolytic therapy can also be enhanced with newer devices such as the ultrasonic EKOS catheter (EKOS Inc., Bothell, WA). The EKOS EndoWave catheter system (EKOS Corporation, Bothell, WA) is a catheter-based drug delivery system utilizing high-frequency, low-power ultrasound. Its therapeutic applications include deep venous thrombosis, acute stroke, and peripheral arterial disease. Use in the central venous and pulmonary arterial tree is in its infancy, and short-term data is unavailable.

Role of HeRO catheter

There is a subset of patients with CVO and ESRD who also have non-existent peripheral venous access for hemodialysis(HD), but have adequate arterial inflow peripherally. These patients need intervention for CVO, plus some manner in which to perform HD without a prolonged indwelling HD catheter. (Figure 38–15)

The HeRO (Hemodialysis reliable outflow) catheter (Hemosphere, Eden Prairie, MN) consists of a 6 mm inner diameter ePTFE upper arm graft anastomosed to an arterial source that is fitted on the other end with a titanium connector that is coupled to a subcutaneous 5mm inner diameter nitinol reinforced silicone outflow catheter placed into either the IJ or subclavian veins and enter into the right atrium. Thus, in these difficult patients, the procedure is either a one-stage PTA+/–Stent/Pharmacomechanical Thrombectomy and HeRO catheter placement or two stage open surgical bypass to create a new channel into SVC/right atrium, followed by HeRO catheter placement.

Results of Endovascular Repair

The effect of Endovascular interventions for CVO is somewhat difficult to judge as most studies are retrospective and single-center and combine both malignant and benign causes of CVO. An early study in terms of endovascular intervention for CVO in hemodialysis patients was Haage et. al, who performed a retrospective review of primary stent placement with the Wallstent in 50 patients.[29] The 3,6,12, and 24 month primary patency were

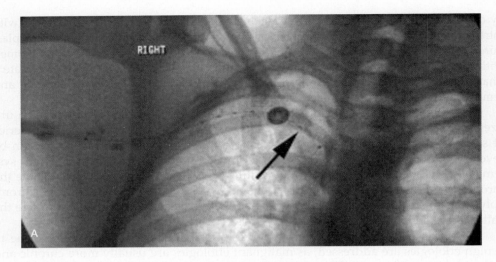

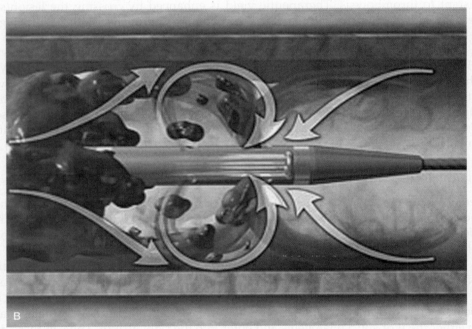

Figure 38–14. A EKOS catheter in central veins B Angiojet catheter (Courtesy of Medrad, Inc.)

92%, 84%, 56%, and 28%. Overall stent patency (primary, assisted, and secondary) was 97% at 12 months, 89% after 24 months, and 81% after 48 months. Bakken and colleagues reviewed their data over a 8 year period and compared primary PTA to PTA + stenting.[30] Primary patency, secondary patency, and ispilateral hemodialysis access survival were equivalent between groups. In fact, stenting actually performed slightly worse (primary patency 12 months 29% PTA vs 21% stenting, p=0.48 and assisted primary patency

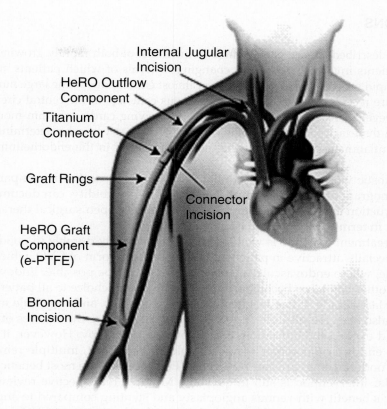

Internal Jugular
Incision

HeRO Outflow
Component

Titanium
Connector

Graft Rings

Connector
Incision

HeRO Graft
Component
(e-PTFE)

Bronchial
Incision

Figure 38–15. HeRO catheter (Courtesy of Hemosphere, Inc.)

12 months 73% PTA vs 46% stenting, p=0.08) Studies by Oderich et. al[31], and Quinn[32], have results more in line with the Bakken study. Why stenting does slightly worse or is equivalent to PTA alone for CVO in patients with hemodialysis is unknown. It could be due to stent thrombosis, increased inflammatory response to a stent, or injury to endothelium with stent struts or architechure. Further studies with larger number of patients and using newer stents are required.

With regards to benign causes of SVC syndrome due to mediastinal fibrosis and CRMD's, Rizvi, et al compared EVR with open repair in 70 patients over a 23 year time period.[33] In the open group, primary, primary assisted, and secondary patency was 44%, 68%, and 75% at 3 years. In the EVR group, primary, primary assisted, and secondary patency was 44%, 96% and 96% at 3 years. This study showed that both open repair and EVR are excellent for treatment of benign causes of CVO/SVC syndrome not involving hemodialysis patients.

In patients with CVO due to malignant SVC syndrome, Lanciego, et al. treated 149 patients with that profile with primary stenting with the Wallstent.[34] Immediate resolution of symptoms occurred within 72 hours in 123 patients (82%). Median symptom free survival was 6 months. Barshes et al. reported 1 year primary patency rates of 64%.[35] Given the patient population in these series with end stage malignancies and life expectancies no more than 1 year, longer studies are not feasible.

CONCLUSIONS

CVO is a well-described clinical entity that is in the midst of both rapidly growing in the number of patients involved, as well as changing in terms of which patients are most affected. The rapid growth in this patient base is almost entirely due to the large number of patients who are receiving chronic indwelling venous catheters in the central circulation, as well as the ever increasing numbers of patients receiving cardiac rhythm monitoring devices. While the exact pathophysiologic cause of CVO has yet to be determined, it is likely due to inflammatory changes at the microscopic level in the endothelium of the venous vessel.

The diagnostic workup for CVO is relatively simple, as no test is comparable to the central venogram. It can be accomplished with little morbidity, can document the extent of obstruction and collateralization, can plan further open surgical therapies, or be therapeutic in terms of endovascular interventions.

Surgical treatment for CVO is well tested and remarkably durable in good candidates. It is especially attractive in patients with the severest form of CVO, which is the SVC syndrome, where endovascular management may not be possible. Endovascular repair, on the other hand, has become the initial treatment of choice to all patients with CVO over the last decade. It has excellent procedural success, and very little morbidity. There has also been a multitude of new devices that increase the chances of technical success and expand the indications for endovascular therapy. However, it should be noted that endovascular repair is not durable and frequent, multiple reinterventions must be undertaken to prevent recurrence. Furthermore, the most beneficial type of endovascular intervention is still in question. Multiple retrospective reviews have failed to show a benefit with venous angioplasty and stenting compared to angioplasty alone. Further understanding of the underlying pathophysiology of CVO, improved stent technology, and further clinical research all will play a role in the future management of central venous obstruction.

REFERENCES

1. Hunter W: The history of an aneurysm of the aorta with some remarks on aneurysms in general. *Med Obs Inq* (Lond) 1757;1:323.
2. Parish JM, Marschke Jr RF, Dines DE, Lee RE: Etiologic considerations in superior vena cava syndrome. *Mayo Clin Proc* 1981;56:407.
3. Rice TW, Rodriguez RM, Light RW: The superior vena cava syndrome: clinical characteristics and evolving etiology. *Medicine* (Baltimore) 2006;85:37.
4. Kundu, S. Review of Central Venous Disease in Hemodialysis Patients. *J Vasc Interv Radiol* 2010;21:963–968.
5. Stoney WS, Addlestone RB, Alford WC, et al. The incidence of venous *thrombosis following long-term transvenous pacing.* Ann Thorac Surg 1976;22:166–70.
6. Spittell PC, Hayes DL. Venous complications after insertion of transvenous pacemaker. *Mayo Clin Proc* 1992;37:258–65.
7. Korzets A, Chagnac A, Ori Y, Katz M, Zevin D: Subclavian vein stenosis, permanent cardiac pacemakers and the haemodialysed patient. *Nephron* 1991;58:103–105.
8. Albers, EL, et al: Percutaneous Vascular Stent Implantation as Treatment for Central Vascular Obstruction Due to Fibrosing Mediastinitis. *Circulation.* 2011;123:1391–1399.
9. Weiss MF, Scivittaro V, Anderson JM: Oxidative stress and increased expression of growth factors in lesions of failed hemodialysis access. *Am J Kidney Dis* 2001;37:970–980.

10. Agarwal AK, Patel BM, Haddad, NJ: Central Vein Stenosis: A Nephrologist's Perspective. *Semin Dialysis* 2007;20(1):53–62.
11. S.C. Rose, T.B. Kinney and W.P. Bundens et al., Importance of Doppler analysis of transmitted atrial waveforms prior to placement of central venous catheters, *J Vasc Interv Radiol* 1998;9:927–934.
12. Thornton MJ, Ryan R, Varghese JC, et al: A three-dimensional gadolinium-enhanced MR venography technique for imaging central veins. *AJR Am J Roentgenol* 1999;173:999.
13. Vincze K, Kulka F, Csorba L: Saphenous-jugular bypass as palliative therapy of superior vena cava syndrome caused by bronchial carcinoma. *J Thorac Cardiovasc Surg* 1982; 83:272.
14. Jost CJ, Gloviczki P, Cherry KJ, et al: Surgical reconstruction of iliofemoral veins and the inferior vena cava for nonmalignant occlusive disease. *J Vasc Surg* 2001;33:320.
15. Doty DB: Bypass of superior vena cava: six years' experience with spiral vein graft for obstruction of superior vena cava due to benign and malignant disease. *J Thorac Cardiovasc Surg* 1982;83:326.
16. Chiu CJ, Terzis J, MacRae ML: Replacement of superior vena cava with the spiral composite vein graft: a versatile technique. *Ann Thorac Surg* 1974;17:555.
17. Doty JR, Doty DB: Spiral saphenous vein bypass graft for superior vena cava obstruction. In Yang SC, Cameron DE, editors: Current Therapy in Thoracic and Cardiovascular Surgery, 2004 Philadelphia, Mosby, p 184–186.
18. Alimi YS, Gloviczki P, Vrtiska TJ, et al: Reconstruction of the superior vena cava: benefits of postoperative surveillance and secondary endovascular interventions. *J Vasc Surg* 1998; 27:287.
19. Dartevelle PG, Chapelier AR, Pastorino U, et al: Long-term follow-up after prosthetic replacement of the superior vena cava combined with resection of mediastinal-pulmonary malignant tumors. *J Thorac Cardiovasc Surg* 1991;102:259.
20. Rizvi AZ, Kalra M, Bjarnason H, et al: Benign superior vena cava syndrome: stenting is now the first line of treatment. *J Vasc Surg* 2008;47:372.
21. S. Glanz, D. Gordon and K.M.H. Butt et al., Dialysis access fistulas: treatment of stenoses by transluminal angioplasty, *Radiology* 1984;152:637–642.
22. R.W. Gunther, D. Vorwerk and K. Bohndorf et al., Venous stenoses in dialysis shunts: treatment with self-expanding metallic stents, *Radiology* 1989;170:401–405.
23. M.R. Sapoval, L.A. Turmel-Rodrigues, A.C. Raynaud, P. Bourquelot, H. Rodrigue and J.C. Gaux, Cragg covered stents in hemodialysis access: initial and midterm results, *J Vasc Interv Radiol* 1996;7:335–342.
24. Oscar C. Munoz, MD, FACC, Ediberto Soto-Cora, MD, FACC, FSCAI, Kamran Ali, MD, FACC, Szymon L. Wiernek, MD, Barbara K. Wiernek, MS, R. Stefan Kiesz, MD, FACC, FSCAI, FESC: Successful Treatment of Chronic Total Occlusions with the Wildcat Catheter, *Vascular Disease Management* 2010;7:E159–E165.
25. Nael K, Kee ST, Solomon H, Katz SG: Endovascular Management of Central Thoracic Veno-Occlusive Disease in Hemodialysis Patients. *J Vasc Interv Radiol* 2009;20:46–51.
26. Courtheoux P, Alkofer B, El Refai M, et al: Stent placement in superior vena cava syndrome. *Ann Thorac Surg* 2003;75:158.
27. Trerotola, et al: Comparison of Gianturco Z stents and Wallstents in a hemodialysis access graft animal model. *J Vasc Interv Radiol* 1995;6(3):387–96.
28. Gerard J. O'Sullivan, Jennifer Ni Mhuircheartaigh, David Ferguson, Eithne DeLappe, Conor O'Riordan and Ann Michelle Browne (2010) Isolated Pharmacomechanical Thrombolysis Plus Primary Stenting in a Single Procedure to Treat Acute Thrombotic Superior Vena Cava Syndrome. *J Endovasc Ther*: 2010;17(1):115–123.
29. Haage P, Vorwerk D, Piroth W, Schuermann K, Guenther RW: Treatment of hemodialysis-related central stenosis or occlusion: results of primary Wallstent placement and follow-up in 50 patients. *Radiology* 1999;121:175–180.
30. Bakken AM, Protack CD, Saad WE, Lee DE, Waldman DL, Davies MG: Long-term outcomes of primary angioplasty and primary stenting of central venous stenosis in hemodialysis patients. *J Vasc Surg* 2007;45:776–83.

31. Oderich GSC, Treiman GS, Schneider P, Bhirangi K. Stent placement for treatment of central and peripheral venous obstruction: a long-term multi-institutional experience. *J Vasc Surg* 2000;32:760–9.
32. Quinn SF, Schuman ES, Demlow TA, Standage BA, Ragsdale JW, Green GS, et al: Percutaneous transluminal angioplasty versus endovascular stent placement in the treatment of venous stenosis in patients undergoing hemodialysis: intermediate results. *J Vasc Interv Radiol* 1995;6:851–5.
33. Rizvi AZ, Kalra M, Bjarnason H, et al: Benign superior vena cava syndrome: stenting is now the first line of treatment. J Vasc Surg 2008;47:372.
34. Lanciego, C, et al: Endovascular Stenting as the First Step in the Overall management of Malignant Superior Vena Cava Syndrome. *AJR* 2009;193:549–558.
35. Barshes NR, Annambhotla S, El Sayed HF, et al: Percutaneous stenting of superior vena cava syndrome: treatment outcome in patients with benign and malignant etiology. *Vascular* 2007;15:314.

39

Endovascular Strategies to Prolong Hemodialysis Access Patency

William D. McMillan, MD

INTRODUCTION

Hemodialysis access remains a challenge for all practicing vascular specialists. Maintenance of existing access typically accounts for 1/3 of peripheral endovascular procedures in both academic and private hospital settings. While recent advances in endovascular therapies have revolutionized the treatment of peripheral vascular disease, challenges related to venous hyperplasia have limited the success of similar technology in the hemodialysis patient. This chapter will attempt to review the options for endovascular salvage of existing hemodialysis access and also provide some data related to the relative success and cost effectiveness of various treatment options.

EPIDEMIOLOGY

While incident rates of end stage renal disease have plateaued in recent years, ongoing U.S. demographic shifts make octogenarians the fastest growing decile of the dialysis population.[1,2] In addition, recent data suggests that some subpopulations of patients are initiating dialysis at an increasing rate, in particular hypertensive, diabetic African Americans[2]. These two patient populations fare particularly poorly with regard to fistula placement, and the vast majority use nonautogenous AV grafts for access.[1,2] Despite the relative success of the fistula first initiative in increasing the proportion of new fistulas placed, functional patency (patency allowing for successful dialysis) remains a problem.[3,4] Consequently the majority of US patients still use nonautogenous grafts for access. The average cumulative functional patency (including both primary and secondary patency) of an arterio-venous graft is 18 months. On average, 2.7 declot procedures are preformed before a new site is initiated and more than 90% of these are done percutaneously. Unfortunately efforts to improve patency rates with antiplatelet agents or other medical treatments have proved futile.

TRADITIONAL ENDOVASCULAR APPROACHES

Despite efforts to monitor flow rates and dialysis pressures, the majority of patients present with a clotted access rather than a stenotic, poorly functioning av graft. The culprit lesion is almost always related to stenosis of the venous outflow. Consequently traditional approaches toward declotting are centered on evaluation and treatment of outflow stenosis.

For patients presenting with a thrombosed AV graft, a combination of thrombolysis and/or mechanical thrombectomy is coupled with angioplasty in an effort to restore flow. Proponents of thrombolysis typically inject 3–6 mg of TPA into the clotted access prior to initiating endovascular treatments.[5,6] Others favor mechanical thrombectomy using either an Arrow-Trerotola device (Arrow International) or a Helix Clot Buster (EV3/Covidien) over pharmacological thrombolysis arguing superior patency outcomes. There are only a few published trials of mechanical thrombectomy devices. Outcomes from these trials are conflicting with some favoring mechanical thrombectomy and others suggesting no difference between mechanical thrombectomy and lyse and wait strategies.[7–9] A single randomized trial of angiojet rheolytic thrombectomy failed to demonstrate clinical efficacy and consequently this technique has largely been replaced.[10]

Regardless of technique for clot management, the principles of percutaneous declotting are the same.[11] The first step is to obtain access to both limbs of the AV graft and to place a wire across the venous anastomosis. Once across, a venogram may be obtained to understand the central and peripheral venous anatomy. After successful thrombolysis, a second venogram is done to evaluate the venous anastomosis. It is typically at this point that angioplasty is done. Finally the arterial plug is cleared using a Fogarty catheter or MTD and arterial flow is restored. By waiting to restore arterial flow until after thrombolysis and initial treatment, the incidence of hematoma is lowered. With flow restored additional treatments, including repeat angioplasty, bare metal stenting or covered stent grafting are performed.

ENDOVASCULAR APPROACHES AND OUTCOMES

Angioplasty

Angioplasty alone remains the treatment of choice for the vast majority of patients. Simple, safe and cost effective this technique is the benchmark by which others are measured. Unfortunately, while initial success rates are high, recurrent stenosis is the rule rather than the exception. The society of interventional radiology defines a successful percutaneous declot as one which lasts for at least one dialysis run. More than 60% of patients return for additional treatment within three months and half are no longer using the access 6 months after the first declot.[12–14] Several strategies have been attempted to prolong the patency rates of these interventions. Cutting balloon angioplasty was offered as an alternative that might theoretically decrease the incidence of recurrent stenosis. However, two randomized trials failed to show benefit of this technique over standard angioplasty.[15,16] Similarly, cryotherapy balloons were thought to have a potential role in preventing recurrent hyperplasia in a few isolated reports.[17] However, early enthusiasm waned, as randomized trials demonstrated no advantage over traditional angioplasty. In addition, both techniques were substantially more expensive owing to the additional device cost and have largely been abandoned. Today, most refractory lesions are treated with prolonged inflation (2–3 minutes) using high-pressure angioplasty balloons sized to the native outflow vessel.

Nitinol Stents

When angioplasty is not able to restore adequate lumen to maintain patency, some favor nitinol stents. In fact, recent sporadic reports extol the virtue of nitinol stents as a primary treatment option for outflow anastomotic stenosis.[18] Despite this, most find that recurrent hyperplasia is as much, if not more, of a problem with nitinol stents as with plasty alone. In our practice these bare metal stents are typically only used for longer segment refractory outflow stenosis in the arm and occasionally at the cephalic arch. However, they remain a good option for central venous stenosis refractory to angioplasty. Large diameter nitinol stents are typically used in the brachiocephalic veins and occasionally even in the SVC. Regardless of location, the failure mode is typically recurrent hyperplasia and is often more difficult to treat with the stent in place.

Covered Stents

Initial reports of covered stents in dialysis access grew out of necessity. Covered stents were used as a bail out technique following vein rupture. Others reported using stent grafts to treat pseudo-aneurysms.[19] Initial reports of stent grafts for recurrent stenosis centered on refractory lesions. Among the first successful applications was recurrent stenosis in the cephalic arch. Viabahn stent grafts were reported to have improved patency as compared to either bare metal stents or plasty alone in this anatomically challenging location.[20]

The most significant report regarding stent grafts for dialysis access with published in the NEJM by Trerotola and others.[21] In this prospective randomized controlled trial (acronym), Fluency stent grafts (C.L. Bard) were used to treat anastomotic outflow stenosis in upper arm AV grafts and compared to angioplasty alone. The Fluency stents demonstrated improved six month patency as compared to plasty alone (51% Fluency vs 23% angioplasty) as well as an even greater benefit for in-stent restenosis (78% angioplasty vs 28% Fluency). This was and is the only randomized controlled trial to date of covered stent grafts in dialysis access. Obviously, the patient population was limited to nonclotted patients with upper arm grafts- a small percentage of patients treated in typical practice. Significant questions remain regarding the patency of stent grafts in other anatomic locations, for instance across the elbow. Also, many question whether the results can be extrapolated to patients presenting with thrombosed access or to patients with long segment stenosis of native outflow veins. The REVISE trial attempts to answer these and other real life questions. The trial uses Viabahn stent grafts (W.L. Gore) to treat a variety of venous outflow stenosis and recently completed enrollment with 291 patients. The results of this trial are expected within the next 18 months. In our practice stent grafts are used for patients with quickly recurring outflow stenosis (2 treatments within three months), recurrent cephalic arch lesions and in the case of rupture refractory to prolonged balloon inflation.

Hybrid stent grafts

In September of 2010 W.L Gore released a hybrid stent graft, incorporating the traditional ePTFE 7 mm graft and a nitinol covered stent graft on one end. The graft was approved as a 510K extension of existing technology and the company positioned it as an option for

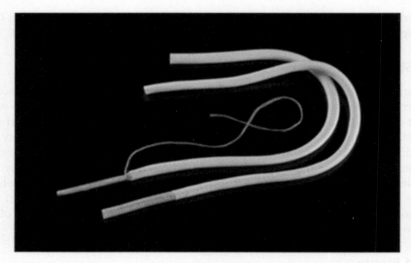

Figure 39–1. Hybrid graft pre and post deployment (with permission W.L. Gore)

failing dialysis access. (Figure 39–1) To date, the grafts have been used in a number of applications including treatment of outflow stenosis, primary AV graft placement for challenging anatomy and for salvage of failing upper arm grafts or fistulae. The technique for placement will be reviewed along with typical failure mechanisms.

For treatment of recurrent venous anastomotic stenosis, a surgical cut down is preformed under local anesthesia. The outflow vein is punctured, typically through the hood of the venous anastomosis using Seldinger technique. A more proximal portion of the venous limb is then dissected free. An appropriately sized peel away sheath is then passed over the wire (14 fr for 8 mm, 12 fr for 6 mm) and the hybrid graft is placed over the wire through the peel away sheath into the recipient vessel. The peel away sheath is then removed and the stent graft is deployed leaving approximately 4 cm within the vessel and 1 cm outside. An appropriately sized angioplasty balloon is then used over the wire to fully expand the stent and a completion venogram obtained. The proximal portion of the graft is then sewn end to end into the existing AV graft. (Figure 39–2)

Two particular failure modes of this device merit discussion. First, the compliance between the stent and the graft is relatively mismatched. As a result, if there is a sharp angle at the insertion site, the graft is prone to kinking. Another problem we encountered early in our experience was that of pseudoaneurysm formation at the distal aspect of the stent. In retrospect, we believe that by pushing the large diameter peel away sheath well into the native vessel, we induced a tear in the vessel distally which was not covered by the stent graft. In each of these cases we simply extended with a second Viabahn. Currently we are careful not to place the end of the sheath more than 3–4 cm into the outflow vein.

Other uses of the hybrid graft include those with completely occluded high brachial veins but an existing upper arm access. In these cases the axillary vein may be accessed percutaneously and the stent graft deployed via a small cut down in the axillary fossa and used to extend the existing graft after an end-to-end proximal anastomosis. Finally, the graft has been used to place primary forearm access in patients with poor outflow veins below the elbow. Here the deep brachial vein is cannulated and the

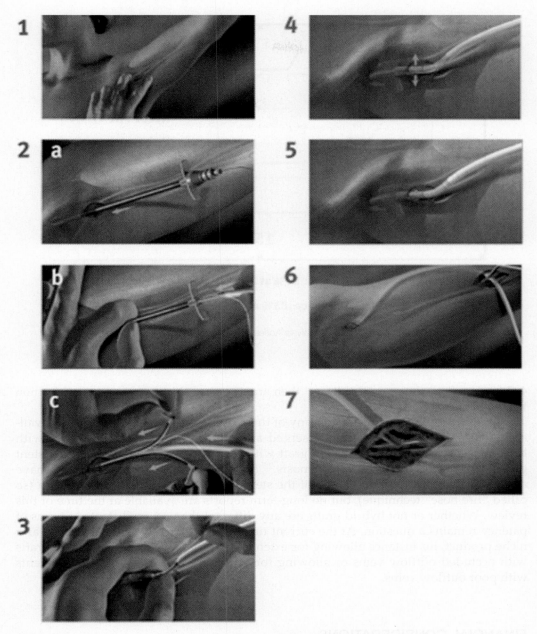

Figure 39–2. Hybrid graft deployment technique (with permission W.L. Gore)

stent graft placed into the deep system with a traditional end to side arterial anastomosis accomplished after placement of the venous portion. These grafts allow use of
brachial veins that would otherwise be too small and or friable for traditional end
to side surgical anastomosis. Early experience with this technique was remarkable
for significant steal syndrome in two patients. In subsequent patients we have used a

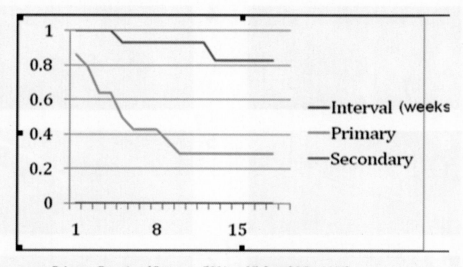

- Primary *Functional* Patency: **50% at 35 days(S.E.<10%)**

- Secondary *Functional* Patency: **83% at 105 days(S.E.<10%)**

Figure 39–3. Hybrid Stent Grafts for Dialysis Access: Primary and Secondary Functional Patency

4x7 mm graft on the arterial side and then anastomosed this in an end-to-end fashion to the hybrid graft.

No formal published results for any of these hybrid graft configurations are available. Our early experience was presented at ISET and demonstrated failures with hyperplasia at the edge of the stent graft with similar patency rates to covered stent grafts for recurrent anastomotic stenosis.[22] (Figure 39–3) More recently some have advocated purposeful under sizing of the stent portion to minimize this problem (so called "fire hose" technique), but no long-term reports are available at the time of this review. Whether or not hybrid grafts are any different than covered stents in terms of patency remains a question. At the current time their primary utility seems to be as a niche product, for instance allowing for extended patency for failing upper arm grafts with occluded outflow veins or allowing for primary forearm AV grafts in patients with poor outflow veins.

FINANCIAL CONSIDERATIONS

As dialysis access procedures increasingly shift from hospital settings to outpatient centers, the financial impact of various treatment options becomes a larger factor in treatment choice. In addition, bundled care for hemodialysis access is expected within two years and the utility of various interventions will be carefully monitored as for-profit dialysis providers will need to split payment with physicians who provide hemodialysis access. While significantly cheaper than hospital settings for total cost, outpatient ambulatory surgery centers and office-based practices are also reimbursed differently than hospitals.

For instance, currently Medicare does not pay for stents of any type in an ambulatory surgery center but will pay for stents in an office based setting. On the other hand, Medicare will only pay for surgical implantation of grafts in an ambulatory surgery center. The degree to which the more expensive endovascular options extend patency with need to be measured against the increased cost associated with their placement. As of today, there is insufficient data to make cost effectiveness comparisons between available devices. In the absence of such data, it is likely that the cheapest techniques will dominate as bundled care dollars are distributed. Obviously longitudinal studies of stent grafts and hybrid grafts need to be completed if they are to be options for future dialysis patients.

CONCLUSION

While percutenous treatment of failing and thrombosed AV access is now accepted as standard, venous outflow stenosis has proven resistant to many endovascular approaches. Covered stents and hybrid stent grafts are exciting new options, but their long-term utility remains questionable. Without data confirming their superiority over angioplasty alone, cost containment will limit the widespread applicability of these or any new endovascular devices for hemodialysis access.

REFERENCES

1. U.S. Renal Data System. USRDS 2009 annual data report: atlas of chronic kidney disease and end-stage renal disease in the United States. Bethesda, MD: National Institute of Diabetes and Digestive and Kidney Diseases, 2009.
2. Vascular Access Work Group. Clinical practice guidelines for vascular access. *Am J Kidney Dis* 2006;48:Suppl 1:S248–S273.
3. NKF-DOQI clinical practice guidelines for vascular access: National Kidney Foundation-Dialysis Outcomes Quality Initiative. *Am J Kidney Dis* 1997;30:Suppl 3:S150–S191.
4. Rakesh Navuluri, M.D.[1] and Sidney Regalado, M.D. The KDOQI 2006 Vascular Access Update and Fistula First Program Synopsis *Semin Intervent Radiol.* 2009 June;26(2):122–124.
5. Cynamon J, Lakritz PS, Wahl SI, Bakal CW, Sprayregen S. Hemodialysis graft declotting: description of the "lyse and wait" technique. *J Vasc Interv Radiol* 1997;8:825–829.
6. Cynamon J, Pierpont CE. Thrombolysis for the treatment of thrombosed hemodialysis access grafts. *Rev Cardiovasc Med* 2002;3[suppl 2]:S84–S91
7. Trerotola SO, Vesely TM, Lund GB, Soulen MC, Ehrman KO, Cardella JF. Treatment of thrombosed hemodialysis access grafts: Arrow-Trerotola percutaneous thrombolytic device versus pulse–spray thrombolysis—Arrow-Trerotola Percutaneous Thrombolytic Device Clinical Trial. *Radiology* 1998;206 : 403–414.
8. Rocek M, Peregrin JH, Lasovickova J, Krajickova D, Slaviokova M. Mechanical thrombolysis of thrombosed hemodialysis native fistulas with use of the Arrow-Trerotola percutaneous thrombolytic device: our preliminary experience. *J Vasc Interv Radiol* 2000;11:1153–1158.
9. Vashchenko N, Korzets A, Neiman C et. Al. Retrospective review of mechanical percutaneous thrombectomy of hemodialysis arteriovenous grafts with the Arrow-Trerotola device and the lyse and wait technique. *AJR* 2010 Jun194(6) 1626–9.
10. Vesely TM, Williams D, Weiss M, Hicks M, Stainken B, Matalon T, Dolmatch B. Comparison of the angiojet rheolytic catheter to surgical thrombectomy for the treatment of thrombosed hemodialysis grafts. Peripheral AngioJet Clinical Trial. *J Vasc Interv Radiol* 1999 Oct;10(9):1195–205.

11. Bent CL, Sahni VA, Matson MB. The radiological management of the thrombosed arteriovenous dialysis fistula. *Clin Radiol* 2011 Jan;66(1):1–12. Epub 2010 Sep 15.

12. Haskal ZJ, Trerotola S, Dolmatch B, et al. Stent graft versus balloon angioplasty for failing dialysis-access grafts. *N Engl J Med* 2010;362:494–503.

13. Lilly RZ, Carlton D, Barker J, et al. Predictors of arteriovenous graft patency after radiologic intervention in hemodialysis patients. *Am J Kidney Dis* 2001;37:945–953.

14. Lumsden AB, MacDonald MJ, Kikeri D, Cotsonis GA, Harker LA, Martin LG. Prophylactic balloon angioplasty fails to prolong the patency of expanded polytetrafluoroethylene arteriovenous grafts: results of a prospective randomized study. *J Vasc Surg* 1997;26:382–390.

15. Wu CC, Lin MC, Pu SY, Tsai KC, Wen SC. Comparison of cutting balloon versus high-pressure balloon angioplasty for resistant venous stenoses of native hemodialysis fistulas. *J Vasc Interv Radiol* 2008 Jun;19(6):877–83. Epub 2008 May 2.

16. Kariya S, Tanigawa N, Kojima H, Komemushi A, Shomura Y, Shiraishi T, Kawanaka T, Sawada S. Primary patency with cutting and conventional balloon angioplasty for different types of hemodialysis access stenosis. *Radiology* 2007 May;243(2):578–87. Epub 2007 Mar 30.

17. Gray RJ, Varma JD, Cho SS, Brown LC. Pilot study of cryoplasty with use of PolarCath peripheral balloon catheter system for dialysis access. *J Vasc Interv Radiol* 2008 Oct;19(10):1460–6. Epub 2008 Aug 9.

18. Kakisis JD, Efthimios D, Averinos et al. Balloon angioplasty verses stent placement of venous anastomotic stenosis of hemodialysis grafts following thrombectomy Society of Vascular Surgery Annual Meeting, June 17 2011 Chicago IL.

19. Vesely TM. Use of stent grafts to repair hemodialysis graft-related pseudoaneurysms. *J Vasc Interv Radiol* 2005;16:1301–1307.

20. Shemesh D, Goldin I, Zaghal I, et al. Angioplasty with stent graft versus bare stent for recurrent cephalic arch stenosis in autogenous arteriovenous access for hemodialysis: a prospective randomized clinical trial. *J Vasc Surg* 2008;48:1524–1531.

21. Haskel Z, Trerotola S, DolmatchB, et.al. Stent graft versus balloon angioplasty for failing dialysis access grafts. *NEJM* 2010, 362;404–503.

22. McMillan WD, Long T, Leville C, Hile C, Groffsky J, Schultz S. Initial experience with a hybrid vascular graft for dialysis access. Presented at the International Society of Endovascular Therapy Annual Meeting Jan 2011.

40

Role of the Distal Revascularization and Interval Ligation (DRIL) for Access-related Hand Ischemia

Salvatore T. Scali, MD and Thomas S. Huber, MD, PhD

INTRODUCTION

Access-related hand ischemia (ARHI), commonly known as "steal syndrome," is one of the most challenging complications for the access surgeon. The construction of an anastomosis between an artery and a vein (i.e. arteriovenous fistula) results in a predictable decrease in the perfusion pressure distal to the anastomosis that can lead to ischemia if the compensatory mechanisms are inadequate. Several clinical predictors have been identified, but their collective positive predictive value is not sufficient to identify scenarios when the hemodialysis access should not be attempted. The diagnosis of ARHI is largely a clinical one that can be aided in equivocal cases with noninvasive vascular laboratory studies. The treatment goals are to reverse the hand ischemia and to preserve the access with the paramount concern to avoid any long-term hand disability. There are a variety of remedial treatment strategies and they should be viewed as complementary with the choice contingent upon the responsible underlying mechanism, the severity of the symptoms, the patient comorbidities and the utility (or potential utility) of the access itself. The distal revascularization and interval ligation procedure (DRIL) is our preferred treatment because it reverses the ischemic symptoms and salvages the access in approximately 90% of the cases. The chapter will review the management of ARHI including the pathophysiology, clinical presentation and treatment options along with outlining our current treatment algorithm.

PATHOPHYSIOLOGY AND RISK FACTORS

The construction of an anastomosis between an artery and a vein creates a high flow, low resistance circuit with the blood preferentially directed towards the venous outflow as a

443

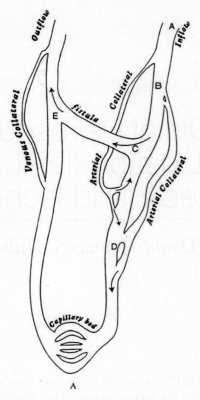

Figure 40–1. A representative diagram of an autogenous arteriovenous hemodialysis access is shown. Note the retrograde blood flow through the anastomosis from the arterial segment immediately distal to the anastomosis. The perfusion of the tissues distal to the anastomosis is supplied predominantly by the arterial collaterals. (Reproduced with permission from Wixon CL et al. Understanding strategies for the treatment of ischemic steal syndrome after hemodialysis access. *J Am Coll Surg* 2000;191:301–310).

result of the pressure gradients (Figure 40–1). The blood flow in the axial artery immediately distal to the anastomosis can be retrograde, antegrade or 'to and fro' depending on these gradients and the timing of the cardiac cycle. Perfusion of the tissue distal to the access is typically augmented through vasodilation of the inflow arteries, collateral recruitment and an increase in the cardiac output. Indeed, Papasavas et al.[1] reported that the construction of an arteriovenous access results in a decrease in the ipsilateral digital pressures in approximately 80% of patients. This 'physiologic steal' is usually well tolerated, but can become clinically significant when the compensatory mechanisms are inadequate. The presence of significant occlusive disease within the inflow (e.g. subclavian) or outflow (e.g. ulnar) arteries can further exacerbate the hemodynamic changes resulting from the access, potentially leading to ischemia. Specifically, the increased blood flow in the extremity resulting from the access can cause an energy loss and pressure decrease in a "sub-critical" proximal lesion similar to the response of an aortoiliac lesion to a vasodilator. Occlusive disease in the forearm or hand, commonly seen in the diabetic population, can further exacerbate the drop in arterial pressure from the access alone.

ARHI occurs in approximately 20% of brachial artery-based access procedures with roughly half (i.e. 10% of all brachial-artery based procedures) classified severe (grade 1 – mild, grade 2 – moderate, grade 3 – severe)[2] and meriting some type of remedial treatment.[1, 3-7] ARHI can occur after distal radial artery-based procedures, but the incidence is significantly less (2%) than the other access procedures and treatment is rarely required.[8,9] The underlying hemodynamic changes with radial artery-based accesses are similar to those outlined above (i.e. decreased arterial pressure distal to the anastomosis). ARHI can also occur after radial artery-based procedures as a result of retrograde flow through the palmar arch and this is potentially reversible by occluding the distal radial artery with a suture or coil.

A variety of clinical factors have been identified as *preoperative* predictors of ARHI. These include age, female gender, diabetes, coronary artery disease, hypertension, tobacco abuse peripheral vascular arterial occlusive disease, brachial artery-based accesses, previous episodes of ARHI, large conduits, and multiple prior access procedures.[5-7,10] Indeed, it has been our anecdotal impression that patients who develop ARHI are at extremely high risk for recurrence with each subsequent access attempt, thereby emphasizing the limitations of ligating an access on one extremity with the intention of placing a new access on the contralateral side. This list of clinical predictors is very extensive and reflects a large percentage of patients with end stage renal disease. Unfortunately, there are no predictive models that are sufficiently accurate to preclude constructing an access in an "at risk" patient. Similar to the clinical predictors, preoperative finger pressure or digital brachial indices (DBIs) measured in the vascular laboratory have also been inconclusive. They can be used in concert with the clinical predictors, but the absolute threshold values are unclear (i.e. DBI < 0.45, < 0.6, < 1.0).[10]

CLINICAL PRESENTATION AND DIAGNOSIS

Patients with ARHI can present with the typical features of either acute or chronic extremity ischemia. In our own DRIL experience, the presentation was bimodal with half of the patients presenting within 7 days of the index procedure and the other half presenting after 30 days[11] The signs and symptoms associated with acute ARHI include the classic "6 P's"- pain, paresthesia, paralysis, pulselessness, poikilothermia, and pallor. Similar to acute lower extremity ischemia, a motor deficit is particularly worrisome and merits emergent treatment. Chronic ARHI can present with either rest pain or tissue loss. Notably, this can manifest months to years after the index procedure, particularly in diabetic patients with advanced forearm vascular disease.

The diagnosis of ARHI is predominantly a clinical one based upon the history and physical examination with imaging (both non-invasive and invasive) reserved for equivocal cases. The differential diagnosis of hand complaints after an access procedure includes diabetic peripheral neuropathy and carpal tunnel syndrome, but ARHI should be considered first and foremost. It is important to ask patients about their dialysis session since the associated hypotension and hypovolemic can often precipitate hand complaints in patients that are otherwise asymptomatic. The physical exam may occasionally confound the diagnosis in the presence of a palpable pulse. Although it may seem contradictory to have a palpable pulse and an "ischemic" hand, all postoperative symptoms must be attributed to ischemia until proven otherwise. It has been our anecdotal impression that the threshold for ischemic symptoms in the upper extremity may be different than for the lower extremity with symptoms developing at a much higher absolute pressure in the upper extremity. Access-related neuropathy can lead to pain, weakness, and paralysis of the muscles in the hand and forearm without significant tissue necrosis. This entity, known as ischemic monomelic neuropathy, is seen almost exclusively in older, diabetic patients.[12,13] Nerve conduction studies demonstrate axonal loss and reduced sensory and motor nerve conduction velocities.[12, 13] The selective involvement of the nerves likely results from their greater metabolic requirements and tenuous blood supply (relative to the muscle tissue). Definitive treatment to reduce the underlying ischemia is mandatory to present long-term disability.

Non-invasive vascular laboratory studies can help corroborate the diagnosis for patients with equivocal symptoms. The diagnosis of ARHI may be excluded if the pressure measurements and the corresponding Doppler waveforms are completely normal (i.e. symmetric wrist/digital pressures, triphasic radial/ulnar waveforms, normal finger PPGs). However, this scenario is quite rare with the more common one being a patient with equivocal symptoms, diminished wrist/digital brachial indices and monophasic Doppler waveforms at the wrist. Not surprisingly, compression of the access usually results in the normalization of the wrist pressures and waveforms. We have taken an aggressive approach in these equivocal cases, assuming that all of the hand complaints were due to ARHI, and have treated them accordingly. Catheter-based arteriography has been used as a diagnostic study, but it is important to remember that ARHI is a hemodynamic problem and arteriography is largely an anatomic study albeit an important part of the treatment algorithm to rule out any significant inflow lesions.

INDICATIONS AND TREATMENT STRATEGIES FOR ARHI

The treatment goals for patients with ARHI are to reverse the hand ischemia and salvage the access although the paramount concern is to prevent any long-term hand disability. The natural history of ARHI is poorly documented, although all patients with moderate to severe ischemia (i.e. grades 2 and 3) likely merit intervention. It has been our anecdotal impression that patients with mild symptoms (i.e. grade 1) may improve over time although they merit close observation. Papasavas et al.[1] reported no additional decreases in the digital pressures after a month postoperatively despite the significant early drop noted above. In contradistinction, it has been our impression that patients with moderate symptoms rarely improve.

There are a variety of different treatment options for patients with ARHI (Table 40-1). Although we favor the DRIL procedure (Figure 40–2), the various treatments should be viewed as complementary since they may afford advantages in specific cases. It is important to remember that the ultimate goal of the remedial procedures is to correct the adverse hemodynamic changes resulting from the access. Zanow et al.[14] constructed a pulsatile flow circuit of an upper extremity arteriovenous access, complete with collateral channels, to examine these changes. Not surprisingly, they found a decrease in the flow through the access (i.e. "flow limiting" strategy) improved the distal perfusion. Siting the arteriovenous anastomosis more proximally on the arterial tree (i.e. PAI - proximalization of the arterial inflow, Figure 40–3) also improved the distal perfusion while ligating the axial artery immediately distal to the anastomosis in an attempt to limit the retrograde perfusion had little effect. Both the DRIL and PAI resulted in a dramatic improvement in the distal perfusion with the PAI having the greatest benefit. Interestingly, the ligation component of the DRIL only increased

TABLE 40–1. TREATMENT OPTIONS FOR ACCESS-RELATED HAND ISCHEMIA

Access ligation

Correction of arterial inflow stenosis/occlusion

Flow limiting procedures (i.e. banding, outflow reduction, anastomosis reduction)

Proximalization of arterial anastomosis (PAI)

Revision using distal inflow (RUDI)

Ligation of artery distal to anastomosis

Distal revascularization and interval ligation (DRIL)

distal flow 10% and the overall benefit of the DRIL was reduced at higher access flow rates. Illig et al.[15] measured arterial pressures and flow rates in 9 patients undergoing the DRIL procedure. They reported that there was a "pressure sink" in the brachial artery with a mean pressure of 102 ± 17 mmHg in the proximal brachial artery that decreased to 47 ± 38 mmHg at the anastomosis and that the flow in the brachial artery distal to the anastomosis was retrograde when the fistula was open. Following the

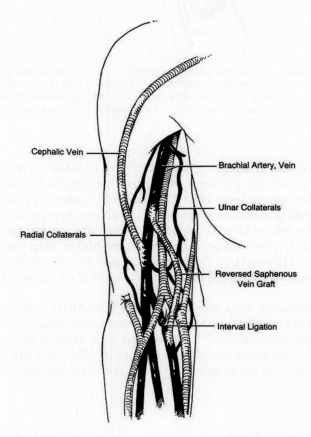

Figure 40–2. A diagram of a distal revascularization and interval ligation (DRIL) procedure is shown for a patient with an autogenous brachial-cephalic access. Note the brachial–ulnar saphenous vein graft and the ligature on the proximal ulnar artery. (Reproduced with permission from Berman SS et al. Distal revascularization-interval ligation for limb salvage and maintenance of dialysis access in ischemic steal syndrome. *J Vasc Surg* 1997;26:393–404).

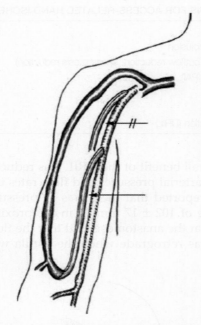

Figure 40–3. Proximalization of the arterial inflow (PAI) is shown for a brachial-cephalic autogenous access. Note that the autogenous access has been dissembled and an interposition graft (4 or 5 mm PTFE) inserted between the more proximal brachial artery and the proximal segment of the original autogenous access. (Reproduced with permission from Zanow J et al. Proximalization of the arterial inflow: A new technique to treat access-related ischemia. *J Vasc Surg* 2006;43:1216–21).

DRIL procedure, the pressure gradient in the brachial artery was essentially unchanged. However, the pressure in the brachial artery bypass and the brachial artery distal to the ligation were 104 ± 27 mmHg (i.e. systemic pressure) and that these values did not change with compression of the access. Reifsnyder and Arnaoutakis[16] also measured the inflow arterial pressures in a small group of patients (N = 9) with ARHI and found that the axillary pressures were higher than the proximal brachial pressures (153 vs 116 mmHg). These data suggest that the pressure drop resulting from the arteriovenous fistula may start more proximal on the arterial tree than previously suspected.

Several investigators have attempted to classify ARHI into "high flow" or "low flow" although the absolute threshold for differentiating these states and their clinical significance remain unresolved.[17-19] Clearly, the flow rates in the access contribute to the hemodynamic changes although it is unclear whether they are independent of the other factors involved in the adaptive (or maladaptive) responses.[17]

LIGATION

Ligating the access eliminates the arteriovenous access and reverses the hemodynamic changes. It should eliminate the ischemic symptoms provided that it is performed in a timely fashion. However, it has been our experience that a small percentage of patients will have some residual paresthesia, presumably from an ischemic neuropathy. The obvious disadvantage of ligation is the loss of the access, a major concern for patients with limited options. However, it is a reasonable approach for patients with acute ARHI after a prosthetic access given its limited patency. Notably, Scheltinga et al.[20] reported that prosthetic accesses were more often associated with acute symptoms (< 24 hrs) while autogenous accesses were associated with chronic symptoms (> 1 month) in their systematic review of the literature. Ligation may also be an appropriate treatment option for patients with severe comorbidities that prohibit a more significant operation, those with limited conduit that preclude a DRIL, and those with persistent ischemic symptoms that have failed another remedial procedure (e.g. prior DRIL or banding). In the small subset of patients that develop ischemic symptoms after a distal radial-cephalic autogenous access from retrograde perfusion through the palmar arch, occlusion of the radial artery distal to the anastomosis can reverse the symptoms while preserving the access.

CORRECTION OF ARTERIAL INFLOW STENOSIS

A stenosis in the inflow vessels proximal to the arteriovenous access may contribute to the development of ARHI as outlined above. Ideally, these should be identified and corrected prior to the index access procedure. The incidence of inflow lesions as a contributing factor has been somewhat variable in the literature, occurring less than 10% of the time in our own experience.[11] This variability is likely due to differences in the preoperative evaluation. In our own practice, we obtain upper extremity arterial pressure measurements and Doppler waveforms in the noninvasive vascular laboratory as part of our preoperative algorithm and our criteria for a suitable inflow artery include an adequate diameter (i.e. brachial artery ≥ 3 mm, radial artery ≥ 2 mm) and the absence of a hemodynamically significant inflow lesion based upon the pressures and waveforms. Regardless, a catheter-based arteriogram should be performed as part of the diagnostic and treatment algorithm for all patients with ARHI to exclude a proximal lesion.

FLOW LIMITING PROCEDURE

There are a variety of "flow limiting strategies" designed to improve distal perfusion while maintaining the access. These approaches are based on the hemodynamic principle that increased resistance in the access will increase distal perfusion through a decrease in the relative resistance through the peripheral arterial bed. These various approaches include arterial inflow reduction, anastomotic narrowing, and venous outflow reduction. The most popular technique is "banding" or narrowing a proximal segment of the vein used for the access. Notably, these techniques have been around for long period of time, but remain somewhat controversial. Gupta et al.[7] recently reported their experience with a variety of remedial therapies for ARHI and concluded that "banding" had a low success rate and a high likelihood of reintervention. The fundamental problem with all of these strategies is finding the tenuous balance between the relative resistance that achieves adequate distal perfusion yet maintains access patency and facilitates effective dialysis. Furthermore, the biologic behavior and the associated hemodynamics of the access may change over time (e.g. inflow artery dilation, outflow vein dilation) and, therefore, the assumptions and modifications made intraoperatively may not be sustained. Notably, the flow through a *large* arteriovenous access is independent of the extent of the communication between the vessels once the anastomosis exceeds 75% of the arterial diameter. This hemodynamic principle underscores the futility of trying to reduce the size of the anastomosis since reducing the anastomotic length of a 3 mm brachial artery to less than 2.25 mm (i.e. < 75% diameter) would likely result in early thrombosis.

Part of the recent enthusiasm for these flow limiting approaches has been predicated upon the use of objective measurements to quantify distal perfusion and access flow.[18, 19] Zanow et al.[19] reported a series of 95 patients with "high flow" accesses (autogenous > 800 mL/min, prosthetic > 1200 mL/min) that underwent flow-directed narrowing of their access using a combination of a plication suture and a prosthetic cuff (Figure 40–4). Long-term relief of symptoms was achieved in 86% of the patients. They used target flow rates of 400 mL/min for the autogenous accesses and 600 mL/min for the prosthetic ones although they stated in the discussion of their manuscript that a target of 750 mL/min may be more appropriate for the prosthetic accesses. Scheltinga et al.[18] performed a systematic review of "banding" as a "flow reduction" procedure and reported that the success rate was < 50% if performed without the guidance of flow measurements or digital pressures. However, they concluded it was very effective when flow rate was monitored and concluded that it was the procedure of choice for "high flow" accesses (i.e. > 1.2 mL/min). Thermann et al.[21] reported that flow-directed banding was effective in the setting of mild, short duration skin lesions, but ineffective for longer-term lesions and those with more extensive tissue

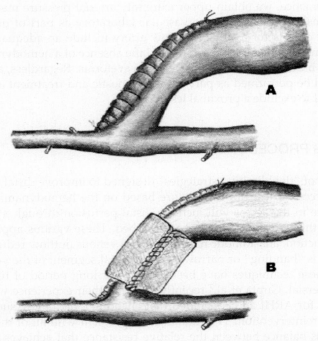

Figure 40–4. The technique described by Zanow et al.[27] to narrow the proximal autogenous access is illustrated. **A** A continuous suture is used to plicate and narrow the proximal portion of the access. **B** A ePTFE "cuff" is placed around the access at the proximal portion of the suture line to prevent further access dilation. (Reproduced with permission from Zanow J et al. Flow reduction in high-flow arteriovenous access using intraoperative flow monitoring. *J Vasc Surg* 2006;44:1273-8).

loss. They concluded that more complex surgical solutions may be required in the setting of these more chronic, extensive lesions.

Miller et al.[22] have described a minimally invasive variant coined the MILLER banding procedure (Minimally Invasive Limited Ligation Endoluminal-Assisted Revision) and have reported fairly impressive results. The technique involves narrowing the access over an angioplasty balloon using a suture. They reported successful relief of symptoms in 109/114 (96%) patients with ARHI with a 6 month patency rate of 75%. Shemesh et al.[23] described a novel "banding" variant in which the restrictive band is place in the mid portion of the access between the "arterial" and "venous" cannulation sites. This creates a pressure gradient between the "arterial" and "venous" sites that maintains adequate access flow and effective dialysis, a scenario which the authors claim is effective for ARHI and "low flow" states. This approach has a significant amount of theoretical appeal, but needs to be further validated.

PROXIMALIZATION OF ARTERIAL INFLOW (PAI)

Resiting the access anastomosis more proximal on the arterial tree (e.g. resiting from the brachial artery at antecubital fossa to the brachial artery near the axilla) may improve the perfusion to the hand. Theoretically, this is based upon the larger caliber of the proximal vessel, the smaller concomitant pressure drop from the arteriovenous access, and the more extensive collateral network. In reality, the technique may represent a variant of the flow limiting approaches given the described approach of using a 4 or 5 mm ePTFE interposition graft. Notably, Zanow et al.[24] reported that the PAI procedure was associated with the resolution of symptoms in 84% of their cases (N = 30) and that the patency rates were excellent. They concluded that it was a good alternative to the DRIL procedure and recommend its use for ARHI resulting from lower flow states (i.e. autogenous access < 800 mL/min, prosthetic access < 1000 mL/min). Thermann and Wollert[25] reported complete resolution of symptoms in 65% of their cases encompassing both radial (N = 5) and brachial artery-based access procedures (N = 18). They reported that the procedure was associated with increased radial artery flow and decreased access flow, but concluded that it was not effective for patients with severe tissue loss. Jennings et al.[26] have reported using the PAI approach "prophylactically" with good results in small group of patients (N = 4) deemed high risk for ARHI

The PAI technique has some appeal since it does not require ligating an axial artery and the hemodynamic models suggest that it is comparable to the DRIL. Furthermore, it may be suitable for patients that do not have adequate autogenous conduit for a DRIL procedure. However, the published experience is fairly limited, and it requires converting an autogenous access to a composite prosthetic/autogenous access and, thereby, increases the infectious and thrombotic complications with the latter particularly worrisome given the small caliber of the graft (i.e. 4 or 5 mm ePTFE).

REVISION USING DISTAL INFLOW (RUDI)

The RUDI involves resiting the arteriovenous anastomosis further distal on the arterial tree by disconnecting the original anastomosis and interposing a vein bypass graft (Figure 40–5). This essentially converts a brachial artery-based access to a radial artery-based

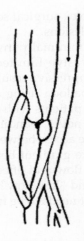

Figure 40–5. Revision using distal inflow is illustrated. Note that the brachial artery anastomosis to the brachial-cephalic access was ligated. An interposition graft was constructed using saphenous vein from the radial artery to the proximal aspect of original access. (Reproduced with permission from Scali ST et al. Treatment strategies for access-related hand ischemia. *Sem Vasc Surg* 2011;24:128–136)

access. Notably, either the proximal (i.e. antecubital) or distal (i.e. wrist) radial artery may be used as the inflow source for the access. As noted above, the incidence of ARHI is dramatically lower for distal radial artery-based access procedures when compared to the brachial artery-based procedures and is also likely lower for proximal radial artery- based procedures. Although this seems somewhat counterintuitive given the close proximity of the brachial artery and the proximal portion of the radial artery (and the potential for retrograde flow from both the radial and ulnar artery through the fistula), the limited clinical experience seems to support the RUDI.[27, 28] Notably, Callaghan et al.[28] reported that the RUDI relieved the precipitating ischemic symptoms and was associated with favorable hemodynamic changes although it was associated with a high access failure rate. Further justification for the RUDI is provided by the lower incidence of ARHI for the de novo proximal radial artery-based procedures when compared to the brachial artery based ones. Both Whitaker[29] and Gupta et al.[7] have reported a 2% incidence of ARHI with the de novo proximal radial artery-based procedures. Indeed, Gupta et al.[7] report that they have changed their practice more recently by incorporating more proximal radial artery-based procedures. One potential advantage to the RUDI is that it maintains perfusion through the axial artery. Paradoxically, the major disadvantage is that it converts a brachial artery-based access to a radial artery-based one. This is potentially problematic, despite the favorable reports above, given the smaller caliber of the radial artery and the high prevalence of occlusive disease in the forearm vessels that can limit their ability to vasodilate and increase flow in a response to the access. Indeed, the presence of significant forearm arterial occlusive disease is likely one of the explanations for the inferior success rates for distal radial-cephalic autogenous accesses that are particularly poor in the elderly, diabetics and women.

DISTAL REVASCULARIZATION WITH INTERVAL LIGATION (DRIL)

The DRIL procedure likely represents the best option for most patients with ARHI. However, it is worth emphasizing that Schanzer et al.[30] described the procedure in 1988 and the overall published experience is somewhat limited given the overwhelming number of patients on hemodialysis. The hemodynamic basis for the technique is the low resistance arterial bypass that overcomes the high resistance collateral circulation and the ligation that prevents retrograde flow from the distal vessels through the fistula. Interestingly, these components that afford the hemodynamic advantage (i.e. arterial bypass, ligation) have been cited as limitations. Concerns have been raised that the DRIL creates a scenario in which perfusion of the hand is dependent upon the bypass and that graft thrombosis could be catastrophic. However, this logic may be flawed since it is the collateral network (i.e. profunda brachial) rather than antegrade flow past the anastomosis that is responsible for the distal perfusion in the absence of the brachial bypass that comprises the DRIL. Despite these concerns, the patency rates for the brachiobrachial bypass that comprise the DRIL are remarkably good with a secondary patency rate > 80% in our series, one of the largest published experiences (Figure 40–6).[11] Among the 7 graft failures in our series, 2 patients developed Grade 3 ischemia (severe), 1 developed Grade 2 ischemia (moderate) and the remaining 3 were asymptomatic. Furthermore, the DRIL provided a marked hemodynamic benefit with a mean increase of 0.34 ± 0.26 and 0.41 ± 0.21 for the wrist brachial indices (WBIs) and DBIs respectively (Figure 40–7). Gupta et al.[7] echoed our enthusiastic support for the procedure in their recent publication concluding that the "DRIL is particularly effective". Unfortunately, the 2 year survival rate in our series was only 30%, suggesting that the annual mortality rate for patients with ARHI may exceed the 23% annual rate reported in the United States for the larger cohort of patients on hemodialysis.[11, 31]

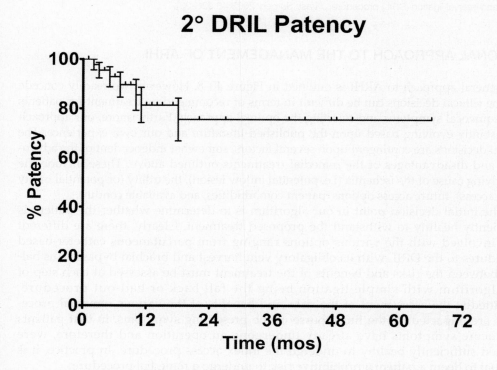

2° DRIL Patency

Figure 40–6. The Kaplan-Meier curve for the secondary patency of the DRIL bypass is shown with the standard error bars. The standard errors were < 10% throughout the time interval analyzed. (Reproduced with permission from Huber TS et al. Midterm outcome after the distal revascularization and interval ligation (DRIL) procedure. *J Vasc Surgery* 2008;48:926–33).

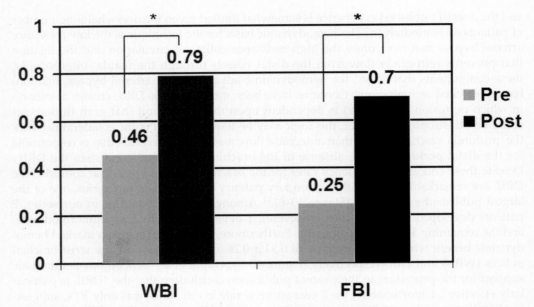

Figure 40–7. The mean preoperative (Pre) and postoperative (Post) wrist/brachial (WBI) and finger/brachial (FBI) indices are shown (alternative name for DBI). Significant increases (p < .05) were noted for both indices after the DRIL procedure. (Reproduced with permission from Huber TS et al. Midterm outcome after the distal revascularization and interval ligation (DRIL) procedure. *J Vasc Surgery* 2008;48:926–33).

RATIONAL APPROACH TO THE MANAGEMENT OF ARHI

Our general approach to ARHI is outlined in Figure 40–8. However, we readily concede that the clinical decisions can be difficult in terms of recommending treatment for patients with equivocal symptoms and selecting the optimal approach. Furthermore, our approach is constantly evolving based upon the published literature and our own experience. The clinical decisions are contingent upon several factors, somewhat independent of the advantages and disadvantages of the remedial treatments outlined above. These include the underlying cause of the ischemia (i.e. potential inflow lesion), the utility (or potential utility of the access), future access options, patient comorbidities, and available conduit.

The initial decision point in our algorithm is to determine whether the patient is sufficiently healthy to withstand the proposed treatment. Clearly, there are different risks involved with the various options ranging from percutaneous catheter-based procedures to the DRIL with its obligatory vein harvest and brachial bypass. This balance between the risks and benefits of the treatment must be assessed at each step of the algorithm with simple ligation being the fall back or bail-out procedure. Admittedly, the assessment of the risks and benefits of the various remedial procedures are impacted by the time course of the presenting symptoms, in that patients with acute symptoms have already undergone an operation and therefore, were deemed sufficiently healthy to undergo the index access procedure. In practice, it is unusual to deem a patient a prohibitive risk to undergo a remedial procedure.

The next step in the algorithm is to determine whether there is a potential inflow lesion. As mentioned above, the incidence of a significant inflow lesion in our experience is quite low, but this has not been the experience of others. An arteriogram (either

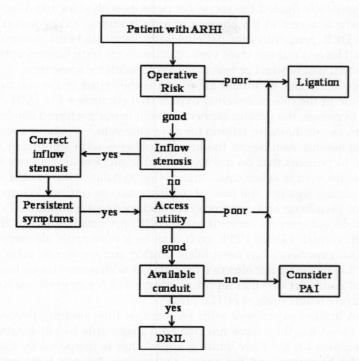

Figure 40–8. Our current treatment algorithm for patients with ARHI is illustrated. A full description of the flow diagram is described in the text. (Reproduced with permission from Scali ST et al. Treatment strategies for access-related hand ischemia. *Sem Vasc Surg* 2011;24:128–136).

catheter-based or CTA) should be obtained to rule out a proximal lesion. It is our preference to perform a catheter-based arteriogram in our hybrid operating room and correct any significant lesions at the same time. These lesions usually occur at the origin of the subclavian artery and are amenable to angioplasty in combination with stenting. In the absence of a significant inflow lesion, we proceed down the outlined algorithm, but it is worth emphasizing that it is important to work through the various steps and potential outcomes before embarking on a specific treatment. Notably, we obtain a catheter-based arteriogram at the time of our DRIL procedures, but it would be unusual for us to correct the lesion and abort the DRIL hoping that correcting the inflow lesion would be sufficient to relieve the presenting symptoms.

An important consideration in the treatment algorithm is the utility or potential utility of the access. Admittedly, this concern is somewhat irrelevant for patients with a functional autogenous access and chronic hand ischemia. However, it is very pertinent for patients with acute symptoms and either a prosthetic or autogenous access and for those with chronic symptoms and a prosthetic access. The treatment choice represents a balance between the likelihood (and potential duration) of the access being functional and the added morbidity associated with the remedial procedure. In our own DRIL experience, the successful autogenous access maturation rate for procedures performed emergently was comparable to our larger cohort of access procedures.[32] However, the autogenous access maturation rates reported from the Dialysis Access Consortium, a randomized controlled NIH-funded trial, were a sobering a

38%.[33] We have generally ligated the access for patients with acute hand ischemia secondary to a prosthetic access in the absence of a contributory inflow lesion. We have performed a few DRIL procedures for patients with chronic ischemic symptoms and a prosthetic access. However, these were very select patients with limited options and a prosthetic access that had worked or was expected to work for some time.

The final decision in our treatment algorithm is the status of the conduit and the feasibility of its use in the brachiobrachial bypass that comprises the DRIL. Similar to lower extremity bypasses, the greater saphenous vein is our preferred conduit and we have used ≥ 3 mm as our diameter criteria for a suitable vein.[32] We have been reluctant to harvest the saphenous vein below the knee in patients with significant peripheral vascular disease. In patients that do not have suitable saphenous vein, we have used the cephalic or basilic vein in select cases, attempting to balance the benefit of preserving the current access against the loss of a future access option. We recommend against the use of prosthetic and cryopreserved cadaveric vein conduits. For patients that lack a suitable autogenous conduit for a DRIL, proximalization of the arterial inflow (PAI) with a small caliber PTFE graft may be a reasonable alternative to ligation. However, our experience has been fairly limited and we would echo the report cited above that it is probably not effective for patients with severe tissue loss.[25] Unlike the description of Zanow et al.[24] that reported using a 4 or 5 mm graft, we have used a 4–7 tapered graft or a 6 mm straight ePTFE graft.

We have had limited experience with the various flow limiting procedures and the RUDI, and, therefore, they have not played a major role in our treatment algorithm. Our enthusiasm for the flow limiting approaches is tempered by the inconsistent reports in the literature and the requisite, tenuous balance between adequate distal perfusion and sufficient access flow to sustain effective dialysis. However, the various flow limiting strategies may be effective for patient that have very high flow rates, particularly those with cardiac dysfunction. The RUDI has a tremendous amount of theoretical appeal, particularly in patients with limited conduit in which a DRIL procedure may not be feasible. Although the published results are very limited, the consistent observation that the de novo proximal radial artery-based access procedures have a lower incidence of ARHI than brachial artery-based procedures is compelling. Our enthusiasm for the RUDI has been tempered by our large diabetic population and relatively poor experience with radial-cephalic autogenous accesses in this cohort. In contrast, we have had an excellent experience with the DRIL procedure and this success has both reinforced our approach and diminished our enthusiasm for the other alternatives.

It is worth emphasizing that the management or treatment of ARHI really begins during the preoperative evaluation. The likelihood of hand ischemia should be determined with each access procedure based upon the clinical predictors outlined above and all preventative strategies to reduce the incidence should be implemented. All potential inflow arterial stenoses should be identified and corrected. The operative procedure should be selected or designed to minimize the risk of ischemia in patients deemed "at risk". This potentially includes using a small diameter conduit (e.g. 3 mm cephalic vein vs. 6 mm basilic vein) where applicable and/or siting the arterial anastomosis at a location less likely to lead to hand ischemia. As noted above, the incidence of ARHI appears to decrease as the anastomosis is sited either further distal (i.e. proximal radial artery, distal radial artery) or proximal (i.e. proximal brachial artery) from the brachial artery at the antecubital fossa. For example, we would construct an upper arm loop using the proximal brachial artery near the axilla in high risk patients that require a prosthetic brachial-axillary access rather than using the brachial artery at the antecubital fossa.

A remedial plan should be generated in the operating room at the time of the index procedure to address any potential hand ischemia. Occasionally, we will obtain a saphenous vein survey during the preoperative workup to identify all potential conduits for a DRIL. In the most extreme circumstances, we have performed a pre-emptive DRIL procedure at the time of the index access creation although these have been reserved for patients with significant ipsilateral tissue loss or prior ARHI.

ADDITIONAL CONSIDERATIONS

DRIL Failures – Despite our enthusiasm for the DRIL procedures, we have had a few cases in which the procedure was ineffective in terms of relieving the initial symptoms. In these instances, it has been difficult to determine whether the persistent symptoms were a result of the initial ischemic nerve injury or frank ongoing ischemic complaints. Our generic approach in these setting is to obtain upper extremity arterial pressures and Doppler wave-forms along with a graft scan of the brachial artery bypass that comprises the DRIL proce-dure. We have a low threshold for obtaining a catheter-based arteriogram since it can help identify potential problems in the arterial inflow, the bypass conduit, and the forearm out-flow. Remedial treatment is often dictated by abnormalities on the arteriogram. In the absence of an identifiable problem, the remedial options include access ligation and some type of flow limiting strategy as previously outlined. Unfortunately, PAI and RUDI are not practical options after a DRIL procedure.

ARHI After Radial Artery-based Procedures - Hand or digital ischemia can occur after distal radial artery-based procedures. The underlying hemodynamic changes are similar to those outlined for the brachial artery-based procedures and result in a pres-sure drop distal to the anastomosis. This is not usually a problem given the dual nature of the circulation to the hand and the dominance of the ulnar artery in the majority of individuals. However, it can become problematic in patients with signifi-cant forearm or hand arterial occlusive disease and for those individuals with a domi-nant radial artery. The dominant artery to the hand should be identified preoperatively with an Allen's test and this is included among the noninvasive studies performed in the vascular laboratory in our algorithm. Access procedures should gen-erally not be performed using the dominant artery to the hand, either the radial or the ulnar, despite the favorable report by Bourquelot et al.[34]due to the risk of hand ischemia associated with the functional access and the potential for the artery to thrombose when/if the access fails. Hand ischemia can also occur after radial artery-based procedures as a result of retrograde flow from the ulnar artery and palmar arch.

The treatment options for patients with hand ischemia secondary to a radial artery-based access are theoretically similar to those outlined above for the brachial artery-based procedures with the exceptions of the DRIL and RUDI. However, ligation remains the most common definitive treatment. Any hemodynamically significant inflow lesions can be corrected, particularly those in the dominant ulnar artery. The radial artery distal to the fistula can be interrupted using either ligatures or coils for individuals with significant retrograde flow through the palmar arch.[9, 35] Notably, Chemla et al.[8] documented hemodynamic improvement in terms of hand perfusion after balloon occlusion of the distal radial artery.

REFERENCES

1. Papasavas PK, Reifsnyder T, Birdas TJ, Caushaj PF, Leers S. Prediction of arteriovenous access steal syndrome utilizing digital pressure measurements. *Vasc Endovascular Surg* 2003 May;37(3):179–84.

2. Sidawy AN, Gray R, Besarab A, Henry M, Ascher E, Silva M, Jr., et al. Recommended standards for reports dealing with arteriovenous hemodialysis accesses. *J Vasc Surg* 2002 Mar;35(3):603–10.

3. Keuter XH, Kessels AG, de Haan MH, Van Der Sande FM, Tordoir JH. Prospective evaluation of ischemia in brachial-basilic and forearm prosthetic arteriovenous fistulas for hemodialysis. *Eur J Vasc Endovasc Surg* 2008 May;35(5):619–24.

4. Lazarides MK, Staramos DN, Kopadis G, Maltezos C, Tzilalis VD, Georgiadis GS. Onset of arterial 'steal' following proximal angioaccess: immediate and delayed types. *Nephrol Dial Transplant* 2003 Nov;18(11):2387–90.

5. Morsy AH, Kulbaski M, Chen C, Isiklar H, Lumsden AB. Incidence and characteristics of patients with hand ischemia after a hemodialysis access procedure. *J Surg Res* 1998 Jan;74(1):8–10.

6. Suding PN, Wilson SE. Strategies for management of ischemic steal syndrome. *Semin Vasc Surg* 2007 Sep;20(3):184–8.

7. Gupta N, Yuo TH, Konig G, Dillavou E, Leers SA, Chaer RA, et al. Treatment strategies of arterial steal after arteriovenous access. *J Vasc Surg* 2011 Jul;54(1):162–67.

8. Chemla E, Raynaud A, Carreres T, Sapoval M, Beyssen B, Bourquelot P, et al. Preoperative assessment of the efficacy of distal radial artery ligation in treatment of steal syndrome complicating access for hemodialysis. *Ann Vasc Surg* 1999 Nov;13(6):618–21.

9. Miller GA, Khariton K, Kardos SV, Koh E, Goel N, Khariton A. Flow interruption of the distal radial artery: treatment for finger ischemia in a matured radiocephalic AVF. *J Vasc Access* 2008 Jan;9(1):58–63.

10. Valentine RJ, Bouch CW, Scott DJ, Li S, Jackson MR, Modrall JG, et al. Do preoperative finger pressures predict early arterial steal in hemodialysis access patients? A prospective analysis. *J Vasc Surg* 2002 Aug;36(2):351–6.

11. Huber TS, Brown MP, Seeger JM, Lee WA. Midterm outcome after the distal revascularization and interval ligation (DRIL) procedure. *J Vasc Surg* 2008 Oct;48(4):926–32.

12. Miles AM. Vascular steal syndrome and ischaemic monomelic neuropathy: two variants of upper limb ischaemia after haemodialysis vascular access surgery. *Nephrol Dial Transplant* 1999 Feb;14(2):297–300.

13. Wilbourn AJ, Furlan AJ, Hulley W, Ruschhaupt W. Ischemic monomelic neuropathy. *Neurology* 1983 Apr;33(4):447–51.

14. Zanow J, Krueger U, Reddemann P, Scholz H. Experimental study of hemodynamics in procedures to treat access-related ischemia. *J Vasc Surg* 2008 Dec;48(6):1559–65.

15. Illig KA, Surowiec S, Shortell CK, Davies MG, Rhodes JM, Green RM. Hemodynamics of distal revascularization-interval ligation. *Ann Vasc Surg* 2005 Mar;19(2):199–207.

16. Reifsnyder T, Arnaoutakis GJ. Arterial pressure gradient of upper extremity arteriovenous access steal syndrome: treatment implications. *Vasc Endovascular Surg* 2010 Nov;44(8):650–3.

17. Malik J, Tuka V, Kasalova Z, Chytilova E, Slavikova M, Clagett P, et al. Understanding the dialysis access steal syndrome. A review of the etiologies, diagnosis, prevention and treatment strategies. *J Vasc Access* 2008 Jul;9(3):155–66.

18. Scheltinga MR, van Hoek F, Bruyninckx CM. Surgical banding for refractory hemodialysis access-induced distal ischemia (HAIDI). *J Vasc Access* 2009 Jan;10(1):43–9.

19. Zanow J, Petzold K, Petzold M, Krueger U, Scholz H. Flow reduction in high-flow arteriovenous access using intraoperative flow monitoring. *J Vasc Surg* 2006 Dec;44(6):1273–8.

20. Scheltinga MR, van Hoek F, Bruijninckx CM. Time of onset in haemodialysis access-induced distal ischaemia (HAIDI) is related to the access type. *Nephrol Dial Transplant* 2009 Oct;24(10):3198–204.

21. Thermann F, Ukkat J, Wollert U, Dralle H, Brauckhoff M. Dialysis shunt-associated steal syndrome (DASS) following brachial accesses: the value of fistula banding under blood flow control. Langenbecks Arch Surg 2007 Nov;392(6):731–7.

22. Miller GA, Goel N, Friedman A, Khariton A, Jotwani MC, Savransky Y, et al. The MILLER banding procedure is an effective method for treating dialysis-associated steal syndrome. *Kidney Int* 2010 Feb;77(4):359–66.

23. Shemesh D, Goldin I, Olsha O. Banding between dialysis puncture sites to treat severe ischemic steal syndrome in low flow autogenous arteriovenous access. *J Vasc Surg* 2010 Aug;52(2):495–8.

24. Zanow J, Kruger U, Scholz H. Proximalization of the arterial inflow: a new technique to treat access-related ischemia. *J Vasc Surg* 2006 Jun;43(6):1216–21.

25. Thermann F, Wollert U. Proximalization of the Arterial Inflow: New Treatment of Choice in Patients with Advanced Dialysis Shunt-Associated Steal Syndrome? *Ann Vasc Surg* 2008 Jul-Aug;23(4):185–90.

26. Jennings WC, Brown RE, Ruiz C. Primary arteriovenous fistula inflow proximalization for patients at high risk for dialysis access-associated ischemic steal syndrome. *J Vasc Surg* 2011 Aug;54(2):554–8.

27. Beecher BA, Taubman KE, Jennings WC. Simple and durable resolution of steal syndrome by conversion of brachial artery arteriovenous fistulas to proximal radial artery inflow. *J Vasc Access* 2010 Oct;11(4):352–5.

28. Callaghan CJ, Mallik M, Sivaprakasam R, Iype S, Pettigrew GJ. Treatment of dialysis access-associated steal syndrome with the "revision using distal inflow" technique. *J Vasc Access* 2011 Jan;12(1):52–6.

29. Whittaker L, Bakran A. Prevention better than cure. Avoiding steal syndrome with proximal radial or ulnar arteriovenous fistulae. *J Vasc Access* 2011 Mar 31;BADFD2EF-44D1.

30. Schanzer H, Schwartz M, Harrington E, Haimov M. Treatment of ischemia due to "steal" by arteriovenous fistula with distal artery ligation and revascularization. *J Vasc Surg* 1988 Jun;7(6):770–3.

31. Goodkin DA, Bragg-Gresham JL, Koenig KG, Wolfe RA, Akiba T, Andreucci VE, et al. Association of comorbid conditions and mortality in hemodialysis patients in Europe, Japan, and the United States: the Dialysis Outcomes and Practice Patterns Study (DOPPS). *J Am Soc Nephrol* 2003 Dec;14(12):3270–7.

32. Huber TS, Ozaki CK, Flynn TC, Lee WA, Berceli SA, Hirneise CM, et al. Prospective validation of an algorithm to maximize native arteriovenous fistulae for chronic hemodialysis access. *J Vasc Surg* 2002 Sep;36(3):452–9.

33. Dember LM, Beck GJ, Allon M, Delmez JA, Dixon BS, Greenberg A, et al. Effect of clopidogrel on early failure of arteriovenous fistulas for hemodialysis: a randomized controlled trial. *JAMA* 2008 May 14;299(18):2164–71.

34. Bourquelot P, Van-Laere O, Baaklini G, Turmel-Rodrigues L, Franco G, Gaudric J, et al. Placement of wrist ulnar-basilic autogenous arteriovenous access for hemodialysis in adults and children using microsurgery. *J Vasc Surg* 2011 May;53(5):1298–302.

35. Plumb TJ, Lynch TG, Adelson AB. Treatment of steal syndrome in a distal radiocephalic arteriovenous fistula using intravascular coil embolization. *J Vasc Surg* 2008 Feb;47(2):457–9.

SECTION **X**

Miscellaneous Vascular Issues

41

Visceral Artery Dissection

*William H. Pearce, MD, Cheong J. Lee, MD and
Heron E. Rodriguez, MD*

INTRODUCTION

Visceral artery dissections (VAD) are uncommon, but, with the widespread use of CT imaging in Emergency Rooms, many more are being found. Patients with VAD present with a range of symptoms varying from rupture and death to an incidental radiographic finding. VADs occur in middle age individuals without known vascular diseases or pre-existing conditions. When asked to care for these patients, there is little literature to guide the physician. This chapter will review existing literature and provide general guidelines on the evaluation and treatment of VADs.

CELIAC ARTERY DISSECTIONS

While the literature is incomplete, and most are case reports, isolated celiac artery dissections are the rarest of all VADs.[1-8] Many of the reported celiac artery dissections occur in conjunction with dissections of the superior mesenteric artery (SMA). Patients with isolated celiac artery dissection present with upper abdominal pain consistent with the location of the artery and visceral nerve distribution. However, 50% of patients are asymptomatic. In 7 of 8 patients reported in one series, the celiac artery dissection involved branch vessels (hepatic, splenic).[4] In these cases, the patients presented with both abdominal and flank pain. In one patient, the dissection involved the common hepatic artery resulting in fulminant hepatic failure. In a second patient, the dissection involved the splenic artery, which resulted in splenic rupture and death. In a report by Amabile, which entailed multiple vessel dissections, all of the patients were male, all were smokers, and all had symptoms for more than 10 days. In this report, more than 75% did not require operative treatment and were treated medically.[9] It is interesting to note that, in one report, an isolated celiac artery dissection occurred following a fall from a height of 900 cm.[2] Review of the trauma literature also revealed two other patients with traumatic injuries to the celiac artery involving motor vehicle accidents. The etiology of the other dissections was unknown.

SUPERIOR MESENTERIC ARTERY DISSECTIONS

Isolated spontaneous dissections of the superior mesenteric artery are the most common of the visceral vessel dissections. More than 100 reports have been made in the literature regarding this entity. The most recent report by Oppat, at the Northwestern December Symposium two years ago, detailed the natural history and prognosis of this process.[10] Generally, the patients present with symptoms classic for intestinal ischemia, consisting of abdominal pain out of proportion to abdominal findings with nausea and vomiting. Patients may or may not have had prior symptoms. In a few case reports, the event may be related to exercise or strenuous activity. Similar to celiac artery dissection, the patients present in the middle-age to elderly patient population. The distribution between men and women is equal. In review of the literature, the majority of SMA dissections have been treated nonsurgically. Surgery has been used for those with end organ ischemia or rupture.[11,12] Here, the mortality rate is high. Unfortunately, most of these cases were reported prior to CT scanning and the diagnosis was made at autopsy. The pathology of the disease revealed involvement of the first few centimeters of the artery with extension distally into the terminal jejunal branches. Surgical and endovascular treatment of these lesions is difficult due to the location. At surgery with a fully dissected superior mesenteric artery, it is difficult for the surgeon to discern the true lumen from the false lumen. Furthermore, attempting to sew to these lesions may be difficult due to friability of the tissue. Similarly, endovascular treatment, while it has been effective in an occasional case, is fraught with the same complications. Even though the proximal flap may be tacked with a stent, a distal dissection may thrombose important jejunal and intestinal branches. Medical treatment includes control of blood pressure and anticoagulation.[9, 13-15]

RENAL ARTERY DISSECTIONS

Renal artery (RA) dissections are very uncommon and most commonly occur as part of an aortic dissection or complications of an endovascular procedure.[16] The overall instance of spontaneous renal artery dissection is between 0.036% and 0.049% in a large angiographic study.[17] However, this incidence is probably much lower than what occurs since many dissections are asymptomatic and may never be detected. While it has been suggested that spontaneous renal artery dissections occur as an underlying manifestation of fibromuscular disease (FMD), recent literature suggests that it is an independent entity not associated with FMD.[18] Spontaneous renal artery dissections occur in the fourth and fifth decades of life and have a male preponderance (4-1). This is unlike FMD, which affects women in the second and third decades of life. Bilateral dissections occur in 10% to 15% of cases. Furthermore, there is no evidence that one artery is more susceptible to dissections. For many years, it was thought that the right renal artery was more commonly affected because of its long length. Conditions that are associated with spontaneous renal artery dissection have included FMD, malignant hypertension, atherosclerosis and inherited connective tissue disease such as Marfan's or Ehlers–Danlos, cystic medial necrosis, segmental arterial mediolysis (SAM), and extreme physical activity.[17-19] There is one case report of bilateral RA dissection following marathon running.[17] In a study by Kanofsky, arteriography in multiple areas did not demonstrate any evidence of fibromuscular disease, suggesting that there was no relationship between the two.[18]

The clinical manifestation of spontaneous RA dissection is generally flank pain associated with hypertension. Flank pain may also be associated with renal dysfunction and hematuria. Many patients may have only mild symptoms and the diagnosis initially is missed since the symptoms are variable in severity and silent infarcts and unexplained hypertension may be late findings. There are fewer than 200 cases of spontaneous renal artery dissection reported in the literature. There is no clear data on outcomes or appropriate treatment.

The diagnosis of RA dissection is made by CTA or MRA. Both of these noninvasive imaging studies show the defect clearly. However, angiography is important when the decision is made to proceed with an intervention. Frequently, RA dissections occur in the mid-portion of the renal artery with extension into the branch vessels. The treatment of spontaneous renal artery dissection has included anticoagulation, antihypertensive medication, surgical intervention, and endoluminal therapies.[20-25] Rarely, an infarcted kidney may require nephrectomy.

Because of the rarity of the condition, there are no large series of either surgical or endovascular treatment of RA dissection. Prior to endoluminal therapies, surgery was the only option. Surgery (bypass or repair) is associated with between 8% and 27% risk of nephrectomy, 6% to 12% of renal artery stenosis, and a 15% risk of anastomotic restenosis.[22,24] Endoluminal therapies have had much better results reported. Pellerin and colleagues reported 16 consecutive patients treated between 1991 and 2006 with spontaneous renal artery dissections in 17 arteries.[20] All of these patients presented with uncontrolled hypertension, 9 with lower back pain, and 12 with progressive renal insufficiency. All of these patients underwent angiography with stent placement. After a mean follow-up of 8.6 years, 7 patients (40%) were off hypertensive medication, 9 were taking either a single or double antihypertensive medication. The most recent follow-up showed that patients' renal function was normal and imaging of the renal arteries did not demonstrate restenosis. Thus, it appears that in patients in whom it is difficult to control blood pressure or who have deteriorating renal function, renal artery stenting is appropriate. The stent must be placed in the main renal vessel to tack down the dissection flap. Unfortunately, placing the stent into the branches may compromise segments of the kidney with resultant renal infarction.

COMMENT

VADs are an uncommon clinical entity. However, with the more common use of CT and MR imaging, these lesions are being diagnosed more frequently. In the past, VADs were only diagnosed when clinical complications occurred such as rupture, abdominal pain, or end organ ischemia. Since many of the patients have been treated nonoperatively or underwent surgical procedures in which histology was not available, it is difficult to understand the etiology of these dissections. The lesions tend to appear in middle age to elderly patients. It also appears there is a slight male predominance and many of the patients have a history of smoking. There are several possible mechanisms to account for these dissections. The first is traumatic with an abrupt stretching of the vessel. The second may be related to segmental arterial mediolysis (SAM). And, finally, these patients may have a form of connective tissue disease. In our own experience 3 of our patients had recent strenuous activities. Two patients developed SMA dissections and one had multiple visceral dissections. The remainder of our patients did not describe any antecedent activity that may have produced increased shear or stress to visceral arteries. All of our patients did not have an underlying connective tissue defect such as Ehlers–Danlos or Marfan's nor was it

TABLE 41–1 ABDOMINAL DISTRIBUTION IN 24 CASES OF SEGMENTAL ARTERIAL MEDIOLYSIS*

Location	Percentage of Cases
Celiac and major branches	52%
Superior mesenteric artery and major branches	28%
Inferior mesenteric artery and major branches	7%
Renal artery	13%

Adapted from Slavin RE, Inada K. Segmental arterial mediolysis with accompanying venous angiopathy: a clinical pathologic review, report of 3 new cases, and comments on the role of endothelin-1 in its pathogenesis. *Int J Surg Pathol.* Apr 2007;15(2):121–134.

reported in the literature. Furthermore, there does not appear to be a particular association with an underlying vasculitis including polyarteritis nodosa.

In all likelihood, many of these patients may have segmental arterial mediolysis even though histology is not available. Segmental arterial mediolysis has a predilection for abdominal visceral arteries. (Table 41–1) SAM was first described by Slavin and Gonzalez-Vitale in 1976.[26] This is a nonatherosclerotic, noninflammatory disease with unknown etiology that affects visceral vessels. The characteristic lesion is mediolysis in the outer media, which may extend inward to involve almost all of the inner media. The mediolysis is produced by expanding vacuoles within the cytoplasm of the smooth muscle cells.[27,28] The vacuoles enlarge to a point that the cell ruptures and the media is lost. Slavin and colleagues have described a process of healing following this injury. Granulation tissue fills the areas of media, which may lead to hemorrhage from ruptures, dissecting hematomas, and aneurysmal enlargement. In addition, there may be separation of the outer media from the adventitia that fills the vessel with granulation tissue forming a fibrous organization that is not dissimilar from medial FMD. Slavin and colleagues believe that segmental mediolysis is a precursor for fibromuscular dysplastic disease. The arterial lesions are segmental and may involve part or the entire arterial wall circumference. The early phases of the process are asymptomatic and only become evident when a complication occurs. Several reports have detailed multiple artery involvement. Ro described a 70-year-old gentleman who had rupture of a gastroepiploic aneurysm, but was also found to have recent arterial dissections in the left gastric artery and both intracranial vertebral arteries.[29] While it appears that in many instances the disease is self limiting, one report by Hashimoto describes a 59-year-old male with a rupture of a splenic artery aneurysm who developed a superior mesenteric artery dissection $1^1/_2$ years later, a gastroepiploic aneurysm 3 weeks later, a right internal carotid artery aneurysm one month later, and splenic artery aneurysms 3 weeks later.[30] We have recently cared for 2 patients with multiple visceral vessel dissections simultaneously. First is a 60-year-old gentleman who presented with abdominal pain and hypertension. The patient was an avid runner. Arteriography, CTA, and MRs all demonstrated the lesions. The patient was treated conservatively and has done well to date. The second patient was a 79-year-old male who was found to have multiple visceral artery dissections with left flank pain. The left flank pain has resolved and the patient has remained stable over the past $1^1/_2$ years.

Mechanisms that produce SAM are unknown. Arterial vasospasm plays a predominant role in the etiology. The visceral circulation is known for its vasoreactivity. The application of norepinephrine to the surface of a vessel may produce experimental SAM, which demonstrated identical histologic findings. In a histologic study, Slavin reported the presence of endothelin one (ET-1) surrounding these vessels and in adjacent veins.[27] He suggests that the segmental nature of the lesions is related to the location of visceral nerves. He suggested ET-1 potentiates the vasoconstrictive effect of the neurotransmitters. His theory would account for why the lesion is scattered and may explain why dissections occur after marathon running. Marathon running produces marked intestinal ischemia from intense vasoconstriction.

Slavin believes that this lesion is a precursor to FMD. However, in is difficult to reconcile the fact that FMD is much more common in young women than in elderly to middle-aged men. He suggests that with aging the arterial structure changes, which allows easier separation between the media and adventitia than in the younger individuals. Thus the disruption of the arterial wall is less likely to occur in the young than it does in the old. However, he does not have an explanation why female patients are more common in the young.

The treatment of arterial dissections of the visceral vessels is tailored to the patient's symptoms. Patients with uncontrolled hypertension, bowel ischemia, and hemorrhage mandate immediate intervention. Interventions may range from surgical bypass, resection, and ligation, to intraluminal treatments such as coiling and stenting. In general, stable patients should be treated with antihypertensive agents and anticoagulation. If the symptoms persist, arteriography should be performed with the option of endovascular intervention. Stenting of renal lesions has shown to provide effective long term relief of renal vascular symptoms. Here it is feasible to tack the proximal tear and avoid branch vessels. There is little literature or experience with any procedures on the celiac or SMA. In conclusion, medical management is recommended for patients without a catastrophic complication. Anticoagulation and blood pressure control is recommended while surgery and endovascular procedures are reserved for arterial rupture or end organ ischemia.

REFERENCES

1. Glehen O, Feugier P, Aleksic Y, et al. Spontaneous dissection of the celiac artery. *Ann Vasc Surg* 2001;15(6):687–692.
2. Gorra AS, Mittleider D, Clark DE, et al. Asymptomatic isolated celiac artery dissection after a fall. *Arch Surg* 2009;144(3):279–281.
3. Kang TL, Teich DL, McGillicuddy DC. Isolated, spontaneous superior mesenteric and celiac artery dissection: case report and review of literature. *J Emerg Med* 2011;40(2):e21–5.
4. Nordanstig J, Gerdes H, Kocys E. Spontaneous isolated dissection of the celiac trunk with rupture of the proximal splenic artery: a case report. *Eur J Vasc Endovasc Surg* 2009;37(2):194–197.
5. Oh S, Cho YP, Kim JH, et al. Symptomatic spontaneous celiac artery dissection treated by conservative management: serial imaging findings. *Abdom Imaging* 2011;36(1):79–82.
6. Poylin V, Hile C, Campbell D. Medical management of spontaneous celiac artery dissection: case report and literature review. *Vasc Endovascular Surg* 2008;42(1):62–64.
7. Woolard JD, Ammar AD. Spontaneous dissection of the celiac artery: a case report. *J Vasc Surg* 2007;45(6):1256–1258.
8. Zeina AR, Nachtigal A, Troitsa A, et al. Isolated spontaneous dissection of the celiac trunk in a patient with bicuspid aortic valve. *Vasc Health Risk Manag* 6:383–386.
9. Amabile P, Ouaissi M, Cohen S, et al. Conservative treatment of spontaneous and isolated dissection of mesenteric arteries. *Ann Vasc Surg* 2009;23(6):738–744.
10. Oppat WF, Boules TN, Subhas G. Spontaneous isolated superior mesenteric artery dissection. In Eskandari MK, Morasch MD, Pearce WH, Yao JST, eds., Vascular surgery:

Therapeutic strategies. Shelton CT: People's Medical Publishing House—USA, 2010, pp 383–391.

11. Lacombe M. Isolated spontaneous dissection of the renal artery. *J Vasc Surg* 2001;33(2): 385–391.

12. Tameo MN, Dougherty MJ, Calligaro KD. Spontaneous dissection with rupture of the superior mesenteric artery from segmental arterial mediolysis. *J Vasc Surg* 2011;53(4):1107–12.

13. Zhang WW, Killeen JD, Chiriano J, et al. Management of symptomatic spontaneous isolated visceral artery dissection: is emergent intervention mandatory? *Ann Vasc Surg* 2009;23(1): 90–94.

14. Takayama T, Miyata T, Shirakawa M, et al. Isolated spontaneous dissection of the splanchnic arteries. *J Vasc Surg* 2008;48(2):329–333.

15. Takach TJ, Madjarov JM, Holleman JH, et al. Spontaneous splanchnic dissection: application and timing of therapeutic options. *J Vasc Surg* 2009;50(3):557–563.

16. Bauersfeld SR. Dissecting aneurysm of the aorta; a presentation of 15 cases and a review of the recent literature. *Ann Intern Med* 1947;26(6):873–889.

17. Iqbal FM, Goparaju M, Yemme S, et al. Renal artery dissection following marathon running. *Angiology* 2009;60:122–126.

18. Kanofsky JA, Lepor H. Spontaneous renal artery dissection. *Rev Urol* Summer 2007;9(3): 156–160.

19. Soga Y, Nose M, Arita N, et al. Aneurysms of the renal arteries associated with segmental arterial mediolysis in a case of polyarteritis nodosa. *Pathol Int* 2009;59(3):197–200.

20. Pellerin O, Garcon P, Beyssen B, et al. Spontaneous renal artery dissection: long-term outcomes after endovascular stent placement. *J Vasc Interv Radiol* 2009;20(8):1024–1030.

21. Ramamoorthy SL, Vasquez JC, Taft PM, et al. Nonoperative management of acute spontaneous renal artery dissection. *Ann Vasc Surg* 2002;16(2):157–162.

22. Reilly LM, Cunningham CG, Maggisano R, et al. The role of arterial reconstruction in spontaneous renal artery dissection. *J Vasc Surg* 1991;14(4):468–477; discussion 477–469.

23. Shmorgun D, Claman P, McGregor P, et al. Renal artery dissection during an in vitro fertilization/intracytoplasmic sperm injection cycle. *Fertil Steril* 2009;92(4):1498 e1491–1493.

24. Slavis SA, Hodge EE, Novick AC, et al. Surgical treatment for isolated dissection of the renal artery. *J Urol* 1990;144(2 Pt 1):233–237.

25. Tsai TH, Su JT, Hu SY, et al. Spontaneous renal artery dissection complicating with renal infarction. *Urology* 2010;76(6):1371–2, 1372.e1.

26. Slavin RE, Gonzalez-Vitale JC. Segmental mediolytic arteritis: A clinical pathologic study. *Lab Invest* 1976;35:23–29.

27. Slavin RE, Inada K. Segmental arterial mediolysis with accompanying venous angiopathy: a clinical pathologic review, report of 3 new cases, and comments on the role of endothelin-1 in its pathogenesis. *Int J Surg Pathol* 2007;15(2):121–134.

28. Slavin RE. Segmental arterial mediolysis: course, sequelae, prognosis, and pathologic-radiologic correlation. *Cardiovasc Pathol* Nov-Dec 2009;18(6):352–360.

29. Ro A, Kageyama N, Takatsu A, et al. Segmental arterial mediolysis of varying phases affecting both the intra-abdominal and intracranial vertebral arteries: an autopsy case report. *Cardiovasc Pathol* 2010;19(4):248–51.

30. Hashimoto T, Deguchi J, Endo H, et al. Successful treatment tailored to each splanchnic arterial lesion due to segmental arterial mediolysis (SAM): report of a case. *J Vasc Surg* 2008;48(5):1338–1341

42

Management of Vascular Thoracic Outlet Syndrome

Douglas Miller, MS and Heron E. Rodriguez, MD

INTRODUCTION

The term Thoracic Outlet Syndrome (TOS) was first coined by Peet *et al* in 1956 to encompass a group of signs and symptoms related to the compression of the brachial plexus, subclavian artery or subclavian vein as they pass from the thorax into the axilla.[1] TOS can be subdivided according to the structures which are affected: neurogenic for compression of the brachial plexus, arterial for compression of the subclavian artery and venous for symptoms related to compression of the subclavian vein. In order to treat patients effectively it is important to keep in mind several important considerations. First, compression of the nerve, artery or vein may occur individually but any combination may occur concomitantly. Second, compression at the thoracic outlet is a dynamic phenomenon that may only occur when the arm is abducted and externally rotated and not with the arm in neutral position. Third, the diagnosis of TOS is a clinical one. There is no single diagnostic test or imaging study that unmistakably confirms or rules out the condition.

EPIDEMIOLOGY

The majority of patients with TOS suffer from neurogenic compression (85%- 95% of cases) whereas vascular TOS is less common. Estimates for venous TOS however suggest an incidence of 1-2 per 100,000 population.[2, 3] Only in 1% of all cases of TOS, the artery is the structure compressed.[4]

Overall, females are affected more often than males, with several studies specific to arterial TOS showing roughly 60% of their cohorts being women[5, 6, 7], although for venous TOS there appears to be a slight preponderance towards males.[8, 9]

ANATOMIC CONSIDERATIONS

The subclavian structures pass from the thorax into the axilla through a narrow gap formed by the clavicle superiorly, first rib inferiorly, the subclavius muscle anterior and superiorly and the insertion of the scalene muscles posteriorly. The anterior and middle scalene muscles arise from the upper portions of the cervical vertebrae. They then insert into the first or the second rib. Although typically the anterior scalene inserts on the first rib and the middle scalene into the first and second rib, great variability is often present. Importantly, the anterior scalene produces interdigitations through which the brachial plexus penetrates. These interdigitations are particularly prominent in the presence of a cervical rib. Cervical ribs are present in up to 2% of the population and are more common in females; however it is important to note that only 10% of this population develop symptoms of TOS.[10] Thus, compression of the subclavian vessels and brachial plexus can occur at the interscalene triangle, the costoclavicular space or more distally by the pectoralis minor muscle. (Figure 42–1)

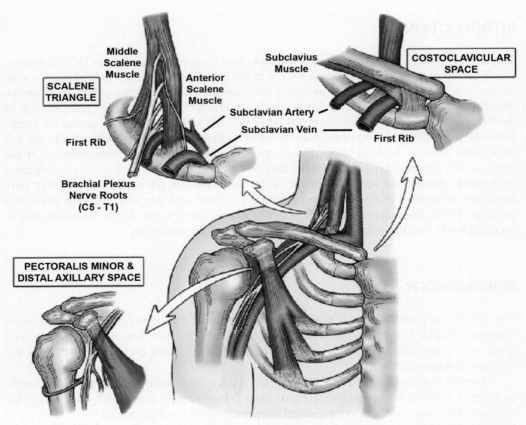

Figure 42–1. Compressive zones of the thoracic outlet. The subclavian structures can be compressed at the costoclavicular space, the scalene triangle or distally at the border of the pectoralis minor muscle. Reprinted with permission.

DIAGNOSIS OF VASCULAR THORACIC OUTLET SYNDROME

History and Physical Examination

A thorough history and physical examination remains the cornerstone of the evaluation of patients with suspected TOS. Any previous trauma to the neck which could have resulted in a fracture of the clavicle or first rib should be noted. Prior history or family history of hypercoagulability or thromboembolic issues should also be inquired. Occupational and recreational activities that require the use of overhead arm motion or recent changes to exercise regimens should be taken into consideration.

Arterial TOS is often asymptomatic, however patients may present with a range of signs and symptoms from fatigue or pain of the affected arm on exertion and Raynaud's phenomenon to critical ischemia of the upper extremity as a consequence of emboli arising from the chronically injured artery or from mural thrombus in a post-stenotic aneurysm sac. Evidence of distal embolism in the hand is often present.

Venous TOS can result in pain, swelling and cyanosis of the arm. This typically occurs in athletes or workers who regularly have their arms elevated or in patient that recently changed their level of activity with a recent abnormally intense use of their arms. When subclavian vein thrombosis occurs in such circumstances the term "effort thrombosis" or Paget-Schroetter syndrome is commonly used.

Adson's test/provocative maneuvers

This test was initially described in the early 20th century and described how in the presence of a cervical rib or large anterior scalene tendon insertion peripheral pulses would become weaker upon performing specific movements. In the case of Adson he asked patients to turn their heads to the affected side after full inspiration whilst sitting upright.[11] The true value of this test has been questioned since, however, as studies using healthy volunteers have shown that performing this maneuver can cause reduction or result in absence of peripheral pulses in those without signs or symptoms of TOS.[12] Several other tests have been developed, some of which are alterations of Adson's, each claiming to be more useful in identifying patients who suffer with TOS.[4] Overall, despite their popularity, they lack sensitivity or specificity in confirming or ruling out the diagnosis of TOS.

X-rays

A chest x-ray is mandatory during the initial evaluation for potential TOS. It will reveal anomalous first ribs. Additionally, the vast majority of cervical ribs are found incidentally on chest x-ray. Cervical spine views allow for more detailed visualization of cervical ribs. Radiographs would also be of use in identifying abnormalities of the clavicle or first rib, such as an old, poorly healed fracture.

Duplex ultrasonography

Ultrasound duplex studies of the arterial and venous systems in the upper extremity are the best initial tests and provide the essential information needed to diagnose vascular TOS. For arterial TOS, although the vessels immediately below the clavicle are not optimally visualized, post-stenotic dilation just distal to the clavicle can be seen. More importantly, the flow characteristics of the vessels distal to the outlet can be diagnostic for proximal flow restriction or distal embolic complications. Additionally, vessel insonation and the acquisition of waveforms and pressures can be obtained both during neutral positions and provocative maneuvers. For venous TOS duplex is excellent in visualizing non-compressibility and echogenic intraluminal material diagnostic for thrombosis in the axillary vein.

Plethysmography

Digital plethysmography is another non-invasive investigation which is capable of giving a relatively accurate indication of blood flow to a patient's digits. Its main value relies on the ability to detect pressure differences caused by provocative maneuvers. For example, when abducted to 90° or 180°, the reduction in blood flow to the upper extremity can be measured if there is compression of the subclavian artery.

CTA

Arterial compression can be clearly demonstrated on a CTA with the arm alongside the body and then with arm elevation. Injection of contrast via the contralateral extremity is recommended to minimize artifacts created by contrast opacification of the ipsilateral venous system. Tumours in the apex of the lung are also visualized optimally with computed tomography.

MRA

Many experts consider MRA the study of choice for the evaluation for TOS. It provides multidimensional views of all the anatomic elements of the thoracic outlet. Excellent visualization of the arteries, veins, nerves, muscles and bones is achieved. Images can be obtained in neutral position and also during arm elevation. The images can be observed in both the arterial and venous phases, and 3D reconstructions of images allow clinicians to observe the patient's anatomy in detail.

Angiography

Angiography should not be used as an initial investigation but it is very valuable when complications of thoracic outlet have occurred and when intervention is being considered. In the case of venous TOS without thrombosis, venography allows clinicians to assess the patency of the vein, the extent of occlusion with positional changes, and determine whether the patient only requires decompressive surgery or will also require venous reconstruction. If a thrombus is present catheter-directed thrombolysis, mechanical thrombectomy and venoplasty can be used during venography.

THERAPY

There is little controversy about the management of patients with arterial TOS. Untreated arterial injury due to repetitive torsion and compression leads to stenosis, post-stenotic aneurismal dilation and distal embolism. In the majority of cases, evidence of distal embolism with compromise of the arteries of the hand is already present by the time of presentation. Thus, thoracic outlet decompression and/or arterial reconstruction is mandatory. Since the subclavian artery can be compressed at any point from the root of the neck to the pectoralis minor tendon, the decompressive approach depends on the specific anatomy of the patient. The surgical plan depends on the details obtained by imaging studies and the experience of the surgeon. In the absence of anatomic anomalies and with compression demonstrated only during arm abduction and elevation, first rib resection via the supraclavicular approach appears to be the wisest choice. If chronic compression has caused arterial damage, revascularization is needed. Interposition grafts from the ipsilateral common carotid to the axillary artery are commonly used. This can be achieved best by a combination of supra and infraclavicular exposure. Eight mm PTFE grafts tunnelled underneath the clavicle have excellent patency rates. Excision of a cervical rib is usually done whereas full thoracic outlet decompression with scalenectomy is only necessary if concomitant neurogenic TOS is demonstrated.

On the other hand, the management strategies for venous TOS and the choice of approach to decompress the thoracic outlet are a matter of heated debate. It is generally agreed that patients with axillo-subclavian vein thrombosis should be anticoagulated. This can be done initially with unfractionated or low molecular weight heparin followed by oral anticoagulation for 3 to 6 months. Most vascular practitioners today favor an attempt of lysis using a combination of catheter directed thrombolytics complemented by suction catheter thrombectomy and balloon angioplasty. This strategy is particularly successful if the thrombus is fresh, preferably less than 1 week old.[13] Stents in the proximity of the thoracic outlet should be avoided, given the very high incidence of stent thrombosis, compression and fractures.[14]

The main controversy resides on whether or not and when to decompress the thoracic outlet after an episode of axillo-subclavian thrombosis. Proponents of mandatory surgical decompression use two strong arguments to justify their position. First, the need to remove a mechanical obstruction to flow that is an essential element in the pathophysiology of this condition. Second, the excellent results reported by several groups after thoracic decompression immediately after successful thrombolysis.[15] However, more recent series have reported encouraging results with aggressive protocols of early catheter directed thrombolysis followed by anticoagulation without immediate surgical decompression. These studies have shown that 80% to 90% of patients treated in such way do extremely well without the need for surgical decompression.[16, 17]. This approach avoids the risks of pneumothorax, hemothorax, lymphatic leaks, nerve injury and postoperative pain associated with thoracic decompression in the vast majority of patients and suggests that a policy of mandatory decompression is associated with unnecessary surgery in 80% to 90% of patients. An algorithm of such strategy is presented in Figure 42–2.

Patients that remain symptomatic after thrombolysis and anticoagulation undergo surgical decompression. For the treatment of venous thoracic outlet syndrome, many prefer the transaxillary approach.[18] This approach removes a large portion of the first rib, much of the floor of the scalene triangle as well as the scalene muscle and affords the best view of the inferior border of the subclavian vein. The cosmetic advantage of avoiding surgical scars in the neck or chest is obvious. Alternatively, decompression of the thoracic outlet can be done using a supraclavicular approach.[19] This approach allows for removal of the anterior and middle scalene muscles and the first rib from posterior to the brachial plexus to anterior to the subclavian vein. When the anterior aspect of the rib cannot be removed from this approach, a separate infraclavicular incision is used.[20]

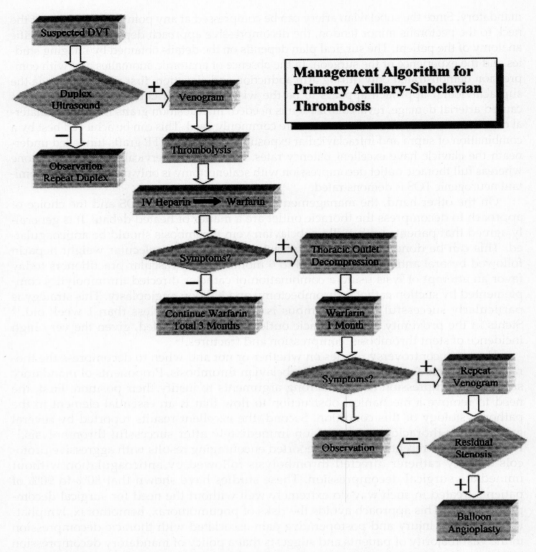

Figure 42–2. Treatment algorithm for patients with primary subclavian vein thrombosis. From Lee WA, Hill BB, Harris EJ Jr. Surgical intervention is not required for all patients with subclavian vein thrombosis. *J Vasc Surg* 2000;32:57–67. Reprinted with permission.

COMPLICATIONS

Re-thrombosis can occur after successful thrombolysis and also after surgical decompression. Interestingly, some authors have noticed that some patients treated with thrombolysis and anticoagulation alone remain asymptomatic even in the event of partial or complete re-thrombosis of the subclavian vein.[17]

Common postoperative complications after decompression include pneumothorax, lymphocele and phrenic nerve dysfunction. Injury to the subclavian artery or vein or injury to the brachial plexus is, fortunately, less common. In our own practice we have abandoned the use of anticoagulation immediately after decompression if venoplasty is performed after witnessing two episodes of severe hemothorax.

CONCLUSIONS

Management of vascular thoracic outlet syndrome requires a thorough understanding of the anatomic basis of the syndrome. Establishing the diagnosis is challenging and relies on a thorough history and physical exam supplemented with imaging studies. Several management options exist, especially for the treatment of venous thoracic outlet syndrome.

REFERENCES

1. Peet RM, Henriksen JD, Anderson TP, Martin GM. Thoracic-outlet syndrome: Evaluation of a therapeutic exercise program. *Proc Staff Meet Mayo Clin* 1956 May 2;31(9):281–7.
2. Lindblad B, Tengborn L, Bergqvist D. Deep vein thrombosis of the axillary-subclavian veins: Epidemiologic data, effects of different types of treatment and late sequele. *Eur J Vasc Surg* 1988 6;2(3):161–5.
3. Illig KA, Doyle AJ. A comprehensive review of Paget-Schroetter syndrome. *J Vasc Surg* 2010;51(6):1538–47.
4. Sanders RJ, Hammond SL, Rao NM. Diagnosis of thoracic outlet syndrome. *J Vasc Surg* 2007;46(3):601–4.
5. Durham JR, Yao JST, Pearce WH, Nuber GM, McCarthy III WJ. Arterial injuries in the thoracic outlet syndrome. *J Vasc Surg* 1995;21(1):57–70.
6. Gelabert HA, Machleder HI. Diagnosis and management of arterial compression at the thoracic outlet. *Ann Vasc Surg* 1997;11(4):359–66.
7. Criado E, Berguer R, Greenfield L. The spectrum of arterial compression at the thoracic outlet. *J Vasc Surg* 2010;52(2):406–11.
8. Lee JT, Karwowski JK, Harris EJ, Haukoos JS, Olcott IV. Long-term thrombotic recurrence after nonoperative management of Paget-Schroetter syndrome. *J Vasc Surg* 2006;43(6): 1236–43.
9. Guzzo JL, Chang K, Demos J, Black JH, Freischlag JA. Preoperative thrombolysis and venoplasty affords no benefit in patency following first rib resection and scalenectomy for subacute and chronic subclavian vein thrombosis. *J Vasc Surg* 2010;52(3):658–63.
10. Brewin J, Hill M, Ellis H. The prevalence of cervical ribs in a London population. *Clin Anat* 2009;22(3):331–6.
11. Adson AW, Coffey JR. Cervical rib: A method of anterior approach for relief of symptoms by division of the scalenus anticus. *Ann Surg* 1927;85(6):839.
12. Rayan G, Jensen C. Thoracic outlet syndrome: Provocative examination maneuvers in a typical population. *J Shoulder Elbow Surg* 1995 4;4(2):113–7.
13. Wilson JJ, Zahn CA, Newman H. Fibrinolytic therapy for idiopathic subclavian-axillary vein thrombosis. *Am J Surg* 1990;159:208–21014.
14. Meier GH, Pollak JS, Rosenblatt M, Dickey KW, Gusberg RJ. Initial experience with venous stents in exertional axillary-subclavian vein thrombosis. *J Vasc Surg* 1996;24:974–8115.
15. Azakie A, McElhinney DB, Thompson RW, Raven RB,Messina LM, Stoney RJ. Surgical management of subclavian vein effort thrombosis as a result of thoracic outlet compression. *J Vasc Surg* 1998;28(5):777–86.
16. W. Anthony Lee, MD, Bradley B. Hill, MD, E. John Harris, Jr, MD. Surgical intervention is not required for all patients with subclavian vein thrombosis. *J Vasc Surg* 2000;32:57–6717.
17. Lokanathan R, Salvian AJ, Chen JC, et al. Outcome after thrombolysis and selective thoracic outlet decompression for primary axillary vein thrombosis. *J Vasc Surg* 2001;33:783–818.

18. Leffert RD, Perlmutter GS. Thoracic outlet syndrome: Results of 282 transaxillary first rib resections. *Clin Orthop* 1999;368:66.

19. Geven LI, Smit AJ, Ebels T. Vascular thoracic outlet syndrome: Longer posterior rib stump causes poor outcome. *Eur J Cardiothorac Surg* 2006;30(2):232–6.

20. Thompson RW, Hernandez IA. The thoracic outlet syndrome: a second look. *Am J Surg* 1979;138:252–3

43

Splanchnic Artery Aneurysms: Minimally Invasive Treatment

Grant T. Fankhauser, MD and
Samuel R. Money, MD, FACS, MBA

Splanchnic artery aneurysms encompass aneurysms of the celiac artery, superior mesenteric artery, inferior mesenteric artery, and their branches. In the literature, fewer than 5,000 cases have been reported.[1] They vary in presentation, etiology, and indication for repair. The prevalence of splanchnic artery aneurysms is quite variable. Different series have suggested a prevalence of 0.1 to all the way up to 2% of the population.[2]

Overall, splanchnic artery aneurysms account for approximately 2-8% of all intra-abdominal aneurysms.[3] The diagnosis of splanchnic artery aneurysms is increasing. This is due to the extended use of sophisticated imaging techniques such as computed tomography, magnetic resonance imaging, and ultrasound.

Splenic artery aneurysms are the most common of the splanchnic artery aneurysms. They account for 40-70% in most major series. Hepatic and celiac aneurysms are next, accounting for anywhere between 10-40%. They are followed by superior mesenteric, gastric, and branch vessel aneurysms.[4] Splanchnic artery aneurysms may be associated with other aneurysms such as aortic, renal, iliac, lower extremity or intra-cranial.

The rupture rate of aneurysms varies based on where the aneurysm is located anatomically.[5] The rupture rate for splenic artery aneurysms is well studied and averages approximately 2%.[6] However, the rupture rate of other splanchnic artery aneurysms is variable based on location, etiology, rate of growth, and how extensively they are sought.[7]

The first successful repair of a splanchnic artery aneurysm was done in 1953 by DeBakey and Cooley.[8] They repaired a superior mesenteric artery aneurysm. Over the past 50 years, most surgery performed on splanchnic artery aneurysms has been open surgery. This has ranged from simple ligation to ligation and bypass. Clearly, the open technique depends upon the need for end organ perfusion and collateralization. Today most splanchnic aneurysms are repaired endovascularly. We will concentrate on endovascular repair for the duration of this discussion.

The theory of endovascular repair for aneurysms where end organ perfusion does not need to be preserved is a simple one. Imagine a room with multiple doors – the aneurysm being the room. One can either fill the room so tight that nothing flows in and out of it, or one can close all the doors and therefore nothing can get in and out of the room. By using coiling, particle injection, gel-foam injection, or gluing, the room can be filled or the doors closed. End-organ perfusion is not preserved except through collaterals. The issue of how to treat a splanchnic artery aneurysm when end-organ perfusion must be maintained is an interesting one and usually employs covered-stent aneurysm exclusion.

In a large clinical review, the Mayo Clinic Vascular Research Center Consortium evaluated the minimally invasive treatment of splanchnic aneurysms.[9] In this series there were 185 splenic artery aneurysms in 176 patients. Fifty-six percent (99 patients) were male with a mean age of 58 years (range 18-89 years). The cause of the aneurysm was varied. Forty-nine patients had aneurysms secondary to previous trauma. Thirty-eight of these were iatrogenic trauma. Eleven were secondary to blunt or non-iatrogenic trauma. The rate of iatrogenic trauma causing splenic artery aneurysms is increasing because of the growing use percutaneous biopsy, drainage, and intervention. Regardless of the intended target organ, percutaneous techniques can traumatize a splanchnic artery, possibly leading to the development of an aneurysm.

There was a wide distribution of splanchnic artery aneurysms in the Mayo Clinic experience (Table 43–1). As one would expect, the splenic artery aneurysms are the most common followed by hepatic and gastroduodenal. It is interesting to note that the aneurysms vary as to whether they are true aneurysms or pseudoaneurysms based on location (Table 43–2). Also notable is that a majority of the splenic artery aneurysms were true aneurysms whereas the vast majority of the hepatic and gastroduodenal artery aneurysms were pseu doaneurysms. This is likely attributable to higher rates of intervention in and around certain arteries like the hepatic. The indication for repair was usually based on size or symptoms in true aneurysms. The majority of patients with an aneurysm greater than 2 cm were offered repair of those with symptoms from the aneurysm size. Pseudoaneurysms on the other hand were repaired mainly based on diagnosis with approximately two-thirds of them having bleeding episodes.

Numerous endovascular techniques are employed in visceral artery aneurysm treatment. The vast majority of patients had coiling (filling the room). Coiling was either used alone or in combination with other techniques (Table 43–3).

TABLE 43–1. TRUE ANEURYSMS AND PSEUDOANEURYSMS BY ARTERIAL LOCATION

Aneurysm Location	True Aneurysm (%)	Pseudoaneurysm (%)
Splenic artery	40 (63%)	23 (37%)
Hepatic artery	11 (20%)	45 (80%)
Gastroduodenal artery	3 (11%)	25 (89%)
Pancreaticoduodenal artery	5 (31%)	11 (69%)
Superior Mesenteric artery	2 (33%)	4 (67%)
Gastric artery	1 (25%)	3 (75%)
Celiac artery	0 (0%)	4 (100%)
Gastroepiploic artery	2 (50%)	2 (50%)
Inferior Mesenteric artery	1 (50%)	1 (50%)
Middle Colic artery	0 (0%)	1 (100%)

TABLE 43–2. INDICATION FOR INTERVENTION BY LOCATION

Aneurysm Location	Bleeding	Size
Splenic artery	17 (27%)	46 (73%)
Hepatic artery	31 (55%)	25 (45%)
Gastroduodenal artery	21 (75%)	7 (25%)
Pancreaticoduodenal artery	7 (44%)	9 (66%)
Superior Mesenteric artery	2 (33%)	4 (67%)
Gastric artery	3 (75%)	1 (25%)
Celiac artery	1 (25%)	3 (75%)
Gastroepiploic artery	3 (75%)	1 (25%)
Inferior Mesenteric artery	0 (0%)	2 (100%)
Middle Colic artery	1 (100%)	0 (0%)

The approach used in a majority of patients for access to the aneurysm was through the femoral artery (148/181). Twenty-eight patients were approached with the brachial approach and 5 patients had direct percutaneous access. The brachial approach was selected based at the operator's discretion as some splanchnic arteries have a downward slope and are best approached from above.

The 30-day mortality in the series was 6.2%, with 3.4% of the patients having aneurysm-related death. Two patients suffered persistent or recurrent bleeding and 4 had withdrawal of care by the family. Immediate success was obtained in 181 of 185 patients (98%). Four aneurysms demonstrated persistent flow. These patients returned to the interventional suite and all were successfully treated by repeat intervention.

There were some complications. First, 12 of 185 patients had access complications, either prolonged pain or hematoma. However, none of these patients required re-intervention. At thirty day follow-up, 2% of the patients had recurrent flow in their aneurysms. They were taken back to the angiography suite and treated successfully with repeat intervention. Long-term follow-up was obtained for mean of 524 days (range 7-3,808). There were 10 additional deaths though none were aneurysm-related. There was one active recurrence in a splenic artery aneurysm that required repeat treatment with coiling.

TABLE 43–3. TECHNIQUES EMPLOYED IN ANEURYSM TREATMENT

Technique	Number of Aneurysms Treated
Coiling*	162
Covered stent placement	10
Particle injection	2
Gelfoam injection	5
Plug deployment	1
Polyvinyl alcohol (PVA) injection	2
Gluing	1
Endoluminal thrombin injection	1
Percutaneous coiling	2
Percutaneous thrombin injection	3

*Coiling was used in combination with other techniques in 20 aneurysms

Long-term morbidity was also present. Two patients required open laparotomy. One patient developed bile duct ischemia following gastroduodeanal artery coiling and required a hepaticojejunostomy. One patient sustained a splenic infarct leading to sepsis that required splenectomy. There were 15 minor intra-abdominal complications. Eight of 56 patients whose hepatic arteries were embolized suffered partial hepatic infarct. Most of these were self-limited and with analgesia and supportive care. Seven of 63 patients who had splenic artery aneurysm coiling sustained splenic infarcts and again these were all treated conservatively.

The Mayo Clinic study discussed a sub-set of aneurysms in which end-organ perfusion needed to be maintained. Ten patients had superior mesenteric aneurysms treated with covered stents. Long-term follow-up (greater than 1 year) was available in 9 of 10 of these patients. There were no in-stent stenoses or complications during the follow-up period. The covered stent sealed the aneurysm; however, additional coiling was required in a few of these cases.

In conclusion, most common hepatic or celiac aneurysms can be treated with coils or glue if a patient has an adequately sized gastroduodenal artery present. Jordan et al. found that the presence of a gastroduodenal artery 3mm or greater is sufficient not to cause any hepatic ischemia.[10] One caveat to this is this can never be used in advanced liver disease or post-hepatic transplant.

Clearly, minimally invasive treatment is successful in a majority of cases but may not be appropriate in all cases. Patients-specific considerations must be taken into account including anatomy and collaterals. Numerous techniques may be used alone or in combination to suit aneurysms in varied locations. Minimally invasive techniques can safely be used to treat splanchnic artery aneurysms in a vast majority of patients.

REFERENCES

1. Tessier DJ, Abbas MA, Fowl RJ, Stone WM, Bower TC, McKusick MA,et al. Management of rare mesenteric arterial branch aneurysms. *Ann Vasc Surg* 2002;16:586–90.
2. Kasirajan K, Greenberg RK, Clair D, Ouriel K. Endovascular management of visceral artery aneurysm. *J Endovasc Ther* 2001;8:150–5.
3. LM Messina, Visceral artery aneurysms, *Surg Clin North Am* 77 (1997), pp. 425–442.
4. Tulsyan N, Kashyap VS, Greenberg RK, Sarac TP, Clair DG, Pierce G, et al. The endovascular management of visceral artery aneurysms and pseudoaneurysms. *J Vasc Surg* 2007;45: 276–83.
5. Ristow AV. Visceral Artery Aneurysms: Role of Open and Endovascular Treatments. VEITH Symposium Presentation November 2010, New York, NY.
6. Pescarus R, Montreuil B, Bendavid Y. Giant splenic artery aneurysms: case report and review of the literature. *J Vasc Surg* 2005;42:344–7.
7. Saltzberg SS, Maldonado TS, Lamparello PJ, et al. Is endovascular therapy the preferred treatment for all visceral artery aneurysms? *Ann Vasc Surg* 2005;19:507–515.
8. DeBakey ME, Cooley DA: Successful resection of mycotic aneurysm of superior mesenteric artery; case report and review of literature. *Am Surg* 1953;19:202–212.
9. Fankhauser GF, Stone WM, Money SR, et al: The minimally invasive management of visceral artery aneurysms and pseudoaneurysms. *J Vasc Surg* 2011;53:966–70.
10. Vaddineni SK. Taylor SM. Jordan WD Jr. Outcome after celiac artery coverage during endovascular thoracic aortic aneurysm repair: preliminary results. *J Vasc Surg* 2007; 45(3):467–71.

44

Laparoscopic Median Arcuate Ligament Release

Kyle Zanocco, MD and Eric S. Hungness, MD, FACS

INTRODUCTION

Celiac artery compression syndrome (CACS), also known as median arcuate ligament syndrome or celiac band compression syndrome, is a rare disorder caused by extrinsic compression and narrowing of the celiac artery by the median arcuate ligament (MAL) of the diaphragm and/or fibrous periaortic ganglionic tissue. CACS was first described in the 1960s, and considerable controversy continues to surround the pathophysiology, diagnosis, and treatment of this rare disorder.[1-3]

PATHOPHYSIOLOGY

Extrinsic compression of the celiac axis by surrounding structures was described as early as the beginning of the 20th century by the anatomist Lipshutz.[4] The takeoff of the celiac artery is most commonly between the level of the 11th thoracic vertebrae and the first lumbar vertebra. Several anatomic scenarios acting alone or in concert have been identified that can lead to celiac artery compression: celiac mesenteric trunk compression by the diaphragmatic crura and MAL, an abnormally cephalad point of origin of the celiac artery with compression by normal diaphragmatic crura and the MAL, a normal takeoff of the celiac artery with long diaphragmatic crura and MAL, or a large fused celiac and/or superior mesenteric ganglia causing compression.[5] Other causes of external compression have been described including aortic dissection, post-operative changes following pancreaticoduodenectomy, aneurysms of small pancreatic arteries, sarcoidosis, duodenal carcinoma, abdominal trauma, and papillary neoplasms of the pancreas.[5-7]

Several theories attempt to explain the mechanism of pain in CACS. The most widely accepted mechanism is that of foregut ischemia during increased demand caused by compromised flow through a compressed celiac artery. Another theory suggests that the pain is caused by a steal syndrome with resulting midgut ischemia when blood from the superior mesenteric artery territory is diverted to the foregut through collaterals during periods of high demand. Others hypothesized that the pain is from overstimulation or chronic irritation of the celiac plexus by the MAL causing splanchnic vasoconstriction and subsequent pain.[8]

SYMPTOMS AND SIGNS

While the clinical presentation of CACS is highly variable, most patients have symptoms of chronic mesenteric ischemia, including weight loss, postprandial abdominal pain, nausea, vomiting, and diarrhea. In several reports, deep expiration has been demonstrated to increase abdominal pain, while deep inspiration tends to alleviate pain.[3,9] Strenuous exercise has also been shown to produce severe abdominal pain in athletes with CACS.[10] On physical examination, an epigastric ejection bruit is commonly audible and may be altered by position and respiration; however, epigastric bruit is not specific to CACS and has been reported to occur in 15.9% of the general population.[9,11]

DIAGNOSIS

Identification of CACS is elusive because its symptoms and signs produce extensive differential diagnoses. Many patients undergo exhaustive workups for their abdominal pain before the diagnosis of CACS is entertained. Clinical algorithms have been constructed to guide the diagnostic workup of a patient with possible CACS.[8,12] These algorithms include performance of esophagogastroduodenoscopy, upper gastrointestinal fluoroscopic contrast imaging, right upper quadrant abdominal ultrasound, and abdominal CT scanning. Any abnormalities discovered in this workup should be addressed and the patient should be subsequently monitored for symptom resolution. If the above tests are normal, gastric emptying time can be measured, which, if abnormally prolonged, can then be followed by vascular imaging studies to confirm the diagnosis of CACS.

Invasive and non-invasive vascular imaging studies can be used to support the diagnosis of CACS. Catheter-based angiography of the celiac axis is the gold standard for the diagnosis of celiac artery compression and typically demonstrates a superior indentation along the proximal celiac axis approximately 5mm from its origin at the abdominal aorta.[13] This indentation is more apparent during expiration. Post-stenotic dilation can be seen in patients with severe compression. Computed tomography (CT) angiography with three-dimensional image reconstruction can demonstrate celiac compression with the added benefit of identifying the median arcuate ligament in relation to the celiac axis.[13] Similarly, magnetic resonance angiography (MRA) with dynamic contrast material-enhanced three-dimensional imaging can be used to demonstrate celiac artery narrowing.[14] An MRA demonstrating celiac artery compression during expiration is shown in Figure 44–1. Ultrasonography can also aid in diagnosis. Some clinicians advocate duplex scanning of the celiac, superior mesenteric and inferior mesenteric arteries in all patients with suspected CACS.[3] The "Doppler Duplex Sign" has been described as a sensitive test for CACS where Doppler ultrasonography performed during deep expiration causes a significant increase in flow velocities at the compressed region of the celiac artery.[15] 13%-50% of healthy patients

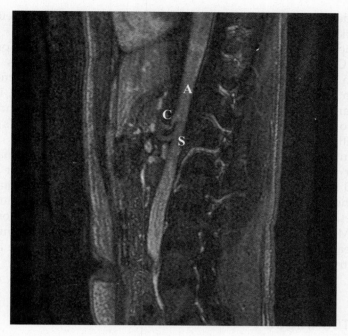

Figure 44–1. Sagital reconstruction of an MRA in a CACS patient showing compression of the celiac artery during expiratory phase (C). A, abdominal aorta; S, superior mesenteric artery.

have been noted to exhibit celiac artery compression during expiration, and most of these patients are asymptomatic.[13,14] Therefore it is important to note that the radiographic feature of celiac axis compression is not independently clinically significant without accompanying symptoms of CACS.

Gastric tonometry has emerged as a useful diagnostic test for gastric ischemia in CACS. This catheter-based procedure measures mucosal pH as a marker of gastric mucosal perfusion. The normal range of gastric mucosal pH is 7.38-7.48 and a gastric mucosal pH of <7.32 indicates significant ischemia.[16] Gastric exercise tonometry incorporates a period of treadmill or stationary bicycle exercise with measurement of gastric mucosal pH before, during, and after exercise.[17] Improvement to normal gastric mucosal pH and a corresponding relief of symptoms after surgical treatment for CACS has been reported by several groups.[17,18]

TREATMENT OPTIONS

A variety of surgical and endovascular procedures have been reported as treatment options for CACS.[19] The open surgical technique for arcuate ligament release consists of exposure of the celiac trunk with dissection and resection of the median arcuate ligament, overlying fibrous bands, and ganglionic periaortic tissue causing external compression of the celiac artery.[3,19] A recent series of open surgical procedures to treat CACS demonstrated that 39% of these procedures included further intervention on the celiac artery including aorto-celiac and aorto-hepatic interposition grafting with greater saphenous vein. Other adjuncts included patch angioplasty, resection of a stenotic segment of celiac artery, and aorto-mesenteric loop bypass.[19]

Laparoscopic MAL release has recently emerged as a successful approach to treatment of CACS with reported advantages of less blood loss and shorter hospitalization.[8,19-22] There is no immediate ability to perform reconstructive vascular procedures on the celiac trunk when laparoscopy is used. However, intraoperative ultrasound can identify instances of persistent inadequate flow and appropriate endovascular or reconstructive measures can be pursued if the patient's symptoms do not resolve with MAL release.[8,19]

Endovascular treatment of MALS using percutaneous transluminal angioplasty (PTA) with or without insertion of stents has been reported, however a high rate of restenosis and stent related complications has been observed.[8] If primary stenting is undertaken, the use of self-expanding Nitinol stents has been recommended to withstand the repetitive mechanical forces generated by external compression on the celiac artery by the MAL.[3] Endovascular treatment modalities appear have a more successful role in the treatment of persistent symptoms following MAL release as opposed to being an effective primary treatment for this condition.[8]

SURGICAL TECHNIQUE

Pre-operative antibiotics is not required for this "clean" operation, but should be dictated by local hospital guidelines. Pneumatic compression boots are used for mechanical deep venous thrombosis prophylaxis, and a urinary catheter and orogastric tube should be inserted.

Similar to that for laparoscopic Nissen fundoplication, the patient is positioned supine with split legs, and a bean bag mattress used for stabilization. After Veress needle insertion and creation of carbon dioxide pneumoperitoneum, the first abdominal trocar is placed in the supraumbilical region approximately 12-14cm inferior to the xiphoid and serves as the camera port. Three to four additional ports are placed in the upper abdomen. (Figure 44–2) The right lateral port is used for the liver retractor, with the right mid-abdominal port used for the surgical assistant. If laparoscopic ultrasound is to be used, the left mid-abdominal port should be 12mm to accommodate the US probe. Laparoscopic exploration of the entire abdominal cavity is performed.

The left lobe of the liver is elevated with a laparoscopic self-retaining "snake" liver retractor. The stomach is then pulled inferiorly to expose the gastrohepatic ligament of the lesser omentum. The pars flacida of the gastrohepatic ligament is divided allowing access to the diaphragmatic crura, which are unroofed by dividing the overlying peritoneum with harmonic shears. (Figure 44–3)

Prior to and throughout dissection of the celiac axis, intraoperative ultrasound is useful to help identify the celiac artery and its branches. A laparoscopic ultrasound probe is placed through the left lateral port and is run gently along the surface of the lesser curve of the lesser omentum. Starting from the base of the right crus of the diaphragm, and moving the probe caudally, ultrasound visualization of the origin of the celiac artery can be seen. Following this vessel caudally reveals its branches more inferiorly. The splenic, left gastric and common hepatic branches of the celiac can be seen ultrasonically at the most caudal extent of the celiac artery.

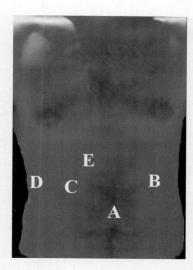

Figure 44–2. The positions of the ports for laparoscopic MAL release are labeled: A, camera; B, ultrasound probe/operating port; C operating port; D, liver retractor; E optional additional operating port.

Once orientation and arterial branches are identified, dissection of the lesser curve fat is initiated. A combination of electrocautery and ultrasonic shear dissection is used to maintain hemostasis during the dissection. Great care must be taken to avoid injury to major arterial branches. As this dissection continues, the left gastric artery gradually comes into view running along the lesser curve of the stomach. This dissection is carried up to the base of the right crus, and extended toward the left where the right and left crus meet. Individual crural muscle fibers are then divided

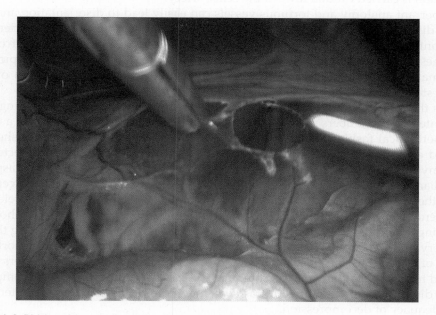

Figure 44–3. Division of the pars flacida to obtain entry into the lesser sac.

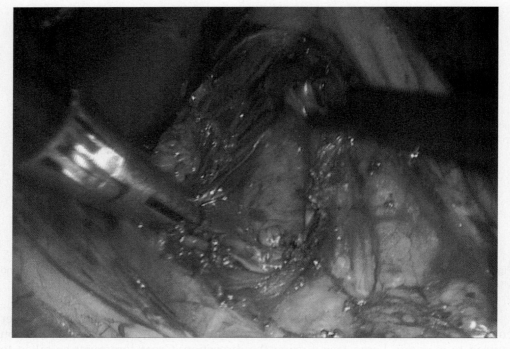

Figure 44–4. Exposure of the supraceliac abdominal aorta.

with hook electrocautery to expose the anterior aspect of the aorta. (Figure 44–4) This dissection is carried caudad toward the celiac artery.

Aberrant anatomy and tortuous vessels can easily lead to disorientation and erroneous dissection. Ultrasound can be used throughout this procedure for reorientation and confirmation of anatomy. Retrograde dissection starting proximally from the branches of the celiac can also be performed to prevent disorientation. Typically, a combination of antegrade and retrograde dissection will meet in the area of most severe stenosis.

As the celiac is approached, entrapping fibers of the MAL and celiac ganglia are encountered. These fibers must be dissected off the artery and its branches in a careful and methodical fashion. Many of these fibers are vascular and ultrasonic shears or hooked electrocautery should be used. (Figure 44–5) As each fiber is dissected, the anatomy of the vessels becomes clearer. As dissection continues, the distal aspect of the celiac artery and its branches can be seen. The dissection is then carried cephalad along the entire length of the celiac artery. It is important to dissect free and release all of the entrapping fibers along the entire length of the celiac artery, including those surrounding the origin of its branches. As the dissection is carried cephalad along the celiac artery, it joins the original dissection plane on the anterior aspect of the aorta. The origin of the celiac artery is visualized and dissection of all surrounding fibers is performed to ensure that the artery is completely released. (Figure 44–6) Upon completion of the dissection, intraoperative ultrasound may be used to demonstrate patent flow and adequacy of decompression.

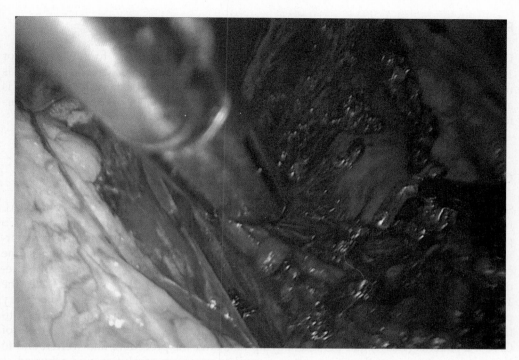

Figure 44–5. Division of constricting bands of the MAL overlying the celiac artery using the hook cautery.

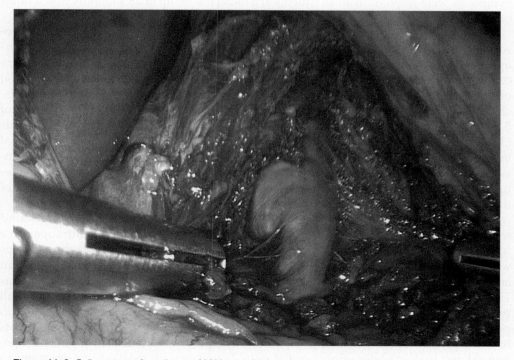

Figure 44–6. Celiac artery after release of MAL and division of all surrounding fibers and paraganglionic tissue.

POST-OPERATIVE CARE

Patients undergoing laparoscopic MAL release are typically admitted to the hospital for 1 or 2 days, and typically kept NPO the night of surgery. Intravenous narcotic analgesia is usually required for pain control and switched to PO pain medication once the diet is advanced and tolerated. Repeat mesenteric duplex exam 4-6 weeks post-surgery is performed to assess the anatomic effectiveness of the MAL release.

OUTCOMES

Several case series documenting single institutional experiences with laparoscopic MAL release have been recently published. Baccari et al describe the treatment of 16 CACS patients with laparoscopic MAL release between 2002 and 2008.[20] All procedures were performed by the same surgeon using either a 4 or 5-port technique to completely expose the celiac artery and free it from all structures causing external compression. The mean procedure length was 90 minutes with average postoperative length of stay of 3 days. 2 of the 16 patients (12.5%) required conversion to an open approach for hemostasis with primary pledgeted suture repair of the celiac artery. No other operative complications were identified. 14 patients (87.5%) experienced complete and durable relief of their symptoms of CACS. 2 patients (12.5%) had persistent symptoms after the procedure and were found to have early restenosis of the celiac artery. Complete symptom resolution was achieved in one case with PTA and stenting and in the other with aortoceliac bypass grafting. Symptoms were resolved in all 16 patients at a mean follow-up of 28.3 months with a range of 2-83 months.

A similar case series has been published by Roseborough, who performed laparoscopic MAL on 15 consecutive CACS patients from 2002 to 2007.[21] Operating time averaged 189 minutes and varied from 96 to 395 minutes. 4 of 15 (27%) cases were complicated by arterial injury requiring conversion to an open procedure. One (6.7%) of the patients who required conversion also developed pancreatitis shortly after discharge requiring readmission and ultimately 6 months of hospitalization with a total of 8 months of total parenteral nutrition before restoring her ability to eat. Four patients (33%) required additional angioplasty to treat persistent stenosis following initial laparoscopic decompression and one patient (6.7%) underwent celiac bypass for intrinsic stenosis that was recognized during the initial operation. On intermediate follow-up, 14 of the 15 (93.3%) patients in the series reported complete or significant relief of their original symptoms. One patient (6.7%) reported no improvement in symptoms.

We have reported on our institutional experience using intraoperative ultrasound to facilitate laparoscopic MAL release on three patients with CACS.[22] Intraoperative ultrasound was used in both the identification of the celiac artery and its branches as well as to confirm adequate decompression following release of the arcuate ligament and surrounding structures. The mean operating room time for these procedures was 151 minutes. All three patients were discharged on the first postoperative day and all procedures were technically successful with normalization of celiac artery velocity on postoperative mesenteric duplex ultrasound examination. Two of the three patients had complete resolution of their preoperative symptoms, while the third patient experienced residual episodes of abdominal pain, however with marked improvement in postprandial epigastric pain and ability to gain weight.

In conclusion, laparoscopic MAL release is a safe and effective treatment for CACS. Endovascular dilational therapy should be employed in refractory cases only after extrinsic compression of the celiac artery is surgically treated. While the laparoscopic approach to CACS is becoming more common, direct comparison between open and laparoscopic MAL release in the form of randomized trials is lacking and unlikely to be performed due to the low incidence of this order. In experienced hands, properly selected patients with CACS will benefit from the minimally-invasive treatment approach with shorter lengths of stay, superior cosmetic outcomes, and less postoperative pain.

REFERENCES

1. Edwards A. Coeliac axis compression syndrome. *Proc R Soc Med* 1969;62(5):488–490.
2. Harjola PT. A Rare Obstruction of the Coeliac Artery. Report of a Case. *Ann Chir Gynaecol Fenn* 1963;52:547–550.
3. Gloviczki P, Duncan AA. Treatment of celiac artery compression syndrome: does it really exist? *Perspect Vasc Surg Endovasc Ther* 2007;19(3):259–263.
4. Lipshutz B. A Composite Study of the Coeliac Axis Artery. *Ann Surg* 1917;65(2):159–169.
5. Loukas M, Pinyard J, Vaid S, Kinsella C, Tariq A, Tubbs RS. Clinical anatomy of celiac artery compression syndrome: a review. *Clin Anat* 2007;20(6):612–617.
6. Fujisawa Y, Morishita K, Fukada J, Hachiro Y, Kawaharada N, Abe T. Celiac artery compression syndrome due to acute type B aortic dissection. *Ann Vasc Surg* 2005;19(4):553–556.
7. Bull DA, Hunter GC, Crabtree TG, Bernhard VM, Putnam CW. Hepatic ischemia, caused by celiac axis compression, complicating pancreaticoduodenectomy. *Ann Surg* 1993;217(3): 244–247.
8. Duffy AJ, Panait L, Eisenberg D, Bell RL, Roberts KE, Sumpio B. Management of median arcuate ligament syndrome: a new paradigm. *Ann Vasc Surg* 2009;23(6):778–784.
9. Kokotsakis JN, Lambidis CD, Lioulias AG, Skouteli ET, Bastounis EA, Livesay JJ. Celiac artery compression syndrome. *Cardiovasc Surg* Apr 2000;8(3):219–222.
10. Desmond CP, Roberts SK. Exercise-related abdominal pain as a manifestation of the median arcuate ligament syndrome. *Scand J Gastroenterol* 2004;39(12):1310–1313.
11. Julius S, Stewart BH. Diagnostic significance of abdominal murmurs. *N Engl J Med* 1967;276(21):1175–1178.
12. Trinidad-Hernandez M, Keith P, Habib I, White JV. Reversible gastroparesis: functional documentation of celiac axis compression syndrome and postoperative improvement. *Am Surg* 2006;72(4):339–344.
13. Horton KM, Talamini MA, Fishman EK. Median arcuate ligament syndrome: evaluation with CT angiography. *Radiographics* 2005;25(5):1177–1182.
14. Lee VS, Morgan JN, Tan AG, et al. Celiac artery compression by the median arcuate ligament: a pitfall of end-expiratory MR imaging. *Radiology* 2003;228(2):437–442.
15. Erden A, Yurdakul M, Cumhur T. Marked increase in flow velocities during deep expiration: A duplex Doppler sign of celiac artery compression syndrome. *Cardiovasc Intervent Radiol* 1999;22(4):331–332.
16. Taylor DE, Gutierrez G. Tonometry. A review of clinical studies. *Crit Care Clin* 1996;12(4): 1007–1018.
17. Mensink PB, van Petersen AS, Kolkman JJ, Otte JA, Huisman AB, Geelkerken RH. Gastric exercise tonometry: the key investigation in patients with suspected celiac artery compression syndrome. *J Vasc Surg* 2006;44(2):277–281.
18. Faries PL, Narula A, Veith FJ, Pomposelli FB, Jr., Marsan BU, LoGerfo FW. The use of gastric tonometry in the assessment of celiac artery compression syndrome. *Ann Vasc Surg* 2000;14(1):20–23.

19. Grotemeyer D, Duran M, Iskandar F, Blondin D, Nguyen K, Sandmann W. Median arcuate ligament syndrome: vascular surgical therapy and follow-up of 18 patients. *Langenbecks Arch Surg* 2009;394(6):1085–1092.

20. Baccari P, Civilini E, Dordoni L, Melissano G, Nicoletti R, Chiesa R. Celiac artery compression syndrome managed by laparoscopy. *J Vasc Surg* 2009;50(1):134–139.

21. Roseborough GS. Laparoscopic management of celiac artery compression syndrome. *J Vasc Surg* 2009;50(1):124–133.

22. Vaziri K, Hungness ES, Pearson EG, Soper NJ. Laparoscopic treatment of celiac artery compression syndrome: case series and review of current treatment modalities. *J Gastrointest Surg* 2009;13(2):293–298.

Index

Information in figures and tables is indicated by *f* and *t*.